T0261630

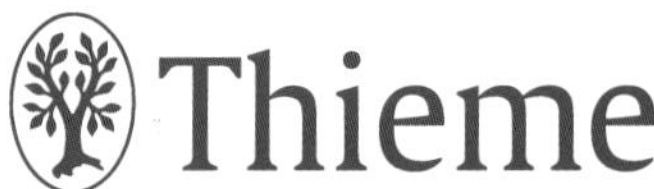
Thieme

Medical Physiology Q&A

Gabi N. Waite, PhD
Professor
Department of Basic Sciences
Geisinger Commonwealth School of Medicine
Scranton, Pennsylvania

Maria Sheakley, PhD
Associate Professor
Department of Biomedical Sciences
Western Michigan University Homer Stryker M.D. School of Medicine
Kalamazoo, Michigan

183 illustrations

Thieme
New York • Stuttgart • Delhi • Rio de Janeiro

Acquisition Editor: Delia K. DeTurris
Managing Editor: Kenneth Schubach
Director, Editorial Services: Mary Jo Casey
Production Editor: Kenny Chumbley
In-House Production Editor: Naamah Schwartz
International Production Director: Andreas Schabert
Editorial Director: Sue Hodgson
International Marketing Director: Fiona Henderson
International Sales Director: Louisa Turrell
Director of Institutional Sales: Adam Bernacki
Senior Vice President and Chief Operating Officer: Sarah Vanderbilt
President: Brian D. Scanlan

Library of Congress Cataloging-in-Publication Data

Names: Waite, Gabi Nindl, author. | Sheakley, Maria, author.
Title: Medical physiology Q&A/ Gabi N. Waite, Maria Sheakley.
Description: New York : Thieme, [2018] | Includes index.
Identifiers: LCCN 2017024887| ISBN 9781626233843 (pbk.) | ISBN 9781626233850 (eISBN)
Subjects: | MESH: Physiological Phenomena | Examination Questions
Classification: LCC QP40 | NLM QT 18.2 | DDC 612.0076--dc23
LC record available at https://lccn.loc.gov/2017024887

Important note: Medicine is an ever-changing science undergoing continual development. Research and clinical experience are continually expanding our knowledge, in particular our knowledge of proper treatment and drug therapy. Insofar as this book mentions any dosage or application, readers may rest assured that the authors, editors, and publishers have made every effort to ensure that such references are in accordance with **the state of knowledge at the time of production of the book.**

Nevertheless, this does not involve, imply, or express any guarantee or responsibility on the part of the publishers in respect to any dosage instructions and forms of applications stated in the book. **Every user is requested to examine carefully** the manufacturers' leaflets accompanying each drug and to check, if necessary in consultation with a physician or specialist, whether the dosage schedules mentioned therein or the contraindications stated by the manufacturers differ from the statements made in the present book. Such examination is particularly important with drugs that are either rarely used or have been newly released on the market. Every dosage schedule or every form of application used is entirely at the user's own risk and responsibility. The authors and publishers request every user to report to the publishers any discrepancies or inaccuracies noticed. If errors in this work are found after publication, errata will be posted at www.thieme.com on the product description page.

Some of the product names, patents, and registered designs referred to in this book are in fact registered trademarks or proprietary names even though specific reference to this fact is not always made in the text. Therefore, the appearance of a name without designation as proprietary is not to be construed as a representation by the publisher that it is in the public domain.

Thieme Publishers New York
333 Seventh Avenue, New York, NY 10001 USA
+1 800 782 3488, customerservice@thieme.com

Thieme Publishers Stuttgart
Rüdigerstrasse 14, 70469 Stuttgart, Germany
+49 [0]711 8931 421, customerservice@thieme.de

Thieme Publishers Delhi
A-12, Second Floor, Sector-2, Noida-201301
Uttar Pradesh, India
+91 120 45 566 00, customerservice@thieme.in

Thieme Publishers Rio de Janeiro, Thieme Publicações Ltda.
Edifício Rodolpho de Paoli, 25º andar
Av. Nilo Peçanha, 50 – Sala 2508
Rio de Janeiro 20020-906, Brasil
+55 21 3172 2297

Cover design: Thieme Publishing Group
Typesetting by Prairie Papers

Printed in India by Replika Press Pvt. Ltd. 5 4 3 2 1
ISBN 978-1-62623-384-3

Also available as an e-book:
eISBN 978-1-62623-385-0

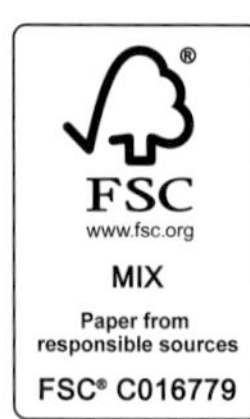

To my mentor and close friend, Dr. Walter Balcavage.

Gabi N. Waite

To the mentors in my life: Dr. Barbara Francois, Dr. Charles “Chuck” Seidel, and Dr. Hashim Shams.

Maria Sheakley

Contents

Preface

A successful student of the medical profession is able to synthesize concepts and principles that govern a human body and apply those concepts and principles to healthy and diseased patients. This requires the ability to integrate basic and clinical science information, such as understanding how the Frank Starling principle applies to cardiac resuscitation and how gastrointestinal physiology can aid in choosing the best diet for a patient.

With this book, it is our goal to provide examples of how to synthesize, integrate, and apply physiological concepts to clinical situations, in a format similar to that used in the United States Medical Licensing Examination (USMLE). Accordingly, we took examples of high-yield concepts that we provide in the classroom and turned them into challenging multiple-choice questions.

This book is a valuable resource for medical students to prepare for the USMLE Step 1 exam. Additionally, it is a book that provides students of any health profession the opportunity to self-assess their level of understanding. Students who need a resource for a condensed review, after completing a medical physiology course, can focus on easy and moderate questions. Students who need to integrate physiological principles with their new understanding of pathology, pharmacology, or other medical topics can select moderate and difficult questions. Nursing and allied health students, who need to perform at a higher level in their area of expertise, will study moderate and difficult questions to prepare for their discipline-specific certifying exams. Even residents and professionals will benefit from a refresher in the mechanistic understanding of medicine.

With the ever-expanding pool of medical knowledge, we see this book as an ongoing project that will continually be revised and updated based on scientific discovery and audience feedback. In this aspect, this book contributes to the new era of electronic publishing, where continuous improvement becomes a necessary reality. We welcome feedback, and look forward to hearing about the ways in which this book is used by aspiring and established medical professionals.

Gabi N. Waite, PhD
Maria Sheakley, PhD

Acknowledgments

We gratefully acknowledge a multitude of colleagues who reviewed materials and answered questions, including David B. Averill, PhD (Geisinger Commonwealth), Roy W. Geib, PhD (Indiana University), David R. Riddle, PhD (Western Michigan University School of Medicine), Dr. Hashim Shams, MD, PhD (Ross University), and Brian Wilcox, MD, PhD (Geisinger Commonwealth).

We are grateful for guidance and support from the entire Thieme staff and for their remarkable editorial and production work. A special thanks to Delia DeTurris (acquisitions), Kenny Chumbley (production), and Kenneth Schubach (management) for their continued help and encouragement throughout the process.

Last, but not least, we are thankful to our wonderful husbands, parents, friends, colleagues, and pets who deserved more attention but accepted our determination to meet the next deadline. Thank you!

How to Use This Series

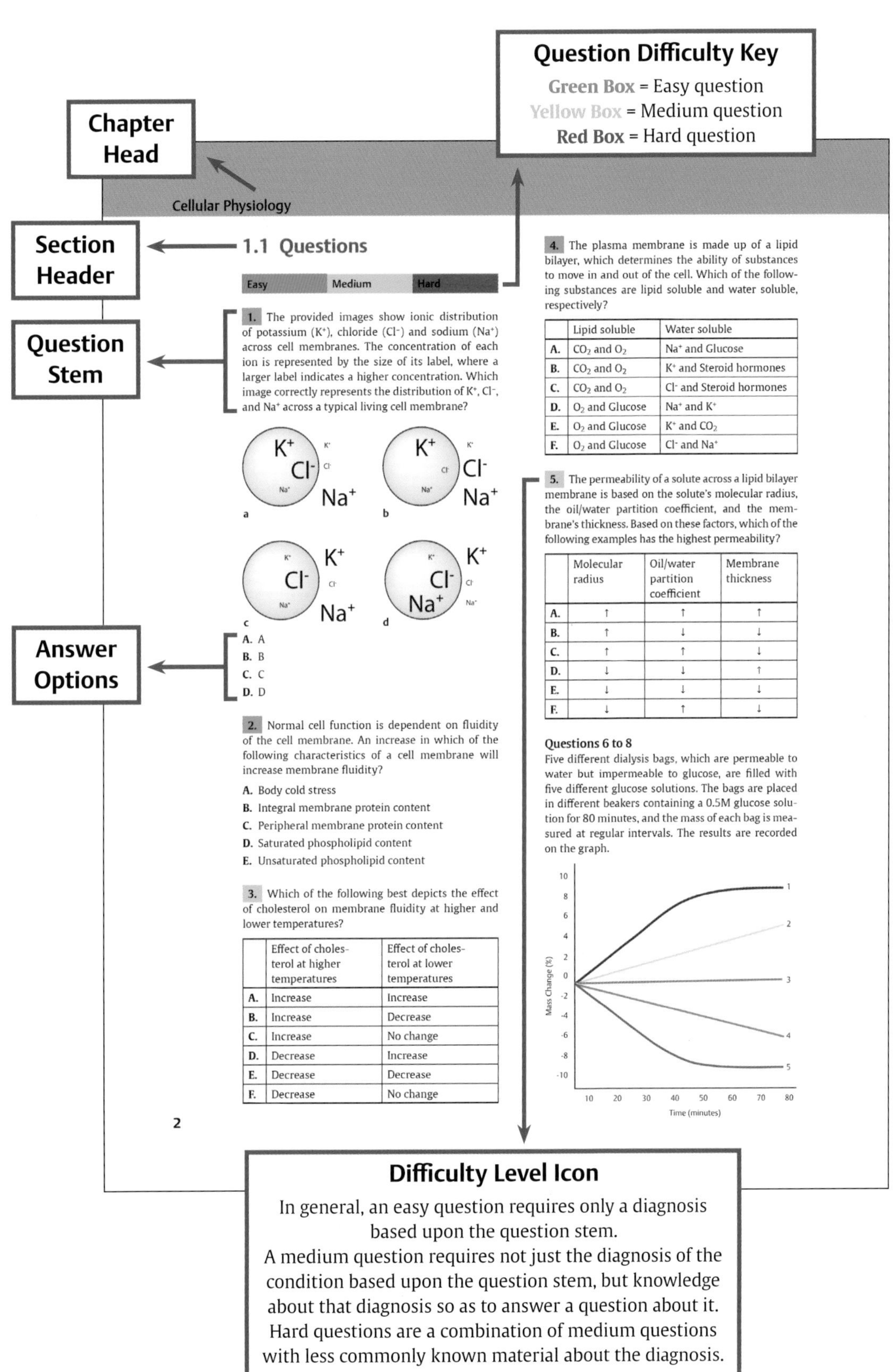

Question Difficulty Key
Green Box = Easy question
Yellow Box = Medium question
Red Box = Hard question
Chapter Head
Section Header
Question Stem
Answer Options
Difficulty Level Icon
In general, an easy question requires only a diagnosis based upon the question stem.
A medium question requires not just the diagnosis of the condition based upon the question stem, but knowledge about that diagnosis so as to answer a question about it.
Hard questions are a combination of medium questions with less commonly known material about the diagnosis.

Cellular Physiology

1.1 Questions

Easy Medium Hard

1. The provided images show ionic distribution of potassium (K^+), chloride (Cl^-) and sodium (Na^+) across cell membranes. The concentration of each ion is represented by the size of its label, where a larger label indicates a higher concentration. Which image correctly represents the distribution of K^+, Cl^-, and Na^+ across a typical living cell membrane?

A. A
B. B
C. C
D. D

2. Normal cell function is dependent on fluidity of the cell membrane. An increase in which of the following characteristics of a cell membrane will increase membrane fluidity?

A. Body cold stress
B. Integral membrane protein content
C. Peripheral membrane protein content
D. Saturated phospholipid content
E. Unsaturated phospholipid content

3. Which of the following best depicts the effect of cholesterol on membrane fluidity at higher and lower temperatures?

	Effect of cholesterol at higher temperatures	Effect of cholesterol at lower temperatures
A.	Increase	Increase
B.	Increase	Decrease
C.	Increase	No change
D.	Decrease	Increase
E.	Decrease	Decrease
F.	Decrease	No change

4. The plasma membrane is made up of a lipid bilayer, which determines the ability of substances to move in and out of the cell. Which of the following substances are lipid soluble and water soluble, respectively?

	Lipid soluble	Water soluble
A.	CO_2 and O_2	Na^+ and Glucose
B.	CO_2 and O_2	K^+ and Steroid hormones
C.	CO_2 and O_2	Cl^- and Steroid hormones
D.	O_2 and Glucose	Na^+ and K^+
E.	O_2 and Glucose	K^+ and CO_2
F.	O_2 and Glucose	Cl^- and Na^+

5. The permeability of a solute across a lipid bilayer membrane is based on the solute's molecular radius, the oil/water partition coefficient, and the membrane's thickness. Based on these factors, which of the following examples has the highest permeability?

	Molecular radius	Oil/water partition coefficient	Membrane thickness
A.	↑	↑	↑
B.	↑	↓	↓
C.	↑	↑	↓
D.	↓	↓	↑
E.	↓	↓	↓
F.	↓	↑	↓

Questions 6 to 8

Five different dialysis bags, which are permeable to water but impermeable to glucose, are filled with five different glucose solutions. The bags are placed in different beakers containing a 0.5M glucose solution for 80 minutes, and the mass of each bag is measured at regular intervals. The results are recorded on the graph.

2

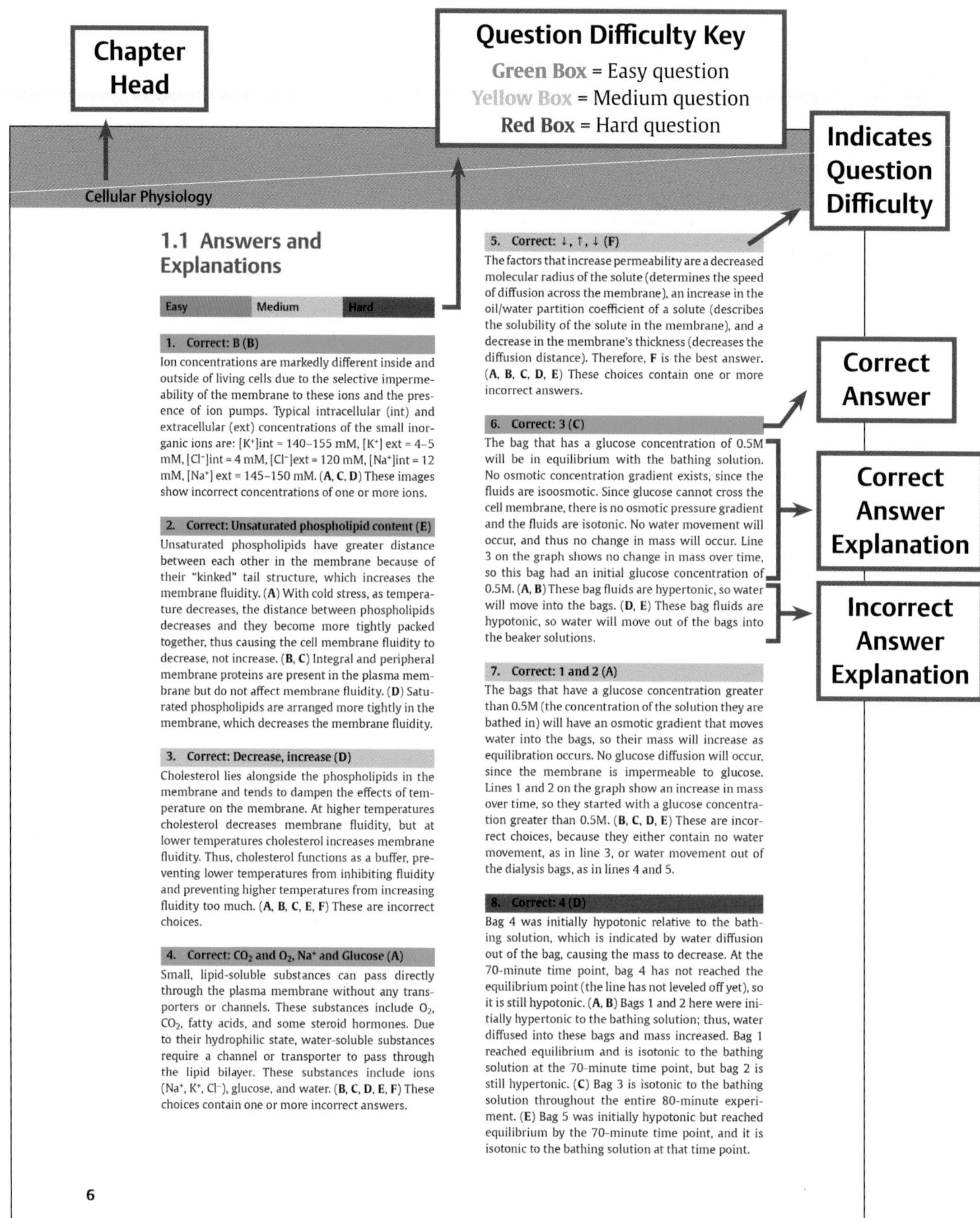

Cellular Physiology

1.1 Answers and Explanations

Easy | Medium | Hard

1. Correct: B (B)

Ion concentrations are markedly different inside and outside of living cells due to the selective impermeability of the membrane to these ions and the presence of ion pumps. Typical intracellular (int) and extracellular (ext) concentrations of the small inorganic ions are: $[K^+]$int = 140–155 mM, $[K^+]$ ext = 4–5 mM, $[Cl^-]$int = 4 mM, $[Cl^-]$ext = 120 mM, $[Na^+]$int = 12 mM, $[Na^+]$ ext = 145–150 mM. (**A**, **C**, **D**) These images show incorrect concentrations of one or more ions.

2. Correct: Unsaturated phospholipid content (E)

Unsaturated phospholipids have greater distance between each other in the membrane because of their "kinked" tail structure, which increases the membrane fluidity. (**A**) With cold stress, as temperature decreases, the distance between phospholipids decreases and they become more tightly packed together, thus causing the cell membrane fluidity to decrease, not increase. (**B**, **C**) Integral and peripheral membrane proteins are present in the plasma membrane but do not affect membrane fluidity. (**D**) Saturated phospholipids are arranged more tightly in the membrane, which decreases the membrane fluidity.

3. Correct: Decrease, increase (D)

Cholesterol lies alongside the phospholipids in the membrane and tends to dampen the effects of temperature on the membrane. At higher temperatures cholesterol decreases membrane fluidity, but at lower temperatures cholesterol increases membrane fluidity. Thus, cholesterol functions as a buffer, preventing lower temperatures from inhibiting fluidity and preventing higher temperatures from increasing fluidity too much. (**A**, **B**, **C**, **E**, **F**) These are incorrect choices.

4. Correct: CO_2 and O_2, Na^+ and Glucose (A)

Small, lipid-soluble substances can pass directly through the plasma membrane without any transporters or channels. These substances include O_2, CO_2, fatty acids, and some steroid hormones. Due to their hydrophilic state, water-soluble substances require a channel or transporter to pass through the lipid bilayer. These substances include ions (Na^+, K^+, Cl^-), glucose, and water. (**B**, **C**, **D**, **E**, **F**) These choices contain one or more incorrect answers.

5. Correct: ↓, ↑, ↓ (F)

The factors that increase permeability are a decreased molecular radius of the solute (determines the speed of diffusion across the membrane), an increase in the oil/water partition coefficient of a solute (describes the solubility of the solute in the membrane), and a decrease in the membrane's thickness (decreases the diffusion distance). Therefore, **F** is the best answer. (**A**, **B**, **C**, **D**, **E**) These choices contain one or more incorrect answers.

6. Correct: 3 (C)

The bag that has a glucose concentration of 0.5M will be in equilibrium with the bathing solution. No osmotic concentration gradient exists, since the fluids are isoosmotic. Since glucose cannot cross the cell membrane, there is no osmotic pressure gradient and the fluids are isotonic. No water movement will occur, and thus no change in mass will occur. Line 3 on the graph shows no change in mass over time, so this bag had an initial glucose concentration of 0.5M. (**A**, **B**) These bag fluids are hypertonic, so water will move into the bags. (**D**, **E**) These bag fluids are hypotonic, so water will move out of the bags into the beaker solutions.

7. Correct: 1 and 2 (A)

The bags that have a glucose concentration greater than 0.5M (the concentration of the solution they are bathed in) will have an osmotic gradient that moves water into the bags, so their mass will increase as equilibration occurs. No glucose diffusion will occur, since the membrane is impermeable to glucose. Lines 1 and 2 on the graph show an increase in mass over time, so they started with a glucose concentration greater than 0.5M. (**B**, **C**, **D**, **E**) These are incorrect choices, because they either contain no water movement, as in line 3, or water movement out of the dialysis bags, as in lines 4 and 5.

8. Correct: 4 (D)

Bag 4 was initially hypotonic relative to the bathing solution, which is indicated by water diffusion out of the bag, causing the mass to decrease. At the 70-minute time point, bag 4 has not reached the equilibrium point (the line has not leveled off yet), so it is still hypotonic. (**A**, **B**) Bags 1 and 2 here were initially hypertonic to the bathing solution; thus, water diffused into these bags and mass increased. Bag 1 reached equilibrium and is isotonic to the bathing solution at the 70-minute time point, but bag 2 is still hypertonic. (**C**) Bag 3 is isotonic to the bathing solution throughout the entire 80-minute experiment. (**E**) Bag 5 was initially hypotonic but reached equilibrium by the 70-minute time point, and it is isotonic to the bathing solution at that time point.

6

Chapter 1

Cellular Physiology

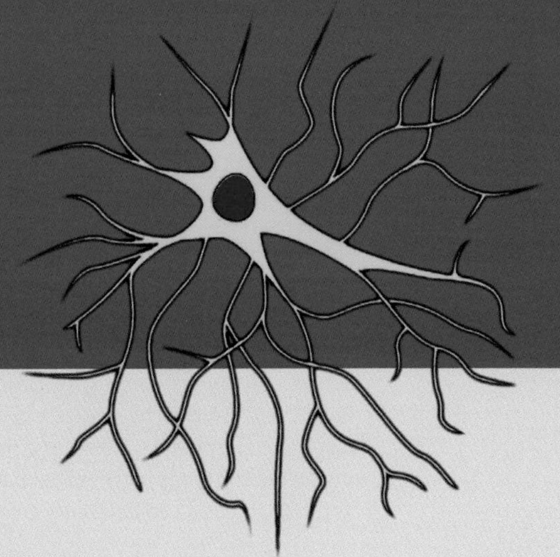

LEARNING OBJECTIVES

- Explain the general physiology of the cellular membrane, including diffusion, membrane transport, intracellular signaling, and feedback.
- Discuss the physiology of osmosis, tonicity, body fluid compartment, Starling forces, and edema formation.
- Discuss the ion channels of the cell membrane and their role in membrane potentials and excitation. Describe the neuronal action potential.

1.1 Questions

Easy	Medium	Hard

1. The provided images show ionic distribution of potassium (K^+), chloride (Cl^-) and sodium (Na^+) across cell membranes. The concentration of each ion is represented by the size of its label, where a larger label indicates a higher concentration. Which image correctly represents the distribution of K^+, Cl^-, and Na^+ across a typical living cell membrane?

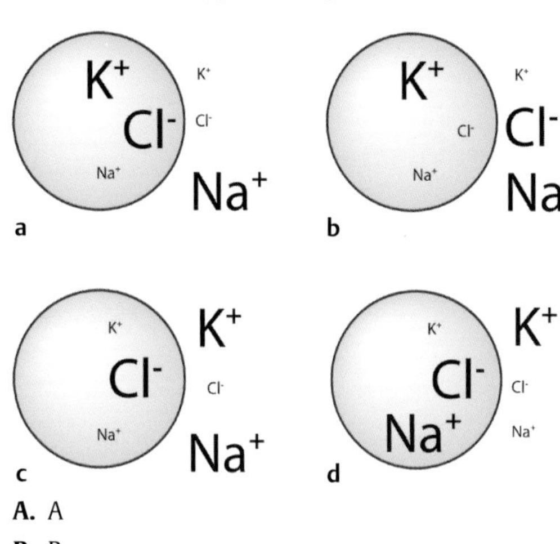

A. A
B. B
C. C
D. D

2. Normal cell function is dependent on fluidity of the cell membrane. An increase in which of the following characteristics of a cell membrane will increase membrane fluidity?

A. Body cold stress
B. Integral membrane protein content
C. Peripheral membrane protein content
D. Saturated phospholipid content
E. Unsaturated phospholipid content

3. Which of the following best depicts the effect of cholesterol on membrane fluidity at higher and lower temperatures?

	Effect of cholesterol at higher temperatures	Effect of cholesterol at lower temperatures
A.	Increase	Increase
B.	Increase	Decrease
C.	Increase	No change
D.	Decrease	Increase
E.	Decrease	Decrease
F.	Decrease	No change

4. The plasma membrane is made up of a lipid bilayer, which determines the ability of substances to move in and out of the cell. Which of the following substances are lipid soluble and water soluble, respectively?

	Lipid soluble	Water soluble
A.	CO_2 and O_2	Na^+ and Glucose
B.	CO_2 and O_2	K^+ and Steroid hormones
C.	CO_2 and O_2	Cl^- and Steroid hormones
D.	O_2 and Glucose	Na^+ and K^+
E.	O_2 and Glucose	K^+ and CO_2
F.	O_2 and Glucose	Cl^- and Na^+

5. The permeability of a solute across a lipid bilayer membrane is based on the solute's molecular radius, the oil/water partition coefficient, and the membrane's thickness. Based on these factors, which of the following examples has the highest permeability?

	Molecular radius	Oil/water partition coefficient	Membrane thickness
A.	↑	↑	↑
B.	↑	↓	↓
C.	↑	↑	↓
D.	↓	↓	↑
E.	↓	↓	↓
F.	↓	↑	↓

Questions 6 to 8

Five different dialysis bags, which are permeable to water but impermeable to glucose, are filled with five different glucose solutions. The bags are placed in different beakers containing a 0.5M glucose solution for 80 minutes, and the mass of each bag is measured at regular intervals. The results are recorded on the graph.

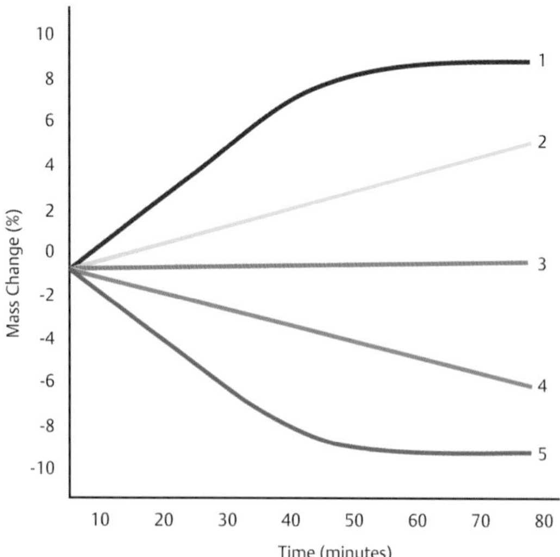

6. Which line on the graph represents the bag that had an initial glucose concentration of 0.5M?

A. 1
B. 2
C. 3
D. 4
E. 5

7. Which lines on the graph represent the bags that had an initial glucose concentration higher than 0.5M?

A. 1 and 2
B. 2 and 3
C. 3 and 4
D. 4 and 5
E. 5 and 1

8. Which line on the graph represents the bag that contains a hypotonic solution at 70 minutes?

A. 1
B. 2
C. 3
D. 4
E. 5

9. Which of the following correctly represents the relationship that governs the diffusion of particles through a cell membrane, not taking into account the electrical force acting on the particle if it is charged?

A. $\Delta P / R$
B. $PA(C_1 - C_2)$
C. $KD/\Delta x$
D. $BT/6\pi r\eta$
E. $(P_c - P_i) - (\pi_c - \pi_i)$

where

A: Surface area (m^2)
B: Boltzmann coefficient (m^2 kg s^{-2} K^{-1})
C: Concentration (M)
D: Diffusion coefficient (m^2/s)
K: Partition coefficient
P: Pressure (N/m^2) or Permeability (m/s)
R: Resistance (Ω)
r: Radius of the particle (m)
T: Temperature (K)
π: Number pi (3.1416) or oncotic pressure (Osm/kg water)
η: Viscosity of medium (Ns/m^2)
Δx: membrane thickness (m)

Questions 10 to 11

The tank shown is divided in half by a lipid membrane. One liter of water is added to each side of the tank, with different concentrations of substance A, as illustrated in the image. The lipid membrane surface area is 2 cm^2 and the solubility of the membrane to substance A is 7×10^{-5} cm/sec.

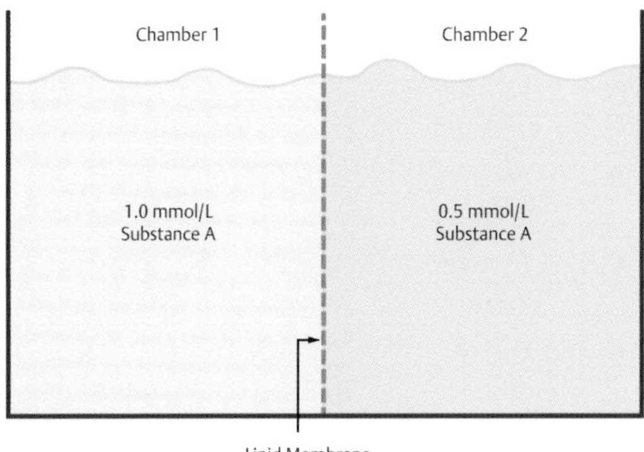

10. What is the net direction of diffusion between chambers 1 and 2, and the net rate of diffusion for substance A?

	Net direction of diffusion	Net rate of diffusion (mmol/sec)
A.	From 1 to 2	7×10^{-5}
B.	From 1 to 2	14×10^{-5}
C.	From 1 to 2	3.5×10^{-5}
D.	From 2 to 1	7×10^{-5}
E.	From 2 to 1	14×10^{-5}
F.	From 2 to 1	3.5×10^{-5}

11. Which of the following changes will increase the net diffusion of substance A?

A. Decrease chamber 1 concentration to 0.7 mmol/L
B. Decrease permeability of substance A
C. Increase chamber 2 concentration to 0.8 mmol/L
D. Increase membrane surface area
E. Increase chambers 1 and 2 to 2 liters of water

12. Which type of transport (passive diffusion, 1° active transport, 2° active transport) is utilized for the three described processes?

	Nitric oxide across a smooth muscle cell membrane	Na^+ and glucose into intestinal cells	Na^+ out and K^+ into cardiac myocytes
A.	Passive diffusion	1° active transport	2° active transport
B.	Passive diffusion	2° active transport	1° active transport
C.	Passive diffusion	1° active transport	1° active transport
D.	Passive diffusion	2° active transport	2° active transport
E.	2° active transport	1° active transport	Passive diffusion
F.	2° active transport	Passive diffusion	1° active transport
G.	2° active transport	1° active transport	2° active transport
H.	2° active transport	Passive diffusion	2° active transport

13. During a routine newborn screening test, an infant tests positive for cystic fibrosis. This is an inherited condition in which the CFTR protein, a membrane chloride channel, is absent or nonfunctional. What effect will this have on water movement in cells with dysfunctional CFTR channels, compared to normal?

A. An increased volume of water will move into cells.
B. An increased volume of water will move out of cells.
C. A reduced volume of water will move into cells.
D. A reduced volume of water will move out of cells.
E. Water movement will not be affected in these cells.

14. A 40-year-old man presents to his primary care physician with a 2-month history of intermittent upper abdominal pain shortly after eating. He is referred to a specialist, and upper gastrointestinal endoscopy is performed. The endoscopy reveals a peptic ulcer. He is prescribed omeprazole, a gastric proton pump inhibitor. What type of cell membrane transport is inhibited by this medication?

A. Facilitated diffusion
B. Osmosis
C. Primary active transport
D. Secondary active transport
E. Simple diffusion

15. In which of the following membrane transport processes is the substance moving by facilitated diffusion?

A. Calcium from sarcoplasm into sarcoplasmic reticulum
B. Glucose from plasma into red blood cells
C. Glucose from gut lumen into intestinal epithelial cells
D. Potassium from extracellular space into striated muscle fibers
E. Sodium from neuronal cytoplasm into extracellular space

16. A circulating hormone binds to an extracellular receptor on a smooth muscle cell and initiates an intracellular response. This hormone most likely has which of the following properties?

A. It is amphipathic.
B. It is fat soluble.
C. It is hydrophilic.
D. It is lipophilic.
E. It is nonpolar.

17. A circulating hormone binds to an extracellular receptor on epithelial tissue and initiates an intracellular response via activation of a second messenger. Which of the following can be classified as a second messenger?

A. Adenylyl cyclase
B. Cyclic AMP
C. Epinephrine
D. G-proteins
E. Guanosine triphosphate

18. The body utilizes negative feedback systems to maintain homeostasis. The flow diagram provided shows the standard components of all negative feedback systems. Which component of the negative feedback system is missing at the point labeled X on the diagram?

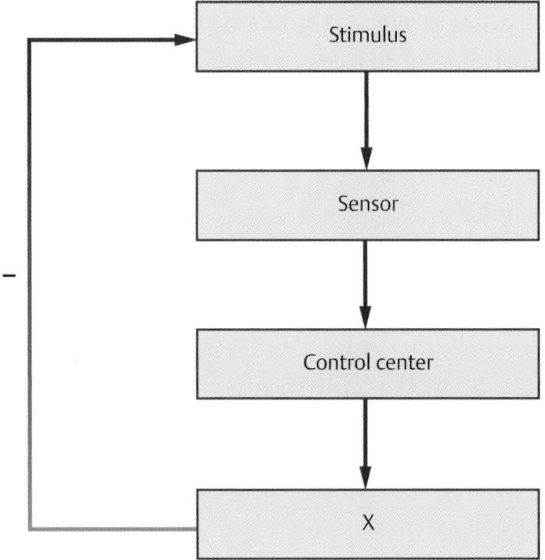

A. Afferent neurons
B. Brain
C. Effectors
D. Efferent neurons
E. Receptors

19. Five drugs are listed in the following table (A–E). If these drug molecules are all equally lipophilic, which of the following conditions would produce the highest rate of transport of the drug molecule into a cell by simple diffusion?

	Molecular weight	Intracellular concentration (mM)	Extracellular concentration (mM)
Drug A	200	0.05	0.5
Drug B	250	1.0	0.4
Drug C	200	0.3	0.9
Drug D	200	0.5	0.5
Drug E	250	0.3	0.9

A. Drug A
B. Drug B
C. Drug C
D. Drug D
E. Drug E

20. In a research study on obesity, it is shown that in the presence of insulin, the transport of d-glucose across the plasma membrane of adipose cells is much faster than the transport of l-glucose. Which of the following best explains the observed finding?

A. Carrier-mediated transport of glucose
B. Exchange transport of glucose
C. Primary active transport of glucose
D. Receptor-mediated endocytosis of glucose
E. Simple diffusion of glucose

21. In the aftermath of an earthquake, humanitarian emergency volunteers handed out isotonic drink solutions containing NaCl and glucose to people with signs of dehydration. These oral rehydration solutions with NaCl and glucose are physiologically more effective than isotonic solutions containing NaCl only. Which of the following is the best explanation?

A. A primary active glucose transporter at the basolateral intestinal cell membrane facilitates Na^+ and water reabsorption from the gut.
B. Oral glucose increases insulin secretion, which then facilitates water reabsorption.
C. The addition of glucose makes it more likely for the person to drink.
D. The cotransport of glucose and Na^+ across the apical membrane of intestinal epithelial cells facilitates Na^+ and water absorption from the gut.
E. The NaCl and glucose solution creates a higher osmotic pressure, which facilitates the uptake of water across the apical membrane of intestinal epithelial cells.

1.2 Answers and Explanations

Easy	Medium	Hard

1. Correct: B (B)

Ion concentrations are markedly different inside and outside of living cells due to the selective impermeability of the membrane to these ions and the presence of ion pumps. Typical intracellular (int) and extracellular (ext) concentrations of the small inorganic ions are: $[K^+]$int = 140–155 mM, $[K^+]$ ext = 4–5 mM, $[Cl^-]$int = 4 mM, $[Cl^-]$ext = 120 mM, $[Na^+]$int = 12 mM, $[Na^+]$ ext = 145–150 mM. (**A**, **C**, **D**) These images show incorrect concentrations of one or more ions.

2. Correct: Unsaturated phospholipid content (E)

Unsaturated phospholipids have greater distance between each other in the membrane because of their "kinked" tail structure, which increases the membrane fluidity. (**A**) With cold stress, as temperature decreases, the distance between phospholipids decreases and they become more tightly packed together, thus causing the cell membrane fluidity to decrease, not increase. (**B**, **C**) Integral and peripheral membrane proteins are present in the plasma membrane but do not affect membrane fluidity. (**D**) Saturated phospholipids are arranged more tightly in the membrane, which decreases the membrane fluidity.

3. Correct: Decrease, increase (D)

Cholesterol lies alongside the phospholipids in the membrane and tends to dampen the effects of temperature on the membrane. At higher temperatures cholesterol decreases membrane fluidity, but at lower temperatures cholesterol increases membrane fluidity. Thus, cholesterol functions as a buffer, preventing lower temperatures from inhibiting fluidity and preventing higher temperatures from increasing fluidity too much. (**A**, **B**, **C**, **E**, **F**) These are incorrect choices.

4. Correct: CO_2 and O_2, Na^+ and Glucose (A)

Small, lipid-soluble substances can pass directly through the plasma membrane without any transporters or channels. These substances include O_2, CO_2, fatty acids, and some steroid hormones. Due to their hydrophilic state, water-soluble substances require a channel or transporter to pass through the lipid bilayer. These substances include ions (Na^+, K^+, Cl^-), glucose, and water. (**B**, **C**, **D**, **E**, **F**) These choices contain one or more incorrect answers.

5. Correct: ↓, ↑, ↓ (F)

The factors that increase permeability are a decreased molecular radius of the solute (determines the speed of diffusion across the membrane), an increase in the oil/water partition coefficient of a solute (describes the solubility of the solute in the membrane), and a decrease in the membrane's thickness (decreases the diffusion distance). Therefore, **F** is the best answer. (**A**, **B**, **C**, **D**, **E**) These choices contain one or more incorrect answers.

6. Correct: 3 (C)

The bag that has a glucose concentration of 0.5M will be in equilibrium with the bathing solution. No osmotic concentration gradient exists, since the fluids are isoosmotic. Since glucose cannot cross the cell membrane, there is no osmotic pressure gradient and the fluids are isotonic. No water movement will occur, and thus no change in mass will occur. Line 3 on the graph shows no change in mass over time, so this bag had an initial glucose concentration of 0.5M. (**A**, **B**) These bag fluids are hypertonic, so water will move into the bags. (**D**, **E**) These bag fluids are hypotonic, so water will move out of the bags into the beaker solutions.

7. Correct: 1 and 2 (A)

The bags that have a glucose concentration greater than 0.5M (the concentration of the solution they are bathed in) will have an osmotic gradient that moves water into the bags, so their mass will increase as equilibration occurs. No glucose diffusion will occur, since the membrane is impermeable to glucose. Lines 1 and 2 on the graph show an increase in mass over time, so they started with a glucose concentration greater than 0.5M. (**B**, **C**, **D**, **E**) These are incorrect choices, because they either contain no water movement, as in line 3, or water movement out of the dialysis bags, as in lines 4 and 5.

8. Correct: 4 (D)

Bag 4 was initially hypotonic relative to the bathing solution, which is indicated by water diffusion out of the bag, causing the mass to decrease. At the 70-minute time point, bag 4 has not reached the equilibrium point (the line has not leveled off yet), so it is still hypotonic. (**A**, **B**) Bags 1 and 2 here were initially hypertonic to the bathing solution; thus, water diffused into these bags and mass increased. Bag 1 reached equilibrium and is isotonic to the bathing solution at the 70-minute time point, but bag 2 is still hypertonic. (**C**) Bag 3 is isotonic to the bathing solution throughout the entire 80-minute experiment. (**E**) Bag 5 was initially hypotonic but reached equilibrium by the 70-minute time point, and it is isotonic to the bathing solution at that time point.

9. Correct: $PA(C_1 - C_2)$ (B)

This is Fick's first law of diffusion, describing the factors influencing the net diffusion rate, J. J is proportional to the membrane permeability (P), the surface area for diffusion (A), and the concentration difference across the membrane ($C_1 - C_2$). The permeability, P, already includes the partition coefficient K, the diffusion coefficient D, and the membrane thickness Δx, as shown in answer **C**. (**A**) This is the bulk flow law. Flow is proportional to a difference in pressure (ΔP) and inversely proportional to resistance (R). (**C**) This is the equation for the permeability, P. P = partition coefficient (K) × diffusion coefficient (D) / membrane thickness (Δx). (**D**) This is the Stokes–Einstein equation, which expresses the relationship for the diffusion coefficient, D. D = [Boltzmann constant (B) × absolute temperature (T)] / [6π × molecular radius (r) × viscosity of medium (η)]. (**E**) This is the Starling equation for transcapillary fluid movement. It is proportional to the difference of the hydrostatic pressure (P_c capillary and P_i interstitial) and the oncotic pressure (π_c capillary and π_i interstitial).

10. Correct: From 1 to 2, 7 × 10⁻⁵ (A)

Substance A will diffuse from high to low concentration down its concentration gradient, so it will diffuse from chamber 1 to chamber 2. Use the Fick law of diffusion to calculate the net rate of diffusion.

$J = PA(C_1 - C_2)$

$J = 7 \times 10^{-5}$ cm/sec × 2 cm^2 × (1.0 mmol/L – 0.5 mmol/L)

$J = 7 \times 10^{-5}$ mmol/sec

11. Correct: Increase membrane surface area (D)

Based on the Fick law of diffusion [$J = PA(C_1 - C_2)$], one of three changes will increase net diffusion across the lipid membrane. (1) An increase in the permeability of the substance, P; (2) an increase in the surface area of the membrane, A; or (3) an increase in the concentration gradient across the membrane, $C_1 - C_2$. Therefore, an increase in membrane surface area is the best answer. (**A**) A decrease in chamber 1 concentration will decrease the concentration gradient across the membrane, which will decrease diffusion rate. (**B**) A decrease in the permeability of substance A will decrease it net diffusion rate. (**C**) An increase in chamber 2 concentration will decrease the concentration gradient across the membrane, which will decrease diffusion rate. (**E**) Increasing the water content in chambers 1 and 2 by equal amounts will not change net diffusion rate.

12. Correct: Passive diffusion, 2° active transport, 1° active transport (B)

Nitric oxide is a gas formed by endothelial cells. It diffuses passively across lipid membranes due to its lipid solubility. Sodium and glucose are cotransported across membranes in the same direction using SGLT1 in the gastrointestinal tract. This cotransport is secondary active transport, since sodium is moving down its concentration gradient while simultaneously cotransporting glucose up its concentration gradient. Sodium and potassium are antiported across membranes using the Na^+/K^+ ATPase, which utilizes ATP to move both cations against their concentration gradients.

13. Correct: A reduced volume of water will move out of cells (D)

Normally, the CFTR moves negatively charged chloride ions out of the epithelial cells. Positively charged sodium ions follow passively, increasing the total electrolyte concentration in the extracellular space, which results in the movement of water out of the cell via osmosis. Hence, if the CFTR channels are dysfunctional, less water will move out of cells. (**A, B**) Decreased electrolyte flow will limit (not increase) osmotic water movement. (**C**) In epithelial cells, the CFTR channel is part of a mechanism to move water out of (not into) cells. (**E**) Water movement will be affected, evident in that cystic fibrosis patients suffer from symptoms due to extracellular fluids with a low water content, such as sweat, digestive juices, and mucus.

14. Correct: Primary active transport (C)

Proton pump inhibitors reduce stomach acid by blocking acid production. They work by inhibiting the gastric H^+/K^+-ATPase (proton pump), which is a primary active transport mechanism because it requires ATP to move the ions against their electrochemical gradients. (**A**) Facilitated diffusion is a type of passive diffusion that does not require ATP, but involves a membrane protein for substances to pass through down their electrochemical gradient. (**B, E**) Osmosis and simple diffusion are passive transport mechanisms that do not require ATP. (**D**) Secondary active transport utilizes energy stored in an electrochemical gradient to cotransport substances. One substance is transported with its gradient, while the other is transported against its gradient.

15. Correct: Glucose from plasma into red blood cells (B)

Movement of glucose occurs via the GLUT1 transporter into red blood cells. Because glucose will be metabolized inside the cells, there is always a gradient that drives glucose into the cells. (**A**) Calcium is transported by a calcium pump into the sarcoplasmic reticulum via primary active transport. (**C**) Glucose is transported into intestinal epithelial cells by secondary active transport via the SGLT transporter. This is necessary so that glucose is always transported toward the blood, despite varying gut glucose concentrations. (**D, E**) Sodium and potassium are either moving by simple diffusion through channels, or transported by the Na-K ATPase, i.e., primary active transport.

16. Correct: It is hydrophilic. (C)

Circulating hormones are typically water soluble. They bind to extracellular receptors on cellular membranes because they are hydrophilic (water loving) and lipophobic (lipid fearing); thus they cannot pass directly through the lipid membrane. (**A**) Amphipathic substances have both hydrophilic and lipophilic properties. Common amphipathic substances are soaps, detergents, and lipoproteins. (**B, D**) Fat-soluble substances are lipophilic and can pass freely thorough a lipid membrane and directly activate intracellular mechanisms without a membrane transporter or intracellular second messenger system. (**E**) Molecules that have partially charged positive and negative areas are polar, and water-soluble substances are polar.

17. Correct: Cyclic AMP (B)

Second messengers are intracellular signaling molecules that are released by the cell in response to exposure to extracellular signaling molecules. They initiate an intracellular signaling cascade and trigger a physiological change. Some examples are cyclic AMP, calcium, inositol triphosphate (IP_3), and diacylglycerol. (**A**) Adenylyl cyclase is an enzyme that catalyzes the conversion of ATP to cyclic AMP and pyrophosphate. (**C**) Epinephrine is a hormone that is derived from the amino acid tyrosine and secreted by the medulla of the adrenal glands. (**D**) G-proteins are enzymes that are bound to G-protein-coupled receptors and are involved in transmitting signals from a variety of stimuli from the outside to the inside of a cell. (**E**) Guanosine triphosphate (GTP) is essential to G-protein signaling in second-messenger systems, but it is not a second messenger itself.

18. Correct: Effectors (C)

Negative feedback is a key regulatory mechanism for physiological function in living things. It is a regulatory mechanism in which a change or stimulus is sensed by a sensor (receptor) and sends a message to the control center (usually the central nervous system). The control center then activates effectors, which will produce an effect to restore the initial change back toward normal. (**A**) Afferent neurons are involved in this pathway; they are indicated by the arrow between the sensors and the control center. (**B**) The brain or central nervous system is usually the control center. (**D**) Efferent neurons are involved in this pathway; they are indicated by the arrow between the control center and the X (effectors). (**E**) The receptors are the sensors.

19. Correct: Drug C (C)

Based on the Fick law, the concentration gradient and molecular weight of a substance both play a role in diffusion across a membrane. The concentration gradient is greatest in drugs C and E, but since the size of the particle is considered in the permeability coefficient, the smaller particles pass through the membrane easier than large particles, so drug C is the best answer. (**A**) Drug A has the same molecular weight as drug C, but it has a smaller concentration gradient across the membrane (recall that the concentration gradient is the difference in concentration, not the ratio of concentrations), which reduces the diffusion rate. (**B**) Drug B has a negative concentration gradient, so it will diffuse out of the cell, not into it. (**D**) Drug D has the same molecular weight has drug C, but it has a zero concentration gradient, so it will not diffuse across the membrane either way. (**E**) Drug E has the same concentration gradient as drug C, but a larger molecular weight, which reduces its diffusion rate.

20. Correct: Carrier-mediated transport of glucose (A)

Glucose transport across adipose cell membranes is mediated by the carrier protein GLUT4 (the insulin-dependent glucose transporter). Carriers have specificity, and the glucose carrier is stereo-selective for D-glucose. (**B**) Exchange transport of glucose occurs in the kidneys, but not in adipose tissue. (**C**) Primary active transport of glucose occurs in the gut, but not in adipose tissue. (**D**) Glucose is not transported via receptor-mediated endocytosis. (**E**) Glucose molecules are too large to pass through the cell membrane via simple diffusion. (Note: a small amount of glucose can diffuse across the membrane via simple diffusion if given adequate time, but it is minimal.)

21. Correct: The cotransport of glucose and Na^+ across the apical membrane of intestinal epithelial cells facilitates Na^+ and water absorption from the gut. (D)

The presence of glucose in the solution greatly increases the absorption of Na^+ and water because Na is cotransported with glucose into the intestinal epithelial cells by SGLT proteins. (**A**) Glucose is not transported with the help of an ATPase to provide a drag for water. (**B**) Insulin is not related to water reabsorption. (**C**) A better taste of the solution is not the reason for adding glucose. (**E**) Both solutions (with and without glucose) are isotonic. In addition, a hypertonic solution would facilitate diarrhea, not water reabsorption.

1.3 Questions

22. At low concentrations, sodium chloride (NaCl) is a salt that completely dissociates in water. However, at very high concentrations some Na^+ and Cl^- ions will reassociate into NaCl. If a 1.0M solution of NaCl represents a very high NaCl concentration, what will the osmolarity (in osmoles/L) of this solution be?

A. Less than 1.0
B. Equal to 1.0
C. Between 1.0 and 2.0
D. Equal to 2.0
E. Greater than 2.0

23. A quantity of red blood cells from a healthy person is placed in a solution of water containing a nondissociable solute at a concentration of 500 millimolar. All of the red blood cells swell and lyse. Which of the following is the best explanation?

A. The cell membrane is impermeable to the solute.
B. The cell membrane is permeable to the solute.
C. The solute is a large and polar molecule.
D. The solution is hypertonic compared to the cell interior.
E. The solution is hypoosmotic compared to the cell interior.

24. As part of plasmapheresis, a technician normally separates the patient's blood cells from plasma and places them in a solution with fresh plasma. This time, erroneously, she places the cells in a solution of plasma with urea added. Which of the following statements best describes what happens to the red blood cells?

A. Will shrink and undergo hemolysis
B. Will shrink and undergo apoptosis
C. Will initially shrink, but then swell
D. Will swell and eventually lyse
E. Will swell and undergo apoptosis

25. Which of the following will initially lead to a decrease in the intracellular volume of a typical mammalian cell, before counterbalancing mechanisms start to regulate the cell's volume?

A. Exposure to a 300 mM urea solution
B. Exposure to 150 mM $MgCl_2$ solution
C. Exposure to a 100 mM NaCl solution
D. Blockade of the Na/K-ATPase in the cell membrane
E. Exposure to distilled water

26. A 19-year-old male patient presents with blood loss due to a stab wound. His blood pressure is low and pulse rate is high. The estimated blood loss is 500 mL. Approximately how much intravenous saline should be administered to replace the blood volume and restore the patient's blood pressure to normal?

A. 0.5 L
B. 1.0 L
C. 1.5 L
D. 2.0 L
E. 2.5 L

27. An 85-year-old man receives intravenous (IV) fluids for three days following a stroke. After the third day, he presents with ankle edema and elevated jugular venous pressure. His charts reveal a total fluid input of 9 L and a urine output of 6 L over these three days. How much excess fluid is this patient carrying?

A. 1.5 L
B. 2.0 L
C. 2.5 L
D. 3.0 L
E. 3.5 L

28. Which of the following will occur if red blood cells are bathed in a solution that is hyperosmotic, relative to plasma?

A. NaCl will diffuse across the plasma membrane into the red blood cells.
B. NaCl will be transported into the red blood cells by active transport.
C. NaCl will be transported out of the red blood cells by facilitated diffusion.
D. Water will move from the extracellular space to the intracellular space.
E. Water will move from the intracellular space to the extracellular space.

29. A 32-year-old man is injured in a car accident and is bleeding profusely. When the ambulance arrives, the man is hypotensive and tachycardic. The paramedic starts intravenous fluid replacement but accidentally infuses 800 mL of sterile pure water instead of normal saline solution. What effect will this infusion have on his plasma osmolarity and on the shape of his red blood cells (RBC)?

	Plasma Osmolarity	RBC shape
A.	Hyperosmotic	Swollen
B.	Hyperosmotic	Crenated
C.	Hypoosmotic	Swollen
D.	Hypoosmotic	Crenated
E.	Isoosmotic	Swollen
F.	Isoosmotic	Crenated

Questions 30 to 31

The tank shown is divided in half by a membrane that is permeable to water and glucose but not fructose. One liter of water is added to each side of the tank, with different concentrations of glucose and fructose, as illustrated in the image.

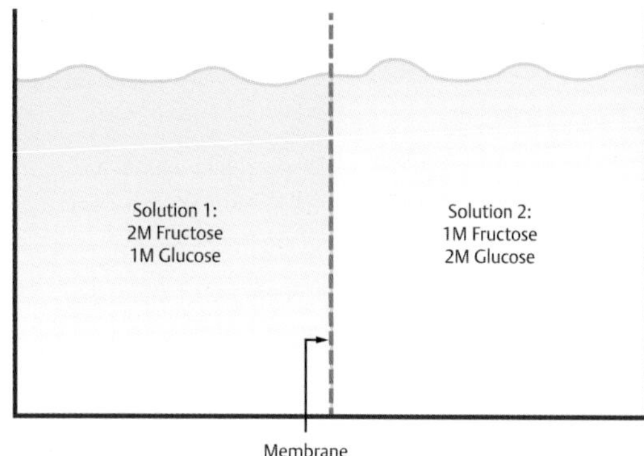

30. At time point zero, before any equilibration occurs, how does solution 1 compare to solution 2?

A. It is hyperosmotic.
B. It is hypoosmotic.
C. It is isoosmotic.
D. It is more saturated.
E. It has more volume.

31. After one hour the system has reached equilibrium. At this time point, how does solution 1 compare to solution 2?

A. It has a greater glucose molarity.
B. It has a smaller glucose molarity.
C. It has a greater volume of water.
D. It has a smaller volume of water.
E. It has a higher number of glucose particles.

Questions 32 to 34

A 42-year-old female patient has an annual exam. She weighs 60 kg. She complains of fatigue. Her hematocrit is 35%.

32. What is the patient's estimated total body water in liters?

A. 25
B. 28
C. 31
D. 34
E. 36

33. What are the patient's estimated extracellular fluid volume and intracellular fluid volume in liters?

	Extracellular fluid volume (in liters)	Intracellular fluid volume (in liters)
A.	12	24
B.	12	36
C.	24	12
D.	24	36
E.	36	12
F.	36	14

34. What is the patient's estimated blood volume in liters?

A. 3.5
B. 4.6
C. 5.4
D. 6.5
E. 7.1

35. Five volunteers of the same weight, height, and total body water are injected with 1 L of different solutions. The infusions are allowed to equilibrate, and no fluid is excreted. Which of the following solutions would cause the greatest increase in extracellular fluid volume?

A. Hypertonic saline
B. Isoosmotic urea
C. Isotonic saline
D. Plasma
E. Water

36. Antidiuretic hormone (ADH) regulates water retention by acting to increase water reabsorption in the kidneys. If the ADH receptors are antagonized, what effects on intracellular fluid volume, extracellular fluid volume, and hematocrit are expected?

	Intracellular fluid volume	Extracellular fluid volume	Hematocrit
A.	↑	↑	↑
B.	↑	↑	↓
C.	↑	↓	↓
D.	↓	↓	↓
E.	↓	↓	↑
F.	↓	↑	↑

37. Antidiuretic hormone (ADH) regulates water retention by acting to increase water reabsorption in the kidneys. If the ADH receptors are antagonized, what effect will this have on extracellular fluid osmolarity and extracellular fluid Na^+ concentration?

	Extracellular fluid osmolarity	Extracellular fluid Na^+ concentration
A.	↑	↑
B.	↑	↓
C.	↑	↔
D.	↓	↑
E.	↓	↓
F.	↓	↔

38. Different tracer substances are used to measure the volumes of different body compartments. Which tracers are used to measure total body water, extracellular fluid volume, and plasma volume, respectively?

	Total body water	Extracellular fluid volume	Plasma volume
A.	Mannitol	^3H_2O	Evans blue dye
B.	Mannitol	Evans blue dye	^3H_2O
C.	^3H_2O	Mannitol	Evans blue dye
D.	^3H_2O	Evans blue dye	Mannitol
E.	Evans blue dye	Mannitol	^3H_2O
F.	Evans blue dye	^3H_2O	Mannitol

39. 300 mL of a 2,500 mg/L mannitol solution is given to a patient intravenously. Two hours later a blood sample is taken, and the concentration of mannitol in the plasma is 100 mg/L. Given the patient has a total body water volume of 25 L, what is the patient's intracellular fluid volume in liters?

A. 7.5
B. 15
C. 17.5
D. 20
E. 25

40. Subjects 1 and 2 are both 70-kg male subjects with the same total body water; depicted by the "normal state" in the image. Subject 1 drinks a hyperosmotic saline solution, while Subject 2 drinks a hypoosmotic saline solution. After steady-state equilibrium is achieved, which diagram best represents the volume and osmolarity shift for each subject?

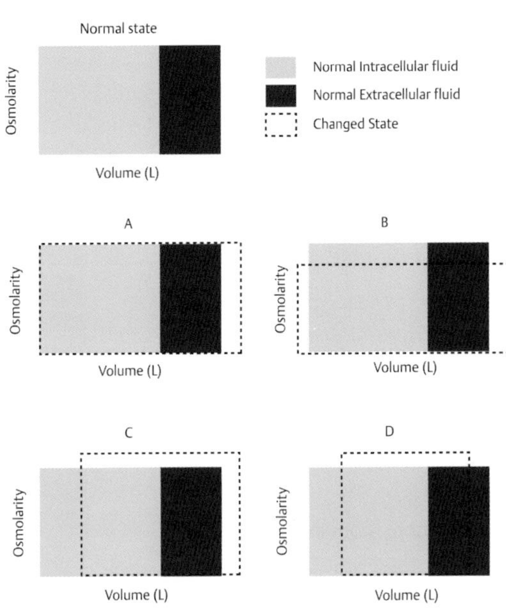

	Subject 1	Subject 2
A.	A	B
B.	A	C
C.	A	D
D.	B	A
E.	B	C
F.	B	D
G.	C	A
H.	C	B
I.	C	D
J.	D	A
K.	D	B
L.	D	C

41. A 30-year-old woman is lost in the woods for 15-hours while hiking on a hot day in June. She has no food and little water, and she walks approximately 15 miles before she is rescued. She is sweating profusely from the exertion. At the time of her rescue, which diagram best represents the relative volume and osmolarity of her fluid compartments, compared to the "normal state" diagram?

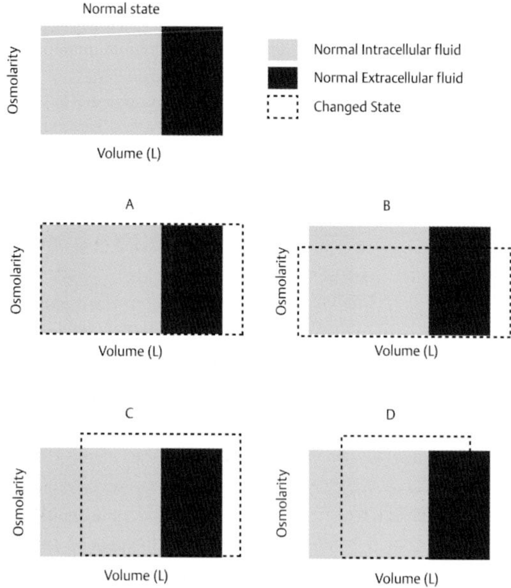

A. A
B. B
C. C
D. D

42. 100 mL of a 5 mg/mL Evans blue dye solution is injected into a patient intravenously. Twenty minutes later, a blood sample is taken and the concentration of Evans blue dye in the plasma is 100 mg/L. What is the patient's estimated plasma fluid volume in liters?

A. 3
B. 5
C. 7
D. 9
E. 10

43. A 68-year-old woman with a history of heart disease presents with peripheral edema and difficulty breathing. She is diagnosed with congestive heart failure. Which tracer substance(s) are required to determine her interstitial fluid volume?

A. ^3H_2O
B. Evans blue dye
C. Inulin
D. Mannitol
E. Mannitol and Evans blue dye
F. ^3H_2O and Mannitol

44. A 63-year-old man presents with abdominal ascites and lower extremity edema. He is diagnosed with liver cirrhosis due to an undiagnosed hepatitis B infection. A deficiency of protein in the blood due to reduced liver function will *most directly affect* which of the Starling forces?

A. Capillary colloid osmotic pressure
B. Capillary hydrostatic pressure
C. Filtration coefficient
D. Interstitial colloid osmotic pressure
E. Interstitial hydrostatic pressure

45. A 23-year old woman received a knife wound to the abdomen and suffered severe blood loss. On arrival of the first responders, her pulse was 115 bpm and blood pressure was 80/65 mm Hg. Intravenous infusion of 0.9% saline was started immediately. Which of the following pressures will be *most directly affected* by this injury?

A. Capillary hydrostatic pressure
B. Capillary colloid osmotic pressure
C. Interstitial hydrostatic pressure
D. Interstitial colloid osmotic pressure
E. Lymphatic pressure

46. A 46-year-old man presents with edema of the right leg following a surgical procedure to repair a torn calf muscle on the right side. The edema is unilateral. His serum proteins and electrolytes are normal. Which of the following pressures will be *most directly affected* by this edema?

A. Capillary hydrostatic pressure
B. Capillary colloid osmotic pressure
C. Interstitial hydrostatic pressure
D. Interstitial colloid osmotic pressure
E. Mean arterial pressure

47. A 15-year-old boy reports blood in his urine 10 days after having a sore throat. He has elevated blood urea and a blood pressure of 170/90 mm Hg with peripheral edema. The fluid volume in which of the following body fluid compartments is increased in this patient?

A. Intracellular

B. Interstitial

C. Plasma volume

D. Intracellular and interstitial

E. Interstitial and plasma

48. A change to which of the following determinants of net filtration pressure favors a fluid shift from the plasma to the interstitium?

A. Decreased capillary hydrostatic pressure

B. Decreased filtration coefficient

C. Increased capillary colloid osmotic pressure

D. Increased interstitial colloid osmotic pressure

E. Increased interstitial hydrostatic pressure

1.4 Answers and Explanations

22. Correct: Between 1.0 and 2.0 (C)

Sodium chloride (NaCl) dissociates in water to give Na^+ and Cl^-, two osmotically active particles. Hence, 1M of fully dissociated NaCl would have an osmotic pressure of 2 osmoles/L. However, since at high concentrations some NaCl will not dissociate, the osmolarity will be lower, somewhere between 1.0 and 2.0. (**A**, **B**, **D**, **E**) Based on the explanation above, these answers are incorrect.

23. Correct: The cell membrane is permeable to the solute. (B)

With a membrane-permeable solute, (reflection coefficient $\sigma = 0$), there is no osmotic pressure created, and the cell behaves as if nothing had been dissolved in water surrounding the cell. The solute enters the cell and produces an osmotic gradient across the cell membrane, and water enters the cell and increases its volume, eventually leading to lysis. (**A**, **C**) Water would leave the cell if the membrane was impermeable to the solute. Large, polar molecules are not likely to cross the cell membrane. (**D**) For the cells to swell and lyse, water must move into the cell, which would happen with a hypotonic (not hypertonic) solution. (**E**) The extracellular solution is hyperosmotic (500 mosmoles/L) compared to the inside of a normal human red blood cell (~300 mosmoles/L).

24. Correct: Will swell and eventually lyse (D)

Urea does not produce osmotic pressure. Urea entering the cell produces an osmotic gradient across the cell membrane, and water enters the cell and increases its volume. The influx of water dilutes the urea inside the cell and more urea enters, followed by more water and increased swelling of the cell. The cell eventually lyses. (**A**, **B**, **C**) Based on the explanation just given, the cell will swell, not shrink. (**E**) Apoptosis is a programmed cell death, which is not initiated by osmosis.

25. Correct: Exposure to 150 mM $MgCl_2$ solution (B)

$MgCl_2$ dissociates into three particles, which gives an overall osmotic pressure of 450 mOsm/kg. This is higher than the 300 mOsm/kg normal value; therefore water will move outward, and the cell shrinks. (**A**) Urea will diffuse into the cell, creating an osmotic gradient across the cell membrane, and water will enter the cell and increases its volume (swell). (**C**) NaCl dissociates into two particles, which gives an overall osmotic pressure of 200 mOsm/kg. This is lower than the 300-mOsm/kg normal value; therefore, water will move inward, and the cell swells. (**D**) When the Na/K-ATPase is blocked, Na^+ accumulates in the cell and it swells. (**E**) Distilled water is hypotonic, which will cause diffusion of water into the cell, causing the cell to swell.

26. Correct: 2.0 L (D)

Typically, about four times the blood volume lost is the volume of saline needed to restore blood volume and pressure back to normal after hemorrhage. For this patient, 500 mL of blood was lost, so 2L of saline should be administered. This is true because of the infused fluid, only about 25% remains in the intravascular space. The other 75% diffuses to the other extracellular spaces. (**A**, **B**, **C**, **E**) These choices are incorrect.

27. Correct: 1.5 L (A)

This man is hypervolemic with interstitial edema and intravascular excess, because he has received 3 liters more fluid than he has passed out in his urine. Remember, however, that he loses approximately 500 mL/day in insensible losses, which is 1.5 L over the three days. Therefore, his total fluid excess is around 1.5 L. (**B**, **C**, **D**, **E**) These choices are incorrect.

28. Correct: Water will move from the intracellular space to the extracellular space. (E)

When cells are placed in a hyperosmotic solution, water moves toward the hyperosmotic region, from the intracellular space to the extracellular space. (**A**) The plasma membrane is not permeable to ions such as Na^+ and Cl^-, so NaCl cannot passively diffuse in or out of the red blood cells. (**B**) The movement of NaCl into the red blood cells would be down the concentration gradient; therefore, active transport would not be required for this movement. (**C**) The movement of NaCl out of the red blood cells would be against the concentration gradient, which would require active transport, not facilitated transport. (**D**) When cells are placed in a hyperosmotic solution, water diffuses toward the hyperosmotic region, not away from it; therefore, water will move from the intracellular space to the extracellular space, not the opposite.

29. Correct: Hypoosmotic, swollen (C)

Normal saline, a 0.9% sodium chloride solution, is isotonic with blood and is most commonly used for fluid resuscitation. Pure water is hypotonic to blood and therefore reduces the plasma osmolality, making it hypoosmotic compared to normal. In this state, water will diffuse into the red blood cells until NaCl concentration is equal inside and outside of the cells. This will cause the cells to swell and possibly lyse. (**A, B**) Adding pure water to an isotonic solution (blood) will dilute the solution and make it hypoosmotic, not hyperosmotic. (**D**) Bathing red blood cells in a hypoosmotic solution will cause swelling and lysis, not crenation, which is shriveling of the cell. (**E, F**) Adding pure water to an isotonic solution (blood) will dilute the solution and make it hypoosmotic, not isoosmotic.

30. Correct: It is isosmotic. (C)

Both solutions have one liter of water and 3M of solute, so they are isoosmotic to each other because they have the same concentration of solute per volume. (**A**) Solution 1 must have a greater concentration of solute per volume to be hyperosmotic. (**B**) Solution 1 must have a reduced concentration of solute per volume to be hypoosmotic. (**D**) Because the solutions are isoosmotic, they have the same level of saturation. (**E**) Because no equilibration has occurred yet, both solutions have one liter of volume; this will change after equilibration occurs.

31. Correct: It has a greater volume of water. (C)

Because the membrane is permeable to glucose, and the concentration of glucose is not the same on both sides of the membrane, glucose will diffuse across the membrane from solution 2 to solution 1 until its concentration is equal on both sides. Because the membrane is impermeable to fructose, the diffusion of glucose will create an osmotic gradient between solutions 1 and 2 because solution 1 will become hypertonic to solution 2 as glucose diffuses. This osmotic gradient will drive water from solution 2 to solution 1 to correct the osmotic gradient, thus increasing the volume of solution 1. (**A, B, E**) At equilibrium, the glucose molarity is 1.5M in both solutions, and water will have moved to solution 1 until both have the same number of particles. (**D**) The water volume of solution 1 is greater as just explained.

32. Correct: 36 (E)

Because total body water makes up approximately 60% of a person's weight, the equation to estimate total body water is 60% of a person's weight. In this case, total body water = 60 kg × 0.6 = 36 L. (**A, B, C, D**) These choices do not contain the correct answer.

33. Correct: 12, 24 (A)

Because extracellular fluid volume (ECFV) makes up approximately 20% of a person's weight, the equation to estimate ECFV is 20% of a person's weight. In this case, ECFV = 60 kg × 0.2 = 12 L. Since intracellular fluid volume (ICFV) makes up approximately 40% of a person's weight, the equation to estimate ICFV is 40% of a person's weight. In this case, ICFV = 60 kg × 0.4 = 24 L. (**B, C, D, E, F**) These choices do not contain the correct answers.

34. Correct: 4.6 (B)

To calculate blood volume from a person's weight and hematocrit, plasma volume must be calculated first. Plasma volume is approximately 5% of the total body weight (plasma volume = 60 kg × 0.05 = 3 L). Next, blood volume is calculated using plasma volume and hematocrit. Blood volume = (Plasma volume) / (1 – hematocrit) = (3 L)/(1 – 0.35) = 3 L/0.65 = 4.6 L. (**A, C, D, E**) These choices do not contain the correct answer.

35. Correct: Hypertonic saline (A)

Although all of these solutions will increase the total body water volume by 1 liter, the hypertonic saline solution will increase the extracellular fluid osmolarity, causing a fluid shift from the intracellular space to the extracellular space. This will increase extracellular fluid by 1 L plus the volume of fluid shifted out of the intracellular space. (**B, E**) Iso-osmotic urea and water are both hypotonic, which will lower the extracellular fluid osmolarity, causing a fluid shift from the extracellular space to the intracellular space. (**C, D**) Isotonic saline and plasma are isotonic, so the entire volume of fluid will remain in the extracellular compartments but will not cause fluid shifts in either direction.

36. Correct: ↓, ↓, ↑ (E)

If ADH receptors are blocked, then more water is excreted in the urine. This will lead to a decrease in the volume of fluid in both the intracellular and extracellular compartments. The loss of water will concentrate the red blood cells, thus increasing the hematocrit. (**A, B, C, D, F**) These answers contain one or more incorrect changes.

37. Correct: ↑, ↑ (A)

If ADH receptors are blocked, then more water is excreted in the urine. This will lead to a decrease in plasma volume, which will concentrate the ions in the plasma and increase both extracellular fluid osmolarity and Na^+ concentration. (**B, C, D, E, F**) These answers contain one or more incorrect changes.

38. Correct: ^3H_2O, mannitol, Evans blue dye (C)

To measure total body water, a tracer that equilibrates into all fluid compartments, such as ^3H_2O, must be used. To measure extracellular fluid (ECF) volume, a tracer that equilibrates into all ECF compartments is ideal. The known crystalloid tracers, such as mannitol, are not perfect because they do not diffuse equally throughout the ECF, but since they do not enter the cells, they can be used as a close estimate of ECF (they underestimate ECF volume). A tracer that binds to albumin, a protein that remains in the plasma, is ideal for measuring plasma volume. Evans blue dye binds to albumin, so it is the most common tracer for plasma volume.

39. Correct: 17.5 (C)

Use the equation (Volume A) (Concentration A) = (Volume B) (Concentration B). The injected volume and concentration of mannitol is A, and the concentration of the blood sample is B. First, solve for Volume B to determine the patient's extracellular fluid volume (ECFV).

Volume B = (Volume A) (Concentration A) / (Concentration B)
Volume B = (300 mL × 2500 mg/L) / (100 mg/L)
Volume B = (750 mg/L)/(100 mg/L)
Volume B = 7.5 L = ECFV

Next, determine the intracellular fluid volume (ICFV) by subtracting the ECFV from the total body water. ICFV = TBW – ECFV = 25 L – 7.5 L = 17.5 L

40. Correct: C, B (H)

Drinking a hyperosmotic solution will first increase extracellular fluid (ECF) volume and osmolarity. The hyperosmolarity of the ECF will promote water diffusion from the intracellular fluid (ICF) compartment to the extracellular compartment until the osmolarity of both compartments is equal, thus reducing intracellular volume and increasing intracellular osmolarity. All of these shifts are represented by box C (increased osmolarity of ICF and ECF, increased volume of ECF, and decreased volume of ICF). Drinking a hypoosmotic solution will first increase extracellular fluid (ECF) volume but decrease extracellular fluid osmolarity. The hypoosmolarity of the ECF will promote diffusion of water from the extracellular compartment to the intracellular compartment until the osmolarity of both compartments is equal, thus increasing intracellular volume and but decreasing intracellular osmolarity. All of these shifts are represented by box B (decreased osmolarity of ICF and ECF, increased volume of ICF and ECF).

41. Correct: D (D)

Since relatively more water than salt is lost during sweating (i.e., sweat is hypotonic), the osmolarity of the hiker's extracellular fluid (ECF) will increase as she sweats, but the ECF volume will decrease because of the loss of water in sweat. The high ECF osmolarity will cause water to shift out of the intracellular fluid (ICF) compartment until ICF osmolarity is equal to ECF osmolarity. This results in a decrease in ICF volume. All of these shifts are represented by box D (increased osmolarity of ICF and ECF, decreased volume of ICF and ECF).

42. Correct: 5 (B)

The indicator dilution principle utilizes Evans blue dye to estimate plasma volume. The dye is injected at a known volume and concentration; then, after an equilibrium period, the plasma concentration of the dye is measured. These three values are used to calculate plasma volume:

Plasma volume = (vol injected)(concentration injected) / (plasma concentration)
Plasma volume = (100 mL)(5 mg/mL)/(100 mg/L)
Plasma volume = (500 mg) / (100 mg/L) = 5 L

43. Correct: Mannitol and Evans blue dye (E)

There is no tracer that is distributed only throughout the interstitial fluid compartment. It is determined indirectly as the difference between measured extracellular fluid (ECF) volume and plasma volumes (Interstitial fluid volume = ECF – plasma volume). To measure ECF volume, a tracer that equilibrates into all ECF compartments is ideal. The known crystalloid tracers, such as mannitol, are not perfect because they do not diffuse equally throughout the ECF, but because they do not enter the cells, they can be used as a close estimate of ECF (they underestimate ECF volume slightly). A tracer that binds to albumin, a protein that remains in the plasma, is ideal for measuring plasma volume. Evans blue dye binds to albumin, so it is most common tracer for plasma volume. (**A**) ^3H2O is used to measure total body water because it equilibrates into all fluid compartments. (**B**) Evans blue dye alone will only give a measurement of plasma volume, not interstitial fluid. (**C**) Inulin is another tracer used to measure ECF. (**D**) Mannitol alone will only give a measurement of ECF, not interstitial fluid. (**F**) This combination of tracers is incorrect as just explained individually.

44. Correct: Capillary colloid osmotic pressure (A)

Plasma proteins are responsible for the osmotic forces that draws water from the interstitial space to the capillaries. With liver cirrhosis, fewer plasma proteins are produced, which reduces capillary colloid osmotic pressure, and thus decreases the net reabsorption of fluid into the capillaries. (**B**) Capillary hydrostatic pressure is produced by the volume of blood in the capillaries. This patient has a decreased capillary hydrostatic pressure due to reduced fluid reabsorption from the interstitial space. (**C**) The filtration coefficient is not affected by changes in capillary colloid osmotic pressure. (**D**) The capillaries are relatively impermeable to proteins, so this value will not be changed much. (**E**) Interstitial hydrostatic pressure is produced by the volume of blood in the interstitium. This patient has an increased interstitial hydrostatic pressure, but it is secondary to the decrease in capillary colloid osmotic pressure, so is not the best answer.

45. Correct: Capillary hydrostatic pressure (A)

The loss of blood will directly affect the capillary hydrostatic pressure, which is altered by changes in blood volume. The loss of blood will cause a decrease in capillary hydrostatic pressure. (**B, D**) Since the stab wound results in the loss of whole blood, the osmotic pressures will not change. Proteins are lost in the same proportion as fluid, so protein concentration remains constant. (**C, E**) Interstitial hydrostatic pressure and lymphatic pressure will decrease as fluid shifts from the interstitium to the plasma, as a result of the drop in capillary hydrostatic pressure. However, these drops are secondary to the change in capillary in hydrostatic pressure, so they are not the best answer.

46. Correct: Interstitial hydrostatic pressure (C)

The surgical procedure most likely disrupted the regional lymphatic flow, causing a regional increase in fluid and small protein accumulation in the interstitial space, which directly increase interstitial hydrostatic pressure in that region. This is termed lymphedema. (**A**) The increased interstitial hydrostatic pressure from the disruption of lymphatic flow will increase fluid reabsorption into the capillaries, thus increasing capillary hydrostatic pressure. However, this increase is secondary to the increase in interstitial hydrostatic pressure, so it is not the best choice. (**B, D**) There is no loss or reduced production of plasma proteins, so the osmotic pressures will not change. (**E**) The effect on mean arterial pressure will be negligible.

47. Correct: Interstitial and plasma (E)

This patient has acute poststreptococcal glomerulonephritis, an acute nephritic syndrome that typically affects children. The patient's elevated blood pressure and peripheral edema are suggestive of volume expansion secondary to salt and water retention due to a defect in renal excretion of sodium. The distribution of extracellular and intracellular water is a function of the extracellular osmolality. If the osmolality of the extracellular fluid is above normal, as is the case in this patient from urea in the blood (uremia), the proportion of water in the extracellular fluid increases. The peripheral edema indicates an increase in interstitial fluid, and the hypertension indicates an increase in plasma volume. (**A, D**) Intracellular fluid volume does not increase because the patient's extracellular fluid is hypertonic relative to the intracellular fluid (due to uremia), which draws water out of the intracellular space. (**B, C**) These are both correct, see answer choice **E**.

48. Correct: Increased interstitial colloid osmotic pressure (D)

A fluid shift from the plasma to the interstitium is filtration. Increasing interstitial colloid osmotic pressure (proteins in the interstitial space) will pull water toward the interstitium, thus promoting filtration. (**A**) Decreasing capillary hydrostatic pressure will promote reabsorption of fluid into the capillaries. (**B**) Decreasing filtration coefficient will make the capillaries less permeable, which does not favor filtration. (**C**) Increasing capillary colloid osmotic pressure pulls water toward the capillaries, which is reabsorption, not filtration. (**E**) Increasing interstitial hydrostatic pressure pushes fluid toward the capillaries, which is reabsorption, not filtration.

1.5 Questions

49. If an experimental drug changed the resting membrane potential of a cell from −70 mV to −50 mV, what effect would this have on the rate of sodium and potassium diffusion across the cell membrane when the membrane is permeable to these electrolytes?

	Rate of sodium diffusion into cell	Rate of potassium diffusion out of cell
A.	↑	↑
B.	↑	↓
C.	↑	↔
D.	↓	↑
E.	↓	↓
F.	↓	↔

50. If a resting myocardial cell membrane was altered to be relatively more permeable to sodium than to potassium or any other ion, then the resting membrane potential would be nearest to which of the following values?

A. −96 mV
B. −90 mV
C. −70 mV
D. +52 mV
E. +134 mV

51. Which of the following choices best describes the absolute values of the equilibrium potentials (E) for potassium (E_{K+}), calcium (E_{Ca2+}), and sodium (E_{Na+}) in millivolts in a neuron?

	E_{K+}	E_{Ca2+-}	E_{Na+}
A.	70	90	130
B.	90	130	60
C.	130	60	70
D.	60	70	90
E.	70	130	90
F.	90	60	130
G.	130	70	60
H.	60	90	70

52. The concentration gradient of which of the following ions is primarily responsible for the resting membrane potential of a myelinated nerve cell?

A. Calcium
B. Chloride
C. Magnesium
D. Potassium
E. Sodium

53. A nerve fiber has a resting membrane potential of –75 mV. The intracellular and extracellular fluid concentrations of Na^+, K^+, and Cl^- are shown in the following table (in mmol/L):

Ion	Intracellular fluid concentration	Extracellular fluid concentration
Na^+	20	145
K^+	110	5
Cl^-	4	90

Which of these ions is close to electrochemical equilibrium under these conditions?

A. Na^+
B. K^+
C. Cl^-
D. Both Na^+ and Cl^-
E. Both K^+ and Cl^-

54. Considering the typical K^+ concentration gradient across a neuronal membrane at rest, which of the following correctly describes the K^+ flux and K^+ conductance?

	K^+ flux	K^+ conductance
A.	Influx	High
B.	Influx	Low
C.	Influx	None
D.	Efflux	High
E.	Efflux	Low
F.	Efflux	None

55. Considering the typical Na^+ concentration gradient across a neuronal membrane at rest, which of the following best describes the Na^+ flux and Na^+ conductance?

	Na^+ flux	Na^+ conductance
A.	Influx	High
B.	Influx	Low
C.	Almost no flux	High
D.	Efflux	Low
E.	Efflux	High
F.	Almost no flux	Low

56. A 32-year-old patient presents with severe diarrhea for 36 hours. He is dehydrated and hypokalemic. What effect will hypokalemia have on the K^+ equilibrium potential and K^+ resting membrane potential of the neurons?

	K^+ equilibrium potential	K^+ resting membrane potential
A.	More negative	More negative
B.	More negative	More positive
C.	More negative	No change
D.	More positive	More negative
E.	More positive	More positive
F.	More positive	No change

57. An experimental drug antagonizes voltage-gated potassium channels. If applied to an axon, how will membrane potential voltages change at the end of phase 1 and phase 2 on the action potential image shown, compared to those of an untreated axon?

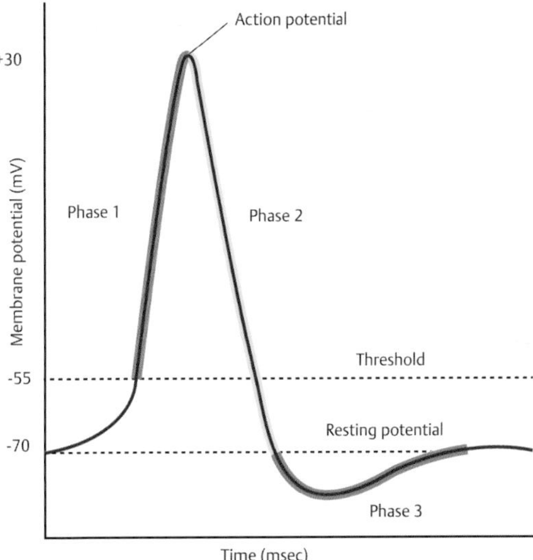

	Voltage at end of phase 1	Voltage at end of phase 2
A.	More positive	More negative
B.	More positive	Less negative
C.	More positive	Same voltage
D.	Less positive	More negative
E.	Less positive	Less negative
F.	Less positive	Same voltage
G.	Same voltage	More negative
H.	Same voltage	Less negative
I.	Same voltage	Same voltage

58. At a node of Ranvier of a myelinated axon, voltage-gated sodium channels are inactivated, voltage-gated potassium channels are activated, and the membrane potential is 10 mV and falling. What phase of the neuronal action potential is occurring at this time?

A. Depolarization
B. Overshoot
C. Repolarization
D. Resting potential
E. Undershoot

59. Six neurons have axons of the same length, but different states of myelination and axon diameter. What combination of axon myelination and nerve fiber diameter would produce the fastest nerve conduction speed?

	Axon myelination	Axon diameter (um)
Nerve 1	Myelinated	15
Nerve 2	Myelinated	10
Nerve 3	Myelinated	3
Nerve 4	Unmyelinated	15
Nerve 5	Unmyelinated	10
Nerve 6	Unmyelinated	3

A. Nerve 1
B. Nerve 2
C. Nerve 3
D. Nerve 4
E. Nerve 5
F. Nerve 6

60. A 39-year-old woman presents with paresthesia of the left hand that resolves 48 hours later. History reveals an episode of weakness in the left leg 6 months prior that lasted for 2–3 days and double vision on several occasions over the past year that lasted for 24 hours. Magnetic resonance imaging (MRI) of the brain and spinal cord reveals lesions that are consistent with a diagnosis of multiple sclerosis. Which of the following is expected in the patient?

A. Increased axon diameter
B. Increased membrane capacitance
C. Increased membrane resistance
D. Decreased number of axonal ion channels
E. Decreased K^+ equilibrium potential
F. Decreased resting membrane potential

61. The image below shows the recording of a neuronal action potential. At which points on the recording (labeled 1–3) are most of the voltage-gated Na^+ channels open, closed, and inactivated?

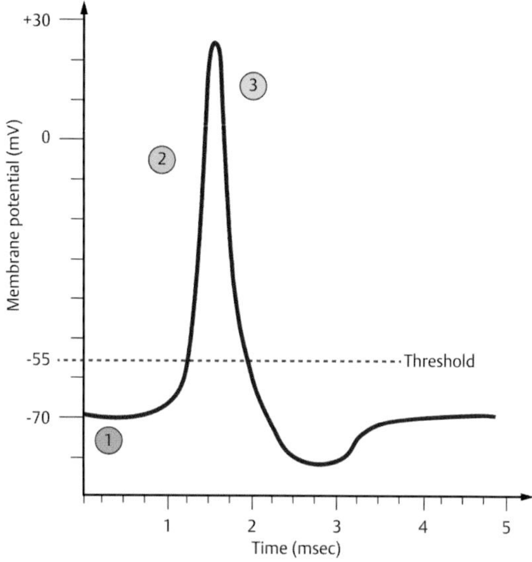

	Na^+ channels open	Na^+ channels closed	Na^+ channels inactivated
A.	Point 1	Point 2	Point 3
B.	Point 1	Point 3	Point 2
C.	Point 2	Point 3	Point 1
D.	Point 2	Point 1	Point 3
E.	Point 3	Point 1	Point 2
F.	Point 3	Point 2	Point 1

62. Which of the following ion channels is involved in propagation of the neuronal action potential and has both an activation and an inactivation gate?

A. Bicarbonate
B. Calcium
C. Chloride
D. Potassium
E. Sodium

Questions 63 to 64

The image shows the phases of a neuronal action potential (labeled 1–4).

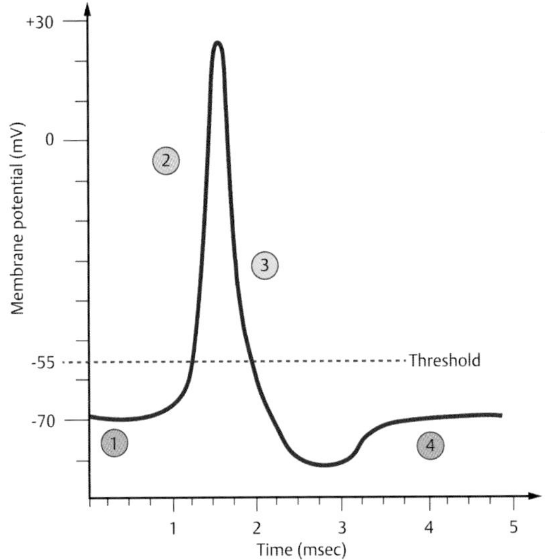

63. If a drug that antagonizes voltage-gated sodium channels is administered to neurons in vitro, and then the cells are stimulated, which phase of the action potential graph would be most directly affected?

A. 1
B. 2
C. 3
D. 4

64. During which phase of the action potential are the potassium leak channels open?

A. 1
B. 2
C. 3
D. 4
E. All phases

65. In comparison to the voltage-gated neuronal sodium channel, which of the following is correct for the voltage-gated potassium channel in regards to opening speed and presence of an inactivation gate?

	Opening speed	Inactivation gate
A.	Similar	No
B.	Similar	Yes
C.	Slower	No
D.	Slower	Yes
E.	Faster	No
F.	Faster	Yes

66. A drug that antagonizes calcium channels is applied to the axon of an unmyelinated motor neuron. What effect will this drug have on the neuronal action potential?

A. Decreases the action potential velocity
B. Depolarizes the neuron
C. Has no effect on the action potential
D. Hyperpolarizes the neuron
E. Increases the action potential velocity

67. A 14-year-old girl presents to the dentist with pain in one of her molars. Tooth decay is detected. When performing the procedure to fill the cavity, the dentist uses as a local anesthetic agent to prevent pain. Which of the following ion channels is most likely blocked by the anesthetic?

A. Bicarbonate
B. Calcium
C. Chloride
D. Potassium
E. Sodium

68. The image shows the phases of a neuronal action potential. At which time points (labeled 1–4) of the neuronal action potential do sodium and potassium have the highest conductance, respectively?

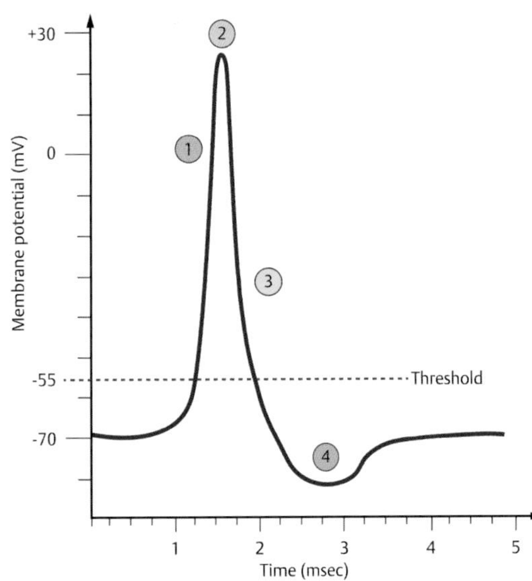

	Highest sodium conductance	Highest potassium conductance
A.	1	3
B.	1	4
C.	2	3
D.	2	4
E.	3	2
F.	3	4
G.	4	2
H.	4	3

69. The image shows a myelinated neuron. At which point along the length of this neuron (labeled A–E) are voltage-gated Na^+ channels most concentrated?

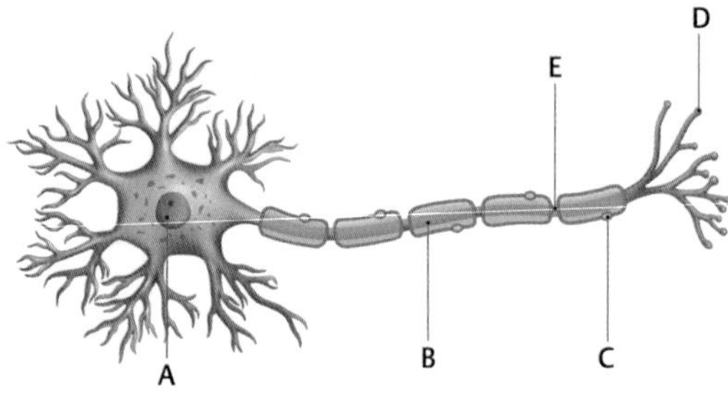

A. A
B. B
C. C
D. D
E. E

70. At which point on the action potential graph of a normal axon is the membrane conductance of Na^+ and K^+ at its lowest?

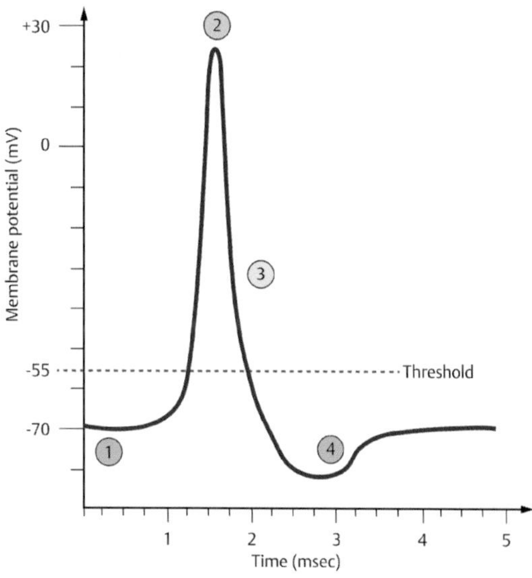

A. 1
B. 2
C. 3
D. 4

71. In an experimental study, isolated motor neurons are placed in various bathing solutions and action potentials are recorded. Which of the following action potentials will most likely be recorded when the extracellular sodium concentration is increased from 140 mM (normal) to 200 mM?

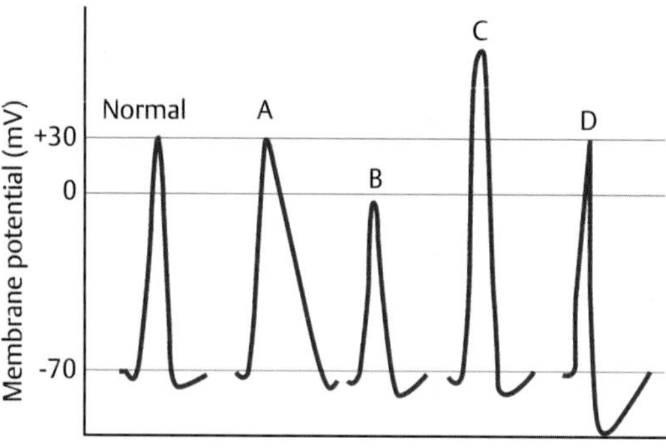

A. A
B. B
C. C
D. D

72. The resting membrane potential of an isolated human cell is –70 mV. The equilibrium potentials for the major ions are as follows:

E_{Na+} = +60mV
E_{K+} = –80mV
E_{Cl-} = –90mV
E_{Ca+} = +125 mV
E_{Mg2+} = 0 mV

Which of the following ions will flow *out of the cell* when the ion channel for that particular ion is opened?

A. Cl^-
B. Mg^{2+}
C. Na^+
D. K^+
E. Ca^{2+}

73. In the 1940s, exposing patients to anoxia for periods of time was considered a possible treatment for schizophrenia. Not considering any compensatory body reactions to anoxia, what happens to the intracellular K^+ and Na^+ concentrations and K^+ equilibrium potential, during an extended period of extreme oxygen deprivation?

	$[K^+]$	$[Na^+]$	K^+ equilibrium potential
A.	Decrease	Decrease	Become less negative
B.	Decrease	Increase	Become less negative
C.	Decrease	Increase	Become more negative
D.	Increase	Decrease	Become more negative
E.	Increase	Decrease	Become less negative
F.	Increase	Increase	Become more negative

74. A second-year medical student joins a neurobiology lab during summer to study the excitability of neurons. The experimental model is the spinal motor neuron. He stimulates the neuron at five different regions and monitors the production of action potentials at the axon. At which of the following regions does he need the lowest stimulus strength to induce an action potential?

A. Cell body

B. Myelin sheath

C. Initial segment

D. Axon terminal

E. Postsynaptic membrane at the synaptic cleft

1.6 Answers and Explanations

49. Correct: ↓, ↑ (D)

Sodium and potassium diffusion is dependent on the electrochemical gradient and the permeability of a membrane. Changing the membrane potential from −70 mV to −50 mV alters the electrical gradient. Sodium normally diffuses into the cell down its electrochemical gradient, but this will be decreased due to the reduced electrical gradient, because the new gradient is closer to the equilibrium potential for sodium. Potassium normally diffuses out of the cell down its electrochemical gradient, and this will be increased due to the larger electrical gradient. (**A, B, C, E, F**) These contain the wrong combination of answer choices.

50. Correct: +52 mV (D)

If a cell membrane is relatively permeable to one ion (i.e., Na^+), and relatively impermeable to the other ions present (i.e., K^+, Ca^{2+}, Cl^-), then the resting membrane potential of the cell will be near the equilibrium potential for the ion that it is more permeable to. In this case, the membrane is most permeable to sodium, so the resting membrane potential will be closest to sodium's equilibrium potential, which is about +52 mV. (**A**) −96 mV is the equilibrium potential of potassium. (**B**) −90 mV is the equilibrium potential of chloride. (**C**) −70 mV is the resting membrane potential of many neurons. (**E**) +134 mV is the equilibrium potential of calcium.

51. Correct: 90, 130, 60 (F)

The equilibrium potential of an ion is determined by E_{ion} = −61 mV log $[Ion]_{inside}/[Ion]_{outside}$. When using typical neuronal ion concentrations, this determines E_{K+} ~ −90 mV, E_{Ca2+} ~ 130 mV, and E_{Na+} ~ 60 mV. However, it has to be noted that the positive or negative sign is switched, when the equation E_{ion} = −61mV log $[Ion]_{outside}/[Ion]_{inside}$ is used. Hence, in medical physiology, rather than memorizing the equation, it makes more sense to estimate absolute values. Because E_{ion} is the electrical potential that counterbalances the ion movement due to its concentration gradient, it tells the force that acts on the ion due to the concentration gradient. This means that at rest the force for K^+ is directed to the outside, and for Ca^{2+} and Na^+ to the inside, respectively. (**A, B, C, D, E, G, H**) These are incorrect absolute values for the equilibrium potentials.

52. Correct: Potassium (D)

Most neurons have a resting membrane potential (RMP) of approximately −70 mV. The RMP is the average of the ion equilibrium potentials, which are determined by the concentrations of the ions in the fluids on both sides of the plasma membrane. The equilibrium potentials are weighted based on the permeability of the cell membrane to the ion. Because potassium has the highest membrane permeability, it contributes the most to the RMP. Because the potassium equilibrium potential is about −90 mV, the potassium concentration gradient is the primary determinant of the RMB in most cells. (**A, B, C, E**) The neuronal cell membrane at rest is relatively impermeable to calcium, chloride, magnesium, and sodium; therefore they are not the primary determinants for the RMP. Moreover, the chloride equilibrium potential is close to the RMP.

53. Correct: Both K^+ and Cl^- (E)

The ions that have the highest conductance will be closest to electrochemical equilibrium. To determine this, first calculate the equilibrium potential for each ion using the Nernst equation. Then compare these values to the membrane potential (–75 mV). The ions that have an equilibrium potential closest to the membrane potential are closest to electrochemical equilibrium. The calculations using the Nernst equation are as follows (assume 2.3 RT/F = –60 mV for ions with one charge):

$E = -60 \times \log$ (concentration inside/concentration outside)

$E_{Na+} = -60 \times \log(20/145) = -60 \times \log(0.14) = -60$ mV $\times -0.86 = +51.6$

$E_{K+} = -60 \times \log(110/5) = -60 \times \log(22) = -60$ mV $\times 1.34 = -80.5$

$E_{Cl-} = -60 \times \log(90/4) = -60 \times \log(22.5) = -60$ mV $\times 1.35 = -81.1$

Based on the equilibrium potential calculations, Na^+ has a low conductance (because the equilibrium potential is not close to the membrane potential), and K^+ and Cl^- have high conductances.

54. Correct: Efflux, high (D)

At rest, neurons have a high intracellular concentration of K^+ relative to the extracellular concentration, which is established by the Na^+/ K^+ ATPase. This favors K^+ efflux, and the net K^+ flux will ultimately depend on the electrical gradient, because any negativity inside will prevent the positive ion from leaving the cell. In addition, resting neurons have a high K^+ conductance, due to K^+ channels that conduct at rest, so-called "leak channels." Because K^+ almost exclusively crosses cell membranes through membrane channels, the permeation of K^+ through membranes can also be termed permeability. These characteristics together promote K^+ efflux. (**A**, **B**, **C**, **E**, **F**) These contain one or more incorrect choices.

55. Correct: Almost no flux, low (F)

At rest, neurons have a high extracellular concentration of Na^+ relative to the intracellular concentration, which is established by the Na^+/K^+ ATPase. This favors Na^+ influx; however, resting neurons have a low Na^+ conductance and permeability, because ions cannot cross the lipid bilayer and because sodium channels are not permeable at rest. Any Na^+ ion that enters the cell due to the imperfection of a biological membrane down its concentration gradient, will immediately be pumped out of the cell by the Na^+/ K^+ ATPase. This combination of low conductivity and Na^+ pump makes it so that there is almost no Na^+ flux at rest. (**A**, **B**, **C**, **D**, **E**) These contain one or more incorrect choices.

56. Correct: More negative, more negative (A)

As the extracellular K^+ concentration decreases (hypokalemia), the concentration gradient of potassium across the membrane increases, and the K^+ equilibrium potential becomes more negative. As the equilibrium potential of K^+ becomes more negative, the resting membrane potential becomes more negative (hyperpolarized) as well, due to the high conductance of K^+ in neuronal cells as rest. (**B**, **C**, **D**, **E**, **F**) These contain one or more incorrect choices.

57. Correct: Same voltage, same voltage (I)

Phase 1 of the action potential is produced by Na^+ influx through voltage-gated sodium channels and will not be affected by a K^+ channel antagonist. Therefore, the membrane potential at the end of Phase 1 will be the same voltage. Phase 2 is produced by K^+ efflux, which will occur at a slower rate if the K^+ channels are antagonized, but repolarization will still occur via the K^+ leak channels due to the electrical gradient produced by depolarization. Thus the voltage will be the same at the end of phase 2. (**A**, **B**, **C**) These are incorrect because voltage at the end of phase 1 will remain the same, not become more positive. (**D**, **E**, **F**) These are incorrect because voltage at the end of phase 1 will remain the same, not become less positive. (**G**, **H**) These are incorrect because voltage at the end of phase 2 will be the same, not more positive or more negative.

58. Correct: Repolarization (C)

During repolarization, the membrane potential moves from a positive 30 mV to negative 70 mV. This is achieved by potassium efflux from the nerve cell through leak channels and opened voltage-gated potassium channels; thus potassium channels are activated. No sodium conduction occurs during this phase, because voltage-gated sodium channels are closed due to their closed inactivation gates. (**A**) Depolarization is the increase in membrane potential from negative 70 mV to positive 30 mV. Sodium influx is responsible for this change in membrane potential. (**B**) The overshoot phase describes the increase in membrane potential above 0 mV and occurs during the depolarization phase. (**D**) The resting potential phase occurs between stimuli, when the membrane potential is steady at negative 70 mV. (**E**) The undershoot phase (or hyperpolarizing afterpotential) occurs at the end of repolarization, when the membrane potential drops below negative 70 mV, which is the resting membrane potential.

59. Correct: Nerve 1 (A)

Action potential conduction velocity increases with myelination and nerve fiber diameter. Myelination permits action potentials to travel at velocities many orders of magnitude higher than an axon of equivalent size and diameter by insulating the axon and increasing conduction. Therefore, the nerve that is myelinated with the greatest diameter will have the fastest conduction speed.

60. Correct: Increased membrane capacitance (B)

The main purpose of a myelin sheath is to increase the speed at which impulses propagate along the myelinated fiber. This is accomplished by decreasing membrane capacitance, which is an inverse function of membrane thickness. In patients with multiple sclerosis, myelination decreases and the membrane becomes "thinner," which increases capacitance. (**A**) Demyelination does not affect axonal diameter. (**C**) Myelination (not demyelination) increases membrane resistance by effectively reducing the number of ion channels along the axon. (**D**) Myelination (not demyelination) causes a reduction in the number of ion channels, concentrating them only at the nodes of Ranvier. (**E, F**) The equilibrium potential of K^+ and the resting membrane potential are not affected by demyelination.

61. Correct: Point 2, point 1, point 3 (D)

(**D**) Voltage-gated Na^+ channels have three main conformational states: closed, open, and inactivated. At resting membrane potential (point 1; –70 mV), the voltage-gated Na^+ channels are closed. When a stimulus initiates an action potential, the voltage-gated Na^+ channels are activated and open, allowing rapid sodium influx, increasing the membrane potential toward +30 mV (point 2). A few milliseconds after activation, the voltage-gated Na^+ channels are inactivated by the closure of an intracellular inactivation gate. (**A, B, C, E, F**) These answers contain the wrong combination of choices.

62. Correct: Sodium (E)

The voltage-gated sodium channel has an activation gate on the extracellular side of the channel and an inactivation gate on the intracellular side. (**A, B, C**) Bicarbonate, calcium, and chloride are not involved in the neuronal action potential. (**D**) Voltage-gated potassium channels have an activation gate on the extracellular side of the channel, but no inactivation gate.

63. Correct: 2 (B)

The phase labeled 2 on the graph is the depolarization phase, which is produced by opening of voltage-gated Na^+ channels to allow Na^+ influx. If this channel is antagonized, depolarization will be slowed or eliminated. (**A, D**) The phases labeled 1 and 4 on the graph are the resting membrane potential, which is maintained by the Na^+/K^+ ATPase. This pump would not be affected by a drug that antagonizes voltage-gated sodium channels. (**C**) The phase labeled 3 on the graph is the repolarization phase, which is produced by opening of K^+ channels for K^+ efflux.

64. Correct: All phases (E)

Potassium leak channels are always open in neurons. The leak channels allow K^+ to move across the cell membrane down its concentration gradient (from a high to low concentration). With the combined ion pumping from the Na^+/K^+ ATPase and leakage of ions, the cell can maintain a stable resting membrane potential. (**A, B, C, D**) These are incorrect choices.

65. Slower, no (C)

Depolarization stimulates the opening of both the voltage-gated sodium channels and voltage-gated potassium channels. However, the sodium channels open rapidly and the potassium channels open slowly. Therefore, depolarization occurs first via sodium influx, then repolarization occurs via potassium efflux. Further, sodium channels have inactivation gates, and potassium channels do not. (**A, B, E, F**) Potassium voltage-gated channels open more slowly that sodium voltage-gated channels. (**D**) Potassium channels do not have inactivation gates.

66. Correct: Has no effect on the action potential (C)

Since there are no calcium channels on the neuronal Because this drug will have no effect on the neuronal action potential. (**A, E**) Velocity of an action potential is determined by the neurons diameter and myelination, not by calcium conductance. (**B**) Depolarization of a neuronal axon is facilitated by sodium influx, not calcium. (**D**) Hyperpolarization of a neuron is facilitated by potassium efflux, not calcium.

67. Correct: Sodium (E)

A local anesthetic, such as lidocaine, acts to prevent pain by altering or blocking the action potentials in sensory neurons. At low concentrations the lidocaine decreases the rate and rise of the neuronal action potential upstroke, and at high concentrations it completely blocks the action potentials, thus preventing sensation. The upstroke of the action potential is produced by the opening of voltage-gated sodium channels. (**A, B, C**) Bicarbonate, calcium, and chloride are not involved in the neuronal action potential. (**D**) Voltage-gated potassium channels are responsible for the repolarization, or downstroke, of the neuronal action potential. Blocking them would prolong the action potential but not disrupt action potential propagation.

68. Correct: 1, 3 (A)

Ions move across the cell membrane through specific ion channels. When these channels open, the permeability and electrical conductance to the respective ion increases. High conductance indicates that electrical charge moves easily through a membrane. For charged particles, such as ions, movement of mass and movement of electrical charge occur simultaneously. So higher permeability indicates higher conductance. Sodium has the highest conductance near the end of the depolarization phase (time point 1), while potassium has the highest conductance during the repolarization phase (time point 3). (**B, C, D, E, F, G, H**) These answers do not contain the correct choices.

69. Correct: E (E)

Myelinated axons have Na^+ channels present only at the unmyelinated nodes of Ranvier; therefore, this is the only part of the axon where Na^+ conductance occurs. This is referred to as saltatory conduction, and it acts to propagate action potentials at rates significantly higher than would be possible without the myelination. (**A**) The nucleus of the neuron does not have voltage-gated Na^+ channels. (**B, C**) The voltage-gated Na^+ channels are predominantly located at the nodes on Ranvier along the neuronal axis, not on the Schwann cells (myelin). (**D**) The presynaptic membrane has a large concentration of voltage-gated Ca^{2+} channels, not voltage-gated Na^+ channels.

70. Correct: 1 (A)

At point 1, the conductance of sodium and potassium is at their lowest because voltage-gated sodium and voltage-gated potassium channels are closed. (**B**) At point 2, sodium is near its highest conductance and potassium conductance is beginning to rise. (**C**) At point 3, sodium conductance is dropping and potassium conductance is at its highest point. (**D**) At point 4, sodium conductance has returned back to its lowest value, since all voltage-gated sodium channels are closed, but potassium conductance is still elevated slightly above its minimum due to the state of hyperpolarization, in which there is still an increase in potassium conductance compared to the resting membrane conductance.

71. Correct: C (C)

Increased extracellular sodium concentration leads to an increased concentration gradient between the inside and outside of the cell, and an increased sodium equilibrium potential, to which the membrane potential is closest at the peak of the action potential. Thus, more sodium will influx during depolarization, causing the nerve action potential to have a higher peak. (**A**) This action potential recording shows delayed repolarization, which would be present with decreased K^+ conductance. (**B**) Decreased extracellular sodium concentration (e.g., 60 mM) would produce an action potential similar to this (lower peak). (**D**) Increased hyperpolarization is caused by an increased K^+ conductance, which is not changed here. (**E**) When extracellular sodium concentration is altered, the shape of the action potential will be altered.

72. Correct: K (D)

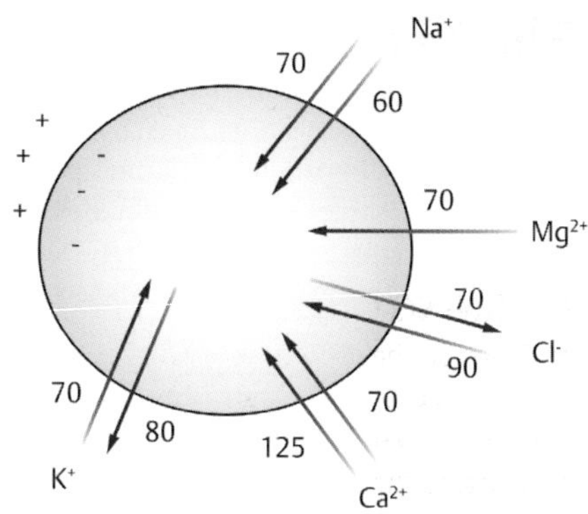

Na^+, K^+, Ca^{2+} and Mg^{2+} are all positive ions. Hence, they are attracted into the cells by a force of 70 mV. The force due to the concentration gradient is 60 for Na^+ (from outside to inside), 80 for K^+ (from inside to outside), 125 for Ca^{2+} (from outside to inside) and 0 for Mg^{2+}. This leaves a resultant force of:

Na^+ = 70 mV + 60 mV = 130mV for Na^+ to move inside

K^+ = 70 mV + (−80 mV) = 10 mV for K^+ to move outside

Ca^{2+} = 70 mV + 125 mV = 195 mV for Ca^{2+} to move inside

Mg^{2+} = 70 mV + 0 mV = 70 for Mg^{2+} to move inside

Cl^- is negative. Hence, it wants to move outside by 70 mV (due to the electric gradient) and to move inside by 90 mV (due to the concentration gradient). The resultant force will be 20 mV to move inside.

73. Correct: Decrease, increase, become less negative (B)

Oxygen deprivation limits the activity of the Na/K-ATPases, which would decrease intracellular K^+ concentration and increase intracellular Na^+ concentration. Potassium equilibrium potential would decrease as the electrochemical gradients for Na^+ and K^+ move to zero. (**A, C, D, E, F**) These choices contain the wrong combination of choices.

74. Correct: Initial segment (C)

The initial segment is the interval between the axon hillock and the point at which myelination begins. The axolemma of this segment has several types of ion channels, which regulate the conversion of graded potentials into nerve action potentials. The excitability is determined by the number of Na^+ channels in a particular area (↑ Na^+ channels = ↑ excitability). The number of Na^+ channels in myelinated mammalian neurons has been estimated to be highest in the initial segment, at 350–500 per micrometer of membrane. (**A, B, D, E**) The number of Na^+ channels per micrometer of membrane in the cell body is 50–75, of the myelin sheath is less than 25, of the axon terminal is 20–75, and of the postsynaptic membrane is less than 20.

Chapter 2

The Nervous System

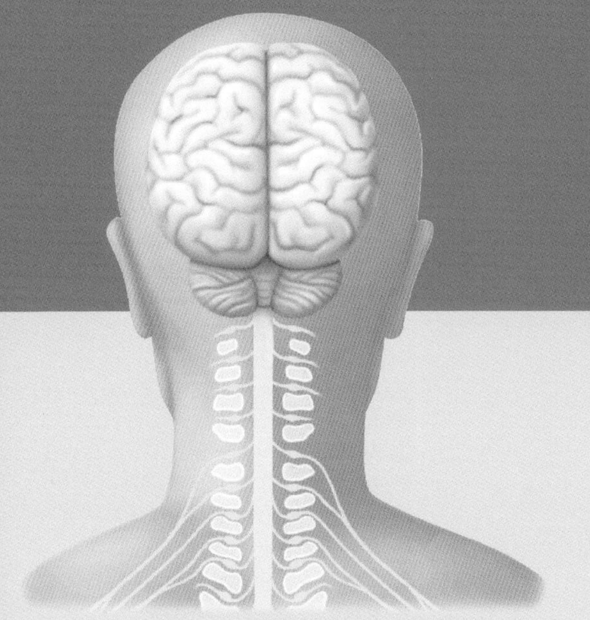

LEARNING OBJECTIVES

- Describe the structure, normal stimuli, transduction at the receptor level, and function of the central nervous system (CNS).
- Describe the structure, normal stimuli, transduction at the receptor level, and function of the autonomic nervous system.
- Describe the structure, normal stimuli, transduction at the receptor level, and function of the senses of vision, hearing, equilibrium, taste, and smell.
- Describe the structure, normal stimuli, transduction at the receptor level, and function of the sensory and motor control systems.

2.1 Questions

Easy	Medium	Hard

1. A 34-year-old woman presents with bladder dysfunction, lower extremity paralysis, and bilateral loss of pain and thermal sensation in her legs for 2 days. Her discriminative touch, vibratory sense, and proprioception is preserved. A magnetic resonance image (MRI) reveals a vertebral bone tumor causing spinal compression. Which of the following best describes the spinal compression responsible for the patient's symptoms?

A. Anterior cord syndrome
B. Cauda equina syndrome
C. Central cord syndrome
D. Compression of exiting roots at C5–C6
E. Compression of exiting roots at L3

2. A 61-year-old male patient with a 10-year history of hypertension suffers a hemorrhagic stroke, disrupting blood flow to the left vagus nerve. Which of the following is most likely to appear in the clinical presentation?

A. The tongue will deviate toward the left.
B. The tongue will deviate toward the right.
C. The uvula will deviate toward the left.
D. The uvula will deviate toward the right.
E. There will be no clinically perceptible deficit.

3. A patient complains of double vision and difficulty walking down steps for 3 months. He is referred to a neurologist for examination. A brain lesion is determined to be responsible for the deficits described. The lesion most likely involves which of the following cranial nerves?

A. Abducens nerve
B. Facial nerve
C. Optic nerve
D. Trigeminal nerve
E. Trochlear nerve

4. Which of the following is a morphine-like neurotransmitter that acts as a natural painkiller?

A. Acetylcholine
B. Dopamine
C. Endorphin
D. Epinephrine
E. Serotonin

5. A 17-year-old boy presents to the emergency department with a cerebellar hemorrhage. On exam, he exhibits jerky eye movements, sways when standing, and has a "drunk-like" gait. Which region of the cerebellum is most likely affected by the hemorrhage?

A. Anterior lobe
B. Dentate nucleus
C. Flocculonodular lobe
D. Interposed nucleus
E. Posterior lobe

6. A 38-year-old mother of three complains of sleeplessness for 6 months. History and physical exam are unremarkable. She agrees to an overnight sleep study, during which normal sawtooth waves are observed on her electroencephalogram (EEG). This EEG pattern is associated with which period of sleep?

A. REM
B. Stage 1
C. Stage 2
D. Stage 3

7. A 48-year-old woman has a stroke that affects the posterior part of Brodmann area 22, resulting in a lesion in the Wernicke area. Which of the following will most likely be observed in the clinical presentation of this patient?

A. Expressive speech deficit
B. Loss of right-sided touch/pressure sensation below the neck
C. Loss of coordinated motor movements
D. Primary visual processing deficit
E. Receptive speech deficit

8. A 39-year old woman presents with progressive weakness in her left hand over several months, and multiple episodes of bladder incontinence. She admits that her vision has been blurry lately, and that all of her symptoms are exaggerated on hot days. She is diagnosed with multiple sclerosis. Damage to which of the following cell types is responsible for this condition?

A. Astrocytes
B. Ependymal cells
C. Microglia
D. Oligodendrocytes
E. Schwann cells

9. A college student presents with signs of meningitis, and a lumbar puncture is performed to collect cerebrospinal fluid (CSF) for analysis. Which of the following cells are responsible for the production of CSF?

A. Astrocytes
B. Ependymal cells
C. Microglia
D. Oligodendrocytes
E. Schwann cells

2.2 Answers and Explanations

Easy	Medium	Hard

1. Correct: Anterior cord syndrome (A)

Anterior cord syndrome is an incomplete spinal cord injury of the anterior regions of the spinal cord. This condition causes paralysis below the level of the lesion, bilateral loss of pain and thermal sensation starting two to three levels below the injury, and bladder and bowel dysfunction. Because the posterior columns are not affected, discriminative touch, vibratory sense, and proprioception are preserved below the lesion. (**B**) Cauda equina syndrome occurs due to compression of the spine at the level of L1/L2 through S2. This condition results in bladder and bowel dysfunction, saddle anesthesia, lower extremity weakness, sexual dysfunction, and lower back pain. (**C**) Central cord syndrome is an incomplete spinal cord injury of the cervical spine that presents with weakness in the extremities, irregular pain and thermal sensation, and urinary retention. (**D**) Compression of exiting roots at C5–C6 would cause weakness of the forearm and wrist extensors and sensory loss of the C6 dermatome. (**E**) Compression of exiting roots at L3 would cause weakness of knee extension, pain over the anterior thigh, decreased sensation over the medial thigh, and a diminished patellar tendon reflex.

2. Correct: The uvula will deviate toward the right. (D)

Lesions of the vagus nerve result in uvular deviation away from the lesion. The left vagus nerve is involved in this patient; therefore the uvula deviates to the right. (**A, B**) The hypoglossal nerve, not the vagus nerve, controls the skeletal muscle of the tongue; therefore A and B are incorrect. (**C**) The uvula deviates away from the lesion, not toward it, as described for answer **D**. (**E**) There is a deficit as explained in answer **D**.

3. Correct: Trochlear nerve (E)

To walk down stairs, the eyes must be able to move downward. Downward movement of the eye involves the inferior rectus muscle, which is innervated by the oculomotor nerve, and the superior oblique muscle, which is innervated by the trochlear nerve. Damage to the trochlear nerve on one side will prevent the affected eye from moving downward. The two eyes will not be able to focus on the same region in the visual field, producing double vision. (**A**) The abducens nerve (CN X) is a somatic efferent nerve that controls movement of a single muscle, the lateral rectus, which abducts the eye. (**B**) The facial nerve (CN VII) controls the muscles of facial expression and conveys taste sensations from the anterior two-thirds of the tongue. (**C**) The optic nerve (CN II) is a sensory nerve for vision, originating at the retina. (**D**) The trigeminal nerve (CN V) has both motor and sensory components and mediates general sensation of the face and scalp, opening/closing of the mouth, and tension of the tympanic membrane.

4. Correct: Endorphin (C)

Endorphins are endogenous opioid neuropeptides produced by the central nervous system and pituitary gland. Their principal function is to inhibit the transmission of pain signals by antagonizing opioid receptors, particularly in the midbrain. (**A, B, D, E**) Acetylcholine, dopamine, epinephrine, and serotonin are common neurotransmitters, and some relationships to pain reduction have been shown, but they are not directly involved in inhibiting pain.

5. Correct: Flocculonodular lobe (C)

Deficits of the flocculonodular lobe can result in loss of oculomotor control, loss of integration of vestibular information for eye and head control, and loss of maintenance of balance equilibrium and muscle tone, as seen in this patient. (**A**) The anterior lobe is responsible for mediating unconscious proprioception. (**B**) The dentate nucleus is responsible for the planning, initiation, and control of voluntary movements. (**D**) The interposed nucleus is responsible for coordinating agonist/antagonist muscle pairs; therefore, a lesion in this area causes tremor. (**E**) The posterior lobe plays an important role in fine motor coordination, specifically in the inhibition of involuntary movement.

6. Correct: REM (A)

In REM sleep, brain waves increase to levels experienced when a person is awake and have a characteristic sawtooth pattern. Heart rate increases, blood pressure rises, and most dreams occur during this stage. (**B**) In Stage 1 (light) sleep, one drifts in and out of sleep and can be awakened easily. Stage 1 sleep is associated with 4–7 Hz theta waves. (**C**) In Stage 2, brain waves become slower with only an occasional burst of rapid brain waves. Stage 2 sleep is associated with 12–14 Hz sleep spindles and K-complexes. (**D**) In Stage 3, extremely slow brain waves called delta waves are interspersed with smaller, faster waves.

7. Correct: Receptive speech deficit (E)

A receptive speech deficit typically results from a lesion in the Wernicke area in the superior temporal gyrus of the cerebral cortex, causing difficulty understanding what others are saying. (**A**) An expressive speech deficit results from a lesion in the Broca area (Brodmann area 44) in the inferior frontal gyrus, causing difficulty expressing thoughts and ideas. (**B**) A loss of touch and pressure sense on the right side below the neck could result from an occlusion of the anterior spinal artery at the level of the medulla affecting the left medial lemniscus, a lesion to the dorsal columns, an infarct of the nucleus cuneatus and nucleus gracilis, or a lesion of the thalamus or somatosensory cortex. (**C**) Loss of coordination and ataxia usually indicate a problem in the cerebellum, not the Wernicke area. (**D**) A primary visual processing deficit would result from a lesion in the occipital lobe.

8. Correct: Oligodendrocytes (D)

Oligodendrocytes myelinate neurons within the central nervous system (CNS). Multiple sclerosis is an autoimmune disease that progressively damages these cells over time, compromising nerve conduction. (**A**) Astrocytes are the most abundant and largest glial cells. They contribute to the blood-brain barrier, metabolize and recycle some neurotransmitters, and buffer extracellular fluid. (**B**) Ependymal cells line the central nervous system ventricles, produce cerebrospinal fluid (CSF), and make up part of the blood-CSF barrier. (**C**) Microglia are innate immune cells of the brain, are activated when the brain is damaged, and also play roles in normal function. (**E**) Schwann cells myelinate the neurons of the peripheral nervous system, not the CNS.

9. Correct: Ependymal cells (B)

Ependymal cells line the central nervous system ventricles, produce CSF, and make up part of the blood-CSF barrier. (**A**) Astrocytes are the most abundant and largest glial cells. They contribute to the blood-brain barrier, metabolize and recycle some neurotransmitters, and buffer extracellular fluid. (**C**) Microglia are innate immune cells of the brain, are activated when the brain is damaged, and also play roles in normal function. (**D**) Oligodendrocytes myelinate neurons within the central nervous system (CNS). (**E**) Schwann cells myelinate neurons of the peripheral nervous system.

2.3 Questions

10. A patient takes a drug that decreases cardiac chronotropy but has little effect on cardiac inotropy. Considering the autonomic pathway most likely affected by this drug, which of the following best describes the neurons, neurotransmitters, and receptors of this pathway?

	Preganglionic neuron	Postganglionic neuron	Postganglionic neurotransmitter	Receptor at target organ
A.	Short and myelinated	Long and myelinated	Norepinephrine	Beta-adrenergic
B.	Short and myelinated	Long and unmyelinated	Acetylcholine	Muscarinic
C.	Short and unmyelinated	Long and myelinated	Norepinephrine	Nicotinic
D.	Short and unmyelinated	Long and unmyelinated	Acetylcholine	Alpha-adrenergic
E.	Long and myelinated	Short and myelinated	Norepinephrine	Beta-adrenergic
F.	Long and myelinated	Short and unmyelinated	Acetylcholine	Muscarinic
G.	Long and unmyelinated	Short and myelinated	Norepinephrine	Nicotinic
H.	Long and unmyelinated	Short and unmyelinated	Acetylcholine	Alpha-adrenergic

11. A medical student breaks out in a cold sweat before presenting a project to her classmates. The postganglionic neurotransmitter responsible for eliciting sweating, if applied to vascular smooth muscle cells, would have what effect on vascular resistance and blood flow through the blood vessels of the gastrointestinal (GI) system?

	Vascular resistance	Blood flow
A.	↓	↓
B.	↓	↑
C.	↓	↔
D.	↑	↑
E.	↑	↓
F.	↑	↔

12. In response to a systemic sympathetic response, epinephrine is released from the adrenal medulla. Which receptor does epinephrine bind to in cardiac muscle cells, bronchial smooth muscle cells, and vascular smooth muscle cells?

	Cardiac muscle cells	Bronchial smooth muscle cells	Vascular smooth muscle cells
A.	β_1	β_2	α_2
B.	β_2	β_1	α_1
C.	α_1	β_1	α_2
D.	β_1	β_2	α_1
E.	β_2	β_1	α_2
F.	α_1	β_2	α_1

13. Which of the following neurons of the autonomic nervous system release norepinephrine?

A. Parasympathetic preganglionic neurons
B. Parasympathetic postganglionic neurons at cardiac muscle
C. Sympathetic postganglionic neurons at cardiac muscle
D. Sympathetic postganglionic neurons at sweat glands
E. Sympathetic preganglionic neurons

14. A 39-year-old woman returns home after eating at a buffet. An hour later she is relaxing in front of the television. Which of the following autonomic responses is most likely occurring at this time?

A. Increased peristalsis
B. Increased sweating
C. Increased circulating epinephrine
D. Decreased blood flow to the skin
E. Dilation of bronchioles

15. While driving, you narrowly avoid a car accident by slamming on the brakes and swerving. Your heart is racing when you come to a stop. Which of the following physiologic parameters will be decreased in response to this experience?

A. Airway resistance
B. Blood glucose concentration
C. Pupil diameter
D. Systolic blood pressure
E. Vascular resistance

16. A 46-year-old woman presents with pain radiating from the left shoulder toward the axilla, ptosis, meiosis, and anhidrosis on the left side of the face. Chest X-ray reveals a tumor in the apex of the left lung, and she is diagnosed with Horner syndrome secondary to a Pancoast lung tumor. Damage or injury to what structure(s) is responsible for the classic Horner syndrome presentation in this patient?

A. Hypothalamic magnocellular cells
B. Preganglionic parasympathetic nerves
C. Preganglionic sympathetic nerves
D. Postganglionic parasympathetic nerves
E. Postganglionic sympathetic nerves

17. A 31-year-old woman presents with episodes of hypertension, nervousness, irritability, panic attacks, and constipation for 4 months. She complains of sweating more than normal, even at night. A computed tomography (CT) scan is performed revealing a functional tumor. Based on the signs and symptoms, where is the tumor most likely located?

A. Adrenal cortex
B. Adrenal medulla
C. Hypothalamus
D. Pancreas
E. Pituitary gland

2.4 Answers and Explanations

10. Correct: Long and myelinated, short and unmyelinated, acetylcholine, muscarinic (F)

This drug is most likely a muscarinic agonist, which would decrease heart rate (chronotropy) but have little or no impact on contractility (inotropy). The pathway for parasympathetic innervation of the heart has long, myelinated preganglionic neurons that synapse with short, unmyelinated postganglionic neurons at the target organ. The postganglionic neurons release acetylcholine, which binds to muscarinic receptors in the sinoatrial node to regulate heart rate. (**A**, **B**, **C**, **D**, **E**, **G**, **H**) These options do not contain the correct combination of answers.

11. Correct: ↓, ↑ (B)

The post-ganglionic neurotransmitter responsible for eliciting sweating is acetylcholine. When applied to vascular smooth muscle tissue of the GI system, it produces a vasodilatory effect, which decreases vascular resistance and increases blood flow. (**A**, **C**, **D**, **E**, **F**) These options do not contain the correct combination of answers.

12. Correct: β_1, β_2, α_1 (D)

Epinephrine binds to: β_1 receptors in cardiac muscle cells to increase heart rate, conduction velocity, and cardiac contractility, β_2 receptors in bronchial smooth muscle cells to produce relaxation, and α_1 receptors in most vascular smooth muscle cells to produce vasoconstriction. (**A**, **B**, **C**, **E**, **F**) These choices do not contain the correct combination of answers.

13. Correct: Sympathetic postganglionic neurons at cardiac muscle (C)

Sympathetic postganglionic neurons release norepinephrine at most target organs, including cardiac muscle tissue. (**A**, **B**) Parasympathetic preganglionic and postganglionic neurons release acetylcholine. (**D**) Sympathetic postganglionic neurons at sweat glands are an exception to the rule for the sympathetic system; they release acetylcholine rather than norepinephrine. (**E**) Sympathetic preganglionic neurons release acetylcholine.

14. Correct: Increased peristalsis (A)

Eating stimulates the parasympathetic nervous system and increases digestive functions (rest and digest); therefore, peristalsis of the intestines will increase. (**B**, **C**, **D**, **E**) These are all sympathetic-mediated actions, which typically will not occur while sitting on the couch after a meal.

15. Correct: Airway resistance (A)

This experience would elicit a sympathetic nervous system response (fight or flight), which increases airway diameter by binding of norepinephrine/epinephrine to β_2 receptors in the smooth muscle of the airways, thus causing relaxation and reducing airway resistance. (**B**) Blood glucose increases in fight-or-flight situations to provide extra energy to the cells. (**C**) Pupil diameter increases to improve vision. (**D**, **E**) Systolic blood pressure and vascular resistance increases due to α_1 receptor activation on the smooth muscle tissue of blood vessels, which induces vascular constriction.

16. Correct: Preganglionic sympathetic nerves (C)

This patient has a lung tumor that is unilaterally compressing the preganglionic nerves of the sympathetic trunk, which arise from the spinal cord in the chest, and ascend to the neck and face. This unilateral disruption of sympathetic nerve activity results in the classic Horner syndrome presentation, which includes meiosis (decreased pupil size), ptosis (drooping eyelid) and anhidrosis (lack of sweating) on the affected side of the face. (**A**, **E**) Injury to the hypothalamus or postganglionic sympathetic nerves can cause Horner syndrome, but they are not indicated in this patient since she has an apical lung tumor, which is most likely responsible for her symptoms. Moreover, magnocellular cells are neuroendocrine cells producing oxytocin and vasopressin, not sympathetic neurons. (**B**, **D**) Horner syndrome results from a sympathetic deficit, not a parasympathetic deficit.

17. Correct: Adrenal medulla (B)

The adrenal medulla secretes epinephrine and norepinephrine in response to sympathetic nervous system stimulation. A tumor here (called pheochromocytoma) can produce uncontrolled secretion of catecholamines, thus increasing sympathetic innervation of all organ systems. This uncontrolled sympathetic innervation explains all of the signs and symptoms of the patient. (**B**, **C**, **D**, **E**) A tumor in the other glands listed would not increase epinephrine or norepinephrine release and thus would not produce all of the patient's signs and symptoms.

2.5 Questions

18. A 13-year-old girl presents to an optometrist with complaints of difficulty seeing the whiteboard from the back of the classroom. She can see her textbooks and computer clearly. Which of the following visual conditions does the girl most likely have, and what is the underlying mechanism of this condition?

	Visual condition	Underlying mechanism
A.	Astigmatism	Increased axial eye length
B.	Astigmatism	Decreased lens elasticity
C.	Hyperopia	Irregular eye shape
D.	Hyperopia	Decreased lens elasticity
E.	Myopia	Increased axial eye length
F.	Myopia	Decreased axial eye length
G.	Presbyopia	Decreased axial eye length
H.	Presbyopia	Irregular eye shape

19. When shifting the eyes from an object that is ten feet (~3 meters) away to an object that is three feet (~1 meter) away, what change occurs to the ciliary muscles and shape of the lens?

	Change to ciliary muscles	Change to shape of lens
A.	Contract	Bulges
B.	Contract	Flattens
C.	Contract	No Change
D.	Relax	Bulges
E.	Relax	Flattens
F.	Relax	No Change

20. A 56-year-old man with hypertension notices difficulty seeing from his right eye but has no other complaints. Neurologic exam reveals a direct response to light in the left pupil without a consensual response in the right pupil. This lack of motor response suggests a deficit from damage to which of the following structures?

A. Right oculomotor nerve
B. Left oculomotor nerve
C. Right optic nerve
D. Left optic nerve

21. An 8-year-old boy was caught playing with matches and is being scolded by his mother. He is embarrassed and his gaze drops down and to the right, as shown in the image. Which muscle, for each eye, is used to achieve this eye movement?

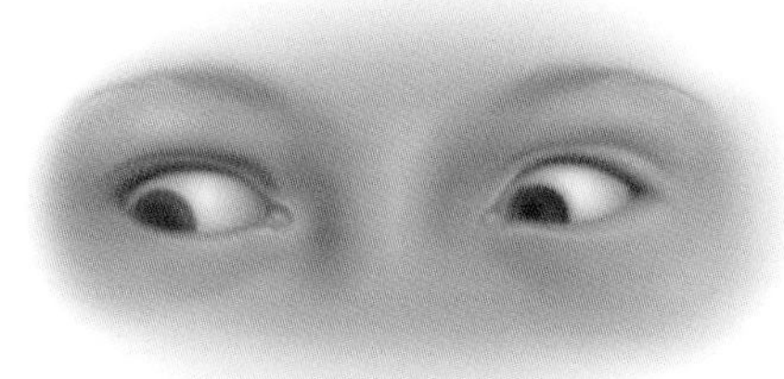

	Muscle for right eye	Muscle for left eye
A.	Inferior rectus	Lateral rectus
B.	Inferior rectus	Superior oblique
C.	Lateral rectus	Inferior rectus
D.	Lateral rectus	Superior oblique
E.	Superior oblique	Lateral rectus
F.	Superior oblique	Inferior rectus

22. A 48-year-old woman presents with a unilateral hearing deficit in the left ear that has progressively developed over the past 10 years. Her history is positive for measles at age 7. Hearing tests reveal a conduction loss but normal nerve function. Dysfunction of which of the following auditory structures is most likely responsible for her hearing loss?

A. Incus
B. Malleus
C. Oval window
D. Round window
E. Stapes

23. A 42-year-old man presents with progressive, moderate, bilateral hearing loss that started at age 32. He has been a factory worker for 20 years and was exposed to loud noise (over 85 decibels) for prolonged periods of time without ear protection. Which of the following terms best characterizes his noise-induced hearing loss?

A. Conductive hearing loss
B. Mixed hearing loss
C. Neural hearing loss
D. Presbycusis
E. Sensory hearing loss

24. A 66-year-old man is referred to an audiologist for complaints of hearing loss following a stroke. Tests reveal deficits in auditory discrimination, acuity, and sound localization. A lesion in what structure of the midbrain would cause these deficits?

A. Cerebral crura
B. Inferior colliculus
C. Periaqueductal gray matter
D. Superior cerebellar peduncle
E. Trochlear nucleus

25. The sense of smell is able to stimulate vivid memories because the olfactory tract projects to which of the following structures in the brain?

A. Amygdala
B. Brainstem
C. Hypothalamus
D. Pituitary gland
E. Thalamus

26. Immediately following a surgical procedure to excise a brainstem tumor, a patient is experiencing dysphagia and a decreased gag reflex. Damage to which of the following combinations of cranial nerves is most likely responsible for the decreased gag reflex in this patient?

A. V and IX
B. IX and X
C. IX and XII
D. X and XII
E. V and XII
F. V and X

27. Which three cranial nerves are responsible for transmitting impulses for the sense of taste to the brainstem?

A. Accessory, olfactory, glossopharyngeal
B. Facial, glossopharyngeal, vagus
C. Glossopharyngeal, hypoglossal, accessory
D. Hypoglossal, facial, olfactory
E. Olfactory, vagus, accessory
F. Vagus, facial, hypoglossal

2.6 Answers and Explanations

18. Correct: Myopia, increased axial eye length (E)

Myopia is nearsightedness due to an increased axial length of the eye, which causes light to focus ahead of the retina. This makes it difficult to focus on distant objects but does not affect focus on nearby objects. (**A**, **B**) Astigmatism is blurred vision due to irregular shape of the eye. (**C**, **D**) Hyperopia is farsightedness due to decreased axial length of the eye. (**F**) Myopia is near-sightedness, but it is due to increased, not decreased, axial length. (**G**, **H**) Presbyopia is farsightedness due to loss of elasticity of the lens.

19. Correct: Contract, bulges (A)

To look at an object that is closer, accommodation for near vision must occur. In this process, the ciliary muscles contract, allowing zona fibers to relax. This causes the lens to bulge (see image). During accommodation for far vision, the ciliary muscles relax, causing zona fibers to stretch and the lens to flatten. (**B**, **C**, **D**, **E**, **F**) These choices do not contain the correct combination of answers.

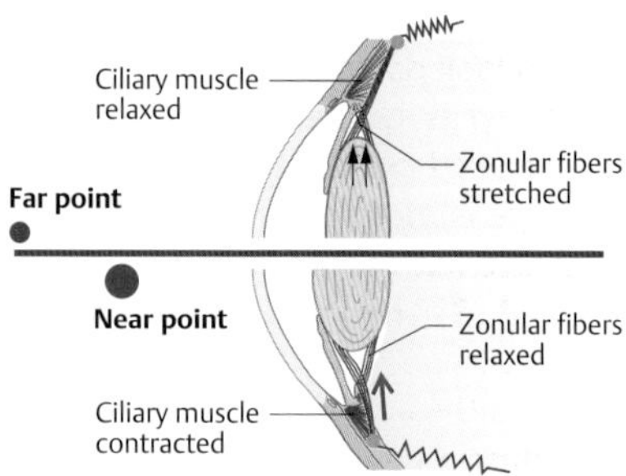

20. Correct: Right oculomotor nerve (A)

Damage to the right oculomotor nerve would cause the contralateral consensual reflex to be lost. Light shone into the left eye can signal to the brain via the normal optic nerve; this normally would cause constriction of both pupils, but since the right oculomotor nerve is damaged, the right pupil cannot constrict. (**B**) Damage to the left oculomotor nerve would cause the opposite response. (**C**, **D**) Following damage to either optic nerve, the direct response would be lost in the eye associated with the damaged optic nerve, but the consensual response would be maintained in that eye.

21. Correct: Superior oblique, inferior rectus (F)

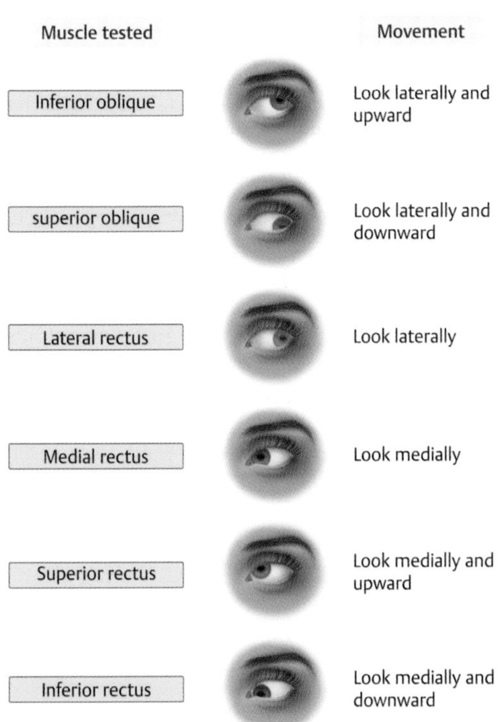

For the boy to look down and to the right with both eyes, his right eye is moving laterally and downward, which is controlled by the superior oblique muscle, and his left eye is moving medially and downward, which is controlled by the inferior rectus muscle (see image). (**A**, **B**) The inferior rectus would move the right eye medially and downward, which would be down and to the left (not right). (**C**, **D**, **E**) The lateral rectus muscle moves the eye laterally, but not downward.

22. Correct: Stapes (E)

The patient has otosclerosis, which causes increased ossification of the stapes and reduces conduction of the ossicles in the middle ear. This condition is progressive, so hearing loss occurs over time. Otosclerosis is linked to previous measles infections, stress fractures of the bones of the middle ear, and immune disorders. (**A**, **B**) In very rare cases, the incus and malleus may be affected by otosclerosis, but normally it is the stapes. (**C**, **D**) Conditions affecting the oval and round windows are typically congenital and do not develop in middle-aged individuals.

23. Correct: Sensory hearing loss (E)

Sensory hearing loss may be from damage to the organ of Corti, an inability of the hair cells to stimulate the nerves of hearing, or a metabolic problem with the fluids of the inner ear. (**A**) Conductive hearing loss is caused by any condition or disease that impedes the mechanical conduction of sound through the middle ear cavity to the inner ear. (**B**) A mixed hearing loss is a sensorineural hearing loss with a conductive component overlaying all or part of the audiometric range tested. (**C**) Neural (or retrocochlear) hearing loss can be the result of severe damage to the organ of Corti that causes the nerves of hearing to degenerate, or an inability of the auditory nerves to convey information. (**D**) Presbycusis is age-related hearing loss. It is a sensorineural hearing loss that is bilateral and irreversible, and it results from degeneration of the cochlea or associated structures.

24. Correct: Inferior colliculus (B)

The inferior colliculus transmits auditory information from the lower brainstem to the cortex. Damage can cause all of the deficits described in the patient. (**A**) The cerebral crura contain nerve tracts that connect the spinal cord to the cerebral hemispheres via the pons. Damage results in upper motor neuron paralysis. (**C**) The periaqueductal gray matter contains enkephalin-positive cells and nerve terminals, which act to regulate pain, cardiovascular functions, and emotional behavior. (**D**) The superior cerebellar peduncle connects the cerebellum to the midbrain. Damage results in ipsilateral deficits in motor coordination. (**E**) The trochlear nucleus (cranial nerve IV) governs the downward movements of the eyes. Damage may cause double vision and flexion of the head toward the lesion.

25. Correct: Amygdala (A)

The amygdala is part of the limbic system, which supports a variety of functions including emotion, behavior, motivation, memory, and olfaction. (**B**) The brainstem regulates basic functions of life, such as cardiac function, respiratory function, and sleep cycles. It also houses motor and sensory tracts from upper portions of the brain to the rest of the body. (**C**) The hypothalamus has many functions, but most importantly it links the nervous system to the endocrine system via the pituitary gland. (**D**) The pituitary is important in controlling growth, development, and the functioning of other endocrine glands. (**E**) The thalamus receives input from other sensory systems, but the olfactory tract projects directly to the olfactory cortex and other regions, without a thalamic relay.

26. Correct: IX and X (B)

The gag reflex involves a brisk and brief elevation of the soft palate and bilateral contraction of pharyngeal muscles. It is mediated by the afferent limb of the glossopharyngeal nerve (CN IX) and the efferent limb of the vagus nerve (CN X). Damage to one or both of these nerves can decrease the gag reflex. (**A**, **C**, **D**, **E**, **F**) The remaining options do not contain the correct combination of cranial nerves. The trigeminal nerve (CN V) has both motor and sensory control and mediates general sensation of the face and scalp, opening/closing of the mouth, and tension of the tympanic membrane. The hypoglossal nerve (CN XII) is a pure motor nerve and controls movements of the tongue.

27. Correct: Facial, glossopharyngeal, vagus (B)

The facial nerve transmits sensory impulses for taste from the anterior two-thirds of the tongue, the glossopharyngeal nerve transmits impulses from the posterior one-third of the tongue, and the vagus nerve conveys taste sensation from the epiglottis and root of the tongue. (**A**, **C**, **D**, **E**, **F**) The hypoglossal nerve is a motor nerve that controls tongue movement. The accessory nerve is a motor nerve that controls the sternocleidomastoid and trapezius muscles. The olfactory nerve is a sensory nerve for smell.

2.7 Questions

28. A 70-year-old woman is admitted to the hospital after waking up with a right facial droop and slurred speech. Stroke is ruled out using a computed tomography (CT) scan, and a neurological exam is used to diagnose the patient with Bell's palsy. Dysfunction of which cranial nerve is most likely responsible for the patient's symptoms?

A. V
B. VI
C. VII
D. X
E. XI

29. A 55-year-old man presents with complaints of acute (i.e., since waking) headache and motor and sensory dysfunction. An angiogram reveals an embolus in the anterior cerebral artery supplying the left hemisphere. Based on the location of this embolus, the patient will likely have a deficit in motor and sensory function in which of the following extremity or extremities?

A. Left lower
B. Right lower
C. Left upper
D. Right upper
E. Left upper and lower
F. Right upper and lower

30. While working out with a trainer, an 18-year-old girl performs biceps curls with progressively heavier weights. When she reaches 40 pounds, she begins to lift the weight then suddenly drops it. Activation of which of the following is most directly responsible for the sudden muscle relaxation that caused her to drop the weight?

A. α-adrenergic receptor
B. β-adrenergic receptor
C. Golgi tendon organ
D. Muscle spindle
E. Stretch receptor

Questions 31 to 32

A 12-year-old boy is hit by a car while riding his bike. X-ray reveals no broken bones, but there is severe bruising and swelling in the left leg, trunk, arm, and back where he was struck by the car. A neurological exam reveals an absent patellar reflex in the left leg.

31. Which nerve roots are assessed with the patellar reflex?

A. C5–C6
B. C7–C8
C. L3–L4
D. S1–S2
E. T9–T10

32. The patellar reflex was tested in the boy by striking the patellar tendon with a reflex hammer. Which of the following responses to the quadriceps and hamstring muscles would indicate a positive (normal) response?

	Quadriceps muscles	Hamstring muscles
A.	Stimulation	Inhibition
B.	Inhibition	Stimulation
C.	Inhibition	Inhibition
D.	Stimulation	Stimulation
E.	Stimulation	No change
F.	No change	Stimulation

33. Compared to a monosynaptic reflex arc, a polysynaptic reflex arc includes which of the following?

A. An afferent neuron
B. An efferent neuron
C. An interneuron
D. A white matter synapse

34. A 17-year-old woman is slammed into a wall while playing hockey. She loses consciousness briefly and is transported to the emergency department. Cognition appears intact, but a neurological exam reveals some muscle weakness and reduced motor control of both lower extremities. Pain and temperature sensations remain intact. She has a positive Babinski sign. Which nervous system tracts are most likely damaged in this patient, and which motor neurons (upper or lower) are primarily affected?

	Damaged nervous system tracts	Primarily affected motor neurons
A.	Extrapyramidal	Lower
B.	Pyramidal	Lower
C.	Spinothalamic	Lower
D.	Extrapyramidal	Upper
E.	Pyramidal	Upper
F.	Spinothalamic	Upper

35. A man with a history of atrial fibrillation presents with an arterial infarct at the level of the cerebral peduncle, which has affected the descending fibers of the corticospinal tract. A neurological exam will reveal which of the following signs?

A. Areflexia
B. Fasciculations
C. Flaccid paralysis
D. Hypotonicity
E. Positive Babinski sign

36. A 59-year-old woman presents with hyperactive reflexes, lower extremity weakness, muscle atrophy, fasciculations, and increased muscle tone. What is her most likely diagnosis, and which treatment affecting the N-methyl-D-aspartate (NMDA) glutamate receptor would be indicated?

	Most likely diagnosis	NMDA receptor drug
A.	Amyotrophic lateral sclerosis	Agonist
B.	Amyotrophic lateral sclerosis	Antagonist
C.	Multiple sclerosis	Agonist
D.	Multiple sclerosis	Antagonist
E.	Primary lateral sclerosis	Agonist
F.	Primary lateral sclerosis	Antagonist

37. A 19-year-old college baseball player is accidentally struck on the right side of the neck with a bat. He is experiencing a loss of fine touch sensation, vibration, and proprioception below cervical spinal nerve 6 (C6) on the right side. He has no loss of pain or thermal sensation on either side. Which of the following findings would most likely be present on magnetic resonance imaging (MRI) of the spinal cord at the site of injury?

A. Complete transection of the spinal cord
B. Damage to the right dorsal white column
C. Damage to the right spinocerebellar tract
D. Damage to the right anteriolateral system
E. Hemisection of the spinal cord

38. Which of the following encapsulated receptors is distributed widely within the skin and fascia and is responsible for the detection of vibration and pressure?

A. Free nerve endings
B. Meissner corpuscle
C. Merkel disks
D. Pacinian corpuscle
E. Ruffini endings

39. A football player is carried off the field after a helmet-to-helmet tackle, and a spinal cord injury is suspected. He is experiencing complete skeletal muscle paralysis of his lower extremities, abdominal region, and intercostal muscles. Most of his arm muscle function is preserved, and he is able to breathe without a ventilator. At which level is the spinal cord most likely injured?

A. C1
B. C4
C. C7
D. L2
E. T10

2.8 Answers and Explanations

28. Correct: VII (C)

Bell's palsy is due to a deficiency in cranial nerve (CN) VII, the facial nerve, which includes the axons of lower motor neurons. CN VII controls the muscles of facial expression, and mediates taste sensation from the anterior two-thirds of the tongue. (**A**) CN V (trigeminal nerve) is responsible for sensations in the face and motor functions such as biting and chewing. (**B**) CN VI (abducent nerve) is a somatic efferent nerve that controls movement of a single muscle: the lateral rectus muscle of the eye. (**D**) CN X (vagus nerve) primarily provides parasympathetic control of the heart and digestive tract. (**E**) CN XI (accessory nerve) controls the sternocleidomastoid and trapezius muscles.

29. Correct: Right lower (B)

The left anterior cerebral artery (ACA) supplies the areas of primary sensory and motor cortex for the lower right extremity. (**A**) The right ACA supplies the areas of primary sensory and motor cortex for the lower left extremity. (**C, D**) The left middle cerebral artery (MCA) supplies the areas of primary sensory and motor cortex for the upper right extremity, and the right MCA supplies those regions for the upper left extremity. (**E, F**) Deficits in both upper and lower extremities would likely involve both the ACA and the MCA.

30. Correct: Golgi tendon organ (C)

In a Golgi tendon reflex, which is mediated by the Golgi tendon organ, excessive skeletal muscle contraction causes the agonist muscle to simultaneously lengthen and relax. This is a protective reflex to prevent muscle damage. (**A, B**) α- and β-adrenergic receptors are generally located on smooth or cardiac muscle, but not skeletal muscle. They indirectly contribute to skeletal muscle function by controlling cardiac output (β-receptors) and regulate blood flow to skeletal muscle (α- and β-receptors). (**D**) Muscle spindles are sensory receptors within the belly of a muscle that primarily detect changes in the length of this muscle for proprioception. (**E**) Stretch receptors in skeletal muscle tissue, such as muscle spindles, are used for proprioception. The stretch receptor reflex leads to muscle contraction, not relaxation.

31. Correct: L3–L4 (C)

The patellar reflex is a myotactic reflex that increases stretch in the muscle and muscle spindles and sends a signal to the L3–L4 level of the spinal cord to initiate a reflex. Damage to the lower motor neurons or spinal cord at or above the level of L3–L4 will result in an absent patellar reflex. (**A**) The nerve roots for the biceps reflex are at C5–C6. (**B**) The nerve roots for the triceps reflex are at C7–C8. (**D**) The nerve roots for the ankle reflex are at S1–S2. (**E**) The nerve roots at T9–T10 are not part of a reflex arc.

32. Correct: Stimulation, inhibition (A)

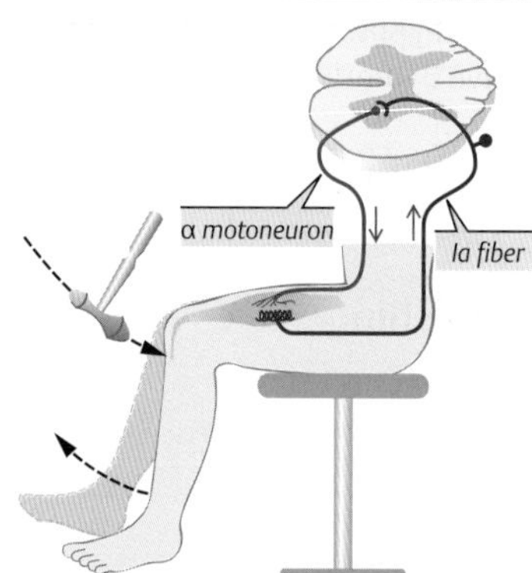

The patellar reflex is a myotactic reflex that causes the knee to jerk when the patellar tendon is struck with a reflex hammer (see image). The hammer strikes the tendon and the tendon stretches, pulling on the muscle spindle and sending information to the spinal cord via the 1a fibers. α-motor neurons carry a message back to the muscle, stimulating the knee extensor muscles (quadriceps) to contract and inhibiting the knee flexor muscles (hamstrings; not shown in the image). (**B, C, D, E, F**) These choices are incorrect based on the previous explanation.

33. Correct: An interneuron (C)

Polysynaptic reflexes (i.e., withdrawal reflexes) have an interneuron in the gray matter of the spinal cord that connects the afferent and efferent signals, so they are three-neuron reflex arcs. In monosynaptic reflexes (e.g., patellar reflex), the afferent and efferent neurons synapse directly in the gray matter without an interneuron. (**A, B**) Both reflexes have an efferent and an afferent neuron. (**D**) The neurons of the reflex arc synapse in the gray matter, not white matter.

34. Correct: Pyramidal, upper (E)

The Babinski sign, along with muscle weakness and reduced motor control, indicates a lesion in the pyramidal tracts (corticospinal), which contain axons of upper motor neurons**.** (**A, B, C**) The Babinski sign indicates an upper motor neuron lesion, so the lower motor neuron options are incorrect. (**D**) Extrapyramidal tracts are indirect, as opposed to the direct pathways of the pyramidal system. They function to selectively activate, suppress, initiate, and coordinate movements. Damage to the extrapyramidal system will result in dyskinesia. (**F**) Damage to the spinothalamic tract leads to a loss of pain and temperature sensation from the contralateral side beginning one or two vertebral segments below the lesion.

35. Correct: Positive Babinski's sign (E)

Corticospinal axons originate from upper motor neurons (UMN). UMN lesions typically result in hyperreflexia, hypertonicity, spastic paralysis, and a positive Babinski sign. (**A**, **B**, **C**, **D**) Lower motor neuron (LMN) lesions produce areflexia, fasciculations, flaccid paralysis, and hypotonicity and are not associated with a positive Babinski sign.

36. Correct: Amyotrophic lateral sclerosis, antagonist (B)

Distinguishing upper from lower motor neuron lesions

Feature	Upper lesion	Lower lesion
Reflexes	Hyperactive	Diminished or absent
Atrophy	Absent*	Present
Fasciculations	Absent	Present
Tone	Increased	Decreased of absent

The patient presents with signs of upper motor neuron lesions (hyperactive reflexes and increased muscle tone) and lower motor neuron lesions (lower extremity weakness, atrophy, and fasciculations), which is consistent with amyotrophic lateral sclerosis (ALS). Since glutamate is the major excitatory neurotransmitter in the central nervous system, and excessive transmission can cause neuronal damage and death, an NMDA antagonist may produce a neuroprotective effect by reducing glutamate excitotoxicty, thus delaying the progression of ALS. (**A**) An NMDA agonist would increase excitotoxicity, leading to more neuronal damage and death. (**C**, **D**) Multiple sclerosis is a demyelinating disease of the central nervous system, which has a different presentation than the patient in this vignette. (**E**, **F**) Primary lateral sclerosis affects upper motor neurons but not lower, so the patient's symptoms are not consistent with this disease.

37. Correct: Damage to the right dorsal white column (B)

The image below shows the tracts of the spinal cord. A lesion to the dorsal column (i.e., fasciculus gracilis and/or fasciculus cuneatus) will result in an ipsilateral loss of vibration and proprioception (sense of body position) as well as loss of all sensation of fine touch, which is what the patient is experiencing. (**A**) Complete transection of the spinal cord would result in complete loss of sensory and motor function below the transection. (**C**) Isolated damage to the spinocerebellar tract rarely occurs and is most commonly associated with more complex syndromes or genetic defects. (**D**) Damage to the anterolateral system could affect the function of one or both tracts that make it up. (1) The anterior spinothalamic tract carries the sensory modalities of crude touch and pressure, and (2) the lateral spinothalamic tract carries the sensory modalities of pain and temperature. The patient does not exhibit any of these symptoms. (**E**) The hemisection of the cord results in a lesion of each of the three main neural systems: the dorsal column, the spinocerebellar tract, and the anterolateral system. This would result in the deficits described for answers **B**, **C**, and **D**.

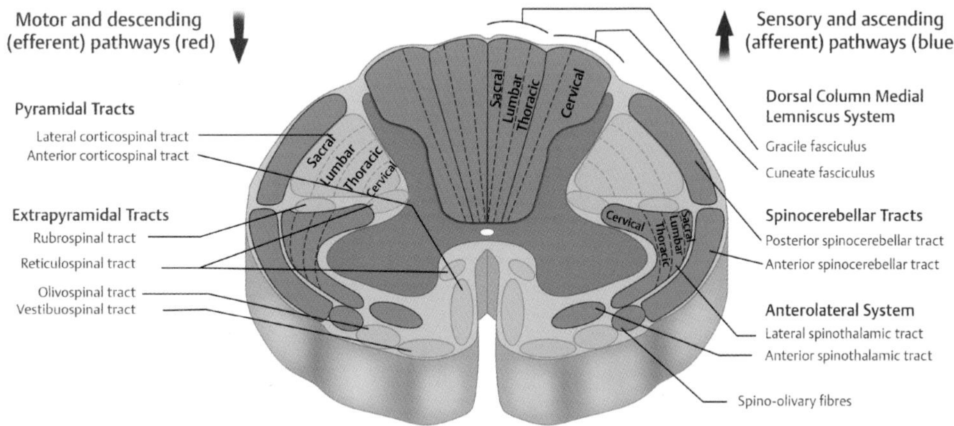

38. Correct: Pacinian corpuscle (D)

Pacinian corpuscles are encapsulated nerve endings in the skin that are responsible for sensitivity to vibration and pressure. They respond only to sudden disturbances and are especially sensitive to vibration. (**A**) Free nerve endings are located in the skin and detect pain and temperature changes. (**B**) Meissner corpuscles detect light touch and vibration; however, they are concentrated in thick hairless skin, especially at the finger pads, and are not widespread throughout the body. (**C**) Merkel disks provide sensory information about pressure, position, and deep static touch. (**E**) Ruffini endings are located in the fingers and are sensitive to skin stretch; they contribute to the control of finger position and movement.

39. Correct: C7 (C)

Damage to the spinal cord at the level of C7 would cause the patient's symptoms because the nerves that innervate the lower extremities, abdominal region, and intercostals are below C7, but the nerves that innervate most upper-extremity muscle and the diaphragm for breathing (phrenic nerve) are above C7. (**A**) Damage at the level of C1 is above the brachial plexus and phrenic nerve and would paralyze the upper extremities and diaphragm as well, requiring a ventilator for respiration. (**B**) Damage at the level of C4 would cause upper-extremity paralysis, but the diaphragm would maintain most of its function, so respiration could occur without a ventilator. (**D**) A person with damage at L2 would have normal respiration, full upper limb, torso and trunk muscle function, and some hip, knee and foot movement. Walking might be possible with assistance. (**E**) A person with damage at T10 would have the full use of the upper body. Partial paralysis of the lower body and legs would be present, and breathing would be normal.

Chapter 3

Musculoskeletal and Integumentary Systems

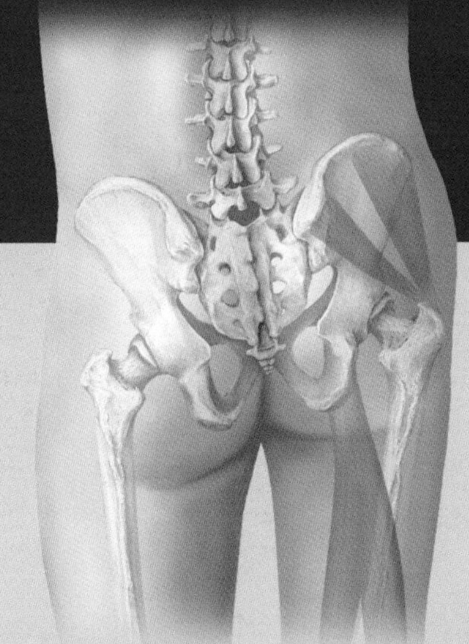

LEARNING OBJECTIVES

- ▸ Explain the general structure-function relationship of skeletal, smooth, and cardiac muscle.
- ▸ Discuss the control of skeletal muscle contraction, excitation-contraction coupling, neuromuscular transmission, and the mechanics and energetics of skeletal muscle contraction.
- ▸ Discuss the control of cardiac muscle contraction, excitation-contraction coupling, and the mechanics and energetics of cardiac muscle contraction.
- ▸ Discuss the control, mechanics, and energetics of smooth muscle contraction.
- ▸ Describe the basic physiology of bone.
- ▸ Describe the basic physiology of the skin.

3.1 Questions

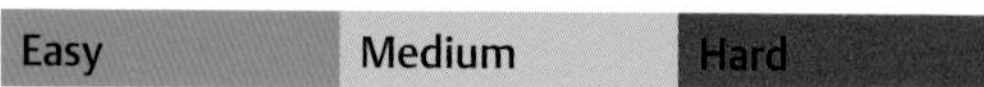

1. A 25-year-old healthy male medical student is doing biceps curls with 20-pound weights in the gym. When his skeletal muscles contract to lift the weight, what change occurs to the sarcomere at the molecular level?

A. The length of the A-band decreases.
B. The length of the I-band decreases.
C. The lengths of the A- and I-bands decrease.
D. The length of the H-band increases.
E. The length of the M-line decreases.

2. During a physiology experiment, a muscle is extracted and suspended in a physiologic solution. The muscle contracts when directly stimulated with an electrode, but it does not contract spontaneously. It continues to contract upon stimulation after being treated with a drug that antagonizes myosin light chain kinase activity, and after it is placed in new salt solution that is calcium-free. Based on the experimental data provided, what type of muscle tissue is most likely being tested?

A. Cardiac muscle
B. Multiunit smooth muscle
C. Skeletal muscle
D. Unitary smooth muscle

3. In the table below, each type of muscle tissue (skeletal, cardiac, smooth) is associated with a functional characteristic that happens exclusively, or most predominantly, in that muscle type. Which of the following choices has the correct associations?

	Absence of pacemaker	Calmodulin as site of Ca^{2+} regulation	Only excitation caused by neuronal stimulation	Relaxation in response to stretch	Voluntary regulation of contraction	Significant amount of anaerobic respiration
A.	Skeletal	Skeletal	Skeletal	Skeletal	Skeletal	Cardiac
B.	Skeletal	Skeletal	Cardiac	Skeletal	Cardiac	Skeletal
C.	Smooth	Smooth	Cardiac	Smooth	Skeletal	Cardiac
D.	Skeletal	Smooth	Skeletal	Smooth	Skeletal	Skeletal
E.	Smooth	Smooth	Smooth	Cardiac	Skeletal	Skeletal

4. Which of the following activities most closely depicts an isometric contraction?

A. Lowering different amounts of weight
B. Passive stretching as a warmup exercise
C. Running downhill then uphill
D. Squeezing gluteal muscles together
E. Walking down a flight of stairs

5. When measuring isotonic contractions in a skeletal muscle preparation, increasing the length of the preparation beyond the resting length (L_0) prior to electrical stimulation would produce which of the following changes to active and passive tension?

	Active tension	Passive tension
A.	↑	↑
B.	↓	↓
C.	↑	↓
D.	↓	↑
E.	↔	↑
F.	↔	↓

6. In a physiology lab, a skeletal muscle is isolated from a frog to conduct muscle function tests. The muscle is stimulated to contract under varying conditions. The solid line on the following afterload–velocity graph represents the contraction of the skeletal muscle at a preload below the muscle's optimal length. Which of the dashed curves (**A–D**) on the force–velocity graph would correlate most closely with the shortening velocity produced by the same muscle for a given afterload, but at a smaller preload?

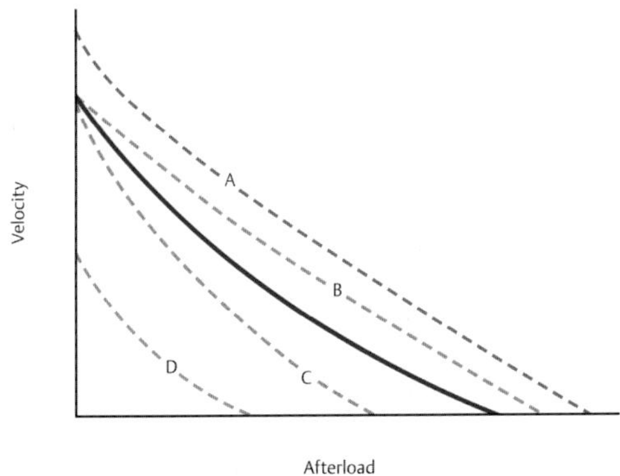

A. A
B. B
C. C
D. D

7. A 45-year-old woman works with a personal trainer to get in shape. After several months of aerobic exercise training, which of the following parameters will be reduced in skeletal muscle tissue?

A. Activity of citric acid cycle enzymes
B. Distance between capillaries
C. Myoglobin concentration per fiber
D. Proportions of fast-twitch fibers
E. Total number of muscle fibers

8. A 15-year-old male high school student begins working with a personal trainer to increase strength and flexibility. The trainer develops a program that includes both weight lifting and yoga. Eight months later, the boy's skeletal muscles now have 25% more sarcomeres in series and 100% more sarcomeres in parallel. Which of the following is the percent increase in the maximum force generation of the boy's muscle?

A. 25
B. 100
C. 125
D. 200
E. 250

9. A 73-year-old man presents with cardiac failure and clinical signs of impaired ability to pump blood forward. Five years ago, he was diagnosed with severe aortic valve stenosis, which chronically increased his cardiac afterload. Three years ago, cardiac ultrasound showed the walls of his left ventricle had thickened all around (concentric hypertrophy). The present ultrasound reveals ventricular walls that are thinner than normal and a dilated left ventricle with a larger volume of blood than normal (eccentric hypertrophy). In the cardiac length–tension curve shown in the image, which of the following combinations best represent the status of his cardiac muscle activity three years ago and at present time?

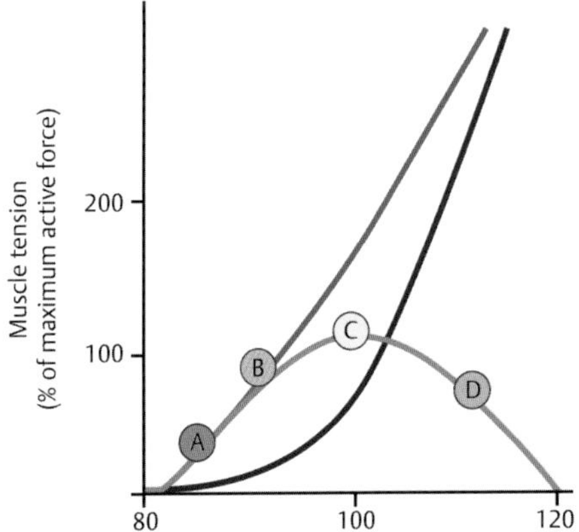

	3 years ago	At present time
A.	A	C
B.	A	D
C.	B	C
D.	B	D
E.	C	D
F.	C	A

3.2 Answers and Explanations

Easy	Medium	Hard

1. Correct: The length of the I-band decreases. (B)

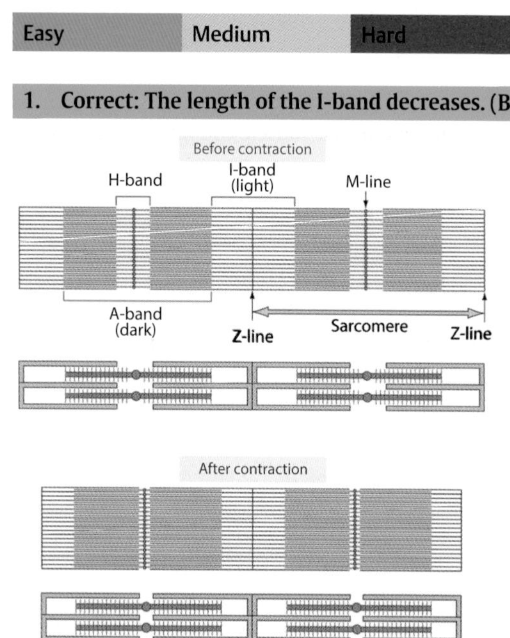

During skeletal muscle contraction, the actin filaments slide over the myosin filaments toward each other, actin and myosin filament overlap increases, and the sarcomere shortens. In this process, the I-band, which represents the actin without myosin overlap, decreases in length as actin and myosin overlap increases (the image). (**A, C**) The A-band remains unchanged since it represents the length of the myosin filaments, which does not change during contraction. (**D**) The H-band, which represents the myosin without actin overlap, decreases in length as actin and myosin overlap increases. (**E**) The M-line, a vertical line made of proteins and located in the center of the sarcomere that anchors the myosin molecules, does not change with contraction.

2. Correct: Skeletal muscle (C)

The muscle tissue being tested contracts when stimulated with an electrode, even in the absence of extracellular calcium, which indicates skeletal muscle tissue. (**A**) Cardiac muscle has automaticity, which allows the muscle to spontaneously contract without any electrical or hormonal stimuli. It also requires extracellular calcium influx through the dihydropyridine receptor (DHP) to open the ryanodine receptors (RyR) on the sarcoplasmic reticulum for substantial cytoplasmic calcium increases (calcium-induced calcium release). Therefore, because the experimental muscle tissue does not contract spontaneously and because it does contract in the absence of calcium, cardiac muscle tissue is excluded. (**B, D**) Smooth muscle tissue requires phosphorylation of myosin light chain (MLC) by myosin light chain kinase (MLCK) for contraction to occur. Because the experimental muscle tissue continues to contract when antagonized by a drug that blocks MLCK, this excludes smooth muscle tissue.

3. Correct: Skeletal, smooth, skeletal, smooth, skeletal, skeletal (D)

Pacemakers are absent in skeletal muscle cells and present in cardiac cells and in single-unit smooth muscle cells. Calmodulin is the site of calcium regulation in smooth muscle, but troponin has this role in skeletal and cardiac muscle. Neuronal stimulation in skeletal muscle exclusively leads to excitation, whereas in cardiac and smooth muscle, it can lead to excitation or inhibition. Smooth muscle has an autoregulatory feature in that stretch leads to muscle relaxation, but in skeletal and cardiac muscle, the contractile strength increases with the degree of stretch over physiological ranges. Skeletal muscle contraction is regulated voluntarily via axon terminals of the somatic nervous system. Cardiac and smooth muscle contraction is involuntary via intrinsic mechanisms, autonomic nerves, hormones, stretch, and local chemicals. Skeletal muscle is the only type with a significant amount of anaerobic respiration and an oxygen debt that can be paid back after contraction. Cardiac and smooth muscle respiration is mainly aerobic. (**A, B, C, E**) These answers have one or more incorrect muscle types associated with the functional muscle characteristic.

4. Correct: Squeezing gluteal muscles together (D)

For an isometric contraction to occur, the muscles need to increase tension without movement. Holding the buttock muscles squeezed together is the closest. A pure isometric contraction is difficult to obtain, though, since typically some stretching of tendons occurs. (**A, C, E**) An isotonic contraction is a controlled shortening of the muscle, in which the tension remains unchanged and the muscle length changes. Lowering weights, running downhill, and walking down stairs are examples that are close to, but not pure isotonic contractions, since the actual load on the muscle will change due to joint movements. (**B**) Passive stretching means holding a position in a relatively relaxed way for a certain amount of time. This is different from isometric stretching, when the held muscle is additionally contracted for some time, for instance by a partner or a wall.

5. Correct: ↓, ↑ (D)

When stretching skeletal muscle beyond its resting length, which is also its optimal length, the passive tension will increase and the active tension will decrease. The passive tension increases because as the sarcomere is stretched, the elastic elements of the sarcomere are passively stretched, and tension increases. The active tension decreases because as the sarcomere is stretched, the actin and myosin overlap decreases, and on stimulation, fewer crossbridges form, and thus less active tension is produced. (**A, B, C, E, F**) These choices do not contain the correct combination of answers.

6. Correct: C (C)

The *x*-intercept in the afterload–velocity relationship represents the point at which the afterload is so great that the muscle fiber cannot shorten, and therefore represents the maximal isometric force (F_{max}). The *y*-intercept represents the maximal velocity of shortening (V_{max}) that would be achieved if there were no afterload. If preload is decreased for a given afterload, the muscle fibers will have a smaller velocity of shortening. This is represented by the downward shift in curve C. It occurs because as preload is decreased, the length–tension relationship dictates that there is a decrease in active tension development. In other words, decreasing the preload causes muscle to contract more slowly against a given afterload. Note that decreasing preload decreases F_{max} and the shortening velocity at a given afterload but does not alter V_{max}. (**A**) Curve A represents contraction of a faster-twitch fiber-type skeletal muscle (i.e., type IIb). (**B**) Curve B represents the changes seen with an increase in preload toward the muscle's optimal length, not a decrease in preload. (**D**) Curve D represents contraction of a slow-twitch fiber–type skeletal muscle (i.e., type I).

7. Correct: Distance between capillaries (B)

The distance between capillaries will be reduced due to a greater number of capillaries (angiogenesis). Aerobic exercise and endurance training stimulates angiogenesis as adaptation to the increased oxygen and nutrient demand. (**A**) Aerobic exercise enhances the muscle oxidative capacity by increasing (not reducing) the activity of citric acid cycle enzymes. (**C**) Aerobic exercise increases (not reduces) the myoglobin concentration per fiber. (**D, E**) The percent number of fast-twitch fibers and the total number of cells are unchanged after endurance training.

8. Correct: 100 (B)

Weight lifting primarily increases skeletal muscle hypertrophy (sarcomeres in parallel), which increase the maximum force development of the muscle. Yoga or other stretching exercises primarily increase the length of skeletal muscles (sarcomeres in series), which increases the shortening velocity and shortening capacity of the muscle but has minimal or no impact on the maximum force generation. Because the sarcomeres in parallel, which are responsible for force development, were doubled (increased by 100%), this would produce an approximate increase in maximum force development by 100% as well. (**A, C, D, E**) These choices do not contain the correct answer.

9. Correct: C, D (E)

The cardiac muscle responded to the chronic increase in afterload with hypertrophy, just as any muscle adapts to training, by creating more myofilaments. More myofilaments allow a greater maximum active force, and three years ago, his site of operation was to the right of normal. Because he was still able to move blood forward effectively into the aorta and because point B is the normal point of operation, point C makes the most sense for his cardiac function three years ago. His cardiac muscle could not continuously produce the higher force and eventually failed. An adaptive increase of blood volume with cardiac failure further stretched his cardiac muscle fibers, but this time to a pathological length, which can produce only submaximal force (point D). (**A, B, C, D, F**) These combinations do not present a gradual increase in fiber length with matching force changes along the bell-shaped active length–tension curve.

3.3 Questions

10. Excitation–contraction coupling is a process in which a muscle cell is stimulated to contract, and this process is followed by muscle cell relaxation. It involves the following events (not necessarily in this order):

1. Action potential
2. Ca^{2+} release into cytoplasm
3. Cross-bridge cycling
4. Cytoplasmic Ca^{2+} removal
5. Depolarization of T tubules

Which of the following lists the correct sequence of events for excitation–contraction coupling in skeletal muscle tissue?

A. 1–2–5–3–4
B. 1–5–2–3–4
C. 1–4–5–3–2
D. 5–1–2–3–4
E. 5–4–3–1–2
F. 5–4–1–3–2

11. At a fitness club, a frequent exerciser and an untrained newcomer run side by side on a treadmill, each at two-thirds of their maximal oxygen uptake (VO_2 max). Which of the following is expected, all else being equal, for the untrained person in comparison to the trained person?

A. Higher bone mineral density
B. Lower maximal heart rate
C. Lower serum lactic acid levels
D. Lower muscle oxidative capacity
E. Shorter time to exhaustion

12. During a physiology experiment, a skeletal muscle is stimulated rapidly, producing an isometric tetanic contraction. If ATP production is inhibited and intracellular ATP levels drop quickly, which of the following processes involved in muscle contraction and relaxation would be directly disrupted by the lack of ATP?

A. Cross-bridge formation
B. Depolarization of the T tubule
C. Opening of ryanodine receptor channels
D. Relaxation of the myocytes
E. The power stroke

13. A researcher accidentally gets stuck in the arm with a syringe of unknown content and experiences profound arm muscle weakness. On arrival at the hospital, electrodiagnostic evaluations show normal frequencies and amplitudes of impulses from α motor neurons innervating the arm muscles that experience weakness. Similarly, normal responses are present when the muscle is directly stimulated by evoked potentials. However, repetitive α motor neuron stimulation leads to weak contractions of the innervated muscle. Which of the following excessive actions is most likely caused by the toxin in the syringe?

A. Activation of postsynaptic acetylcholine receptors
B. Modulation of axonal ion channels
C. Presynaptic inhibition of acetylcholine release
D. Release of calcium from intramuscular calcium stores
E. Release of calcium from presynaptic calcium stores

14. A 45-year-old female experiences episodic double vision while reading in the evening. She first noticed it several months ago, and since then her symptoms have gotten worse. Lately, she also avoids eating tough food, since chewing is difficult. She does not have any leg extremity weakness or sensory complaints. An edrophonium (Enlon, Akorn, Inc., Lake Forest, IL) test is positive. A reduction of which of the following regarding the α motor neuron and the innervated muscle fibers best explains her symptoms?

A. Amplitude of muscle fiber action potential
B. Amplitude of the α motor neuron action potential
C. Amplitude of the end-plate potential
D. Calcium flux into the presynaptic terminal
E. Muscle fiber action potential propagation velocity
F. Muscle fiber myosin ATPase activity
G. Release of acetylcholine into the synaptic cleft

15. A patient with muscle weakness is evaluated, and his arm muscles become progressively weaker during repeated lifting of a weight. Clinical nerve conduction tests indicate that repetitive stimulation of the motor nerve leads to normal action potentials recorded from the nerve, but impaired compound action potentials recorded from the innervated muscle fibers. Direct stimulation of the muscle with needle electrodes produces normal muscle action potentials and contractions. Direct application of acetylcholine to the motor end plate also leads to normal muscle responses. Based on these test results, which of the following is most likely leading to the muscle weakness in this patient?

A. Defect in the contractile mechanism of the muscle
B. Defect in transmission at the neuromuscular junction
C. Defect in acetylcholine receptors on the motor end plate
D. Demyelination of the nerve fibers
E. Depletion of ATP in the muscle cells

16. While a person is carrying a stack of books, another large book is placed on the top of the stack. Which of the following best describes how the skeletal muscles compensate for the increase in the load being carried?

A. Decrease muscle length below the resting length
B. Increase muscle length beyond the resting length
C. Increase the maximum shortening velocity
D. Increase the number of motor units activated
E. Increase the strength of each cross-bridge interaction

17. The image shows a twitch contraction of a skeletal muscle fiber after being stimulated at time zero. If this muscle fiber were stimulated at time zero, and again with a second similar stimulus after 30 milliseconds, which of the following is expected?

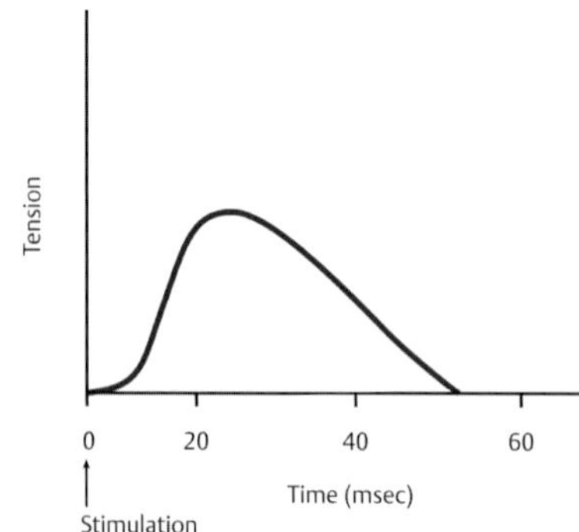

A. A second contraction of higher tension
B. A second identical twitch contraction
C. Failure of the muscle to contract
D. Some period of fused tetanus
E. Two shorter twitch contractions

18. A 35-year-old woman reports muscle weakness when lifting progressively heavier loads. An electromyogram (EMG) measures electrical activity in her biceps muscle as she lifts a 5-pound weight, then a 10-pound weight. While the EMG results look relatively normal for the 5-pound lift, when she is lifting the heavier load, the electrical activity does not increase as expected for a normal contraction. This abnormal electrical activity is most likely due to which of the following physiologic defects?

A. Depletion of sarcoplasmic ATP
B. Impaired cross-bridge cycling
C. Impaired motor unit recruitment
D. Impaired conduction between muscle fibers
E. Reduced sarcoplasmic calcium release

19. A weight of 50 g was used to stretch a skeletal muscle to an initial length (L_0) of 30 cm. After initialization, the muscle was anchored between two nonflexible plates at a fixed distance apart, and a force transducer replaced the 50-g weight. The transducer indicated an initial force (F_0) of 50 g at the L_0 of 30 cm. In this arrangement, shown in the image, the muscle was stimulated to tetanus and a force (F_1) of 150 g was measured. Which of the following is the approximate maximum amount of active force in grams that the muscle is generating?

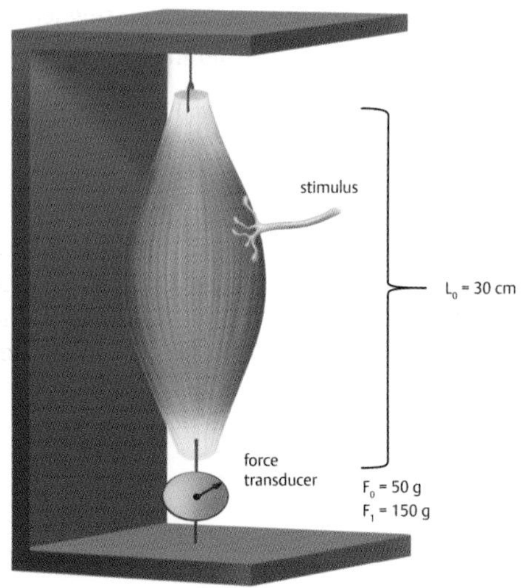

A. 50
B. 100
C. 120
D. 150
E. 170
F. 200

20. The image shown graphically depicts the changes in active and passive tension (in grams) with changes in muscle length (in centimeters). At what length is total tension approximately 20 g with a contribution from actin–myosin interaction only?

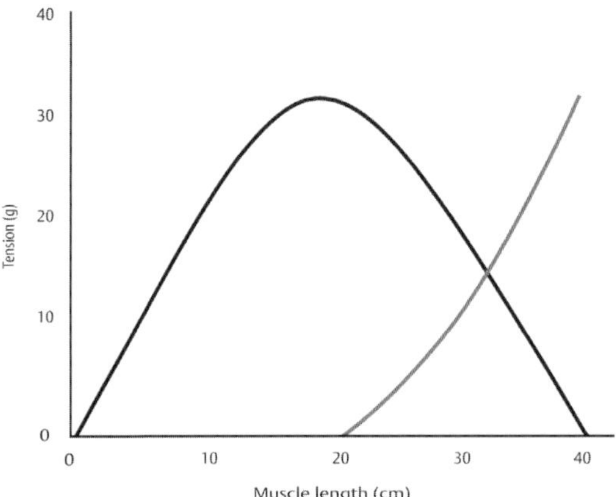

A. 10 cm
B. 15 cm
C. 25 cm
D. 30 cm
E. 35 cm

21. The image shown graphically depicts the afterload–velocity relationship for two muscle fibers at resting length. Curve 1 was generated from a muscle fiber in the gastrocnemius muscle, and curve 2 was generated from a muscle fiber of the same muscle in the same person one year later. Which of the following physiologic changes to the muscle best explains the shift from curve 1 to curve 2?

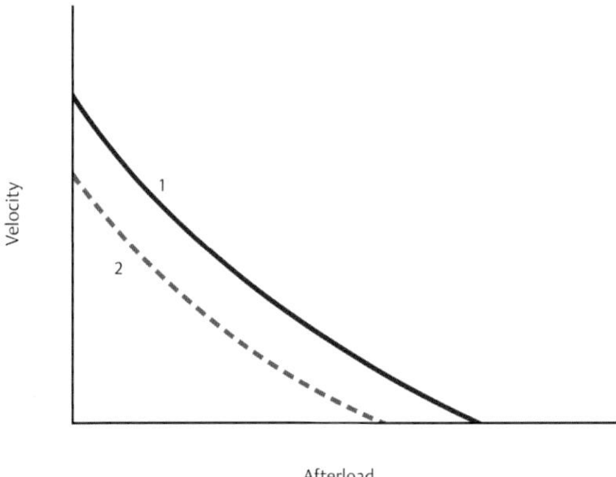

A. A decrease in type IIb muscle fibers
B. A decrease in the number of motor units
C. A decrease in the number of sarcomeres in series
D. An increase in the availability of calcium
E. An increase in the number of sarcomeres in parallel

22. As part of a public health education session, the dietary values of white and red meat are discussed. Which of the following is a correct statement regarding the physiological features of turkey breast and wing muscles (both white meat)?

A. High concentration of myoglobin so that turkeys do not easily fatigue

B. High oxygen requirement since turkeys spend a lot of time walking

C. Many mitochondria so that the birds can fly a long time

D. Rapid development of high tension for activity burst to escape predators

E. Richly perfused so that activity can be sustained for a long time.

3.4 Answers and Explanations

10. Correct: 1–5–2–3–4 (B)

Action potentials travel along the surface of the myocytes and into the T (transverse) tubules, depolarizing the muscle cell membrane. This depolarization opens voltage-sensitive L-type calcium channels located on the sarcolemma and triggers a subsequent release of calcium from the sarcoplasmic reticulum (SR) through ryanodine receptor (RyR) channels. Calcium released by the SR increases the intracellular calcium concentration. The free calcium binds to troponin-C on the thin (actin) filaments and induces a conformational change that shifts troponin-I and exposes a site on the actin molecule that binds to the myosin head, and results in ATP hydrolysis that produces a conformational change in the actin–myosin complex. The result of these changes is cross-bridge cycling, such that the actin and myosin filaments slide past each other, thereby shortening the sarcomere. Finally, calcium entry into the cell slows and calcium is re-sequestered by the SR to allow relaxation to occur. Small amounts of cytosolic calcium are also transported out of the cell by sodium–calcium exchange pumps. (**A, C, D, E, F**) These answer choices have the wrong sequence of events.

11. Correct: Lower muscle oxidative capacity (D)

The untrained person has a lower expression and activity of oxidative enzymes, since endurance training increases virtually the entire enzymatic machinery for energy production from oxygen. (**A**) Bone mineral density could have been slightly improved for the trained (not the untrained) person. While it has been shown that weight-bearing exercise increases bone strength and density, the main determinant is genetics. (**B**) The trained (not the untrained) person has a lower resting and exercise maximal heart rate, since his/her heart adapted to chronic rhythmic exercise by increasing left ventricular volume. The consequent larger stroke volume enables a lower heart rate to satisfy adequate cardiac output. (**C**) The trained (not untrained) person has lower serum lactic acid levels at matched exercise levels, because endurance training shifts from carbohydrate to fat metabolism for energy production, hence decreasing lactic acid accumulation. (**E**) The trained and untrained persons become exhausted at roughly the same time. The trained person runs much faster to reach 75% of $VO_{2\ max}$, and fatigue occurs due to the same underlying physiological reasons.

12. Correct: Relaxation of the myocytes (D)

ATP is directly needed for two specific events during skeletal muscle contraction and relaxation. The first is dissociation of myosin from actin during the cross-bridge cycle. The hydrolysis of this ATP by the myosin ATPase provides the energy for myosin to move along actin filaments. The second ATP is to power the calcium ATPase (SERCA) for calcium reuptake into the sarcoplasmic reticulum (SR), which allows the myocyte to relax between contractions. (**A, B, C, E**) The other events listed do not directly require the presence of ATP for their function.

13. Correct: Presynaptic inhibition of acetylcholine release (C)

Because the muscle and the motor neuron themselves respond normally to direct stimulation, the action of the toxin is most likely at the neuromuscular junction (NMJ). Presynaptic neurotoxins inhibit the release of acetylcholine (ACh), causing a neuromuscular blockade and profound muscle weakness. Some snake venoms act in this way. (**A**) Blocking (not activating) postsynaptic ACh receptors (such as α-neurotoxins) would cause a neuromuscular blockade and muscle weakness. (**B**) Modulation of axonal ion channels (the mechanism of some pain medications) would disrupt neuronal action potential propagation, which is not the case here. (**D**) Excessive intracellular calcium release in skeletal muscle fibers would cause excessive muscle contraction (not muscle weakness), at least at the beginning. (**E**) Excessive intracellular presynaptic calcium increase would lead to excessive Ach release and excessive muscle contraction (not weakness).

14. Correct: Amplitude of the end-plate potential (C)

The woman has the classic symptoms of myasthenia gravis (MG), confirmed by the erdrophonium test. MG patients have autoimmune antibodies against the postsynaptic acetylcholine receptors at neuromuscular junctions. The smaller number of available receptors will reduce the endplate potential (EPP) amplitude so much that not all EPPs reach threshold to cause a muscle fiber action potential and, consequently, muscle contraction. (**A, B**) Action potentials are all-or-none events, and at a particular site their amplitude does not change without extracellular or intracellular ion changes. (**D, G**) Presynaptic calcium influx and, consequently, transmitter release is not affected in MG. (**E, F**) The skeletal muscle fibers of MG patients are intact, so action potentials propagate at normal speed, and myosin ATPase normally hydrolyzes ATP.

15. Correct: Defect in transmission at the neuromuscular junction (B)

Because the nerve action potential generation and conduction appear to be normal, and direct stimulation of the muscle fiber with either electrodes or acetylcholine (ACh) results in a normal muscle contraction, the problem must be at the synapse between the nerve and the muscle, which is the neuromuscular junction. (**A**) The contractile mechanism of the muscle is not defective, because direct stimulation of the muscle fiber elicits a normal muscle contraction. (**C**) The ACh receptors are functional, because application of ACh at the motor end plate leads to a normal muscle response. (**D**) Because direct stimulation of the motor nerve generates normal nerve action potential and conduction, the nerves are not likely demyelinated. (**E**) The cells are not ATP depleted because direct stimulation of the muscle fiber elicits a normal muscle contraction.

16. Correct: Increase the number of motor units activated. (D)

Whole muscles are made up of many muscle fibers organized into motor units. All muscle fibers in a single motor unit are of the same fiber type. Each skeletal muscle fiber is stimulated by one motor neuron only, and as greater force of contraction is required (i.e., to hold a greater load), more motor units are recruited. (**A, B**) Resting length for skeletal muscle is at the peak of the force–tension curve, so changing skeletal muscle length above or below resting length results in a movement down the curve. A less forceful contraction is produced that is less effective to support a heavier load. (**C**) Maximum shortening velocity (V_{max}) is greater in fast-twitch muscle fibers than in slow-twitch fibers, but skeletal muscle cannot change its V_{max} to adjust to different loads. (**E**) The number of cross-bridge interactions can change, but not the strength of those interactions.

17. Correct: A second contraction of higher tension (A)

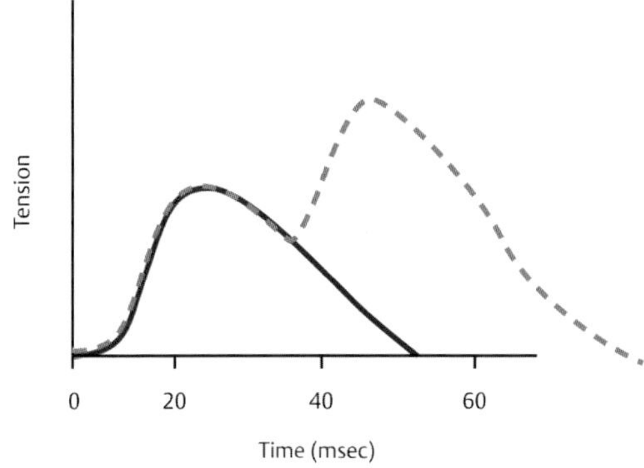

A muscle fiber contraction of higher tension occurs if the second stimulus happens before the first twitch has been completed. The contraction will still be twitch-like, but with increased strength (see image). The principle is called frequency summation. The additional tension is due to a second release of Ca^{2+} from the sarcoplasmic reticulum (SR), which adds to the intracellular Ca^{2+} already there and activates additional actin–myosin cross-bridges. (**B**) For two separate identical twitch contractions to occur, the second stimulus would need to have been given after the first twitch has completely relaxed. (**C**) Two stimuli causing twitch contractions will not cause muscular block. (**D**) Only a series of high-frequency stimuli will lead to fully tetanized (fused) muscle contraction. (**E**) The time of a twitch contraction is determined by the relative rates of calcium release and reuptake from the SR, which is not changed with two sequential stimuli.

18. Correct: Impaired motor unit recruitment (C)

Whole muscles are made up of many muscle fibers organized into motor units. All the muscle fibers in a single motor unit are of the same fiber type. Each skeletal muscle fiber is stimulated by one motor neuron only, and as greater force of contraction is required (i.e., to lift a greater load), more motor units are recruited. (**A, B, D, E**) Depletion of ATP, impaired cross-bridge cycling, impaired conduction, and reduced calcium release would all impact the electrical activity when lifting both the 5- and 10-pound weights, not just the heavier load.

19. Correct: 100 (B)

The experiment describes one data point of the length-tension curve. The passive force necessary to stretch the muscle to 30 cm is 50 g. At this length, the total force that is necessary to keep the muscle from changing its length is 150 g. Hence, the active force that the muscle can exert when stimulated is the difference of 100 g. (**A, C, D, E, F**) These are incorrect values for the active tension.

20. Correct: 10 cm (A)

The active tension curve (blue line) is produced by actin–myosin interaction, whereas the passive tension curve (red line) is produced by passive stretch. Total tension is the sum of the active and passive tension. The muscle length of 10 cm is the only point on the graph where the total tension is 20 g, with contributions from active tension only. (**B**) At a muscle length of 15 cm, the total tension is approximately 25 g, with contributions from active tension only. (**C**) At a muscle length of 25 cm, the total tension is approximately 30 g, with a contribution of 25 g from active tension and 5 g from passive tension. (**D**) At a muscle length of 30 cm, the total tension is approximately 25 g, with a contribution of 15 g from active tension and 10 g from passive tension. (**E**) At a muscle length of 35 cm, the total tension is approximately 25 g, with a contribution of 10 g from active tension and 20 grams from passive tension.

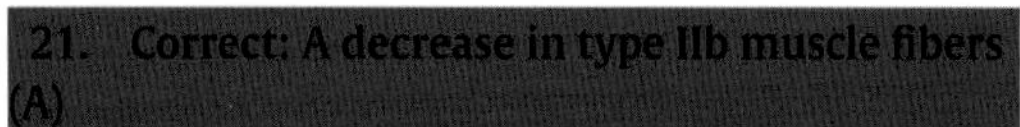

21. Correct: A decrease in type IIb muscle fibers (A)

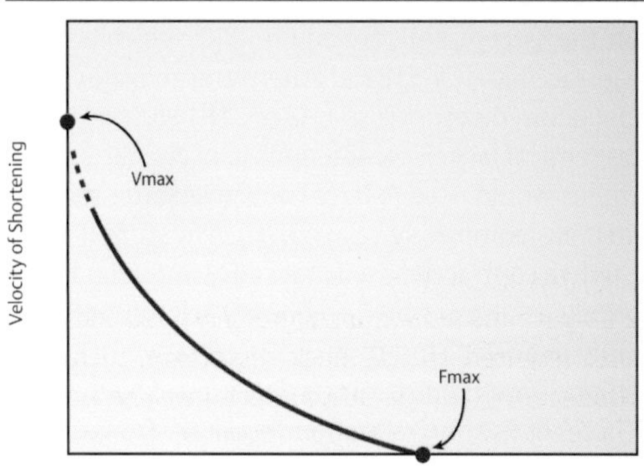

Type IIb muscle fibers have the greatest maximum velocity (V_{max}), followed by type IIa fibers, then type I fibers. Extensive physical training (or lack thereof) can change muscle fibers within the same fiber category (i.e., from type IIb to IIa, and vice versa), thus affecting the V_{max} of the muscle. In this case, the muscle fibers transitioned from type IIb to IIa, resulting in the decrease in V_{max}. (**B**) A decrease in the number of motor units will decrease shortening velocity (shift curve downward), without changing the V_{max}. (**C**) A decrease in sarcomeres in series will decrease shortening velocity (shift curve downward) without changing the V_{max}. (**D**) An increase in calcium will increase shortening velocity (shift curve upward) and V_{max} and will also increase the maximum force developed (F_{max}). (**E**) An increase in the number of sarcomeres in parallel would increase the shortening velocity and V_{max}.

22. Correct: Rapid development of high tension for activity burst to escape predators (D)

Turkey breast and wing muscles consist mainly of white muscle fibers (meat), also called type IIb fibers. These fibers contract quickly and produce a lot of power but fatigue easily. Turkeys use their breast and wing muscles when they need to shoot in the air and escape predators. (**A, B, C, E**) These are all features of red muscle fibers (type I fibers) and are present in turkey legs and thighs (dark meat). They contain a high concentration of myoglobin, have a high oxygen requirement, and are rich in mitochondria and blood vessels in order to produce energy aerobically for long sustained activities without fatigue, such as walking on the ground.

3.5 Questions

23. Which of the following characteristics can be used to differentiate type IIa skeletal muscle fibers from type IIb skeletal muscle fibers?

A. Glycolytic capacity
B. Myoglobin content
C. Myosin ATPase activity
D. Twitch speed
E. Uses of ATP during contraction and relaxation

24. A 48-year-old truck driver was involved in a severe accident and suffered major injuries. He was bedridden for 3 weeks with very restricted movements. After that, both of his legs were in a cast for 8 weeks, during which time he could use a wheelchair. Three months after the accident, he started physical therapy. The physical therapist noted the initial force–velocity features of the patient's leg muscles (curve X on the image) and monitored the changes throughout the therapy. Over 3 months, the patient's force–velocity profile shifted from the curve X to the dotted curve Y. Which of the following is expected to be increased in number in the patient's leg muscles by the end of the training?

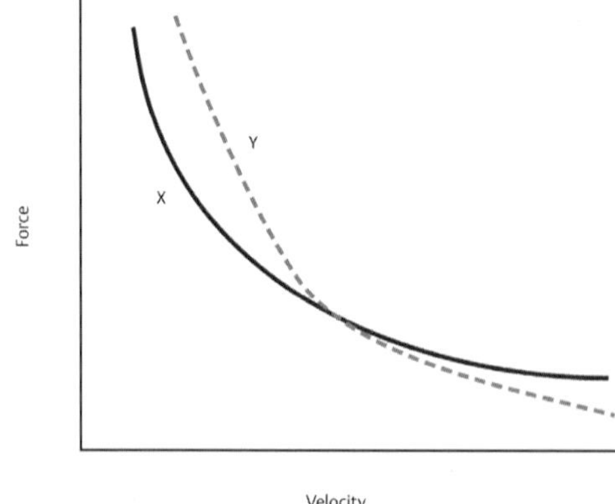

A. Myofibers
B. Myofilaments
C. Myosin ATPase
D. Type I fibers
E. Type IIa fibers
F. Type IIb fibers

25. Three elite athletes volunteer to participate in a clinical research project to investigate differences in skeletal muscle structure and function. The individuals are matched for weight and age, and muscle biopsies from each volunteer's quadriceps muscle is collected and analyzed. The results are reported in the following table:

	Glycogen content	Myoglobin content	Mitochondrial activity	Myofiber size
Volunteer 1	High	Low	Low	Large
Volunteer 2	Low	Low	Low	Small
Volunteer 3	Low	High	High	Small

Which specimens most likely came from an elite marathon runner and an elite weightlifter, respectively?

A. Volunteer 1 is a marathon runner, and volunteer 2 is a weightlifter.
B. Volunteer 1 is a marathon runner, and volunteer 3 is a weightlifter.
C. Volunteer 2 is a marathon runner, and volunteer 1 is a weightlifter.
D. Volunteer 2 is a marathon runner, and volunteer 3 is a weightlifter.
E. Volunteer 3 is a marathon runner, and volunteer 1 is a weightlifter.
F. Volunteer 3 is a marathon runner, and volunteer 2 is a weightlifter.

26. Which of the following changes to calcium handling would prevent cardiac muscle tissue from contracting?

A. Increase the extracellular Ca^{2+} concentration.
B. Increase the opening time of dihydropyridine receptors.
C. Increase the opening time of ryanodine receptors.
D. Inhibit the $Ca^{2+}/3Na^{+}$ exchanger.
E. Sequester all extracellular Ca^{2+}.

27. Over a normal physiologic range, the strength of cardiac muscle contraction increases with increasing number of contractions per minute (i.e., higher heart rate). Which of the following is the correct description that underlies this behavior at higher heart rates?

A. Central muscle fatigue is inhibited.
B. More motor units are recruited.
C. The force is approaching tetanus.
D. There are more action potentials per minute.
E. There is a greater myofilament overlap.

Questions 28 to 29

In a 68-year-old female, an aggressive head and neck cancer required radical neck dissection, including thyroidectomy and parathyroidectomy. The patient is on hormone replacement therapy. Six months later, she presents with muscle weakness, fatigue, and constipation for several weeks. On questioning, she denies feeling cold or not being able to tolerate cold temperatures. Physical examination reveals that her weight has not changed, and her skin has normal appearance, but her nails are brittle. Chvostek sign (hyperexcitability of facial nerve) is positive. Her serum laboratory values, relative to reference ranges, are as follows:

Albumin	Normal
Corrected calcium	Low
Phosphorus	Elevated
Magnesium	Normal
Creatinine	Normal
Parathyroid hormone:	Low
25-(OH)D	Normal
1,25-$(OH)_2$D	Normal
Total T3/T4	Normal
TSH	Normal

28. Based on the woman's clinical presentation, which of the following is expected in her cardiac muscle while at rest, when compared to normal?

	Maximal isometric force	Shortening velocity	Muscle spasms	Dihydropyridine receptor activity	Ryanodine receptor activity
A.	↔	↓	↑	↓	↑
B.	↔	↓	↔	↔	↔
C.	↓	↓	↔	↔	↓
D.	↓	↔	↔	↓	↓
E.	↓	↓	↓	↓	↓

29. In the same patient, cardiac function analyses revealed that the amount of blood ejected from the ventricles per beat was decreased, so there was a greater end-diastolic volume, which is more blood remaining inside the ventricles before systole. The table lists the impact of the increased end-diastolic volume on her cardiac muscle force compared to normal intraventricular blood volume between heartbeats. Which of the following presents the correct impact?

	Passive force	Active force	Total force
A.	↓	↓	↓
B.	↔	↓	↓
C.	↔	↑	↑
D.	↑	↓	↔
E	↑	↔	↑
F.	↑	↑	↑

30. The image depicts the active length–tension curves for skeletal (red line) and cardiac (orange line) muscle tissues. Which points on the curves indicate the lengths at which skeletal and cardiac muscle are at their resting and optimal lengths?

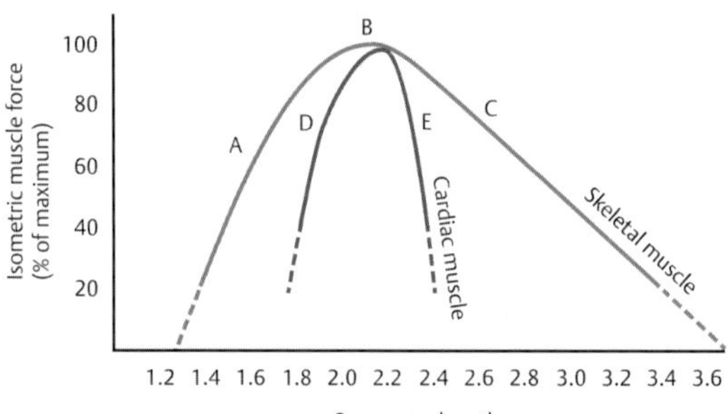

	Skeletal muscle		Cardiac muscle	
	Resting length	Optimal length	Resting length	Optimal length
A.	B	A	D	E
B.	B	B	D	B
C.	B	C	E	D
D.	A	A	E	B
E	A	B	B	D
F.	A	C	B	E

3.6 Answers and Explanations

Characteristics of skeletal muscle fibers			
	Type 1 (slow oxidative)	**Type IIa (fast oxidative)**	**Type IIb/x (fast glycolytic)**
Twitch speed	Slow	Fast	Fast
Myosin ATPase	Slow	Fast	Fast
Color	Red	Red	White
Myoglobin content	High	High	Low
Capillary density	High	High	Low
Mitochondrial content	High	High	Low
Oxidative capacity	High	High	Low
Glycogen content	Low	Intermediate	High
Glycolytic capacity	Low	High	High
Type of exercise	Endurance	Intermediate	Short, forceful

23. Correct: Myoglobin content (B)

The table above shows the characteristics of skeletal muscle fibers. Type IIa fibers are a hybrid between the type I and type IIb muscle fibers, which means they share different characteristics with each type. Type IIa fibers have a high myoglobin content, which gives them a red color like type I fibers, and a greater endurance than type IIb fibers, since the latter have a low myoglobin content and a white color. (**A, C, D, E**) Each of these characteristics is the same for type IIa and IIb muscle fibers.

24. Correct: Myofilaments (B)

Increasing the number of myofilaments increases muscle strength since more cross-bridges can form between thick and thin myofilaments. The total number of cross-bridges is the primary determinant for total muscle force. The image shows the expected change in the force–velocity curve after strength training, which is known to add more sarcomeres and/or cause fiber hypertrophy, dependent on the type of exercise. In contrast, speed training would primarily shift the right side of the curve upward. (**A, D, E, F**) The total number of muscle cells (myofibers) and the relative proportions of fiber types cannot be significantly changed during moderate exercise such as that occurring during rehabilitation. (**C**) Increasing the number/activity of myosin ATPase would increase the maximum velocity of muscle shortening at light loads. Under these conditions, the speed with which the thick and thin filaments slide along each other is determined by the time of the ATP-consuming cross-bridges to occur.

25. Correct: Volunteer 3 is a marathon runner, and volunteer 1 is a weightlifter. (E)

Elite marathon runners generally have a greater proportion of type I skeletal muscle fibers, which are better for endurance, while elite weight lifters generally have a greater proportion of type IIb skeletal muscle fibers, which are better for fast bursts of energy. Type I fibers characteristically have a small myofiber size and lower glycogen content, but high myoglobin content and mitochondrial activity, which is what we see in volunteer 3. Type IIb fibers characteristically have a larger myofiber size and high glycogen content, but low myoglobin content and mitochondrial activity, which is what we see in volunteer 1. While it has traditionally been believed that the proportions of muscle fiber types cannot be significantly changed through training, this issue has recently been revisited, and for now, controversy exists. However, independent of the final answer on fiber type change, people with a genetically determined higher proportion of a given muscle fiber type are more likely to become elite athletes in the sport that is supported by that muscle fiber type. (**A, B, C, D, F**) These choices do not contain the correct answer choices.

26. Correct: Sequester all extracellular Ca^{2+} (E)

In cardiac muscle tissue, calcium influx from the extracellular space through the dihydropyridine (DHP) receptor is essential for cardiac contraction to occur. This is called calcium-induced calcium release. Therefore, sequestering all of the extracellular calcium would eliminate influx through the DHP receptor, and contraction wound not occur. (**A, B, C**) Increasing Ca^{2+} in the extracellular or intracellular space (via DHP or RyR calcium channels) will increase excitation-contraction coupling, which will enhance cardiac muscle contraction, not prevent it. (**D**) The $Ca^{2+}/3Na^{+}$ exchanger removes calcium from cardiac muscle cells, so inhibition of this exchanger would affect relaxation of the cells but would not inhibit contraction.

27. Correct: There are more action potentials per minute. (D)

With an increased heart rate, intracellular Ca^{2+} accumulates and is available to the contractile apparatus, so that tension increases. The phenomenon is called Bowditch or staircase effect. Calcium accumulates because with more action potentials, there is more time for Ca^{2+} to enter the cell. Additionally, more Na^+ enters the cell, which leads to fewer active Na^+–Ca^{2+} exchangers, so intracellular Ca^{2+} builds up. (**A**) Central fatigue is a mechanism that downregulates the motor command to skeletal muscle. It is not a regulatory tool of cardiac muscle. (**B**) In cardiac muscle, the functional syncytium via gap junctions removes the possibility of recruitment of motor units. (**C**) Physiologically, cardiac muscle operates in twitch, not tetanic, fashion. (**E**) Changing the heart rate does not necessarily have any effect on myofilament overlap. Increasing intracellular calcium increases the strength of contraction at any given sarcomere length.

28. Correct: ↓, ↓, ↔, ↔, ↓ (C).

It should be clear that the woman experiences symptoms of hypocalcemia such as weakness, fatigue, and constipation. While these can also be caused by hypothyroidism, lack of cold intolerance and normal values for T3/T4 and TSH eliminate it. A positive Chvostek sign in the presence of hypocalcemia and hypoparathyroidism confirms the diagnosis. Maximal isometric force is decreased, since the intrinsic ability of force development independent of load (contractility) is proportional to intracellular Ca^{2+}. This is decreased, since less Ca^{2+} is released from the sarcoplasmic reticulum due to a smaller amount of trigger Ca^{2+}. The smaller amount of trigger Ca^{2+} is because less Ca^{2+} enters the cell during normal muscle stimulation. The shortening velocity (V_{max}) is decreased in the presence of hypocalcemia. It is a special feature of cardiac muscle that contractility is regulated by intracellular Ca^{2+}. With hypocalcemia the generation of force by actin and myosin filaments and the rate of cross-bridge cycling are decreased. Hypocalcemia-induced muscle spasms are due to hyperexcited nerves (low extracellular Ca^{2+} increases the membrane permeability for Na^+). Hence, it is a feature of skeletal, not cardiac, muscle. Dihydropyridine (DHP) receptors are L-type calcium channels that respond to depolarization and are regulated by neurotransmitters, hormones, and cytokines, not by calcium itself. Ryanodine receptors are activated by the trigger Ca^{2+} that enters the cell through DHP receptors. Hence, their activity is decreased by hypocalcemia. (**A, B, D, E**) These choices have one or more incorrect changes.

29. Correct: ↑, ↑, ↑ (F)

More blood volume in the ventricles between heartbeats (end-diastolic volume) increases the cardiac fiber length and hence increases the passive force. The force is passive because the muscle has not yet contracted (i.e., the heart is in diastole). As in skeletal muscle, an increased cardiac muscle fiber length toward the optimal length increases the degree of overlap of thick and thin filaments, hence increasing cardiac muscle active force. Fiber stretching also increases Ca^{2+} sensitivity of troponin C and Ca^{2+} release from the sarcoplasmic reticulum, which additionally contribute to the active length–force relationship of cardiac muscle. Since active and passive forces increase, total force increases as well. For the condition of the woman, it means that hypocalcemia had decreased the peak force and shortening velocity of her heart muscle, which decreased the amount of blood that was pumped out of her heart. The intrinsic ability of cardiac muscle to contract more strongly with higher preload has a counterbalancing effect, so that after some time, her cardiac function is not as bad as it would have been at the onset of hypocalcemia. (**A, B, C, D, E**) These choices have one or more wrong impacts of cardiac muscle fiber stretch on cardiac muscle fiber force.

30. Correct: B, B, D, B (B)

For skeletal muscle tissue, the resting length (L_0) of the muscle is also the optimal length for force generation. So these points are identical for skeletal muscle tissue, both at the peak of the length–tension curve (point B). Physiologically, this makes sense because the muscle should be able to generate maximum force from its resting position, and if greater force is required, then more motor units can be recruited to increase force. For cardiac muscle tissue, there is no motor unit recruitment. Therefore, the resting length of cardiac muscle is generally about 75% of the optimal length (point D), which allows cardiac muscle to increase its force of contraction by stretching toward its optimal length, which is at the peak of the length–tension curve (point B). (**A, C, D, E, F**) These choices contain the wrong combination of answers.

3.7 Questions

31. Which of the following is a correct distinguishing feature of sustained smooth muscle contraction in comparison to cardiac and skeletal muscle contraction?

A. It can happen independent of an action potential.

B. It has a faster rate of cross-bridge cycling.

C. It is independent of cytosolic calcium.

D. It requires greater amounts of ATP.

32. In a muscle physiology lab, several muscle specimens have been mixed up. To determine its muscle fiber type, a muscle specimen is stimulated to contract, and both force and ATP hydrolysis are measured. Both force and ATP hydrolysis increase on stimulation, but as stimulation is maintained, force remains elevated and ATP hydrolysis decreases to levels just above those seen at rest. What type of muscle is most likely being stimulated?

A. Cardiac muscle
B. Fast-twitch skeletal muscle
C. Multiunit smooth muscle
D. Slow-twitch skeletal muscle

33. An experimental cancer drug is developed that, as a side effect, inhibits smooth muscle cell vasospasms. This drug most likely stimulates which enzyme that normally antagonizes smooth muscle contraction?

A. Myosin light-chain kinase
B. Myosin phosphatase
C. Phospholipase C
D. Protein kinase C
E. Rho-kinase

34. As part of tissue engineering, two tissue preparations are tested. Preparation 1 contains intact blood vessel rings. Preparation 2 contains blood vessels with intact vascular smooth muscle but disrupted vascular endothelium. When acetylcholine is added, the smooth muscle in preparation 1 relaxes, while the smooth muscle in preparation 2 contracts. The presence of which molecule/substance in preparation 1 is responsible for this effect?

A. Calcium
B. Calmodulin
C. Cyclic adenosine monophosphate
D. Cyclic guanosine monophosphate
E. Nitric oxide

35. A 19-year-old woman has an asthma attack. She immediately uses a nebulizer, and after a few minutes she can breathe normally again. Which of the following is the most likely mechanism of action of the medication in the nebulizer?

A. Activating muscarinic acetylcholine receptors
B. Activating nicotinic acetylcholine receptors
C. Blocking adrenergic receptors
D. Enhancing alpha motor neuron activity
E. Enhancing parasympathetic activity
F. Enhancing sympathetic activity

36. A 34-year-old woman presents with recurrent nausea and vomiting. A gastrointestinal motility disorder is suspected, which is confirmed by an electrogastrogram (see image). At rest (trace X), it shows inappropriately large depolarizations of the intestinal smooth muscle membrane potentials. Trace Y shows her smooth muscle membrane potentials after administration of a drug. Which of the following drugs most likely caused trace Y?

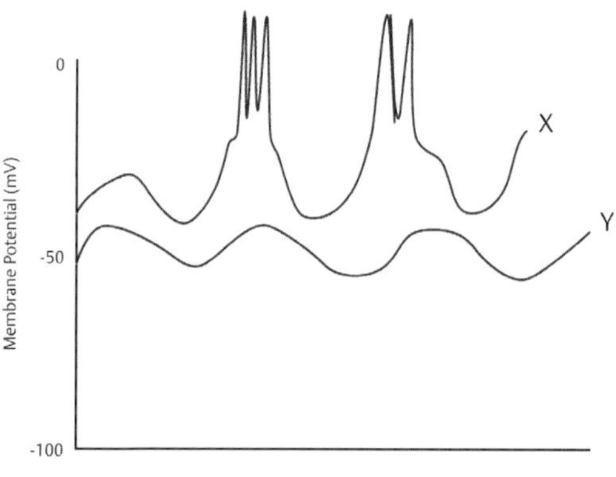

A. Adrenergic reuptake inhibitor
B. Agonist of L-type calcium channel
C. Cholinesterase inhibitor
D. Somatostatin receptor antagonist
E. Sympathetic antagonist

37. A drug is developed that inhibits contraction in pathologically contracted vascular smooth muscle cells, thus reducing blood pressure. This drug directly inhibits the activity of Rho-kinase (ROCK). The action of this drug most likely inhibits smooth muscle contraction via which of the following mechanisms?

A. Activation of myosin light chain kinase
B. Activation of phospholipase C
C. Antagonizing the G-protein-coupled receptor
D. Inhibition of calcium sensitization
E. Inhibition of myosin phosphatase

3.8 Answers and Explanations

31. Correct: It can happen independent of an action potential. (A)

Smooth muscle can be stimulated to contract via any mechanism that increases intracellular calcium, including stimuli such as circulating tissue factors, hormones, and calcium channel agonists. (**B**) Smooth muscle has a slower rate of cross-bridge cycling, leading to fewer cross-bridge cycles per given time.

(**C**) Smooth muscle contraction is dependent on cytosolic calcium. (**D**) Smooth muscle contraction can be sustained long-term with less ATP compared to cardiac and skeletal muscle.

32. Correct: Multiunit smooth muscle (C)

In smooth muscle tissue, phosphorylation of myosin light chains correlates well with the shortening velocity of smooth muscle. There is a rapid burst of energy utilization, which is measured by oxygen consumption; then, within a few minutes, intracellular calcium decreases, myosin light chain phosphorylation decreases, energy utilization decreases, and the muscle can relax. Sustained contraction of smooth muscle occurs as well, particularly in tonically active smooth muscles. This sustained contraction is due to special myosin cross-bridges, termed latch-bridges. The dephosphorylated myosin heads dissociate from actin very slowly, producing slow cross-bridge cycling, which is important for maintaining tension in smooth muscle tissue at low energy costs. (**A, B, D**) The striated muscles (cardiac and skeletal) do not have latch-bridges and thus cannot sustain contraction without constant ATP hydrolysis.

33. Correct: Myosin phosphatase (B)

Myosin phosphatase is normally inhibited in the signaling pathway that leads to smooth muscle cell contraction because otherwise it would dephosphorylate myosin regulatory light chain (MLC), causing inhibition of smooth muscle contraction. Therefore, stimulating myosin phosphatase would dephosphorylate MLC, thus inhibiting the action of MLC, and decrease smooth muscle contraction and the associated vasospasms. (**A**) Myosin light chain kinase (MLCK) directly stimulates myosin in smooth muscle, thus promoting contraction. (**C**) Phospholipase C stimulates MLCK and inhibits myosin phosphatase, thus promoting smooth muscle cell contraction. (**D, E**) Protein kinase C and Rho-kinase are part of a pathway that inhibits myosin phosphatase and thus promotes smooth muscle contraction.

34. Correct: Nitric oxide (E)

D. Mode of action of steroid hormones

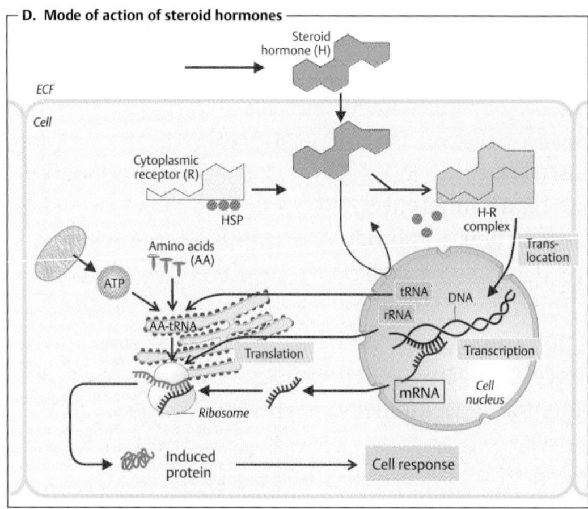

E. Nitric oxide (NO) as a transmitter substance

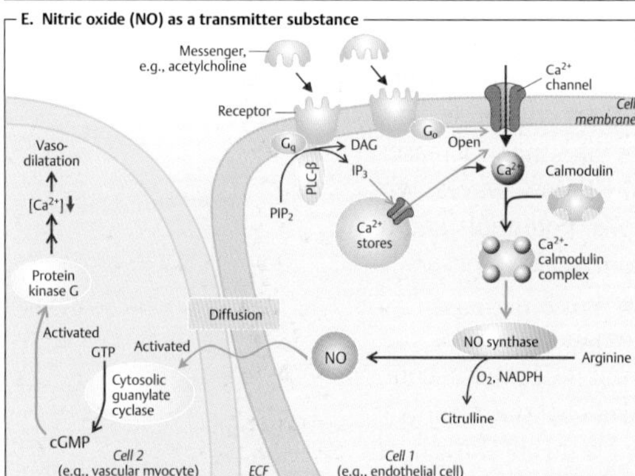

In blood vessels, nitric oxide synthesis is stimulated when acetylcholine (ACh) binds to muscarinic M_3 receptors on endothelial cells. Nitric oxide diffuses to smooth muscle cells, causing their relaxation. In isolated smooth muscle, ACh directly binds to M_3 receptors, which increases intracellular calcium and consequently causes smooth muscle contraction. This can be demonstrated in vascular disease with endothelial dysfunction when smooth muscle receptors are directly activated. (**A, B, C, D**) Calcium, calmodulin, cAMP, and cGMP are present in endothelial cells, smooth muscle cells, or both (see figure), but none of these molecules/substances is responsible for the intercellular communication in preparation 1 from endothelial to smooth muscle cells to cause smooth muscle relaxation.

35. Correct: Enhancing sympathetic output (F)

An asthma attack is due to bronchospasms, and bronchioles contain smooth muscle. Sympathetic stimulation relaxes these muscles in the airways and increases air flow to the lungs, a response that makes biological sense in a fight-or-flight situation. The most common medication in nebulizers is albuterol, which is a short-acting β-adrenergic agonist. (**A, E**) Activating muscarinic acetylcholine (ACh) receptors, or other ways of enhancing parasympathetic output, would aggravate bronchoconstriction. (**B, D**) Activating nicotinic ACh receptors, or enhancing α motor neuron activity, would cause skeletal muscle system spasms, as well as serious central nervous system side effects. (**C**) Blocking adrenergic receptors would prevent, not promote, bronchio-dilation.

36. Correct: Adrenergic reuptake inhibitor (A)

Gastrointestinal (GI) smooth muscle membranes exhibit an inherent spontaneous activity called slow waves. Their amplitudes and plateau phase durations are decreased by the sympathetic, in this case an adrenergic reuptake inhibitor that increases the lifetime of norepinephrine in the varicosity. Decreased slow-wave activity decreases the frequency of spike potential development. This decreases GI smooth muscle contractions. (**B**) Smooth muscle membrane potential changes are mainly driven by calcium flux instead of sodium flux. Hence, an L-type calcium channel agonist stimulates excitation contraction coupling and would aggravate the patient's contractions. (**C**) Acetylcholine (in this case, a drug that increases its lifetime) increases the amplitude and duration of GI slow waves, which increases the frequency of spike potentials and consequently GI smooth muscle contraction. Increasing GI motility makes biological sense with parasympathetic stimulation. (**D**) While a somatostatin receptor agonist (not antagonist) would inhibit GI muscle contraction, the mechanism is most likely not due to slow wave changes. (**E**) A sympathetic agonist (not antagonist) could have caused the effect as explained in answer A above.

37. Correct: Inhibition of calcium sensitization (D)

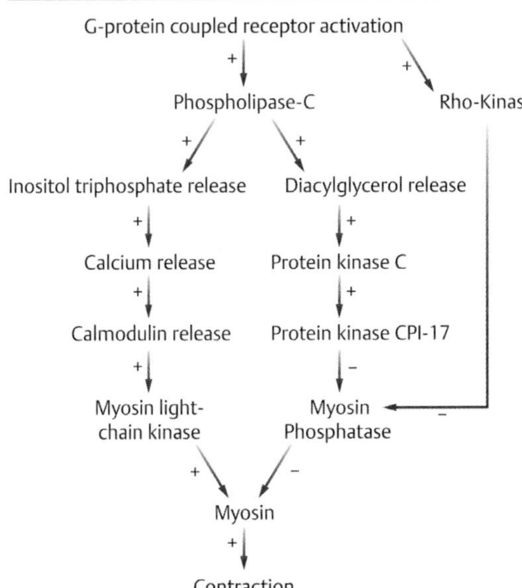

Calcium sensitization is a shift in the calcium dependence of contractility toward a lower cytosolic free calcium value following activation of a G-protein-coupled receptor (GPRC). This occurs normally in smooth muscle tissue by inhibition of myosin light chain phosphatase by Rho-kinase (ROCK). By blocking ROCK, myosin phosphatase is not inhibited, and sensitization of the myofilaments to calcium is inhibited. (**A, B**) Activation of myosin light chain kinase (MLCK) and phospholipase C (PLC) will stimulate, not inhibit, smooth muscle contraction. (**C**) Antagonization of the G-protein-coupled receptor will inhibit the entire pathway responsible for smooth muscle cell contraction; however, this is not the mechanism of action of this drug, since the question states that the drug directly inhibits ROCK. (**E**) Inhibition of myosin phosphatase will stimulate, not inhibit, smooth muscle contraction.

3.9 Questions

38. An 11-year-old girl is brought to her primary care physician after 6 months of complaints of knee pain. She does not recall any acute injury to the knee. She has been a gymnast for five years and claims that the pain is worst when at gymnastics practice, but subsides when she rests. Physical exam reveals a swollen and tender bump on the proximal tibia below the knee, which the girl claims is in the region of her discomfort. The physician suspects Osgood-Schlatter disease and confirms the diagnosis with ultrasound. What is the underlying cause of Osgood-Schlatter disease in adolescent children?

A. Bone and joint degeneration due to loss of blood supply due to injury
B. Degeneration of the patellar cartilage from overuse
C. Fracture of the epiphyseal growth plate of the proximal tibia
D. Inflammation of the attachment point of the patellar tendon to the tibia
E. Separation of the tibial tuberosity from the tibia from overuse

39. A full-term male baby is born to healthy parents. The baby has a long torso, short extremities, and short fingers. In addition, he has a disproportionately large head (macrocephaly) with a prominent forehead (frontal bossing). These features are characteristic of a condition that has which of the following underlying pathologies?

A. Decreased osteoclast activity
B. Defect in conversion of cartilage to bone
C. Defect in the formation of collagen
D. Defect in the formation of cartilage
E. Degeneration of cartilage

40. A 77-year-old white female was admitted to the hospital with a broken hip. Past history revealed that she was in good health prior to the incident. She does not regularly exercise, but is conscious about a healthy diet. She is taking medication for thyroid deficiency. X-ray shows demineralization, but no expanded bone. Calcium pyrophosphate crystals are absent from joints. A bone mineral scan shows reduced bone density. Her laboratory results are as follows:

Calcium: 9.3 mg/dL
Phosphorus: 2.6 mg/dL
Alkaline phosphatase: 45 IU/L
Erythrocyte sedimentation rate: 10 mm/hr
Urinary hydroxyproline: 42 mg/d

Osteoporosis is suspected. Which of the following test results differentiates a diagnosis of osteoporosis from a diagnosis of osteoarthritis?

A. Bone density results
B. Erythrocyte sedimentation rate
C. Serum calcium
D. Serum phosphorus
E. Urinary hydroxyproline

Questions 41 to 42

A 58-year-old obese woman presents with bilateral knee pain. Her knees are "stiff" in the morning and become painful throughout the day with activity. The pain subsides with rest. Physical exam reveals limited range of motion in the affected joints and tenderness on palpation, but no warmth or erythema, and the joint appearance is normal. An X-ray shows narrowing of the medial compartment joint space and osteophyte formation. Laboratory tests reveal elevated plasma alkaline phosphatase.

41. What is the most likely cause of the patient's elevated plasma alkaline phosphatase?

A. Degeneration of articular cartilage in the knee joints
B. Elevated plasma parathyroid hormone
C. Increased osteoblast activity in the knee joints
D. Increased osteoclast activity in the knee joints
E. Inflammation of the knee joints

42. Which of the following is the most likely underlying cause of the patient's disorder?

A. Accumulate of calcium pyrophosphate in the joint fluid
B. Autoimmune disease of the synovial joint lining
C. Chondrocyte injury and articular cartilage degeneration
D. Inflammation of the joint synovium

3.10 Answers and Explanations

38. Correct: Separation of the tibial tuberosity from the tibia from overuse (E)

Osgood-Schlatter disease most often occurs during growth spurts, when bones, muscles, tendons, and other structures are changing rapidly. Because physical activity puts additional stress on bones and muscles, children who participate in athletics are at an increased risk for this condition. A bony bump called the tibial tubercle covers the growth plate at the end of the tibia. The quadriceps muscles attach to the tibial tubercle via the patellar tendon. When a child is active, the quadriceps muscles pull on the patellar tendon, which in turn, pulls on the tibial tubercle. In some children, this repetitive traction on the tubercle leads to inflammation of the growth plate. The prominence, or bump, of the tibial tubercle may become very pronounced and can even separate. (**A**) This answer describes osteonecrosis. (**B**) This answer describes chondromalacia patellae. (**C**) This answer describes a type I fracture of the growth plate of a long bone. (**D**) This answer describes patellofemoral syndrome.

39. Correct: Defect in conversion of cartilage to bone (B)

The baby has all of the characteristic features of achondroplasia, which is caused by a gene mutation in the *FGFR3* gene. The *FGFR3* gene makes a protein called fibroblast growth factor receptor 3, which is involved in converting cartilage to bone. *FGFR3* is the only gene known to be associated with achondroplasia. (**A**) Osteoclasts are bone cells that break down bone tissue. Decreased osteoclast activity would reduce bone remodeling but is not responsible for the defective bone growth seen in achondroplasia. (**C**) Collagen is found in many tissues, such as tendons, ligaments, skin, and cartilage, but is not responsible for the defective bone growth seen in achondroplasia. (**D, E**) The underlying pathology of achondroplasia is the conversion of cartilage to bone, not a defect in cartilage formation or an abnormal degeneration of cartilage.

40. Correct: Bone density results (A)

Bone mineral density would not be affected in osteoarthritis, which is a degenerative joint disease that results in pain rather than fractures. In contrast, osteoporosis presents with bones that are less dense and more likely to fracture, so that a bone density scan reveals signs of demineralization. (**B, C, D, E**) These values are typically in the normal range for both diseases. Urinary hydroxyproline can be elevated in rheumatoid arthritis, not osteoarthritis.

41. Correct: Increased osteoblast activity in the knee joints (C)

Normal alkaline phosphatase (ALP) levels in adults range from 20 to 140 IU/L. Elevated ALP levels can indicate several different physiologic and pathologic processes, including the active formation of bone, since ALP is a byproduct of osteoblast activity. In this case, the development of osteophytes (bony outgrowths) in the joint cavity is the likely occasion of the increased osteoblast activity and cause of the patient's pain and resulting increase in ALP. (**A, B, D, E**) These answer choices do not impact ALP levels in the plasma.

42. Correct: Chondrocyte injury and articular cartilage degeneration (C)

This patient has classic signs of osteoarthritis (OA). The trigger of OA is often unknown, but it is frequently seen in aged people and obese people due to increased wear and tear on the joints, and following mechanical injury of the joint. The tissue damage stimulates chondrocytes to attempt repair, which increases production of proteoglycans and collagen. However, efforts at repair also stimulate the enzymes that degrade cartilage, as well as inflammatory cytokines, which are normally present in small amounts. Inflammatory mediators trigger an inflammatory cycle that further stimulates the chondrocytes and synovial lining cells, eventually breaking down the cartilage. Chondrocytes undergo programmed cell death (apoptosis). Once cartilage is destroyed, exposed bone rubs against bone in the joint cavity. (**A**) Accumulates of calcium pyrophosphate in the joint fluid is associated with pseudogout, not OA. (**B**) Autoimmune disease of the synovial joint lining and inflammation of the synovium is associated with rheumatoid arthritis (RA), not OA . (**D**) Joint inflammation may result from OA, but it is not the cause of OA.

3.11 Questions

43. A 75-year-old man with a long smoking history presents with wheezing, chest tightness, and a chronic cough. He says that he rarely leaves the house anymore since he is already breathless after normal tasks such as dressing. Arterial oxygen saturation is 74% (normal ≥ 98%). His post-bronchodilator forced expiratory volume in one second [FEV_1]/ forced vital capacity [FVC] ratio is 0.5. His FEV_1 is 30% of predicted. Which of the following is expected for his color of skin and nail beds?

A. Bluish
B. Orangey
C. Reddish
D. Whitish
E. Yellowish

44. A patient asks whether her medication is available in the form of a transdermal patch. The clinician denies and explains that the active ingredient cannot penetrate skin due to its molecular size and chemical characteristics. Which of the following medication is most likely being referenced?

A. Estrogen
B. Insulin
C. Nicotine
D. Nitroglycerin
E. Testosterone
F. Scopolamine

45. A mother admits her 2-year-old child for genetic testing because the boy has suffered from heat exhaustion several times on hot summer days, and because she also cannot tolerate heat. Based on the results, anhidrotic ectodermal dysplasia is diagnosed, which presents with absent or greatly reduced number of sweat glands. Which of the following difficulties is most likely an additional clinical feature of the child?

A. Breathing due to respiratory tract malformation
B. Eating due to malformed teeth or anodontia
C. Digesting due to abnormal gastrointestinal tract
D. Hearing due to malformed auditory ossicles
E. Walking due to underdeveloped muscle

46. A clinician explains to a postmenopausal woman that she still produces female sex hormones, but in her adipose tissue and skin rather than her ovaries. Which of the following hormones is produced in her adipocytes and skin cells?

A. Androstenedione
B. Estradiol
C. Estriol
D. Estrone
E. Pregnenolone
F. Progesterone

47. A 68-year-old Muslim woman, wearing a classic black hijab, presents with pain in the lower spinal and pelvic region. She describes the pain as dull and especially prominent when walking or carrying something. X-ray images of the spine show microfractures. Serum calcium and phosphorus concentrations are within reference ranges. Serum alkaline phosphatase and parathyroid hormone levels are elevated. 25-hydroxyvitamin D is decreased. Which of the following is the most likely diagnosis?

A. Excessive urinary phosphate loss
B. Osteogenesis imperfecta
C. Postmenopausal osteoporosis
D. Proximal renal tubular acidosis
E. Senile osteoporosis
F. Vitamin D deficiency

48. During a routine doctor's visit, a 24-year-old man describes his life as antisocial and depressing. On physical examination, he presents with androgenic alopecia. His body mass index is 43. His blood pressure is 145/110 mm Hg. Fasting serum glucose and triglyceride levels are high; high-density lipoprotein is low. In addition to counseling him on a healthier lifestyle, which of the following medication could be considered?

A. 1-α hydroxylase inhibitor
B. 5-α reductase inhibitor
C. 11-β hydroxlyase inhibitor
D. 21-β hydroxylase inhibitor
E. Aromatase inhibitor

3.12 Answers and Explanations

43. Correct: Bluish (A)

The man suffers from severe chronic obstructive pulmonary disease (COPD), consistent with his symptoms, his very low FEV_1/FCV ratio, and his very low predicted FEV_1 value. In such advanced stages of restricted air flow, hemoglobin is depleted of oxygen, at which state it has a deep purplish-blue color. When it can be seen in skin and nail beds, it is called cyanosis. (**B**) Orange skin is most likely from diets with a high amount of carotenoids such as present in carrots, mangoes, and tomatoes. (**C**) Reddish skin, or erythema, is due to extreme filling of the capillaries in the dermis and may be caused by skin injury, exposure to heat, infection, inflammation, or allergy. (**D**) Whitish color is associated with a lack of melanin, such as albinism or vitiligo. Cyanosis could present with greyish skin color, though, when there is very low skin blood flow, such as in cor pulmonale as a COPD complication. (**E**) A yellowish skin is typically due to a buildup of the yellow pigment bilirubin in the blood and is called jaundice.

44. Correct: Insulin (B)

Insulin is a peptide hormone, in which a 21- and a 30-amino-acid chain are joined together. In addition to its large size, it is water soluble and therefore cannot diffuse through epidermal cell membranes to reach blood vessels of the dermis. (**A, E**) Steroid hormones such as estrogen and testosterone are lipid soluble, since they are derived from cholesterol. Transdermal patches can be used for hormone replacement therapy. (**C**) Nicotine is a small two-ring chemical that can pass through skin and mucous membranes and hence is available in many forms including patches, gum, lozenges, and nasal spray. (**D**) Nitroglycerin is an organic nitrate that is converted by mitochondria to the vasodilator nitric oxide, which as a gas can easily penetrate cell membranes. (**F**) Scopolamine is a small lipid-soluble organic compound that acts as a muscarinic antagonist. It was the first drug to be made commercially available as a transdermal patch.

45. Correct: Eating due to malformed teeth or anodontia (B)

Ectodermal dysplasias are inherited disorders that cause abnormal development of ectodermal structures. In the anhidrotic, X-linked form, children have no or a minimal number of sweat glands, as well as symptoms related to other malformed ectodermal structures, such as skin, hair, nails, and teeth, the latter being the only available answer choice. The children's teeth are often malformed or missing, so they have difficulties eating. (**A, C**) The respiratory and the gastrointestinal tract are endodermal derivatives. Hence, difficulties of breathing or digesting are not expected. (**D, E**) Bone (ossicles), cartilage, and muscle are mesodermal derivatives. Hence, difficulties hearing or walking are not expected.

46. Correct: Estrone (D)

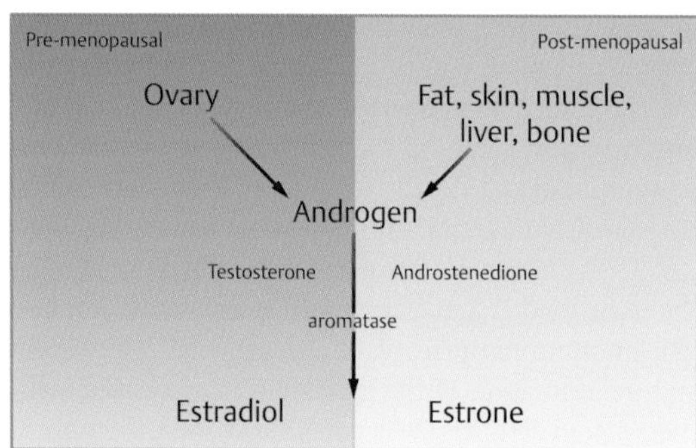

In postmenopausal woman, estrogen production occurs almost exclusively outside of the ovaries. Aromatase in fat, skin, and some other tissues catalyzes the conversion of circulating androstenedione to estrone (see image). (**A**) Androstenedione is an androgen that is produced by the adrenal gland of the postmenopausal woman and converted to estrogen. (**B**) Estradiol is the main estrogen of premenopausal woman. It is produced by ovarian granulosa cells that aromatize testosterone (see image). (**C**) Estriol is produced during pregnancy by the fetoplacental unit. (**E**) Pregnenolone is a key precursor for all steroid hormones, but not a hormone by itself. (**F**) Progesterone is a hormone that supports fertilization and gestation. Hence, it is not produced in postmenopausal women.

47. Correct: Vitamin D deficiency (F)

The woman suffers from vitamin D deficiency, most likely caused by reduced sun exposure due to whole-body clothes. When exposed to sunlight, cutaneous vitamin D (7-dehydrocholesterol) is converted to cholecalciferol, which is metabolized in the liver to 25-hydroxycholecalciferol (25[OH]D). Moreover, cutaneous production of vitamin D decreases with age, and dietary vitamin D intake is often low in older people, both further reducing her 25(OH)D production. At very low levels, there is not enough substrate for its conversion to 1,25-dihydroxyvitamin D, leading to reduced intestinal absorption of calcium and phosphorus. Initially, hypocalcemia leads to increased release of parathyroid hormone (PTH). The consequent bone demineralization can normalize serum calcium and phosphorus but leads to osteomalacia, which presents with bone pain (especially when weight bearing), microfractures, muscle weakness, and difficulty walking. Serum alkaline phosphatase (ALP) is elevated and indicates increased osteoblastic activity and bone turnover in general. (**A, B, C, D, E**) In all these conditions, 25(OH) D and PTH are normal. Moreover, phosphate wasting (present in **A** and **D**) would lead to low serum phosphate, and osteoporosis (**C** and **D**) would present with normal ALP.

48. Correct: 5-α reductase inhibitor (B)

5-α reductase converts testosterone into dihydrotestosterone (DHT), which is responsible for male pattern baldness, known as androgenic alopecia. When experienced prematurely at age 24, it can provide a stressor that contributes to depression. Hence, an inhibitor could be considered. Moreover, high-density lipoprotein (HDL) contains linolenic and linoleic acids, which are known to inhibit 5-α reductase, further justifying the medication. The man's HDL is low as part of his metabolic syndrome (high BMI, elevated glucose and triglycerides, high blood pressure). (**A**) 1-α hydroxylase catalyzes the renal conversion of vitamin D into its active form. Inhibition would not be indicated. (**C, D**) 11-β hydroxylase and 21-β hydroxylase are enzymes in the adrenal cortex as part of steroidogenic hormone production. When inhibited as part of congenital adrenal hyperplasias, patients show signs of virilization due to increased adrenal androgen production. Additional androgen could be converted into additional DHT and aggravate the man's condition. Additionally, inhibiting the 11-β form would further raise blood pressure. (**E**) Aromatase inhibitors disrupt excessive estrogen production and could be used against gynecomastia in men, which is not the case here.

Chapter 4

Blood and Immune Systems

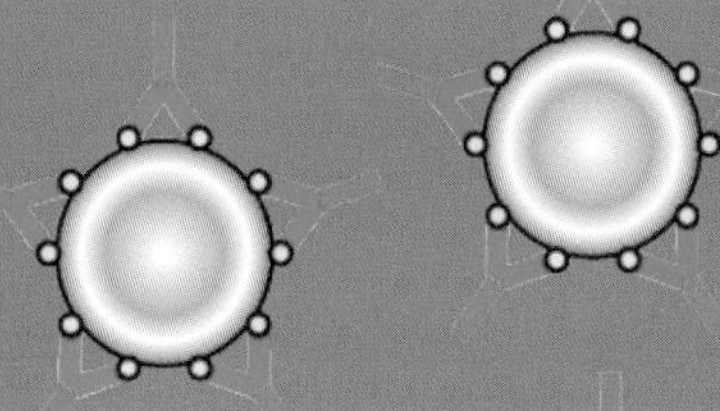

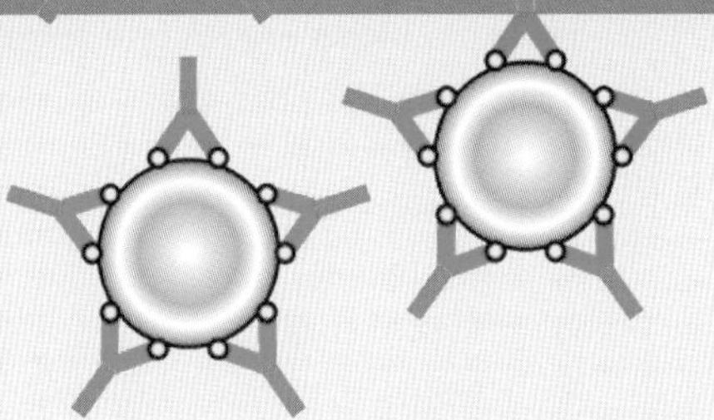

LEARNING OBJECTIVES

- Discuss the basic physiology of the blood
- Discuss the basic physiology of the immune system

4.1 Questions

Easy	Medium	Hard

1. A patient with which of the following conditions is likely to present with a higher blood viscosity and a higher erythrocyte sedimentation rate as compared to normal?

A. Hyperthermia
B. Iron deficiency anemia
C. Polycythemia
D. Sickle cell anemia
E. Systemic lupus erythematosus

Questions 2 to 3

A 43-year-old Caucasian woman visits her gynecologist with complaints of menorrhagia. She admits to feeling tired and short of breath on exertion, and the physician notes that the woman looks pale. When questioned about her diet, she states that she is a vegetarian, but eats fish occasionally. Her family history is unremarkable. A complete blood count (CBC) is ordered and the results are as follows:

RBCs: $3.95 \times 10^6/\mu L$
Hb: 9 g/dL
Hct: 31%
WBCs: $8 \times 10^3/\mu L$
Plt: $250 \times 10^3/\mu L$
RBC shape: normal

2. What is the woman's mean corpuscle volume, and would this finding be described as normocytic, microcytic, or macrocytic?

	Mean corpuscle volume (fL)	Description
A.	22.8	Normocytic
B.	22.8	Microcytic
C.	22.8	Macrocytic
D.	78.5	Normocytic
E.	78.5	Microcytic
F.	78.5	Macrocytic
G.	95.2	Normocytic
H.	95.2	Microcytic
I.	95.2	Macrocytic

3. Based on the woman's history, physical, and lab data, what type of anemia is she most likely suffering from?

A. Aplastic anemia
B. Iron deficiency anemia
C. Pernicious anemia
D. Sickle cell anemia

4. Which of the following conditions most likely leads to anemia but presents with a normal hematocrit and a normal hemoglobin concentration?

A. Acute hemorrhage
B. Aplastic anemia
C. Folate deficiency
D. Hemolysis
E. Iron deficiency
F. Vitamin B_{12} deficiency

5. A 37-year-old woman suffers from recurrent headaches and dizziness. Her hematocrit is 52%, and leukocyte and platelet counts are elevated. A peripheral blood screen for JAK2 V617F is positive, making the diagnosis of polycythemia vera (PV) likely. In order to support the diagnosis and to eliminate other causes of polycythemia, a serum test for which of the following substances is warranted?

A. Albumin
B. Bilirubin
C. Erythropoietin
D. Hemoglobin
E. Haptoglobin

6. A 34-year-old female has noticed a marked decrease in energy over the last few months. She has an overall healthy lifestyle but usually drinks 6 units of alcohol per week, usually on weekends. Her physical exam does not present any abnormalities. Her laboratory blood results are as follows, with abnormal values indicated with an asterisk:

WBCs:	11,000/mL
RBCs:	4.0×10^6/L*
Hb:	9.7 g/dl*
Hct	29.9%*
MCV:	69.7 fL*
MCH	22.6 pg/cell*
MCHC:	28 g/dl*
RDW:	18.4%*
Plt:	450×10^9/L
PT:	13 seconds
aPTT:	28 seconds
Serum iron:	29 g/dL*
Transferrin:	450 mg/dL*
Serum ferritin:	15 ng/mL*
TIBC:	533 g/dL*

What is the most likely diagnosis?

A. Acute bleeding
B. Anemia of chronic disease
C. Iron deficiency anemia
D. Liver disease
E. Vitamin B_{12} deficiency
F. Vitamin K deficiency
G. Von Willebrand's disease

7. The image shows the results of an ABO blood group testing card, on which a drop of a patient's blood was placed on each of the four circles. The first circle from the left contained anti-A antibody; the second circle contained anti-B antibody; the third circle contained anti-D antibody; and the fourth circle did not contain any antibodies. The blood in circles 1 and 3 agglutinated. There was no agglutination in circles 2 and 4. Based on the test result of the patient, which of the following choices are correct in regards to the patient's ability to receive blood and donate blood?

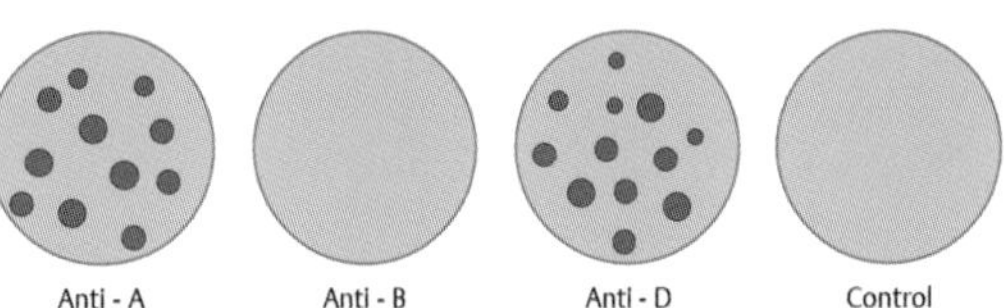

	Patient can donate blood to people with following blood groups	Patient can receive blood from people with following blood groups
A.	A+, A−, B+, B−, O, AB	O+, O−
B.	A+, A−, B+, B−	O+, O−
C.	O+	A+, A−, B+, B−
D.	A+, AB+	A+, O+, O−
E.	A+, AB+	A+, A−, B+, B−, O

8. A 25-year-old woman gives birth to a healthy baby following a nonproblematic pregnancy. This is her second child. Three days later the baby returns with a fever and jaundice. The mother's blood type is AB negative and the father's blood type is A positive. Hemolytic disease of the newborn is suspected. Which of the following combinations of blood types is possible for the first and second child, if the diagnosis of hemolytic disease of the newborn is confirmed?

	First child blood type	Second child blood type
A.	A+	AB+
B.	A−	A+
C.	B−	AB−
D.	AB−	A−
E.	B+	B−
F.	AB+	B−

9. A patient is concerned that her gums have been bleeding when she has brushed her teeth for the past 3 weeks. She recalls digestive problems and episodes of steatorrhea over the past couple of weeks, which she tries to ease by drinking large amounts of herbal tea. Her prothrombin time (PT) is 18 seconds, and her partial thromboplastin time (PTT) is 36 seconds. Her platelet count is normal. Laboratory analysis would most likely indicate a deficiency in which of the following vitamins?

A. Vitamin A
B. Vitamin C
C. Vitamin D
D. Vitamin E
E. Vitamin K

10. A 9-year-old boy presents to the emergency department with a minor cut on his forearm that has been bleeding for 30 minutes. The bleeding is stopped after another 30 minutes, and the physician suspects hemophilia. Several weeks later, additional lab tests confirm a mild form of hemophilia B. A defect in which of the factors of the coagulation cascade shown in the image is responsible for hemophilia B?

A. A
B. B
C. C
D. D
E. E

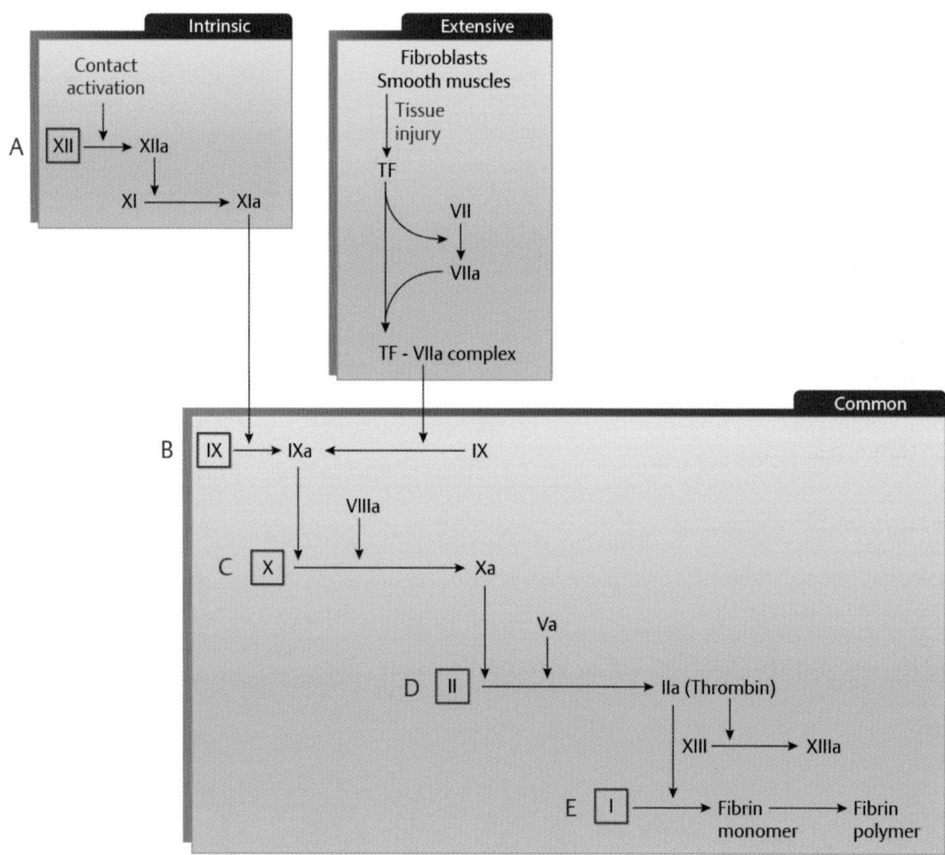

Questions 11 to 12

A 15-year-old girl suffers from recurrent epistaxis (nosebleeds), gingival bleeding when brushing her teeth, and heavy menstrual bleeding. Her mother suffers from similar symptoms, and her 1-year-old brother bruises very easily. All three have been diagnosed with Type 1 von Willebrand's disease.

11. For all three family members, what results would be expected on the following lab tests: platelet count, bleeding time (BT), prothrombin time (PT), and activated partial thromboplastin time (aPTT)?

	Platelet count	BT	PT	aPTT
A.	Decreased	Prolonged	Unaffected	Prolonged
B.	Decreased	Unaffected	Prolonged	Unaffected or prolonged
C.	Decreased	Unaffected	Unaffected	Unaffected
D.	Unaffected	Prolonged	Prolonged	Prolonged
E.	Unaffected	Prolonged	Unaffected	Unaffected or prolonged
F.	Unaffected	Unaffected	Prolonged	Unaffected or prolonged

12. To what protein does von Willebrand factor normally bind to on the surface of platelets?

A. Adenosine diphosphate (ADP)

B. Glycoprotein Ib (GPIb)

C. Platelet factor 3 (PF3)

D. Prostacyclin

E. Thromboxane A_2

13. A 35-year-old woman asks for a thorough checkup because she suffers from heavy menstrual bleeding. She also bruises easily, and her gums bleed easily after brushing her teeth. She denies the use of aspirin except to treat occasional infrequent headaches. Her platelet count is normal, but bleeding time is prolonged. Specific tests show low levels of von Willebrand factor (vWF) and factor VIII procoagulant, and decreased platelet aggregation when ristocetin is added to the plasma. An analogue of which of the following hormones is most likely to be administered for preventing future bleeding episodes?

A. Arginine vasopressin

B. Antidiuretic hormone

C. Cortisol

D. Epinephrine

E. Prolactin

14. A 67-year-old woman with a 5-year history of hypertension has suffered from palmar erythema and facial flushing associated with pruritus (itching) for several years. She has undergone phlebotomy for erythrocytosis on multiple occasions; however, erythrocytosis persists (red blood cells 7 million/μL, hemoglobin 18.9 g/dL, hemocrit 57.7%). She was transferred to the hematology department. Splenomegaly, low plasma erythropoietin (EPO), and a positive genetic test for the *JAK2* mutation confirmed a diagnosis of polycythemia vera. A bone marrow biopsy would most likely reveal which of the following findings?

A. Decreased myeloid progenitor stem cells

B. Increased myeloid progenitor stem cells

C. Decreased lymphoid progenitor stem cells

D. Increased lymphoid progenitor stem cells

E. Decreased pluripotent stem cells

F. Increased pluripotent stem cells

4.2 Answers and Explanations

Easy	Medium	Hard

1. Correct: Systemic lupus erythematosus (E)

Systemic lupus erythematosus (SLE) presents with a high blood viscosity, due to the presence of high-molecular-weight immunoglobulins in plasma, and with a high erythrocyte sedimentation rate (ESR), since the increased amount of protein favors red blood cell (RBC) clumping so that they settle more rapidly than normal. (**A**) Hyperthermia leads to low (not high) blood viscosity, since there is an inverse relationship between "blood thickness" and temperature. ESR might be elevated, since there is increased molecular motion at higher temperatures. (**B, C**) Iron deficiency anemia presents with low viscosity and polycythemia with high viscosity, since blood viscosity is strongly related to the total number of blood cells. It alters the velocity of the upward flow of plasma, so that RBC aggregates fall more rapidly in anemia and more slowly in polycythemia. (**D**) Sickle cell anemia is a special case, since the irregular shape of the sickled RBCs increases cell aggregation, leading to high blood viscosity. Sickled cells settle more slowly, leading to lower ESR than normal.

2. Correct: 78.5, microcytic (E)

Mean corpuscular volume (MCV) is the average volume of red blood cells (RBCs) in a sample. This patient's MCV is 78.5 fL/RBC, which is below the normal range (80–96 fL), so these cells are microcytic, which means they are smaller than average. The calculation for MCV is as follows:

MCV = Hematocrit × 10/red blood cell count (million/μL)
MCV = (31 × 10)/(3.95 million/μL)
MCV = 310/3.95 = 78.5 fL

(**A, B, C, D, F, G, H, I**) These answers have incorrect calculations or cell descriptions.

3. Correct: Iron deficiency anemia (B)

The most common form of anemia is iron deficiency anemia. This can have several causes, such as chronic blood loss (e.g., excessive menstruation), or reduced intake of iron (e.g., vegetarian diet), both of which the patient has. The red blood cells (RBCs) in this condition are microcytic due to low iron. Based on these findings, this is most likely the type of anemia the patient is suffering from. (**A**) Aplastic anemia is a blood disorder in which the body's bone marrow does not make enough new blood cells. The RBCs that are present are normal in size, not microcytic, which rules out this anemia. (**C**) Classic pernicious anemia is caused by the failure of gastric parietal cells to produce sufficient intrinsic factor (a gastric protein secreted by parietal cells) to permit the absorption of adequate quantities of dietary vitamin B_{12}. The RBCs are megaloblasts, which are macrocytic cells, which rules out this anemia. (**D**) Sickle cell anemia is a serious disease in which the RBCs contain abnormal hemoglobin molecules that stick to each other where normal hemoglobin molecules do not, forming long rigid stacks that cause the cells to have a sickle shape that does not move easily through the blood vessels. In sickle cell anemia, the number of RBCs is lower than normal because sickle cells do not last very long. The abnormal shape of these cells rules out this type of anemia, since the patient's RBCs were normal shaped.

4. Correct: Acute hemorrhage (A)

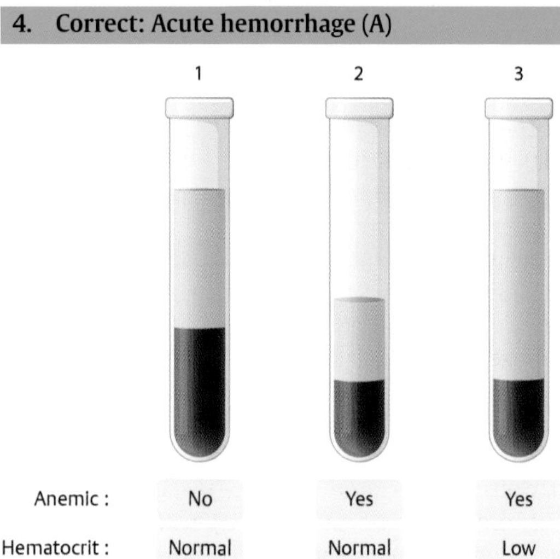

In major acute hemorrhage, fluids and cells are lost by about equal amounts, so that immediately after the blood loss, hematocrit and hemoglobin values remain unchanged (see image, test tube 2). (**B, C, D, E, F**) Anemias that result in a lower number of red blood cells (RBCs), and hence lower total blood O_2 carrying capacity, present with low hematocrit and low hemoglobin, independent of the cause (see image, test tube 3). These may include failure of RBC formation in the bone marrow (aplastic anemia), increased destruction of RBCs (hemolytic anemia), and failure of RBC maturation due to folic acid, iron, or vitamin B_{12} deficiency.

5. Correct: Erythropoietin (C)

Polycythemia vera is a hereditary neoplastic bone marrow disorder, leading to constant overproduction of erythrocytes due to mutated myeloblasts. In response, erythropoietin (EPO), the hormone that normally stimulates bone marrow to produce erythrocytes, is low. On the other hand, any condition that leads to increased production of EPO (such as hypoxia or renal tumors) will cause overproduction of erythrocytes and is defined as secondary polycythemia. (**A, B, D, E**) The serum values of these components do not help to support the woman's diagnosis or help to distinguish primary from secondary polycythemia. Albumin is a nonspecific serum carrier, and bilirubin is the breakdown product of heme proteins. Hemoglobin is elevated in both primary and secondary polycythemia. Haptoglobin binds to hemoglobin and is elevated as an acute-phase reaction.

6. Correct: Iron deficiency anemia (C)

Iron deficiency may lead to microcytic (low MCV, mean cell volume), hypochromic (low MCHC, mean cell hemoglobin concentration) anemia, as evidenced by the low red blood cell count (RBC), hemoglobin concentration (Hb) and hematocrit (Hct). Diagnosis is supported by low serum iron and ferritin. Transferrin, the number of transporters not bound to iron, is high, and the total iron-binding capacity (TIBC) test is high, since more iron is needed to saturate all transferrin molecules. Iron deficiency is the most common cause of anemia in women of childbearing age. When mild, it does not present with any signs other than some degree of weakness or pallor. (**A**) Acute bleeding presents with normal (not low) Hct and Hb. (**B**) Anemia of chronic disease is the next best answer, when just considering the low MCV and MCHC values. However, the clinical vignette does not provide any hints of a chronic inflammatory disorder or cancer. Moreover, ferritin is typically high since it is not only an iron storage molecule, but also an acute-phase reactant that will be elevated in chronic disease. (**D, F, G**) Liver disease, vitamin K deficiency, and von Willebrand's disease present with changes in platelet counts (Plt) or clotting times (prothrombin [PT] and activated partial thromboplastin time [aPTT]), which are normal in this case. (**E**) Vitamin B_{12} deficiency leads to megaloblastic (high MCV) cells due to abnormal RBC DNA synthesis and inhibition of cell division. On the other hand, cells are normochromic (normal MCHC) due to their normal amount of hemoglobin.

7. Correct: A+, AB+, A+, O+, O– (D)

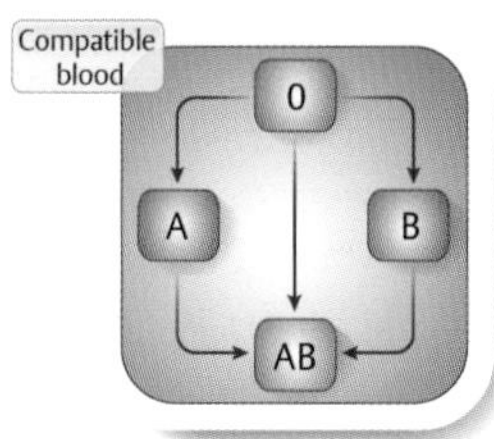

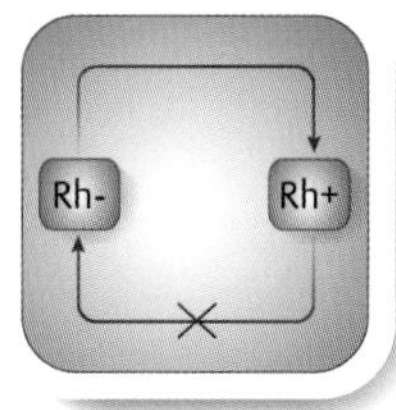

The patient's blood group is type A+, indicating that his/her red blood cells (RBCs) have antigen A, which agglutinates with anti-A antibody (circle 1). It does not agglutinate with anti-B due to the lack of antigen B (circle 2). Agglutination in circle 3 with anti-D means that the patient's blood has Rh (rhesus) antigen and is said to be Rh positive. The patient can donate blood to a person with the same blood group of A+ and to a person with the blood group AB, since that person will not have anti-A antibody, which would cause clumping. The patient's serum has anti-B antibody. Hence, he/she can receive blood from blood groups without antigen B (i.e., type A and type O blood), not type B or type AB blood. The Rh+ patient can receive blood from Rh+ and Rh– donors but cannot donate to Rh– people. (**A, B, C, E**). This makes choice **D** the correct combination (see image) and all other choices incorrect.

8. Correct: A+, AB+ (A)

	Mother
Father	AB
AO	AA, AO, BO, AB ⟶ **A, B, AB**
AA	AA, AB ⟶ **A, AB**

There are two parts to the question; first is determining the children's possible blood types based on the parents' blood types, and second is understanding the circumstances that lead to hemolytic disease of the newborn. Based on the parents' blood types, the children must be Type A, B, or AB (see image). For hemolytic disease of the newborn to occur, some fetal blood must enter the mother's circulation during pregnancy, and the mother must be Rh negative and the baby must be Rh positive. If these occur, then the mother will produce antibodies against the Rhesus D antigen, which is present on the fetus's red blood cells. During a subsequent pregnancy with an Rh-positive fetus, the antibodies enter the fetal circulation and destroy the Rh D positive fetal RBCs, leading to hemolytic disease of the newborn. So, both children in the case must be Rh+. With the widespread use of Rho(D) immune globulin (RhoGAM, Kedrion Biopharma Inc., Fort Lee, NJ), an anti-D immunoglobulin, hemolytic disease of the newborn has almost disappeared. (**B, C, D, E, F**) Each of these answers is incorrect because one or both children are Rh negative, and both children must be Rh positive for hemolytic disease of the newborn to occur.

9. Correct: Vitamin K (E)

Vitamin K acts as a cofactor for the carboxylation reactions in the synthesis of coagulation factors II, VII, IX, and X. Normal values of this fat-soluble vitamin are from diet and intestinal bacteria, so altered gut flora and/or fat malabsorption (resulting in steatorrhea) can lead to vitamin K deficiency and hence impairment of hemostasis (bleeding gums, prolonged PT and PTT). (**A, B, C, D**) These vitamin deficiencies do not present with increased PT and PTT; rather, they result in characteristic clinical symptoms that are not present in this case, such as night blindness (vitamin A deficiency), scurvy (Vitamin C deficiency), rickets or osteomalacia (vitamin D deficiency), or nonspecific neurologic symptoms and red blood cell hemolysis (vitamin E deficiency).

10. Correct: B (B)

Hemophilia B, also called factor IX (FIX) deficiency, is a genetic disorder caused by missing or defective factor IX, a clotting protein. Although it is normally hereditary, about 30% of cases are caused by a spontaneous mutation. (**A, C, D, E**) A defect in these factors does not cause hemophilia B.

11. Correct: Unaffected, prolonged, unaffected, unaffected or prolonged (E)

Type 1 von Willebrand's disease is an intrinsic pathway coagulation defect, not a problem with the number of platelets; therefore, platelet count is normal. Bleeding time (BT), a test performed to assess clotting time and platelet function, is prolonged because von Willebrand factor (vWF), which normally promotes platelet adhesion, is deficient. Prothrombin time (PT) is unaffected because that test is specific for defects in the extrinsic coagulation pathway, not the intrinsic pathway. The activated partial thromboplastin time (aPTT) may be normal or elevated because, depending on the severity of the disease, factor VIII is bound to vWF, which protects the factor VIII from rapid breakdown within the blood. Deficiency of vWF can therefore lead to a reduction in factor VIII levels, which explains the elevation in aPTT time. (**A, B, C, D, F**) These choices have incorrect combinations of blood lab values for individuals with von Willebrand's disease.

12. Correct: Glycoprotein Ib (GPIb) (B)

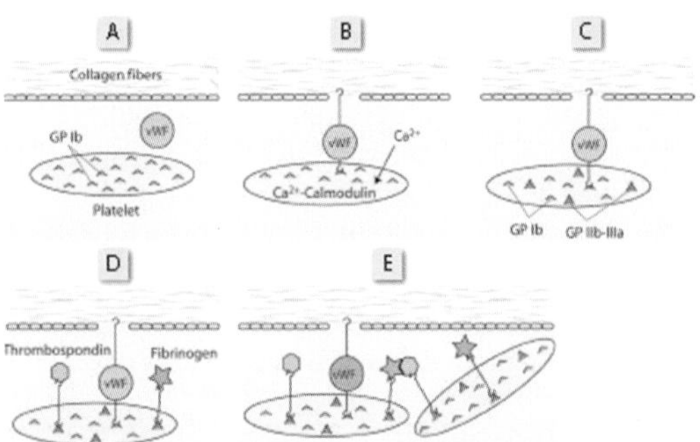

Glycoprotein Ib (GPIb), also known as CD42, is a membrane receptor that binds von Willebrand factor, allowing platelet adhesion and platelet plug formation at sites of vascular injury. (**A**) Adenosine diphosphate (ADP) strengthens platelet plugs by inducing platelet aggregation. It is a nucleotide, not a protein. (**C**) Platelet factor 3 (PF3) is derived from platelets and acts to convert prothrombin to thrombin. (**D**) Prostacyclin is an inhibitor of platelet aggregation. It is a prostaglandin, not a protein. (**E**) Thromboxane A_2 is derived from platelets and promotes platelet aggregation. It is an eicosanoid lipid, not a protein.

13. Correct: Arginine vasopressin (A)

Desmopressin, an analogue of arginine vasopressin, is part of the treatment of von Willebrand's disease (vWD). The woman's easy bruising, prolonged bleeding time, and normal platelet count makes an inherited disorder of platelet function likely. Specific tests for vWD, such as von Willebrand factor (vWF), vWF activity via ristocetin cofactor activity, and Factor VIII activity, confirm the diagnosis of the disease, which causes poor platelet adhesion to vascular walls and deficient factor VIII production. When desmopressin binds to V_2 receptors, it supports the release of stored vWF into the circulation. This is a less known function of V_2 receptor activity, which is better known for its antidiuretic effects. (**B, C, D, E**) These hormones are not part of the treatment of mild to moderate bleeding disorders.

14. Correct: Increased myeloid progenitor stem cells (B)

In polycythemia vera, a mutation in the *JAK2* gene causes uncontrolled proliferation of the myeloid stem cells, resulting in hyperplasia of the erythroid (red blood cell), granulocytic (white blood cell), and megakaryocytic (platelet) cell lines. This results in increased red blood cell mass, leading to a variety of problems, including hypertension and flushing. The high RBC mass also inhibits erythropoietin (EPO) release, because oxygen delivery is adequate. The myeloid stem cells also stimulate production of mast cells, which release histamine; this is responsible for the patient's pruritus. (**A**) Polycythemia vera results from increased myeloid stem cells, not decreased, as just described. (**C, D**) The lymphoid stem cells are progenitors to lymphocytes and natural killer cells, which are not increased or decreased in polycythemia vera. (**E, F**) The pluripotent stem cells are the precursors to both myeloid and lymphoid progenitor cells. The mutation for polycythemia vera occurs at the level of the control of myeloid progenitor cell formation, but not above that.

4.3 Questions

Questions 15 to 16

A 12-year-old girl presents with nausea, vomiting, severe headache, and pain when lowering her chin towards the neck. A white blood cell (WBC) differential count and spinal fluid collection are ordered. Viral meningitis is diagnosed from the spinal fluid specimen, and the WBC differential count shows that one type of white blood cell is greatly elevated above normal.

15. Which white blood cell is expected to be abnormally high in response to the girl's infection, and what substance is released from that cell in response?

	White blood cell type	Substance released
A.	Basophils	Cytotoxic granules
B.	Basophils	Lysozyme
C.	T-lymphocytes	Histamine
D.	T-lymphocytes	Cytotoxic granules
E.	Eosinophils	Lysozyme
F.	Eosinophils	Peroxidase

16. The girl's mother decides to have her other child vaccinated against viral meningitis. What type of immunity will be produced by this vaccination?

A. Artificially acquired active immunity
B. Artificially acquired passive immunity
C. Naturally acquired active immunity
D. Naturally acquired passive immunity

17. The complement system comprises a cascade of proteins, C1–C9, which play an important role in host defense processes. Which of the following components of the complement system are most important for neutrophil chemotaxis, generation of anaphylatoxin, and cytolysis, respectively?

	Neutrophil chemotaxis	Anaphylatoxin	Cytolysis
A.	C5a	C3a, C4a, C5a	C5b, C6, C7, C8, C9
B.	C5a	C5b, C6, C7, C8, C9	C3a, C4a, C5a
C.	C3a, C4a, C5a	C5a	C5b, C6, C7, C8, C9
D.	C3a, C4a, C5a	C5b, C6, C7, C8, C9	C5a
E.	C5b, C6, C7, C8, C9	C3a, C4a, C5a	C5a
F.	C5b, C6, C7, C8, C9	C5a	C3a, C4a, C5a

18. A patient's past history reveals that he suffered from recurrent pyogenic bacterial infections, including pneumococcal disease, between the ages of 3 and 8. He had a normal resistance to other microbes. His clinical status improved with age. He became an immunologist and understands now that he has a specific innate immune defect due to a mutation in the *MYD88* gene. The innate immune defect of this patient is most likely directly affecting the activity of which of the following?

A. Cytotoxic T lymphocytes
B. IgE immunoglobulins
C. Memory B lymphocytes
D. Toll-like receptor signaling
E. Type 2 helper T cells

19. Human vaccination using DNA vaccines is a fast developing approach that aims to prepare people to mount an adequate immune response when confronted in the future with an infectious agent. Which of the following correctly describes the process of human vaccination by DNA vaccines?

A. Bacterial plasmid DNA injection in host animals that produce antibodies given to humans
B. Human injection with factors that prevent mutation of DNA viruses to avoid immune evasion
C. Injection of bacterial plasmid DNA that encodes the antigen of the sought immune response
D. Injection of pretreated bacteria with DNA that encodes human immune system elements
E. Use of recombinant DNA technology to produce an attenuated pathogen to inject in humans

20. A patient presents with a cold sore on her lip due to the herpes simplex virus. Which of the following is the correct antigen-presenting cell, antigen-presenting molecule, and responding effector cell for the herpes simplex virus?

	Antigen-presenting cell	Antigen-presenting molecule	Effector cell
A.	Dendritic cell	MHC class I	T helper cell
B.	Any cell	MHC class I	Cytotoxic T cell
C.	B cell	MHC class I	Any immune cell
D.	Dendritic cell	MHC class II	T helper cell
E.	Any cell	MHC class II	Cytotoxic T cell
F.	B cell	MCH class II	Any immune cell

21. In regards to leukocyte extravasation, which of the following types of leukocyte is normally the first to exit the blood vessel at the injury site in response to an inflammatory stimulus?

A. Basophils
B. Eosinophils
C. Lymphocytes
D. Monocytes
E. Neutrophils

22. A 27-year-old African American woman presents with a low-grade fever, fatigue, decreased appetite, weight loss, and joint stiffness and swelling, especially in her hands and knees. The physician notes a reduced range of motion. A rheumatic condition is suspected, and lab tests are ordered. The interpreted lab results are as follows:

Complete blood count: Normal
Chemistry profile: Suggest impaired kidney function
Thyroid panel: Normal
Urinalysis: Traces of protein, casts, RBCs
Erythrocyte sedimentation rate: Elevated
Antinuclear antibodies: Positive
Rheumatoid factor antibodies: Negative
Hand and knee X-ray: Soft tissue swelling, no joint space narrowing or bone damage.

Which of the following is the most likely diagnosis?

A. Hashimoto's thyroiditis
B. Osteoarthritis
C. Rheumatoid arthritis
D. Scleroderma
E. Systemic lupus erythematosus

23. Two patients, each with hypersensitivity conditions, present in the clinic. The first patient is a 41-year-old woman diagnosed with Graves' disease, and the second is a 38-year-old man with severe rheumatoid arthritis. How are the hypersensitivity disorders in these patients best characterized?

	Patient 1	Patient 2
A.	Type I	Type III
B.	Type I	Type II
C.	Type II	Type I
D.	Type II	Type III
E.	Type III	Type IV
F.	Type III	Type II
G.	Type IV	Type II
H.	Type IV	Type III

24. A 5-year-old boy seeking refuge in North America has been continuously ill with life-threatening bacterial infections and granuloma formation for the past 6 months. The parents confirm that the child has been frequently ill since birth; however, it had gotten significantly worse since their relocation. The mother seems to have some problems as well, but language barriers have to be overcome first to obtain more detailed information. Laboratory assessment reveals a negative (abnormal) nitroblue tetrazolium (NBT) reduction test, which is confirmed by a negative dihydrorhodamine 123 (DHR) oxidation test. Based on this information, which of the following immune cells is most likely functioning abnormally in the boy?

A. B lymphocytes
B. Macrophages
C. Natural killer cells
D. Platelets
E. T lymphocytes

25. A 45-year-old patient presents with diarrhea and blood in his stools. These symptoms started about 2 years ago and became gradually more severe. Three days ago, the man developed fever and extreme fatigue. His gastrointestinal discomfort is now significantly worse, with up to 10 stools per day, accompanied by severe cramps and blood loss. A complete blood count shows a hemoglobin concentration of 11 g/dL, an erythrocyte sedimentation rate of 50 mm/h, and a high-sensitivity C-reactive protein (hs-CRP) level of 4.0 mg/L. A fast-check stool culture reveals the presence of bacteria. An endoscopic picture of the large intestinal wall is shown in the image. Which of the following combinations of inflammatory cells would most likely be present in a colonic biopsy sample?

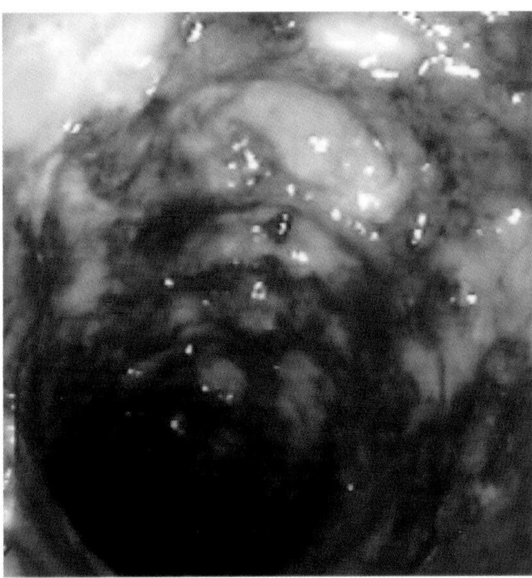

A. Basophils, eosinophils, and mast cells
B. Basophils, eosinophils, and neutrophils
C. Macrophages, basophils, and mast cells
D. Macrophages, lymphocytes, and plasma cells
E. Neutrophils, basophils, and mast cells
F. Neutrophils, macrophages, and lymphocytes

4.4 Answers and Explanations

15. Correct: T-lymphocytes, cytotoxic granules (D)

Meningitis is an infection of the membranes (meninges) surrounding the brain and spinal cord and can have a bacterial, fungal, or viral cause. This question requires you to know that lymphocytes are most elevated in viral infections and that they release cytotoxic granules (containing perforin, granzyme, and granulysin) to fight viruses. (**A, B, C, E, F**) Basophils and eosinophils primarily play a role in parasitic infections and allergies. Basophils release histamine, and eosinophils release peroxidase.

16. Correct: Artificially acquired active immunity (A)

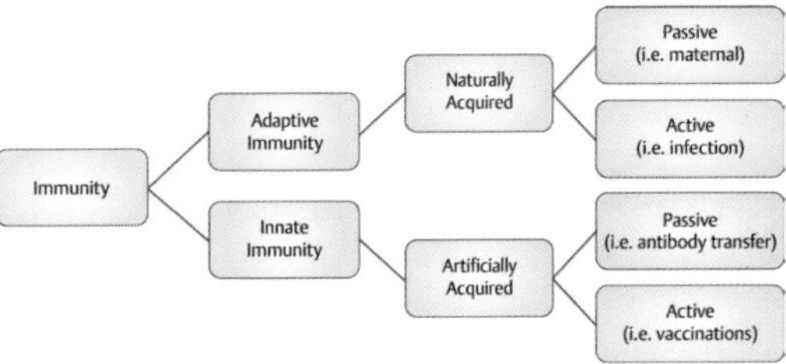

Artificially acquired active immunity is induced by vaccination. A vaccine stimulates a primary response against the antigen without causing symptoms of the disease. (**B**) Artificially acquired passive immunity is a short-term immunization induced by the deliberate transfer of antibodies from one organism to another. (**C**) Naturally acquired active immunity occurs when a person is exposed to a live pathogen in nature (not induced by deliberate exposure) and develops a primary immune response that leads to immunological memory. (**D**) Naturally acquired passive immunity is the transfer of antibodies from one individual to another, such as when maternal antibodies are transferred to the fetus through the placenta.

17. Correct: C5a, C3a, C4a, C5a, C5b, C6, C7, C8, C9 (A)

Neutrophil chemotaxis is mediated by C5a, a potent chemotactic agent, by attracting neutrophils and macrophages to sites of inflammation. Anaphylatoxin production also involves C5a, as well as C4a and C3a, as potent mediators of inflammation. These proteins mediate increases in capillary permeability via degranulation of mast cells and basophils, leading to the release of histamine and vasodilation. Cytolysis involves C5b, C6, C7, C8, and C9 complement cascade proteins, leading to the formation of a membrane attack complex (MAC), which perforates the pathogen's cell membrane and causes major damage to the cell (lysis). (**B, C, D, E, F**) These answer choices contain the wrong combinations of answers.

18. Correct: Toll-like receptor signaling (D)

Patients with specific innate immune system defects have only recently been identified. They present with some abnormal activity of innate immune cells such as neutrophils, monocytes, natural killer cells, basophils, or mast cells. The commonality of these cells is that they bind to unique proteins of microorganisms via pattern recognition receptors, of which Toll-like receptors (TLRs) are a major class. TLR signaling results in the release of cytokines that mediate the immune response. The *MYD88* gene mutation leads to TLR signaling problems and manifests in the patient as a weak defense against bacterial infection. On the other hand, the patient has an intact adaptive immune system, the system that develops with training and through memory. This explains the fact that some children with *MYD88* deficiency can outgrow their illness. (**A, B, C, E**) These are all components of the more advanced adaptive immune system, either the cell-mediated branch (cytotoxic T cells, T helper 2 cells) or the humoral branch (IgE immunoglobulins, memory B cells).

19. Correct: Injection of bacterial plasmid DNA that encodes the antigen of the sought immune response (C)

The general principle of a DNA vaccine is to inject humans with DNA that eventually leads to the production of antigenic protein. The DNA is bacterial plasmid DNA with a promoter for eukaryotic cells (i.e., SV40), which is taken up by human antigen-presenting cells, which then produce the encoded protein. This antigenic protein elicits an immune response just as a conventional vaccine does. It has to be noted that DNA vaccines are already tested that encode immune assistance proteins rather than the antigenic protein itself. (**A**) This is an example of passive immunization, in which the administration of antibodies (in this case produced in a host animal) supports a person's own immune response against a pathogen. (**B**) Viruses (not only DNA viruses) have multiple mechanisms to undergo genetic change in order to avoid recognition by the host's immune system. There are no injectable factors that prevent these virus strategies. (**D**) Pretreated bacteria are injected as part of active immunization, so that the human immune system generates elements that remember the pathogen, not so that the bacterial DNA translates into human immune system elements. (**E**) This describes the current practice of active immunization against viral diseases in that an attenuated (weakened) virus is given to people in order to mount an immune response that does not cause illness but provides long-term protection due to immunologic memory.

20. Correct: Any cell, MHC class I, cytotoxic T cell (B)

The herpes simplex virus initially replicates in epithelial cells but can then spread and exist in a latent form inside most other cells. Such infected host cells enzymatically digest the virus, couple virus pieces to major histocompatibility complex (MHC) class I molecules, and present the peptide complexes on their cell surface to cytotoxic CD8+ T cells. These cells are programmed to kill any cell with such a complex on their surface. In general, class I MHC molecules are expressed by almost all cells in order to deal with intracellular antigens. (**A, C, D, E, F**). These combinations have one or more incorrect components. Dendritic cells and B cells are class II antigen-presenting cells. They couple digested parts of extracellular antigens with MHC class II molecules and present these complexes to CD4+ T Helper cells. However, it should be noted that a virus itself also produces proteins that activate class II pathways, so herpes simplex infections can evoke CD4+ and CD8+ T cell-mediated immune responses.

21. Correct: Neutrophils (E)

In response to an inflammatory stimulus, neutrophils are the first to undergo extravasation (i.e., migration across the endothelium of the blood vessels into the interstitium) at the injury site. (**A, B, C, D**) The neutrophils degranulate at the injury site and attract a second wave of immune cells to the site, which contains mainly monocytes. Recruitment of all the other leukocytes is necessary for a proper immune response, since they all fulfill different functions in the tissue, but they are recruited at later times, depending on the responsiveness to certain chemokines and the expression/activation of adhesion molecules.

22. Correct: Systemic lupus erythematosus (E)

Systemic lupus erythematosus (SLE) is a chronic disease that causes pain, inflammation, and swelling. It has a wide range of symptoms, which makes it difficult to diagnose, but 95% of people affected by SLE will test positive for antinuclear antibody (ANA). If positive for ANA, then several additional antibody tests may be ordered to confirm SLE, such as anti-dsDNA, aPLs, and antibodies to histone. (**A**) Hashimoto's thyroiditis can be ruled out because the thyroid panel was normal. (**B**) Osteoarthritis is not the best choice because it is not an inflammatory disease (although some localized inflammation can occur), and this patient has signs of systemic inflammation (i.e., elevated erythrocyte sedimentation rate) and the X-ray shows soft tissue swelling and no joint space narrowing. (**C**) Rheumatoid arthritis is not the best answer because renal complications are rare with this disease, and the rheumatoid factor antibody test is negative. (**D**) Scleroderma is a chronic connective tissue disease generally classified as one of the autoimmune rheumatic diseases. Hardening and tightening of patches of skin may reduce the range of motion (ROM) in the affected areas. While the patient has reduced ROM, none of the other symptoms fit this diagnosis.

23. Correct: Type II, Type III (D)

Type II hypersensitivity is antibody-mediated. In the case of Graves' disease, thyroid-stimulating immunoglobulins recognize and bind to the thyrotropin receptor (TSH receptor), which stimulates the secretion of thyroxine (T_4) and triiodothyronine (T_3). Type III hypersensitivity is immune complex–mediated. In the case of rheumatoid arthritis, IgG binds to a soluble antigen and forms a circulating immune complex. This complex is deposited primarily in the joints and initiates a local inflammatory reaction. (**A, B, C, E, F, G, H**) These answers all contain an incorrect combination of choices.

24. Correct: Macrophages (B)

The boy has chronic granulomatous disease (CGD), based on severe, recurrent bacterial infections (especially evident under the stress of fleeing the family's home country and being exposed to new pathogens) and the lack of an oxidative immune response (negative NBT and DHR tests). It is most likely the X chromosome–linked form of the disease (patient is male and mother has immune system–related problems). The main defect in CGD is a failure to mount a respiratory burst; hence, it leads to abnormally functioning macrophages (also neutrophils, monocytes, and eosinophils). The macrophages still ingest the bacteria but are not able to kill them, since they do not produce superoxide anion and superoxide-derived reactive oxygen species such as hydrogen peroxide. The intracellular survival of pathogens leads to the development of granulomas in various tissues. (**A**) Abnormal functioning B cells can lead to hypogammaglobulinemias. (**C**) Pure natural killer (NK) abnormality disorders present with severe viral (not bacterial) infections such as herpes and papillomavirus infections, since these cells are primarily involved in cellular, rather than humoral, immunity. Granuloma formation is not seen. NBT and DHR tests are normal. (**D**) Platelets are not directly involved in the immune response. Abnormal functioning leads to bleeding disorders. (**E**) Abnormal T lymphocyte functioning results in severe viral, fungal, and protozoal infections rather than recurrent bacterial infections.

25. Correct: Neutrophils, macrophages, and lymphocytes (F)

The patient has obvious signs of chronic and acute inflammation (elevated erythrocyte sedimentation rate and serum C-reactive protein, pus and mucus overlying the colonic mucosa). Chronic inflammation over years caused gastrointestinal (GI) irritation and wounds, leading to diarrhea and bleeding ulcers. He most likely suffers from ulcerative colitis. It weakened his body so much that he has recently developed anemia (low hemoglobin) and a GI infection (bacteria in stool), leading to significantly worse diarrhea and cramps. In a colonic biopsy sample, one expects the presence of neutrophils as acute inflammatory cells, as well as indicator cells of chronic inflammation such as macrophages and lymphocytes. (**A, B, C, E**) Basophils and mast cells are immune indicator cells of allergies and/or parasitic infections, which is not the case here. Eosinophils may be numerous in chronic disease, although they are more a sign of quiescent ulcerative colitis. (**D**) This answer choice is missing neutrophils. Their presence is expected as indicators of active disease. Moreover, plasma cells are especially present below the base of crypts (basal plasmacytosis), so they might not be present on all endoscopic biopsy samples.

Chapter 5

Cardiovascular and Lymphatic Systems

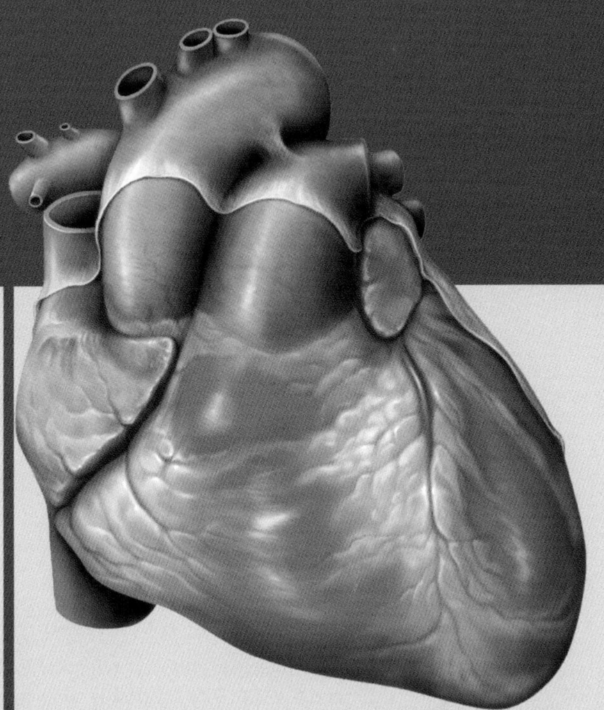

LEARNING OBJECTIVES

- Discuss the circuitry and hemodynamics of the cardiovascular system, including heart and vascular pressures, vascular compliance, and factors affecting blood flow and resistance.
- Discuss the electrophysiology of the heart, including excitation-contraction coupling, the fast- and slow-response action potentials, cardiac conduction system, and conduction velocities.
- Describe the parts of a typical electrocardiogram (ECG) trace and calculate the duration of the PR interval, QRS complex, and QT interval. Describe the 12 ECG leads, and interpret the rate, rhythm, and axis of an ECG trace to identify a conduction block or arrhythmia.
- Describe the phases of the cardiac cycle and pressure–volume loops, including the timing of heart sounds and murmurs. Discuss the jugular venous pulse relative to the right heart cardiac cycle. Identify the heart valve auscultation points on the chest and the common valve pathologies associated with abnormal heart sounds and murmurs.
- Discuss the interdependence of the cardiac and vascular systems by utilizing the cardiac-vascular function curves for changes to blood volume, inotropy, venous compliance, and arterial tone. Discuss Starling's Law of the heart. Describe the relationships between cardiac output, venous return, central venous pressure, and vascular resistance.
- Discuss the local control of microcirculations by hyperemia and autoregulation, particularly for the special circulations of the body. Describe the role of Starling forces in fluid exchange and lymph flow.
- Discuss mechanisms for control of blood pressure, including the baroreceptor reflex and the autonomic nervous system. Describe treatment mechanisms to control blood pressure.

5.1 Questions

Easy	Medium	Hard

1. Right heart catheterization of a 44-year-old man reveals normal right heart pressures. His right atrial pressure is between 2 and 6 mm Hg over 24 hours. Pulmonary arterial pressure is 24/8 mm Hg. Which of the following values is expected for his right ventricular pressure?

A. 30/10 mm Hg
B. 25/2 mm Hg
C. 25/10 mm Hg
D. 20/10 mm Hg
E. 20/2 mm Hg

2. A 38-year-old homeless woman with known alcoholic liver disease presents with melena (black, tarry feces). She initially responds well to intravenous saline administration, but when switched to fresh blood, she suddenly shows signs of decompensated liver cirrhosis and blood clots are passed per rectum. Aggressive fluid resuscitation fails to bring her systolic blood pressure above 100 mm Hg, so a central venous pressure (CVP) line is inserted, which measures a CVP of +1 cm H_2O with a manometer in the mid-axillary line. Which of the following has most likely caused the low CVP?

A. Overaggressive fluid resuscitation
B. Pulmonary artery stenosis
C. Pulmonary hypertension
D. Right-sided heart failure
E. Severe hypovolemia

3. A 1-year-old infant seems to be abnormally weak and frequently fatigued. Electrocardiography shows atrial flutter, and echocardiography reveals shortened chordae tendineae and thickened and sclerotic leaflets of the tricuspid valve. The complete blood count is normal. A rare congenital condition leading to tricuspid valve stenosis is diagnosed. Without treatment, which of the following is most likely present/expected in the near future in this patient?

A. Abdominal discomfort
B. Crackles in the lung
C. Pulmonary hypertension
D. Rheumatic fever
E. Right atrial myocyte wasting

4. In a given arteriolar blood vessel, the pressure is held constant and the radius is decreased. The resultant change in blood flow could also be accomplished by keeping pressure and radius constant and changing which of the following?

A. Decreasing compliance
B. Decreasing flow path length
C. Decreasing resistance
D. Increasing fluid density
E. Increasing viscosity

5. In a laboratory experiment, a blood vessel is perfused with saline at a constant flow rate. The driving pressure along the vessel is 32 mm Hg. After the application of a vasodilator, the vessel radius doubles. Assuming all other hemodynamic parameters are constant, what new driving pressure (in mm Hg) is required to keep the flow rate constant?

A. 2
B. 4
C. 8
D. 16
E. 32

6. The following illustration depicts a vascular bed consisting of vessels organized both in series and parallel. The resistance of each vessel (R_1–R_5) is indicated. The pressure at point A is 80 mm Hg and the pressure at point D is 31 mm Hg. What is the flow (in mL/min) through the system (point A to point D)?

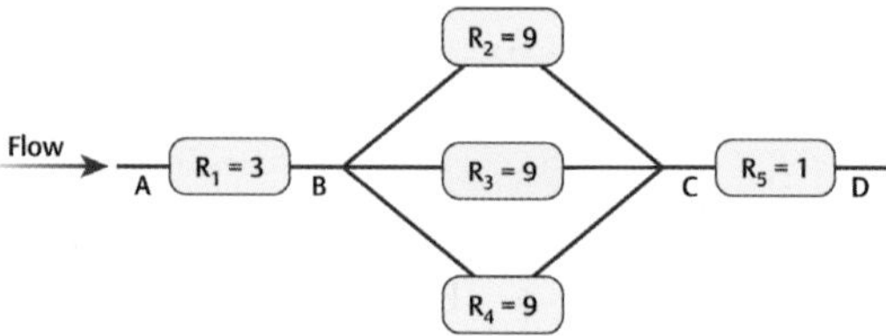

A. 3
B. 7
C. 10
D. 18
E. 20

7. The following illustration shows interconnected capillary beds. If the resistances R_1 through R_6 are equal in magnitude, and flow is constant, which statement about total resistance in Region A and Region B is correct?

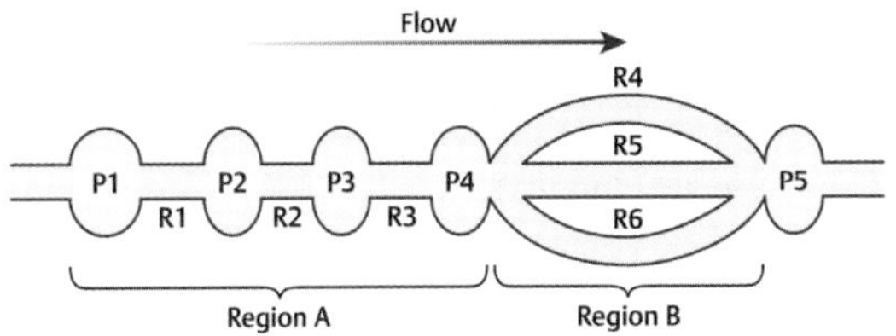

A. A equals B.
B. A is greater than B.
C. A is less than B.

8. In a 40-week old fetus, pulmonary artery pressure is 50 mm Hg and pulmonary vascular resistance is 0.4 mm Hg/mL/min/kg. After the baby is born at term, pulmonary blood flow doubles, and pulmonary artery pressure decreases 2.5-fold. Which of the following is closest to the pulmonary vascular resistance (in mm Hg/mL/min/kg) after birth?

A. 1.00
B. 0.80
C. 0.10
D. 0.04
E. 0.08

9. A 75-year-old man with no serious health complaints is scheduled for a routine cardiovascular checkup. What is expected for his arterial compliance as compared to a healthy 25-year-old man, and what effect will this have on his arterial pressure and cardiac work?

	Change in arterial compliance with age	Effect of compliance change on arterial pressure	Effect of compliance change on cardiac work
A.	↓	↓	↓
B.	↓	↑	↑
C.	↑	↔	↑
D.	↓	↑	↓
E.	↑	↓	↓

10. A patient at rest is given a drug that reduces venous compliance but has no other cardiac or vascular effects. What effect will this drug have on venous return and venous blood capacity?

	Venous return	Venous blood capacity
A.	↓	↑
B.	↓	↓
C.	↓	↔
D.	↑	↑
E.	↑	↓
F.	↑	↔

11. The graph shown depicts two compliance curves for the same vein measured at different times. Which of the following conditions or physiologic changes might cause curve 2 to shift toward curve 1?

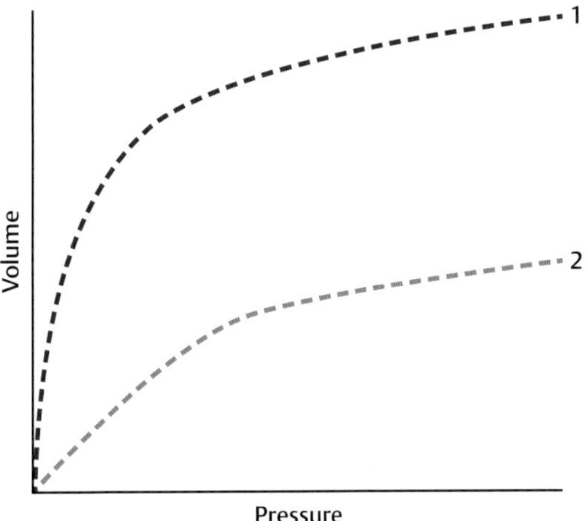

A. Hemorrhage
B. Normal aging
C. Reduced venous tone
D. Sympathetic activation
E. Venous wall calcification

12. A 6-year-old girl is dehydrated due to diarrhea and vomiting for 24 hours. Which of the following volume changes in splanchnic veins and systemic circulation are expected in order to maintain mean circulatory filling pressure?

	% Volume in splanchnic veins	% Volume in systemic circulation
A.	↓	↑
B.	↓	↓
C.	↓	↔
D.	↑	↑
E.	↑	↓
F.	↑	↔

13. An athlete training for a marathon is suspected to have received illegal erythropoietin injections to increase his red blood cell count. If true, which of the following hemodynamic parameters is expected to be decreased?

A. Blood pressure
B. Blood vessel length
C. Capillary blood flow
D. Radius of capacitance vessels
E. Radius of resistance vessels

14. In the systemic circulatory system, as blood flows from arteries to capillaries, what changes occur to the total cross-sectional area of the blood vessels, the velocity of blood flow, and the mean blood pressure?

	Total cross-sectional area	Velocity of blood flow	Mean blood pressure
A.	↑	↑	↑
B.	↑	↓	↑
C.	↑	↓	↓
D.	↓	↓	↓
E.	↓	↓	↑
F.	↓	↑	↑

15. Which of the following are correct features of the pulmonary artery compared to the aorta?

	Pressure in pulmonary vessel	Pulmonary compliance	Pulmonary resistance	Pulmonary capillary flow rate
A.	↑	↑	↓	↓
B.	↓	↑	↓	↓
C.	↓	↑	↓	↔
D.	↓	↓	↑	↔
E.	↑	↓	↑	↔
F.	↑	↓	↑	↓

16. A 56-year-old woman with a history of hyperlipidemia and hypertension is admitted to the emergency room because of shortness of breath and fatigue. She admits that climbing stairs is especially tiring and that she coughs a lot. Her resting heart rate is 142 beats per minute; her arterial blood pressure is 100/70 mm Hg. Bilateral auscultation reveals crackles of the lungs. Heart sound examination reveals an S3 gallop. Her belly is bulged at the flanks, and the percussion sound changes when she is turned to the side. Additionally, there is pitting ankle edema. She is diagnosed with congestive heart failure. Over a year's time, lifestyle changes and pharmacologic therapy help to restore her values towards normal. Which of the following changes to cardiac output and central venous pressure are most likely observed at her recovered state in comparison to her previous symptomatic state?

	Cardiac output	Central venous pressure
A.	↓	↓
B.	↓	↑
C.	↓	↔
D.	↑	↓
E.	↑	↑
F.	↑	↔

17. A medical student builds a model to better understand the relationship between blood vessel arrangement and hemodynamic properties. The student connects four identical tubes (A, B, C, D) in parallel to an inlet tube X and an outlet tube Y and fills the system with a fluid that has a viscosity similar to blood. A pressure gradient is applied between X and Y, which causes a laminar flow of 1 L/min. Which of the following is a correct statement in regards to each tube (A to D), when the pressure gradient is doubled by increasing the pressure in X while the pressure in Y remains constant and the flow remains laminar?

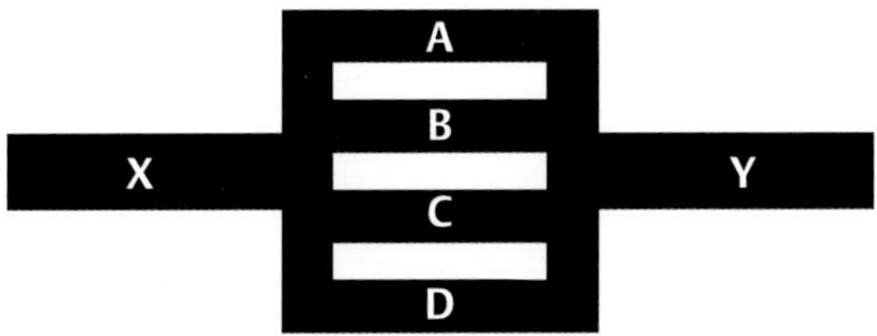

A. Circumferential wall stress will be half.

B. Fluid shear stress will be half.

C. Fluid velocity will be half.

D. Flow rate will be double.

E. Resistance will be one-sixteenth.

18. A 25-year-old man sustained a knife wound to the groin. He received stitches to the wound and was treated with fluids to compensate for blood loss. One month later, he seems to have recovered. He does not complain about any symptoms such as fatigue or difficulty breathing, even with moderate activity. SpO_2 is 98%. However, imaging shows that he developed an arteriovenous shunt between the iliac artery and vein. As a result, which of the following will most likely be decreased in his systemic circulation?

A. Arterial blood pressure

B. Arterial pulse pressure

C. Blood velocity in the shunt

D. Circulation time

E. Turbulence in the shunt

5.2 Answers and Explanations

Easy	Medium	Hard

1. 25/2 mm Hg (B)

Since blood flows down a pressure gradient, from higher to lower pressure, the systolic pressure in the right ventricle needs to be higher than the systolic pressure of 24 mm Hg in the pulmonary artery, so that blood is carried from the heart to the lungs. This excludes choices D and E. On the other hand, the diastolic pressure in the right ventricle needs to be lower than the right atrial pressure of 2–6 mm Hg, so that mixed venous blood can flow into the right ventricle through an open tricuspid valve. During this time, a closed pulmonic valve prevents the backflow from the higher pulmonary artery pressure of 8 mm Hg to the lower pressure of 2 mm Hg in the right ventricle. (**A**, **C**, **D**) The diastolic pressure is not low enough for the right ventricle to fill, and in choice D the systolic pressure is additionally too low to make the blood flow into the pulmonary artery. (**E**) The systolic and diastolic pressures are too low for the right ventricle to empty and fill.

2. Correct: Severe hypovolemia (E)

Severe hypovolemia (most likely as a result of gastrointestinal bleeding and liver failure) leads to low venous return and low central venous pressure (CVP), which is used clinically as an indicator of low right atrial pressure and low cardiac preload. When measured manually with a manometer, it is recorded as centimeters of water column. Normal values are between 4 and 12 cm H_2O. (**A**) Aggressive fluid administration is crucial during active hemorrhage and is not the cause of low CVP. It should be avoided *after* the hemorrhage has subsided to avoid further bleeding. (**B**, **C**, **D**) Pulmonary artery stenosis, pulmonary hypertension, and right-sided heart failure all lead to venous congestion and elevated CVP.

3. Correct: Abdominal discomfort (A)

A stenotic tricuspid valve obstructs flow from the right atrium to the right ventricle. If untreated, it results in increased volume in the venous circulation, which will lead to increased pressure due to vessel wall responses such as thickening and fibrosis, and, eventually, right heart failure. When the hydrostatic pressure exceeds the oncotic pressure, progressively painful abdominal fluid accumulation and ascites would be expected. (**B**) Crackles in the lung indicate pulmonary congestion, which is a result of left ventricular, not right ventricular failure. (**C**) Blood flow to the pulmonary vasculature is hindered, and one expects decreased (not increased) pulmonary blood flow. (**D**) While rheumatic fever is a common cause of tricuspid valve stenosis, the child has a rare congenital valve malformation. Normal blood cell count rules out infection. (**E**) One would expect right atrial myocyte hypertrophy (not wasting) due to the increased blood volume and transmural pressure.

4. Correct: Increasing viscosity (E)

Decreasing blood vessel radius at a given pressure decreases blood flow, which can also be achieved by increasing blood viscosity. This is primarily done by increased hematocrit. (**A**) Blood vessel compliance is not directly related to blood flow. (**B**) Flow path length is inversely related to flow, so that a longer (not a shorter) vessel would have a lower flow rate. (**C**) Resistance opposes flow, so that increasing (not decreasing) resistance would decrease flow. (**D**) Arteriolar fluid density is mainly determined by the plasma protein concentration, and protein changes have no significant impact on flow rate.

5. Correct: 2 (A)

Based on the Poiseuille equation (see image), vascular flow is proportional to the fourth power of the radius. If the radius of a vessel is doubled (e.g., from 1 to 2) with no other hemodynamic changes, then flow increases 16-fold, as can be seen in the following calculation: If a vessel radius is 1, then the flow rate $r = 1^4 = 1 \times 1 \times 1 \times 1 = 1$. If the radius doubles to 2, $r = 2^4 = 2 \times 2 \times 2 \times 2 = 16$. So, if flow rate increases 16-fold, then driving pressure must decrease 16-fold to keep flow constant, or 32 mm Hg/16 = 2 mm Hg. (**B, C, D, E**) These choices do not include the correct driving pressure to keep flow constant.

$$\text{Flow rate} = \frac{\pi(\text{driving pressure})\text{radius}^4}{8(\text{blood viscosity})(\text{vessel length})}$$

6. Correct: 7 (B)

Use the bulk flow equation (flow = driving pressure/resistance) to solve this problem:

Driving pressure = Pressure at point A – Pressure at point D = 80 – 31 = 49 mm Hg.
Resistance from A to B = 3 mm Hg × min × mL^{-1}
Resistance from B to C = 1/(1/9 + 1/9 + 1/9) = 1/(3/9) = 1/(1/3) = 3 mm Hg × min × mL^{-1}
Resistance from C to D = 1 mm Hg × min × mL^{-1}
Total resistance = 3 + 3 + 1 = 7 mm Hg × min × mL^{-1}
Flow = Driving pressure/Resistance = 49 mm Hg/(7 mm Hg × min × mL^{-1}) = 7 mL/min

(**A, C, D, E**) These are incorrect values.

7. Correct: A is greater than B. (B)

If each of the resistances were to be 1, then the total resistance of region A would be 3, and the total resistance of region B would be 1/3, so the resistance of region A is greater than that of region B. When resistances are in series, total resistance is the sum of the individual resistances ($R_{total} = R_1 + R_2 + R_3 = 1 + 1 + 1 = 3$). When resistances are arranged in parallel, total resistance is calculated as follows: $1/R_{total} = 1/R_4 + 1/R_5 + 1/R_6 = 1/1 + 1/1 + 1/1 = 3/1$, or $R_{total} = 1/3$. (**A, C**) These are incorrect statements.

8. Correct: 0.08 (E)

In the fetus, pulmonary blood flow is 125 mL/min/kg (50 mm Hg divided by 0.4 mm Hg/mL/min/kg), which doubles to 250 mL/min/kg in the newborn. Pulmonary artery pressure decreases 2.5-fold, from 50 mm Hg to 20 mm Hg. Hence, pulmonary vascular resistance is 0.08 (20 mm Hg divided by 250 mL/min/kg). The decrease in pulmonary vascular resistance due to lung expansion at birth allows pulmonary blood flow to increase and oxygen exchange to occur in the lungs. (**A, B, C, D**) These are incorrect values.

9. Correct: ↓, ↑, ↑ (B)

In healthy sedentary people, arterial compliance progressively reduces by about half between the ages of 25 and 75. Based on the formula for volume compliance ($C = \Delta V/\Delta P$), for a given stroke volume, arterial pressure is increased when compliance is reduced. Increased arterial pressure leads to increased cardiac stroke work. (**A, D**) Decreased arterial compliance leads to hypertension and increased, not decreased, cardiac work, a common occurrence with increasing age. (**C, E**) With age, arteries become stiffer, which means that arterial compliance (the inverse of stiffness) is decreased (not increased or unchanged).

10. Correct: ↑, ↓ (E).

A reduction in venous compliance is due to an increase in venous tone, which acts like a "constriction" of the veins. Since veins hold ~ 60% of the total blood volume at rest (venous reservoir), a decrease in venous compliance will reduce the venous blood capacity by reducing the cross-sectional area within the veins, and thus drive a portion of the venous reservoir towards the heart, which increases central venous pressure. Increased central venous pressure increases cardiac output through the Frank-Starling mechanism, and this increase in total blood flow through the circulatory system increases venous return. (**A, B, C, D, F**) These choices do not include the correct changes produced by a decrease in venous compliance.

11. Correct: Reduced venous tone (C)

To shift from curve 2 toward curve 1, the vein must increase compliance, since curve 1 shows an increased slope compared to curve 2. By reducing venous tone, the vein relaxes and its compliance increases, so that it can hold a larger volume for a given change in pressure. (**A**) Hemorrhage will initiate a baroreceptor reflex that reduces venous tone in order to displace the venous reservoir into circulation. (**B**) During the normal aging process, venous compliance decreases, largely due to stiffening of the vessel walls. (**D**) Sympathetic activation will cause an increase in venous tone, which reduces compliance. (**E**) Calcification of the venous wall reduces venous compliance by stiffening the vessel wall.

12. Correct: ↓, ↑ (A)

Hypovolemia will initiate a baroreceptor response that will decrease venous compliance, especially of splanchnic and cutaneous veins due to their high α-adrenergic innervation. The splanchnic system contains about 20% of total blood volume and serves as the main reservoir of blood that easily can change volume to maintain filling pressure in the right heart. The mobilization of this venous reservoir enables adequate perfusion of all tissues in the body. In addition, Starling forces will increase reabsorption of fluid from the interstitial space, thus further compensating for the loss of blood volume. (**B**, **C**, **D**, **E**, **F**) These choices do not include the correct cardiovascular responses produced by hypovolemia.

13. Correct: Capillary blood flow (C)

Polycythemia increases blood viscosity, which will reduce capillary blood flow by increasing resistance. (**A**, **B**, **D**, **E**) Blood viscosity will have no direct impact on blood pressure, vessel length, radius of capacitance vessels (veins), or radius of resistance vessels (arterioles).

14. Correct: ↑, ↓, ↓ (C)

As blood flows from arteries to capillaries, the total cross-sectional area of the vessels increases due to massive branching of arterioles and capillaries. The velocity of blood flow decreases due to the smaller individual radius of the arterioles and capillaries. The mean blood pressure decreases due to the high cross-sectional area of the arterioles and capillaries. (**A**, **B**, **D**, **E**, **F**) These choices do not include the correct combination of answer choices.

15. Correct: ↓, ↑, ↓, ↔ (C)

The pulmonary artery operates at a lower pressure compared to the aorta. The pressure is enough for blood to flow to the lung, which provides low resistance due to primarily open capillary beds. The pulmonary artery has a higher compliance, since it can hold more blood at a lower pressure gradient. The pulmonary artery resistance is lower, since the vessel can open wider due to its higher compliance. Blood flow over a minute (flow rate) has to be equal to aortic blood flow since the pulmonary and systemic circulations are arranged in series. (**A**, **B**, **D**, **E**, **F**) These choices list one or more incorrect features of the pulmonary artery.

16. Correct: ↑, ↓ (D)

The woman's heart failed, leading to signs and symptoms of left-sided cardiac dysfunction (dyspnea on exertion, S3 gallop, pulmonary edema) and of right-sided cardiac dysfunction (leg edema, ascites). Her low arterial blood pressure points toward low left ventricular ejection fraction, supported by signs of hypoxia (tiredness). Although a multitude of problems perpetuated by body compensatory mechanisms are typically behind congestive heart failure, they have in common that cardiac output and venous return are low. Hence, the change from the symptomatic to the recovered state includes increase in cardiac output and decrease in central venous pressure. (**A**, **B**, **C**, **E**, **F**) These choices have one or more incorrect statements.

17. Correct: Flow rate will be double. (D)

Since the parallel tubes (A to D) are identical, each tube will carry one-fourth of the total flow. With a pressure gradient of 1 L/min, this will be 0.25 L/min, and with a pressure gradient of 2 L/min, it will be 0.5 L/min, or double the original flow. (**A**) Circumferential wall stress is proportional, at a given radius, to the transmural distending pressure, which is increased (not halved) with increased fluid pressure and unchanged outside pressure. (**B**) Fluid shear stress will be increased (not halved) due to a larger velocity difference between adjacent fluid layers. With double flow, the fluid velocity at the center of each tube will double, while the velocity right at the tube wall remains zero, so that the difference from layer to layer will increase. (**C**) Fluid velocity is proportional to flow rate, and hence will be double (not half). (**E**) The resistance of each tube is given, and without changing tube diameter, tube length, or fluid viscosity, resistance remains the same.

18. Correct: Circulation time (D)

The circulation time is decreased due to the increased blood velocity in the shunt. Velocity is increased due to increased flow as a result of the large pressure gradient between the iliac artery and vein. (**A, B**) The lack of hypoxemia (normal SpO_2) and hypoxia (no fatigue or difficulty breathing) indicates that he can maintain mean arterial blood pressure. To do so, the heart will need to contract more strongly, and systolic blood pressure will be high. Due to the decreased peripheral vascular resistance, diastolic blood pressure will be low. This increases (not decreases) arterial pulse pressure. (**C**) Blood velocity in the shunt is increased as explained in D. The total cross-sectional area at this level of the cardiovascular system might be unchanged or smaller, and hence either does not impact or increases (not decreases) blood velocity. (**E**) Turbulent flow in the shunt will not be decreased. Most likely, it is increased due to the increased blood velocity and the large vessel diameter, which increases the Reynolds number. A bruit or palpable thrill could confirm it.

5.3 Questions

19. Which of the following cells/structures require calcium influx for cell membrane depolarization at the threshold potential?

A. Atrioventricular (AV) nodal cells
B. Cardiac ventricular muscle cells
C. Nerve cell bodies
D. Presynaptic nerve terminals
E. Skeletal muscle cells

20. Cardiac sinoatrial (SA) node cells produce slow-response action potentials like that shown in the image. The upstroke in phase 0 is due to which of the following?

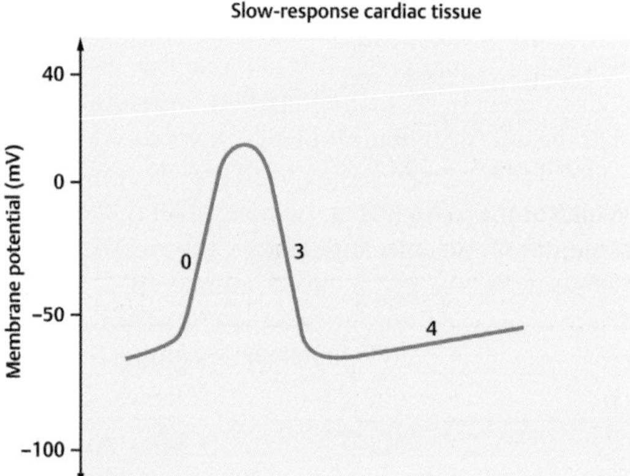

A. Influx of Ca^{2+}
B. Efflux of Ca^{2+}
C. Influx of K^+
D. Efflux of K^+
E. Influx of Na^+
F. Efflux of Na^+

21. The conduction pathway through the heart has a normal physiologic delay. In which of the following cardiac conduction tissues does this delay occur?

A. Atrioventricular node
B. Bundle of His
C. Bundle branches
D. Purkinje fibers
E. Sinoatrial node

22. The conduction velocities of cardiac action potentials are measured in a controlled setting at four different locations in the hearts of ten young healthy adults. The following average results are obtained:

Location 1: 0.035 m/s
Location 2: 0.931 m/s
Location 3: 1.980 m/s
Location 4: 4.152 m/s

Which of the following is the correct cardiac structure of each measured location?

	Location 1	Location 2	Location 3	Location 4
A.	AV node	Atrial myocytes	Bundle branches	Purkinje fibers
B.	AV node	Bundle branches	Atrial myocytes	Purkinje fibers
C.	AV node	Bundle branches	Ventricular myocytes	Purkinje fibers
D.	Atrial myocytes	Bundle branches	AV node	Ventricular myocytes
E.	Atrial myocytes	Purkinje fibers	Bundle branches	Ventricular myocytes

23. A 66-year-old man with hypertension is prescribed a drug that inhibits depolarization of the sinoatrial (SA) node of the heart, thereby decreasing impulse conduction of the atria and ventricles. What is the most likely mechanism of action of this drug?

A. β_1-adrenergic agonist
B. β_2-adrenergic antagonist
C. Funny (F) channel agonist
D. Voltage-dependent Ca^{2+} channel antagonist
E. Voltage-dependent K^+ channel antagonist
F. Voltage-dependent Na^+ channel agonist

24. A new antiarrhythmic drug was designed that partially inactivates fast voltage-gated sodium channels. Which of the following are the correct effects of this drug on the ventricular myocyte action potential (AP) in regard to its rate, upstroke velocity, and amplitude, as well as on the ventricular conduction velocity?

	AP rate	AP upstroke velocity	AP amplitude	Ventricular conduction velocity
A.	↓	↓	↓	↔
B.	↓	↔	↔	↔
C.	↓	↓	↓	↓
D.	↔	↓	↔	↓
E.	↔	↓	↓	↓

25. A patient is given a drug that shortens the duration of phase 4 of the slow-response action potential in the sinoatrial (SA) nodal conduction cells. Which of the following changes to the resultant cardiac contractions would most likely be produced from this drug?

A. Absence of atrial contractions
B. Absence of atrial and ventricular contractions
C. Decreased frequency of ventricular contractions
D. Decreased frequency of atrial and ventricular contractions
E. Increased frequency of atrial and ventricular contractions

26. A 12-year-old girl with paroxysmal supraventricular tachycardia is taught to monitor and interpret her heart rate on a smart watch. When an arrhythmic episode occurs, the girl is to stick her face into a bucket of cold water in order to lower the dangerously high heart rate. The mechanism of action of a successful intervention involves the decrease of which cardiac myocyte ion membrane permeability and affects which cardiac action potential?

	Ion with decreased membrane permeability	Type of affected cardiac action potential
A.	Calcium	Fast response
B.	Calcium	Slow response
C.	Potassium	Fast response
D.	Potassium	Slow response
E.	Sodium	Fast response
F.	Sodium	Slow response

Questions 27 to 29

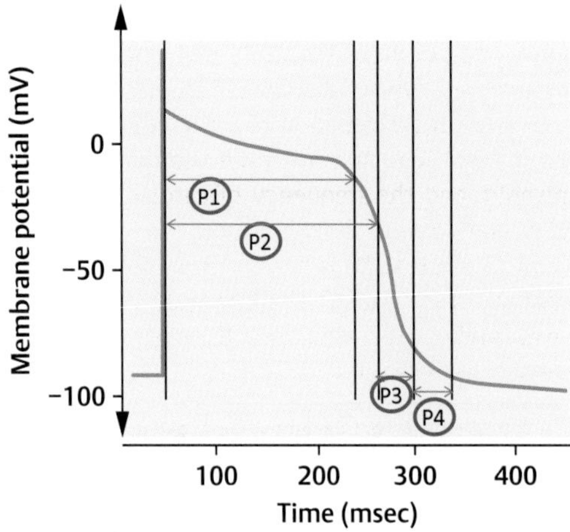

27. As part of a continuing medical education (CME) session for cardiologists, the presenter uses the figure of the ventricular cardiac action potential to explain how functional electrical reentry can lead to arrhythmias in a structurally normal heart. During which of the following periods (labeled P1–P4) of the cardiac action potential are ventricular cardiomyocytes responsive to atypical restimulation and initiation of functional reentry circuits?

A. P1 only
B. P2 only
C. P3 only
D. P4 only
E. P1 and P2
F. P2 and P3
G. P2 and P4
H. P3 and P4

28. Which of the following currents (I) across the ventricular cardiomyocyte plasma membrane best coincides with P4 of the action potential in the image?

A. I_{Ca}
B. I_{K1}
C. $I_{K\text{-}ACh}$
D. I_{Ks}
E. I_{to}

29. The image shows a typical action potential of a ventricular cardiac myocyte when stimulated at time zero. If the cell is stimulated again during the time labeled P3, how will the second action potential differ from the first?

A. Decreased length
B. Faster upstroke
C. No plateau phase
D. Reduced amplitude
E. Slower repolarization

30. Skeletal muscle tissue can undergo tetanic contractions, but cardiac muscle tissue cannot. In comparison to skeletal muscle, what mechanism prevents cardiac muscle tissue from producing a tetanic contraction?

A. Less intracellular Ca^{2+} accumulation
B. Longer absolute refractory period
C. Slower cross-bridge cycling rate
D. Slower decline of intracellular Ca^{2+}
E. Slower repetition rate of stimulation

5.4 Answers and Explanations

19. Correct: Atrioventricular (AV) nodal cells (A)

Atrioventricular (AV) nodal cells are conduction cells in the heart that produce a slow-response action potential. This type of action potential utilizes calcium influx through voltage-dependent, primarily L-type calcium channels for depolarization (as does the sinoatrial node). (**B, C, D, E**) Cardiac ventricular muscle cells, nerve cell bodies, presynaptic nerve terminals, and skeletal muscle cells all utilize sodium influx via fast sodium channels for cell membrane depolarization.

20. Correct: Influx of Ca^{2+} (A)

The upstroke of the slow-response action potential (AP), labeled phase 0, is produced by calcium influx through primarily voltage-dependent L-type calcium channels. (**B**) Phase 0 is produced by calcium influx, not efflux (**C, D**) Potassium efflux is responsible for phase 3 and contributes to phase 4 of the slow response AP. (**E, F**) Sodium influx through funny channels is important during phase 4 for the pacemaker potential (spontaneous depolarization) of conduction cells.

21. Correct: Atrioventricular node (A)

The atrioventricular (AV) node is the junction for conduction from the atria to the ventricles. The physiologic conduction delay occurs here to allow time for the atria to contract fully, and therefore fill the ventricles, before the conduction can spread to the ventricles and stimulate contraction. This provides efficient ventricular filling. (**B, C, D, E**) These conduction tissues do not have a physiologic delay.

22. Correct: AV node, atrial myocytes, bundle branches, Purkinje fibers (A)

Conduction velocity is slowest at the atrioventricular (AV) node, in order to complete atrial depolarization before ventricular depolarization. The velocities can vary between 0.01 and 0.05 m/s, since they are slower with parasympathetic and faster with sympathetic stimulation. Conduction velocity is fastest at the specialized conduction fibers of the heart (about 4 m/sec for Purkinje fibers and about 2 m/sec for bundle branches). Conduction velocities of contractile cells (atrial and ventricular myocytes) are about 1 m/sec, which is faster than the velocities of AV nodal cells and slower than the velocities of the special conduction fibers. (**B**, **C**, **D**, **E**) These choices do not correctly align conduction velocities with the indicated locations in the heart.

23. Correct: Voltage-dependent Ca^{2+} channel antagonist (D)

Depolarization of the sinoatrial (SA) node occurs via opening of voltage-dependent Ca^{2+} channels. A voltage-dependent Ca^{2+} channel antagonist will reduce the number of calcium channels that open, thus reducing the rate of depolarization of the SA node and the impulse conduction velocity of the atria and ventricles. (**A**) A β_1 adrenergic agonist will stimulate β_1 receptors, which are located in the SA node, and will increase impulse conduction of the SA node (not decrease). (**B**) A β_2 adrenergic antagonist will inhibit β_2 receptors, which are primarily located in the airways, and block airway dilation. (**C**) A funny channel agonist will stimulate I_f current, which will reduce the duration of phase 4 of the slow-phase action potential of the SA node, which will increase the rate of impulse conduction of the SA node. (**E**) A voltage-dependent K^+ channel antagonist will block K^+ channels and decrease the rate of depolarization. (**F**) A voltage-dependent Na^+ channel agonist will open more Na^+ channels for depolarization of cardiac muscle cells, but not the SA node, which is depolarized by Ca^{2+} influx.

24. Correct: ↔, ↓, ↓, ↓ (E)

The rate of the ventricular action potential (AP) is not affected because it is set by cardiac sinoatrial nodal cells, which do not have fast voltage-gated sodium channels. The ventricular cells will still create APs, since only a few responsible sodium channels are necessary to depolarize the ventricular cell membrane potential to reach threshold potential, after which an AP is automatically generated (all-or-none principle). The AP upstroke velocity (dV/dT) and the AP amplitude are decreased, since fewer activated channels decrease the size of the inward current per time. The ventricular conduction velocity is decreased, since it is directly related to dV/dT and the size of the inward current. With less inward current, there will be less local currents that spread to adjacent sites and depolarize them to threshold. (**A**, **B**, **C**, **D**) These answers have one or more incorrect choices.

25. Correct: Increased frequency of atrial and ventricular contractions (E)

The duration of Phase 4 of the slow-response action potential determines the frequency of contractions (heart rate). If the duration of phase 4 is shortened, then it takes less time to reach the depolarization threshold, and the frequency of cardiac (atrial and ventricular) contractions increases per minute, and vice versa. (**A**, **B**, **C**, **D**) A shorter phase 4 of the slow-response action potential will increase the number of atrial and ventricular contractions per minute, not decrease or block them.

26. Correct: Sodium, slow response (F)

A successful intervention for a tachycardic episode is that the cold-water immersion decreases the heart rate by stimulating the parasympathetic nervous system (PS). PS stimulation leads to the release of acetylcholine, which binds to M_2 receptors in the sinoatrial (SA) nodal cells and changes the shape and duration of their slow-response action potentials. It decreases the sodium permeability, leading to decreased I_f current and a decreased rate of phase 4 depolarization. (**A**, **C**, **E**) Heart rate is regulated at SA nodal cells, which express slow- (not fast-) response action potentials. (**B**) The PS does not alter the calcium membrane permeability. (**D**) The PS increases (not decreases) potassium membrane permeability, in addition to the changes in I_f just explained. Increased potassium permeability through K^+-ACh channels hyperpolarizes the membrane, which makes the tissue less excitable and hence leads to decreased heart rate.

27. Correct: P3 and P4 (H)

Functional reentry in a structurally normal heart is most likely when cardiac myocytes are restimulated during the relative refractory period (P3) and/or the supernormal period (P4) of their action potentials. During these times, sufficient voltage-gated sodium channels are available for another action potential to occur, and abnormal impulses can reenter the cardiac tissue and cause arrhythmias. For the supernormal period, action potential generation requires an even weaker stimulus than normal, since the membrane is still depolarized and hence closer to the threshold potential. (**A**) P1 is the absolute refractory period, when myocytes cannot initiate new action potentials under any circumstances. (**B**) P2 is the effective refractory period, when normally no new action potentials can be generated. (**C**, **D**) P3 and P4 are the relative refractory period and the supernormal period, respectively. By themselves, they are not the best answer, since they are both times when reentry circuits can start. (**E**, **F**, **G**) Each of these answers includes either the absolute or the effective refractory period, when reentry is impossible or highly unlikely.

28. Correct: I_{K1} (B)

During P4, inward rectifier channels open, causing a potassium outward current (I_{K1}) that contributes to the repolarization of the membrane potential. The full resting membrane potential has not been reached yet, so a cell can be restimulated with a slightly smaller than normal stimulus. This feature gives P4 its name: supernormal period. (**A**) Inward calcium current (I_{Ca}) is present during the cardiac action potential plateau phase and best coincides with P1 and P2. (**C**) The potassium outward current $I_{K\text{-}ACh}$ is part of the sinoatrial (not the ventricular) cell action potential. It is present when acetylcholine binds to membrane receptors and initiates G-protein signaling that leads to the opening of the channel. (**D**) I_{Ks} is an outward rectifying current through potassium channels that open during the plateau and early repolarization phases of the cardiac action potential, so that the current coincides with late P2 and early P3 of the figure. The "s" stands for "slow," because the channels respond more slowly to depolarization than the fast voltage-gated Na^+ channels. (**E**) I_{to} is a transient outward current through potassium channels that cause the first repolarization of the cardiac action potential following the upstroke. It marks the beginning of P1 and P2.

29. Correct: Reduced amplitude (D)

When a ventricular myocyte is restimulated during the relative refractory period (P3 of the image), many Na^+ channels are still inactivated. The resultant smaller-than-normal Na^+ current leads to an action potential (AP) with reduced amplitude. The earlier the stimulus occurs (beginning versus end of P3), the lower the amplitude. (**A**) APs that were initiated during P3 might be slightly longer, because the smaller number of available Na^+ channels leads to a slower rate of rise of the upstroke. However, AP length is primarily affected by the length of the plateau phase and the rate of repolarization. (**B**) The rate of rise of the AP (dV/dT) depends on the number of available Na^+ channels, and a smaller Na^+ inward current leads to a slower (not faster) upstroke. (**C**) The AP plateau phase depends on the balance between inward Ca^{2+} and outward K^+ currents, not the availability of Na^+ channels. (**E**) Repolarization is due to greater outward than inward currents, so that a smaller Na^+ current would cause faster (not slower) repolarization. However, the impact of early AP changes on late AP events is not easily predictable because of the complexity of the involved currents.

30. Correct: Longer absolute refractory period (B)

The long absolute refractory period (ARP) in cardiac muscle is due to the action potential (AP) plateau phase generated primarily by calcium influx. Since the ARP lasts nearly as long as the muscle contraction itself, the membrane is capable of being stimulated again only after twitch force has fallen nearly completely. This means that tetanic contraction is prevented despite the functional syncytium of the heart muscle. In skeletal muscle, the duration of the AP is much shorter than the duration of the muscle twitch contraction. Thus, the membrane is capable of generating another AP before the twitch force of the first stimulus has decayed. (**A, C, D**) The rise of intracellular Ca^{2+} at the beginning of the twitch, the rate of cross-bridge cycling, and the decline of intracellular Ca^{2+} at the end of the twitch contraction are comparable in skeletal and cardiac muscle tissue, or at least not responsible for the different means of force gradation. (**E**) Stimulation frequency can increase to over 300 stimuli per minute in cardiac muscle, so the repetition rate of stimulation is not the limiting factor.

5.5 Questions

31. Which of the following electrocardiographic leads will produce a positive (upward) net QRS-wave deflection if a wave of depolarization is moving through the heart as depicted by the arrow on the image?

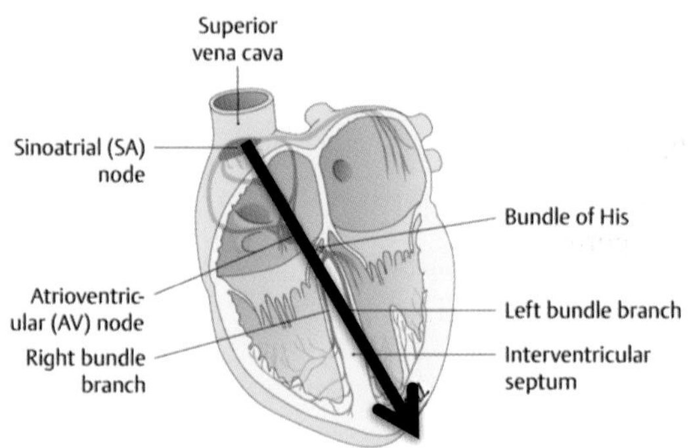

A. II, III, aVR, and V1
B. I, III, V1, and V2
C. I, II, aVR, and V2
D. II, aVF, V4, and V5

32. The cell-to-cell conduction of a wave of depolarization through the atrioventricular (AV) nodal cells of the heart occurs during which segment or interval of the electrocardiogram (ECG) trace?

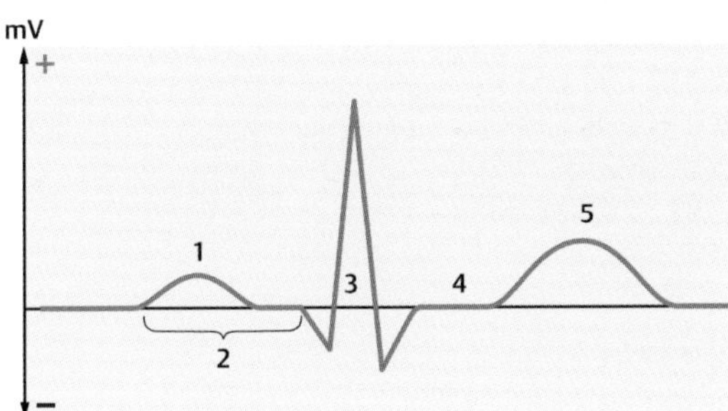

A. 1
B. 2
C. 3
D. 4
E. 5

33. During a semiannual exam, the electrocardiogram (ECG) recording of a trained athlete reveals a cardiac arrhythmia shown in the following trace. The abnormality seen in this lead II trace is due to a change in which of the following electrical event(s) in the heart?

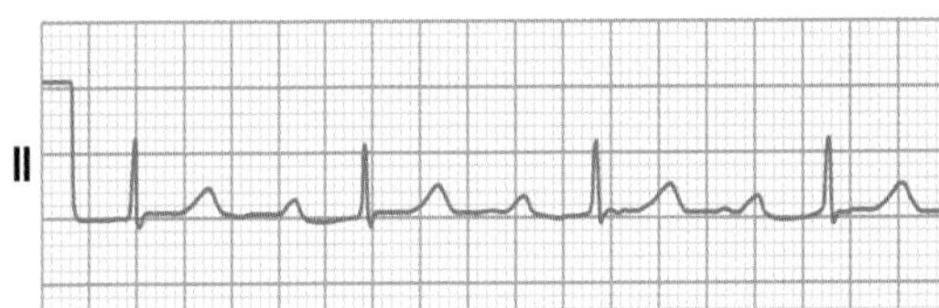

A. Atrial depolarization
B. Atrial repolarization
C. Atrioventricular (AV) conduction time
D. Ventricular depolarization
E. Ventricular repolarization

34. A normal electrocardiogram (ECG) trace of one cardiac cycle, and a normal recording of one ventricular action potential, are shown. The wave on the ECG trace marked with a star most closely corresponds to which phase of the ventricular action potential?

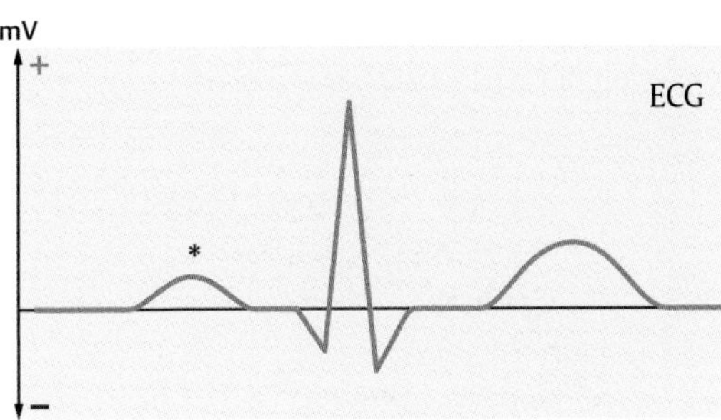

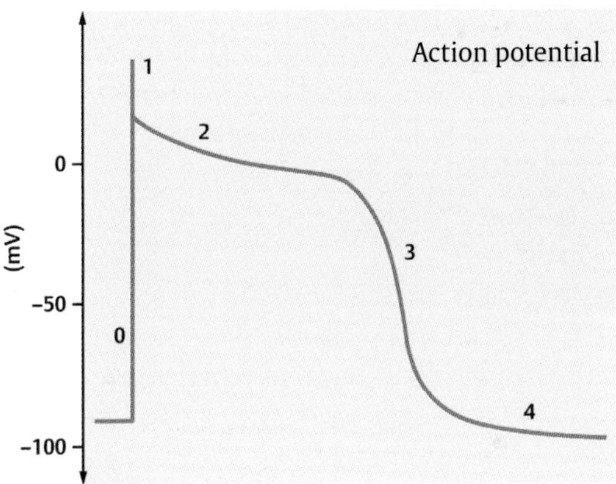

A. Phase 0
B. Phase 1
C. Phase 2
D. Phase 3
E. Phase 4
F. Event is not visible

35. In a healthy person with a heart rate of 60 beats per minute, which of the following periods in the electrocardiogram (ECG) would be the longest?

A. P wave
B. P-R interval
C. QRS complex
D. Q-T interval
E. T wave

36. In low-voltage electrical accidents with more than 45 mA of electricity reaching the heart, circulatory collapse due to ventricular fibrillation is the main cause of death. The probability for random desynchronization of the myocardium is highest when the electrical signal arrives at the myocardium during the vulnerable phase of the cardiac cycle. This phase corresponds with which of the following waves on the electrocardiogram (ECG)?

A. P

B. Q

C. R

D. S

E. T

37. A 61-year-old man with a previous myocardial infarction presents with shortness of breath and fatigue. An electrocardiogram is ordered. The trace reveals wide QRS complexes in all leads. Which of the following changes to cardiac innervation or conduction is most likely responsible for the wide QRS complexes?

A. Decreased parasympathetic innervation to the heart

B. Decreased conduction rate along the bundle branches

C. Decreased conduction rate from the SA node to the AV node

D. Sinus bradycardia

E. Sinus tachycardia

38. A 58-year-old woman complains of shortness of breath on exertion. An electrocardiogram (ECG) is ordered and her lead I trace is shown. Which of the following waves, segments, or intervals on her ECG trace is outside of the normal range?

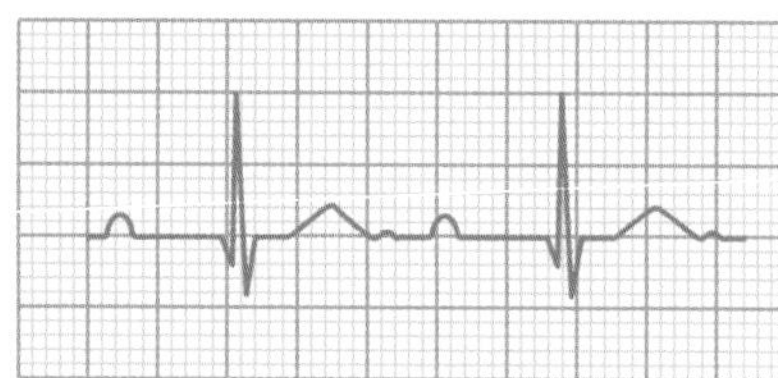

A. P wave

B. P-R interval

C. QRS complex

D. ST segment

E. Q-T interval

39. A 3-year-old boy with a congenital pulmonary artery stenosis has right ventricular hypertrophy. Which of the following QRS mean electrical axes is most consistent with this diagnosis?

A. –70°

B. –40°

C. 0°

D. +50°

E. +110°

40. A 48-year-old male with a history of hypertension presents with shortness of breath for the past 5 days, especially at night while lying flat. A 12-lead electrocardiogram (ECG) is ordered, and the results are shown. Based on the ECG results, what is the man's approximate QRS mean electrical axis?

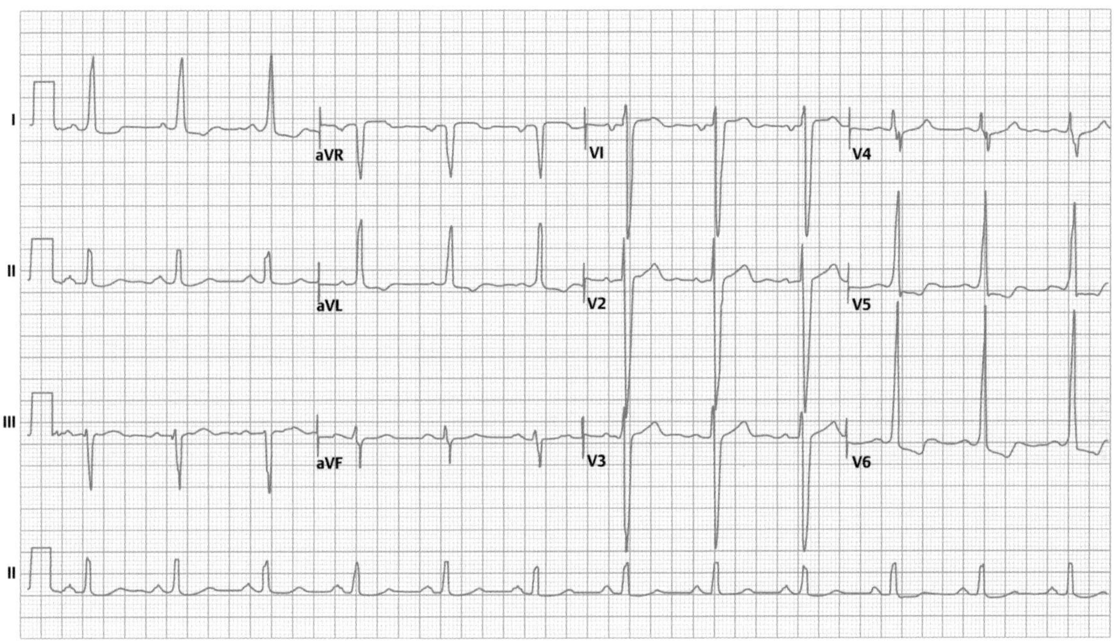

A. –60°
B. –30°
C. 0°
D. +30°
E. +60°

41. The wife of an elderly man, who is recovering normally in the hospital from surgery, nervously shouts for help. She reports that she just looked at the cardiac monitor for the first time and saw that the electrocardiogram (ECG) looks "tiny" and "almost flat." The responding resident does not see any signs of patient distress. The ECG shows sinus rhythm. When the ECG is switched from the currently displayed lead I to leads II or III, the R wave amplitudes increase and are both about the same height. When the ECG is switched to aVF, the R waves are taller than in leads I, II, and III. Which of the following will the resident physician most likely do next?

A. Ask the family member to continue watching
B. Call emergency code blue
C. Consult a cardiologist
D. Explain that the patient's heart is beating normally
E. Explain that occasional ECG oddities are normal
F. Form a rapid response team

42 A 57-year-old male reports to the emergency department with complaints of chest pain, particularly discomfort near his sternum, and says it reminds him of a prior myocardial infarction 5 years ago. A 12-lead electrocardiogram (ECG) is recorded and is shown. Which of the following cardiac irregularities can be determined from the patient's ECG?

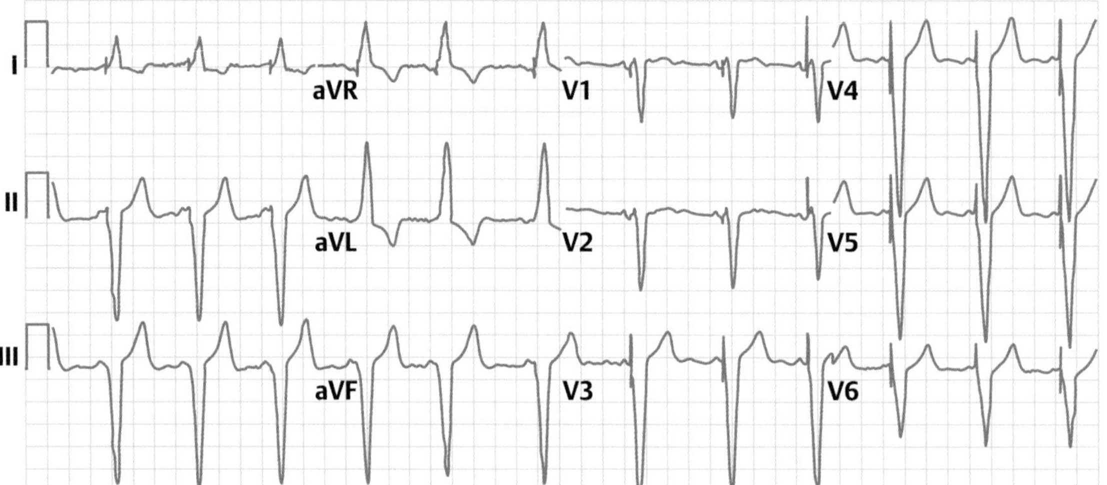

A. Left axis deviation
B. Right axis deviation
C. Right ventricular hypertrophy
D. Sinus bradycardia
E. Sinus tachycardia

43. Which of the following electrocardiogram (ECG) traces shows a regularly irregular rhythm?

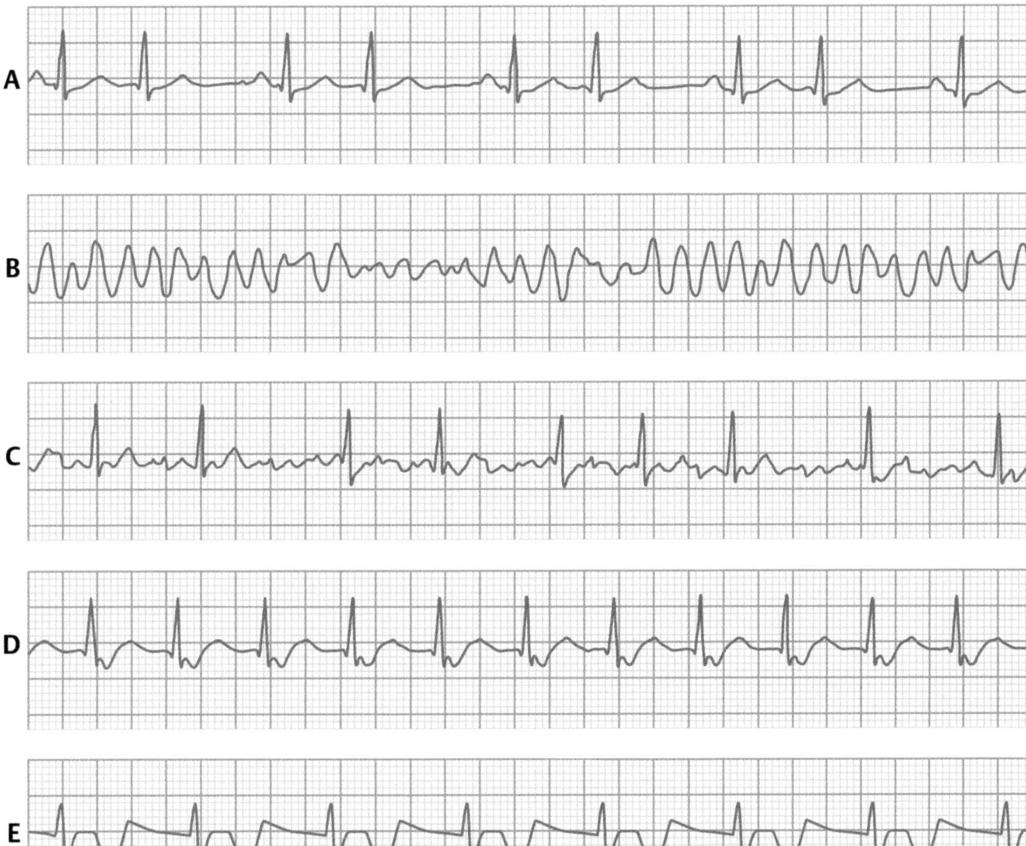

A. A
B. B
C. C
D. D
E. E

44. A 49-year-old smoker with uncontrolled hypertension presents with complaints of shortness of breath for 2 hours, and an electrocardiogram (ECG) is ordered. The results are shown. The patient is diagnosed with atrial flutter. What are this patient's approximate atrial and ventricular heart rates in beats per minute?

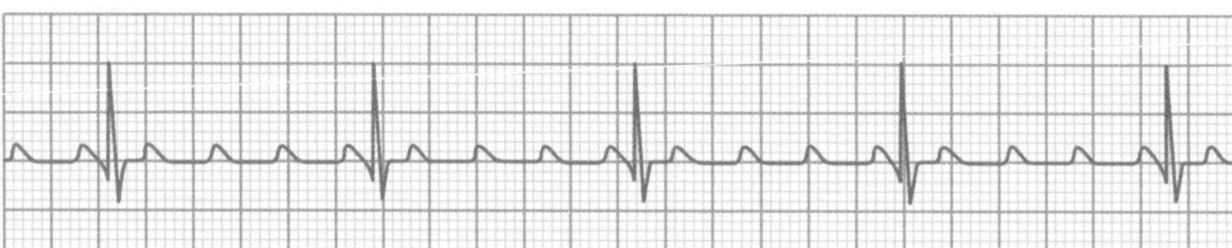

	Atrial heart rate (bpm)	Ventricular heart rate (bpm)
A.	215	100
B.	215	75
C.	215	55
D.	150	100
E.	150	75
F.	150	55
G.	100	100
H.	100	75
I.	100	55

45. A patient presents with complaints of a "racing heart" and "lightheadedness." The symptoms come and go and last for 30 to 60 minutes. The patient experiences such an episode while wearing a 24-hour Holter monitor, which leads to the diagnosis of atrial fibrillation. Which of the following electrocardiogram (ECG) strips belongs to the patient?

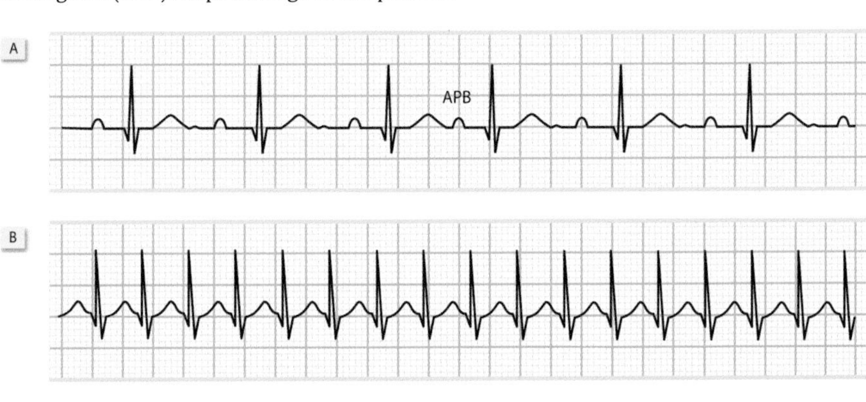

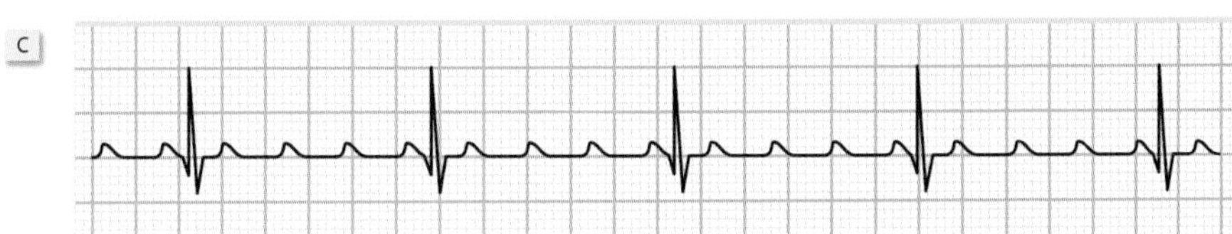

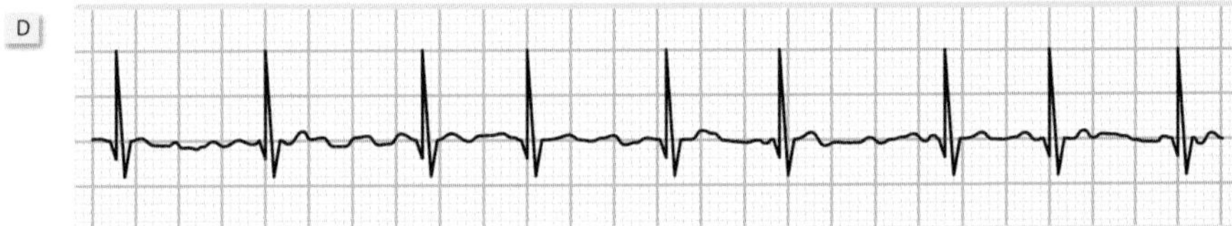

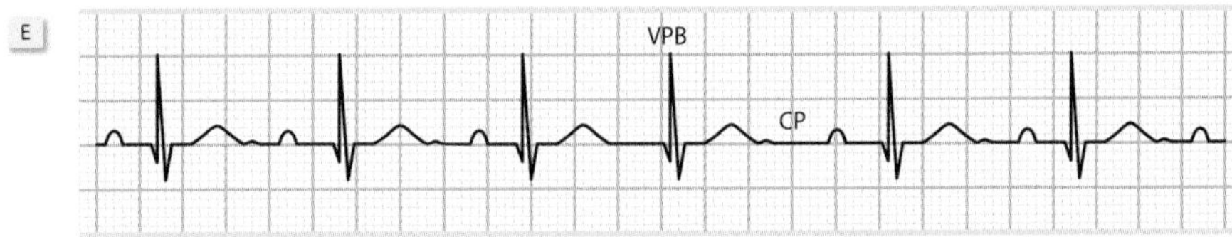

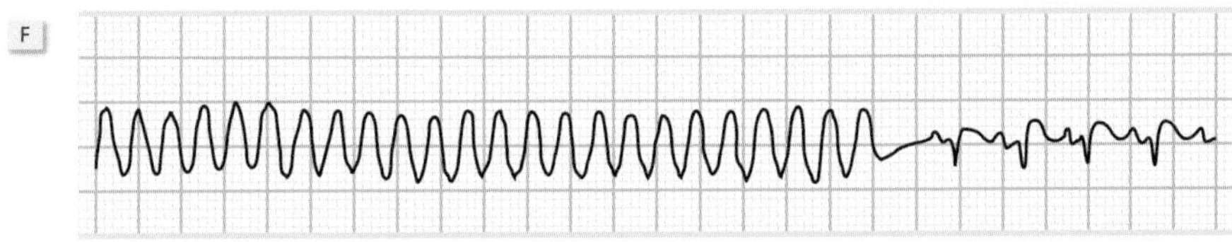

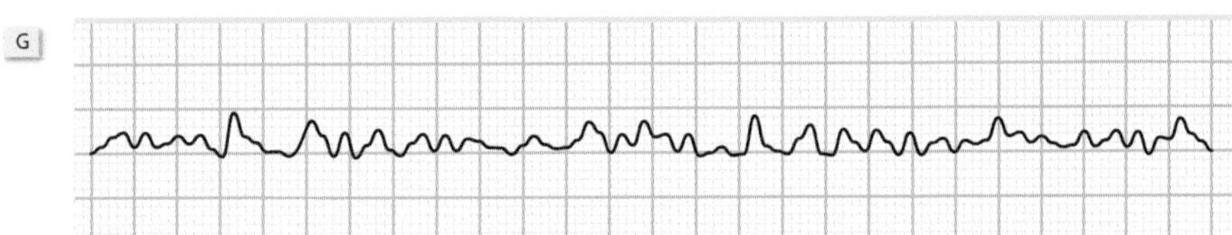

A. A
B. B
C. C
D. D
E. E
F. F
G. G

46. A 13-year-old girl presents with recurrent episodes of syncope, which are induced by bending over (e.g., to tie her shoes). Her electrocardiogram (ECG) reveals a short P-R interval and a delta wave. Based on her presentation, her symptoms are most likely caused by abnormal accessory conduction pathways through which structure of the heart?

A. Atrial septum

B. Atrioventricular node

C. Atrioventricular ring

D. Heart valves

E. Ventricular septum

47. A 53-year-old woman presents at the primary care facility with a chief complaint of tiredness. As part of the differential diagnosis, an electrocardiogram (ECG) is obtained. It shows a normal sinus rhythm with no missed beats, a QRS complex of 110 milliseconds, and a P-R interval of 320 milliseconds. The point-of-care ultrasound shows no signs of left ventricular hypertrophy. The patient is referred to a cardiologist, and her current list of medications is checked. At this time, which of the following drug categories is of least concern for further aggravating her heart condition?

A. Angiotensin-converting enzyme (ACE) inhibitors

B. β blockers

C. Calcium channel blockers

D. Cholinergic stimulants

E. Cholinesterase inhibitors

48. At a routine 2-month checkup, a mother tells the pediatrician that her infant sometimes becomes lethargic and breathes fast and shallow during feeding. The child is referred for cardiovascular assessment, which includes wearing a Holter monitor for 72 hours. The electrocardiogram (ECG) from the Holter monitor during one of the episodes is shown. Which of the following is the most likely cause of the tachycardic episode?

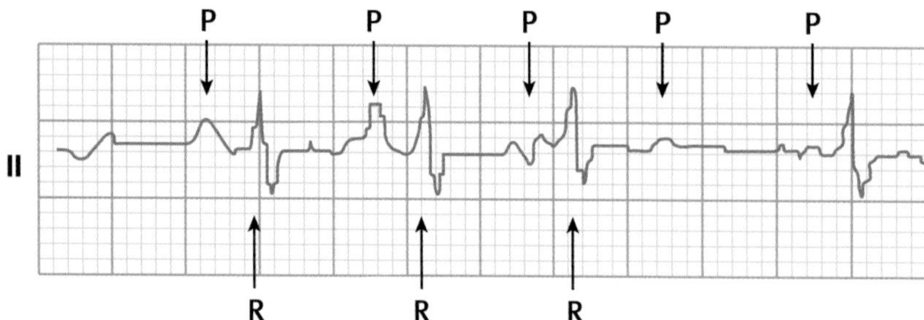

A. Atrial flutter

B. Ectopic atrial tachycardia

C. Enhanced ventricular automaticity

D. Premature ventricular beats

E. Sinus tachycardia

49. Which of the provided images is correctly labeled for the electrode placement and polarity of the three standard limb leads?

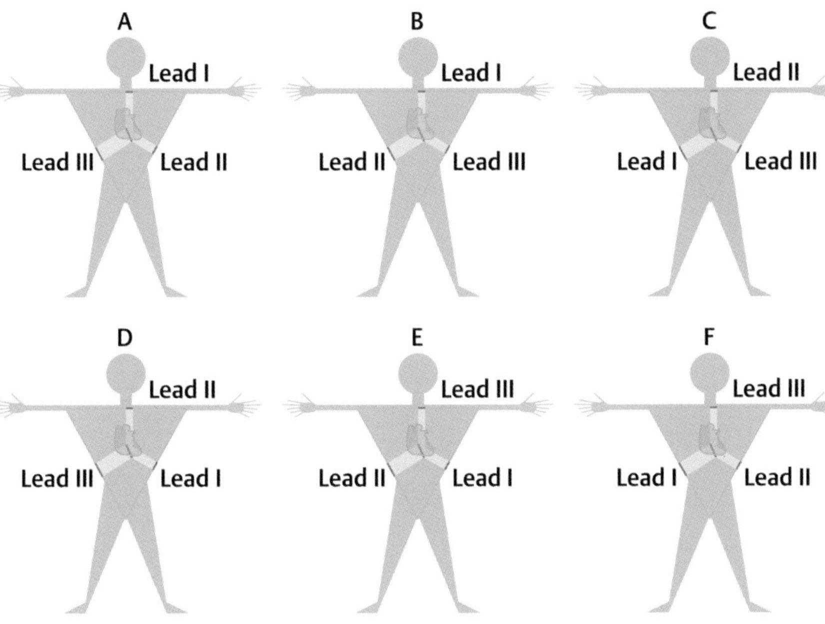

A. A
B. B
C. C
D. D
E. E
F. F

50. A 53-year-old man presents with chest pain on exertion that resolves after a few minutes of rest. He has been experiencing this for two months. He describes the pain as a "squeezing" sensation that sometimes radiates towards his neck and jaw. In which of the following conditions is this clinical presentation most consistent?

A. Anxiety disorder
B. Myocardial infarction
C. Myocarditis
D. Pleuritis
E. Stable angina

51. A 71-year-old male presents to the emergency department half an hour after beginning to experience chest pain on exertion. He describes it as "an elephant is sitting on his chest." His electrocardiogram shows ST segment elevation. Which of the following biomarkers is the earliest to rise in serum after an acute myocardial infarction (MI)?

A. Cardiac troponin
B. Creatine kinase-MB
C. Creatine kinase-MM
D. Lactate dehydrogenase
E. Myoglobin

52. A 50-year-old woman presents with shortness of breath upon exertion for 1 month. Electrocardiogram (ECG) reveals a heart block. During a procedure to implant a pacemaker, the following data are collected:

Heart rate = 80 beats/min
Left ventricular end diastolic volume = 110 mL
Left ventricular end systolic volume = 60 mL
Right atrial pressure = 4 mm Hg
Wedge pressure = 2 mm Hg

What is the cardiac output (L/min) of the patient?

A. 3
B. 4
C. 6
D. 8
E. 9

53. A 31-year-old man is in the cardiac intensive care unit due to complications from excessive and long-term methamphetamine use. His cardiac index is 1.9 L/min/m^2, which is significantly lower than the value recorded in his medical record 2 years ago. Considering only the given information, which of the following could have caused this change in his cardiac index?

A. He had myocardial infarcts.
B. He has lost weight.
C. His heart is racing.
D. He is sweating extensively.
E. His limb has been amputated.

5.6 Answers and Explanations

31. Correct: II, aVF, V4, and V5 (D)

As a wave of depolarization moves toward the positive end of an electrode, it produces an upward deflection on the electrocardiogram (ECG) trace. Therefore, since the depolarization wave is moving downward and leftward through the heart, any lead with the positive electrode inferior or left of the heart will produce a net upward deflection. The positive electrodes of leads II and aVF are on the foot, and the positive electrode of leads V4 and V5 are near the apex of the heart (all inferior to the heart). Thus, each of these leads will produce a net positive (upward) deflection on the ECG trace. (**A**) In this group of leads, the positive electrode of the aVR lead is on the right arm, so it will produce a net negative deflection for this wave of depolarization. (**B**) In this group of leads, the positive electrode of leads V1 and V2 are on the chest wall to the right of the heart, so they will produce a net negative deflection for this wave of depolarization. (**C**) aVR and V2 will produce net negative deflections, for reasons explained in answers A and B.

32. Correct: 2 (B)

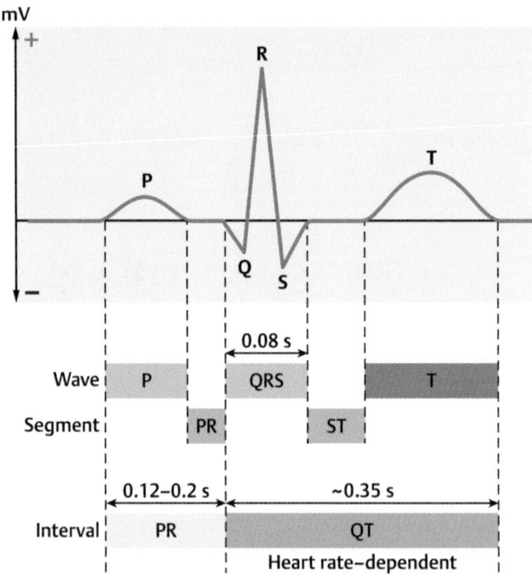

The portion of the ECG trace labeled 2 is the PR interval, which includes the depolarization of the AV nodal cells of the conduction system. (**A**) The portion of the ECG trace labeled 1 is the P-wave, which is produced by depolarization of the atrial muscle cells. Although AV nodal conduction contributes to the downslope of the P wave, this is not the best answer. (**C**) The portion of the ECG trace labeled 3 is the QRS complex, which is produced by depolarization of the ventricular muscle cells. (**D**) The portion of the ECG trace labeled 4 is the ST segment. It is the time when all ventricular muscle cells are depolarized and no vectors are recorded on the ECG. (**E**) The portion of the ECG trace labeled 5 is the T wave, which is produced by the repolarization of the ventricular muscle cells.

33. Correct: Atrioventricular (AV) conduction time (C)

This ECG trace shows a first-degree heart block, which is indicated by long PR intervals without any missing QRS complexes. The PR interval includes the recording of the depolarizations of the conduction tissue from the sinoatrial (SA) node to the Purkinje fibers and indicates how long it takes the conduction cells (not myocytes) to depolarize. The typical duration is 0.12–0.20 seconds, and trained athletes may have a long PR interval due to increased vagal tone to the heart. (**A**) Atrial depolarization is indicated by the P wave of the ECG trace, which has a normal duration on this trace. (**B**) Atrial repolarization is not indicated by a visible wave of the ECG trace, as it occurs during the QRS complex. (**D**) Ventricular depolarization is indicated by the QRS complex and ST segment of the ECG trace, which is normal on this trace. (**E**) Ventricular repolarization is indicated by the T wave of the ECG trace, which is normal.

34. Correct: Event is not visible (F)

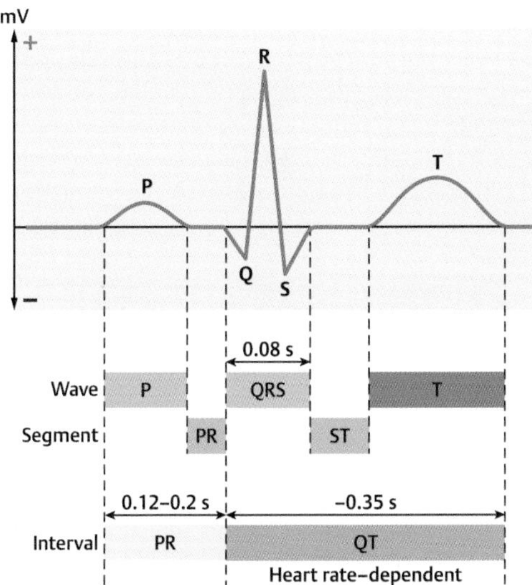

The wave on the ECG trace marked with a star is the P wave and is produced by atrial depolarization. Since the action potential recording shown is for ventricular myocyte depolarization, the atrial depolarization is not visible on this recording. (**A, B**) Phases 0 and 1 most closely correspond with the QRS complex. (**C**) Phase 2 most closely corresponds with the ST segment. (**D**) Phase 3 most closely corresponds with the T wave. (**E**) Phase 4 most closely corresponds with the TP segment. between the end of the T-wave and start of the next P-wave.

35. Correct: Q-T interval (D)

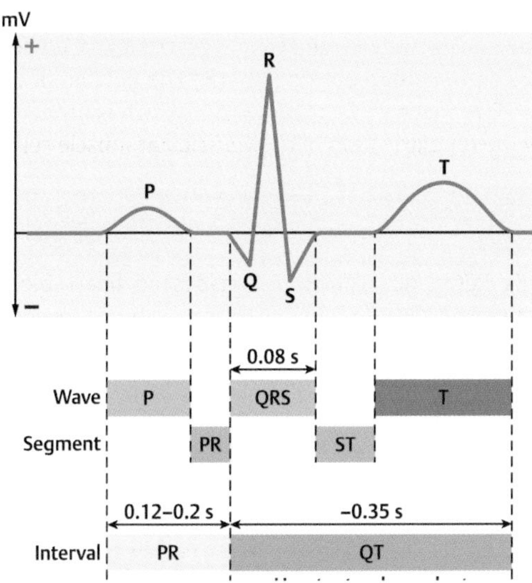

In an ECG of a healthy person with a heartbeat of 60 beats per minute, the longest part of the cardiac cycle is ventricular depolarization and repolarization, represented by the Q-T interval. (**A, B, C, E**) Depolarization of the atria (P wave), atrial contraction until the beginning of ventricular contraction (P-R interval), depolarization of the ventricles (QRS complex), and repolarization of the ventricles (T wave) are all shorter time periods than the Q-T interval.

36. Correct: T (E)

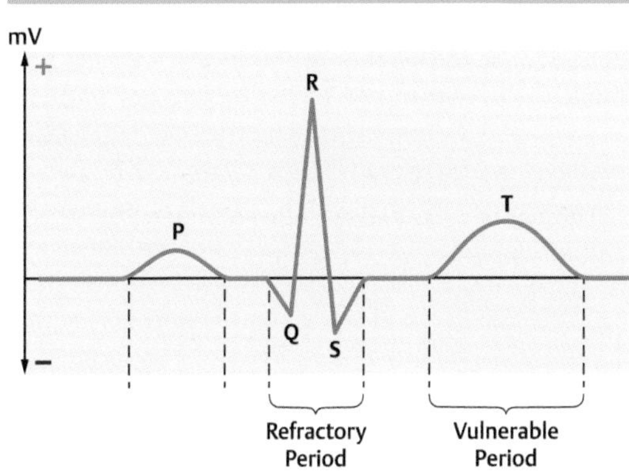

The vulnerable period of the cardiac cycle encompasses the T wave. During this time, the membrane potentials of ventricular myocytes repolarize and are normally not yet reactivated. However, enough Na^+ channels are in a state that allows their reactivation, and when it happens by electrical shock, Na^+ inward currents initiate action potentials that randomly spread through the myocardium and cause ventricular fibrillation. (In addition to the time of interaction, the amount, type, and duration of the current also play a role.) At the beginning of the T wave, the cell is still in the relative refractory phase, meaning that a stronger than normal stimulus is necessary for excitation. The middle and end of the T wave are the true vulnerable period, meaning that only a small electrical stimulus is necessary for excitation. Almost all Na^+ channels are ready to open and the membrane potential is still depolarized (i.e., closer to the threshold potential than at rest). (**A**) Excitation during the P wave, when the ventricular myocyte membrane potential is at rest, will cause ectopic foci and premature heartbeats. Dependent on the interactions of these abnormal pacemakers with the normal intrinsic pacemaker of the heart, it can lead to tachycardia or bradycardia. (**B, C, D**) These represent times when the ventricular cell membranes are at the absolute refractory period of the cardiac cycle, the least sensitive time for excitation.

37. Correct: Decreased conduction rate along the bundle branches (B)

If it takes longer for the cells in the bundle branches to depolarize (e.g., due to damage), then there is a delay in the depolarization of myocytes in the ventricular septum. Since the QRS complex is recorded when ventricular myocytes are depolarizing, any delay will increase the duration of the QRS complex and widen it. (**A**) Decreased parasympathetic innervation to the heart will increase heart rate and increase conduction rate. (**C**) Decreased conduction time from the SA node to the AV node will impact the duration of the P wave. (**D, E**) Sinus bradycardia and tachycardia will primarily alter the length of the T-P interval and have little effect on the QRS complex.

38. Correct: P-R interval (B)

The P-R interval is measured from the beginning of the P wave to the beginning of the QRS complex, and should be between 0.12 and 0.20 seconds in duration, which is 3–5 small boxes on the ECG paper (each small box is 0.04 seconds). This patient's P-R interval is 0.36 seconds (9 small boxes), which is abnormally long, indicating a first-degree atrioventricular block. (**A**) The normal duration of the P wave is shorter than 0.12 seconds (3 small boxes) and is normal for this patient. (**C**) The normal duration of the QRS complex is less than 0.10 seconds (2.5 small boxes) and is normal for this patient. (**D**) The normal duration of the S-T segment is 0.8 to 0.12 seconds (2–3 small boxes) and is normal for this patient. (**E**) The normal duration of the Q-T interval is less than half of one R-R interval. So first calculate the duration between two R waves, which is 0.92 seconds (23 small boxes), then measure the Q-T interval, which is 0.44 seconds (11 small boxes). Since the Q-T interval is less than half of the R-R interval, it is normal for this patient.

39. Correct: +110° (E)

Right ventricular hypertrophy typically causes a right axis deviation of the heart, which typically falls between +90° and +120° on the QRS mean electrical axis, which makes +110° the best choice. (**A, B**) Mean electrical axes of −70° and −40° constitute a left axis deviation. (**C, D**) Mean electrical axes of 0° and +50° are in the normal range.

40. Correct: 0° (C)

The fastest way to estimate the QRS mean electrical axis (MEA) is to find an isoelectric lead. For this trace, lead aVF is approximately net zero, meaning the upward and downward deflections of the QRS complex are approximately equal. This means that the patient's MEA will be perpendicular to the aVF lead, which is lead I. Since lead I has two sides, 0° and ±180°, you have to look at the QRS deflection of lead I to determine the MEA. Since lead I has positive QRS deflections, it indicates that the mean QRS vector is pointed toward the positive electrode of the lead, and that is at 0°. (**A, B, D, E**) These choices do not include the correct MEA for this patient.

41. Correct: Explain that the patient's heart is beating normally. (D)

The equal R wave amplitudes of leads II and III and the largest R wave amplitude in aVF indicate that the patient's mean QRS electrical axis is close to +90°. The "flat" ECG appearance in lead I indicates that it is the isoelectric lead axis, with the QRS vector perpendicular to the lead and hence causing only very small deflections. The sinus rhythm and the absence of any other clinical signs indicate that the heart is beating normally. (**A**) Asking a family member to monitor the ECG is inappropriate. (**B**) Code blue initiates an emergency response for a patient in cardiac arrest. (**C**) An expert cardiologist does not need to be consulted, since every hospital physician understands the basics of a 12-lead ECG. (**E**) This is, on its own, an untrue and dangerous statement. (**F**) A rapid response team is an interdisciplinary team that discusses early signs and symptoms to avoid future deleterious situations. It is not necessary for an asymptomatic patient.

42. Correct: Left axis deviation (A)

When the QRS complex of lead I is net positive and lead aVF is net negative, this puts the mean electrical axis of the patient in the left axis deviation quadrant (−30° to −90°). (**B**) Right axis deviation would be indicated if lead I was net negative and lead aVF was net positive. (**C**) Right ventricular hypertrophy is indicated by right axis deviation, which is not present in this patient. (**D, E**) This patient does have a sinus rhythm (SA node is acting as the pacemaker of the heart), but his heart rate is 75 beats per minute, which is within the normal range (not bradycardia or tachycardia). To calculate the heart rate, count the number of large boxes between two consecutive R-waves (4 large boxes), and multiply by 0.2 seconds (since the time duration of each large box is 0.2 seconds; 4 boxes × 0.2 seconds = 0.8 seconds per beat). Then divide this number into 60 seconds/minute (60/0.8 = 75 beats per minute). For a faster, less accurate approximation, divide 300 by the number of large boxes between consecutive R waves. A result of 3, 4, or 5 is normal. A result of 1 and 2 indicates tachycardia. A result of 6 and more indicates bradycardia.

43. Correct: A (A)

A regularly irregular rhythm is indicated by a pattern that repeats itself within the trace, over and over again. (**B**) This trace is a ventricular fibrillation, and it shows no rhythm. (**C**) This trace shows an irregularly irregular rhythm, which is indicated by a complete lack of pattern within the trace. (**D, E**) Both of these traces show a regular rhythm, which is indicated by evenly spaced R waves throughout the trace.

44. Correct: 215, 55 (C)

To measure atrial heart rate, count the number of small boxes between the peaks of two consecutive P waves (7 small boxes), and multiply by 0.04 seconds (7 × 0.04 sec = 0.28 sec/beat), then divide that number into 60 seconds/minute (60/0.28 ~ 215 beats per minute). To measure ventricular heart rate, count the number of small boxes between the peaks of two consecutive R waves (28 small boxes), and multiply by 0.04 seconds (28 × 0.04 sec = 1.12 sec/beat), then divide that number into 60 seconds/minute (60/1.12 ~ 55 beats per minute). (**A, B, D, E, F, G, H, I**) These answers do not have the correct atrial and ventricular rates.

45. Correct: D (D)

Atrial fibrillation is identified by the absence of definite P waves and an irregularly irregular rhythm. (**A**) This trace shows a premature atrial beat, labeled APB. (**B**) This trace shows an episode of paroxysmal supraventricular tachycardia. (**C**) This trace shows atrial flutter. (**E**) This trace shows a ventricular premature beat, labeled VPB. (**F**) This trace shows ventricular flutter. (**G**) This trace shows ventricular fibrillation.

46. Correct: Atrioventricular ring (C).

The syncope and ECG findings are characteristic of Wolff-Parkinson-White (WPW) syndrome. In this syndrome, the heart has abnormal conduction pathways between the atria and ventricles through the atrioventricular (AV) ring, which normally does not conduct an electrical current; these pathways disrupt the normal conduction pathway and electrical activity of the heart. (**A, E**) The atrial and ventricular septa have normal conduction pathways and are not disrupted by WPW. (**B**) The AV node is the normal conduction pathway from the atria to the ventricles. (**D**) The heart valves do not conduct electrical currents.

47. Correct: Angiotensin-converting enzyme (ACE) inhibitors (A)

The electrocardiogram shows no missed beats, a normal QRS complex (<120 msec), and a long P-R interval (> 200 msec), pointing towards first-degree atrioventricular (AV) nodal conduction delay. The lack of a wide QRS complex and left ventricular hypertrophy makes left bundle branch block not likely. Any drugs that further slow AV conduction velocity are of high concern, which is not the case for ACE inhibitors. They do not directly act on the heart but rather block angiotensin II production, which decreases blood pressure via actions at blood vessels, the kidney, and the posterior pituitary. Eventually, their use will need to be considered as well, since blocking the renin-angiotensin system also slightly damps sympathetic activity and its positive dromotropic effect. (**B, C**) β blockers inhibit the action of the sympathetic nervous system to increase I_{Ca}, while calcium channel blockers directly minimize I_{Ca}. Both lead to decreased inward current during the upstroke of the AV nodal action potential and hence decrease conduction velocity. (**D, E**) Drugs that stimulate (as cholinergic stimulants) or extend (as cholinesterase inhibitors) the action of the parasympathetic nervous system have a negative dromotropic effect, because the parasympathetic decreases calcium inward current and increases potassium outward current.

48. Correct: Ectopic atrial tachycardia (B)

One can see that the most striking feature of the ECG is the fact that each P wave looks different (change in amplitude, inverted), while the QRS complexes following each P wave look normal and narrow. This indicates that there are multiple ectopic foci in the atria that generate action potentials that are all conducted to the ventricles and contribute to the heart rate. The rhythm is benign and might present with respiratory symptoms, either as cause for or as a result of the arrhythmia. (**A**) Atrial flutter would show multiple P waves in front of each QRS complex, typically in a regular pattern. (**C, D**) Enhanced ventricular automaticity is the spontaneous activity of ventricular cells that can cause premature ventricular beats or other arrhythmias, all presenting with abnormal QRS complexes, which is not the case here. (**E**) Sinus tachycardia would present with normal regular P waves, just occurring at a fast rate.

49. Correct: B (B)

Standard limb lead I is between the right arm and the left arm (positive electrode on left arm). Standard limb lead II is between the right arm and the left leg (positive electrode on left leg). Standard limb lead III is between the left arm and the left leg (positive electrode on left leg). (**A, C, D, E, F**) These choices do not depict the correct lead placements.

50. Correct: Stable angina (E)

Angina in men typically causes uncomfortable pressure, fullness, squeezing or pain in the center of the chest and may radiate to the neck, jaw, shoulder, back, or arm. Stable angina occurs during times of physical activity or strong emotions, when narrowed arteries may prevent adequate oxygen perfusion of the heart, and subsides with rest. The episodes are transient, and the symptoms are relieved by rest. (**A, B, C, D**) Anxiety, myocardial infarction, myocarditis, and pleuritis typically do not cause chest pain associated with physical activity that subsides with rest.

51. Correct: Myoglobin (E)

The time of appearance in serum of cardiac proteins released from dying myocardial cells depends on the rate of diffusion through damaged tissue into the circulation. Myoglobin can elevate as early as 30 minutes and hence may be useful in the early detection of MI in the emergency department. However, levels are not very specific to MI. (**A**) Troponin serum levels (assayed as high sensitive troponin I or contemporary troponin I) elevate about 3–4 hours after MI and are currently the preferred marker for the diagnosis of MI. (**B, C**) Creatine kinase levels increase within 3–12 hours. The MB isoform is mainly from cardiac cells; the MM form is found mainly in skeletal muscle. (**D**) Lactate dehydrogenase increases about 18 hours post MI. Isoenzymes 1 and 2 are found in myocardial cells. It is nowadays rarely measured.

52. Correct: 4 (B).

Cardiac output is calculated by heart rate times stroke volume. The stroke volume is the end diastolic volume minus the end systolic volume. So cardiac output = (80 beats/min)(110 mL – 60 mL) = (80)(50) = 4,000 mL/min = 4L/min. (**A, C, D, E**) These choices do not include the correct cardiac output calculation.

53. Correct: He had myocardial infarcts. (A)

Myocardial infarcts decrease cardiac output (CO) and hence cardiac index (CI), which is CO per square meter of body surface area (BSA). The patient's CI is so low that it suggests heart failure as a consequence of long-term abuse of the sympathomimetic methamphetamine, leading to increased myocardial oxygen consumption. (**B**, **E**) Weight loss and limb amputation decrease BSA, which would increase CI, all other being equal. (**C**) Increased heart rate increases CO and CI, all other being equal. (**D**) Excessive sweating indicates sympathetic activation, which would increase (not decrease) his CO and thus CI.

5.7 Questions

54. A 26-year-old heroin addict is transported to the hospital after overdosing. Physical exam reveals a fever and a heart murmur at the lower left sternal border. Infective endocarditis is suspected, and blood cultures are ordered. Which heart valve is most likely involved?

A. Aortic
B. Mitral
C. Pulmonary
D. Tricuspid
E. Both aortic and mitral

55. A 55-year-old man presents with complaints of dizziness and shortness of breath on exertion. The physician detects a heart murmur heard during the portion of the cardiac cycle labeled X on the image. Which of the following heart valve pathologies would most likely produce this murmur?

A. Aortic valve stenosis
B. Mitral valve stenosis
C. Pulmonic valve stenosis
D. Tricuspid valve regurgitation
E. Mitral valve regurgitation

56. A 50-year-old man visits his physician for an annual exam. He complains of mild breathlessness on exertion. Upon cardiac auscultation the physician detects an S3 heart sound. At which point on the cardiac cycle diagram does the S3 heart sound occur?

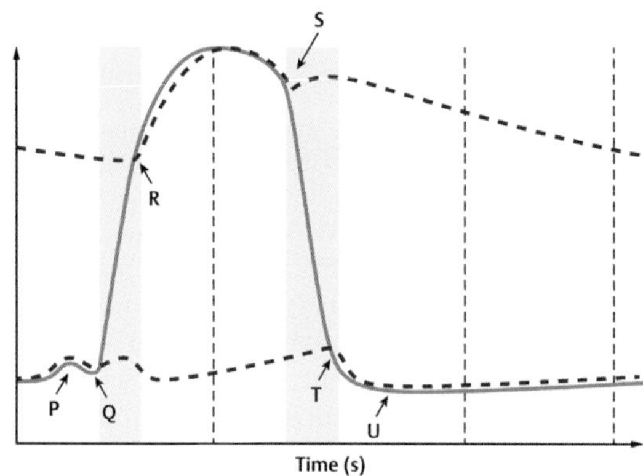

A. P
B. Q
C. R
D. S
E. T
F. U

57. The following diagram shows the changes in left ventricular pressure (red line) and aortic pressure (blue line) during one heartbeat in a person with aortic valve stenosis. At which point does the aortic valve open?

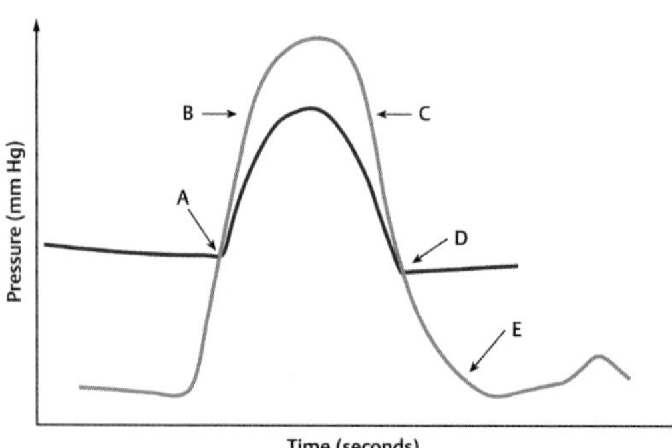

A. A
B. B
C. C
D. D
E. E

58. A 65-year-old patient presents to the emergency department with shortness of breath. She describes being fatigued and weak for months. Echocardiography visualizes a holodiastolic murmur that can be auscultated at the upper right sternal border. Her arterial blood pressure is 154/63 mm Hg. Which of the following pathologies best explains these findings?

A. Aortic valve regurgitation
B. Aortic valve stenosis
C. Mitral valve regurgitation
D. Mitral valve stenosis
E. Pulmonic valve regurgitation
F. Pulmonic valve stenosis
G. Tricuspid valve regurgitation
H. Tricuspid valve stenosis

59. A 31-year-old man presents to the emergency department with shortness of breath and dizziness. His electrocardiogram (ECG) is shown. P and R waves are identified with arrows. Auscultation reveals a normal S1 sound; a wide split S2 sound during inspiration; and a III/IV systolic crescendo-decrescendo murmur that is loudest at the left sternal border. Which of the following changes to ventricular heart rate and central venous pressure (CVP) are most likely present?

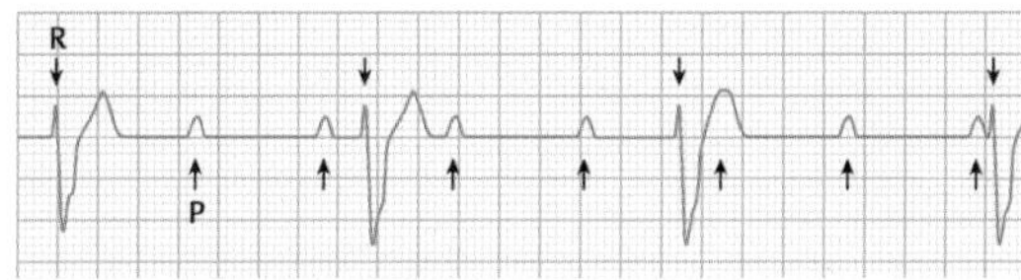

A. Bradycardia and decreased CVP
B. Bradycardia and increased CVP
C. Bradycardia and normal CVP
D. Tachycardia and decreased CVP
E. Tachycardia and increased CVP
F. Tachycardia and normal CVP

60. The figure represents the pressure changes in the jugular vein during a single cardiac cycle. What event produces the "c-wave" on the jugular venous pulse waveform?

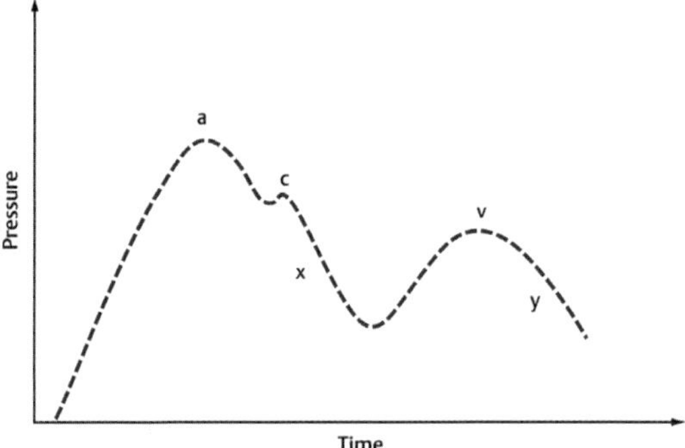

A. Right atrial contraction phase
B. Bulging of tricuspid valve toward the atrium
C. Slow filling phase of the ventricle
D. Opening of the tricuspid valve
E. Rapid ejection of blood from the ventricle

61. A patient undergoes Swan-Ganz right heart catheterization in order to examine his mitral valve hemodynamics. The balloon-tipped, multi-lumen catheter is inflated to occlude the pulmonary artery branch, and the distal catheter port measures pressure fluctuations between 4 and 12 mm Hg during the cardiac cycle. Which of the following cardiac events is responsible for the upstroke of the "v-wave" in this patient's pressure recording?

A. Left atrial contraction
B. Mitral valve bulging
C. Passive left atrial filling
D. Rapid ventricular filling
E. Ventricular contraction

62. A 40-year-old man presents with heart palpitations and fatigue. On auscultation a mid-diastolic murmur is heard and is loudest at the apex of the heart. Ultrasound reveals a moderate tricuspid valve stenosis. On the jugular venous pulse waveform shown, what is the most prominent change expected in this patient?

A. Absent a-wave
B. Cannon a-wave
C. Prominent a-wave
D. Prominent v-wave
E. Steep y-descent

63. A diagram showing pressure changes of the left atrium (LA), left ventricle (LV), and aorta (A) during one cardiac cycle is shown. The seven phases of the cardiac cycle are labeled on the diagram (1–7). During which phase of the cardiac cycle is the largest volume of blood pumped from the left atrium to the left ventricle?

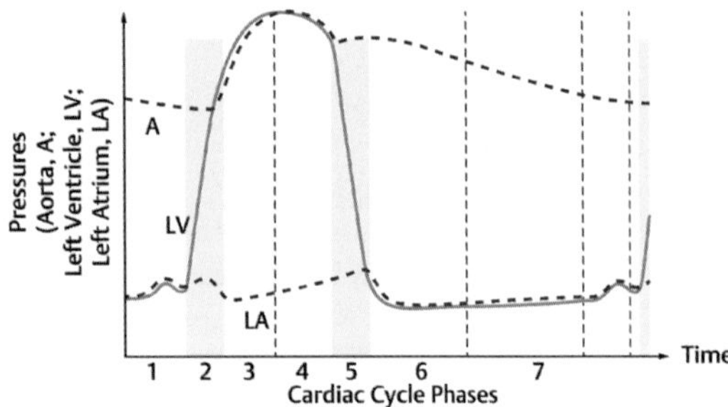

A. 1
B. 2
C. 3
D. 4
E. 5
F. 6
G. 7

64. During the physical exam of a 63-year-old male patient, simultaneous heart sound auscultation and carotid pulse palpitation are performed. A low-pitched heart sound is heard just before the carotid pulse is felt. Which of the following heart sounds is mostly likely heard?

A. S1
B. S2
C. S3
D. S4
E. Split S1

65. A 14-year-old boy is in cardiac arrest after being hit with a baseball in the chest above the left ventricle. This devastating occurrence, called commotio cordis, is very rare, since the impact must occur during the ascending phase of the T wave. During this time, the heart is normally electrically repolarizing. Which of the following events is also occurring at this time?

A. Ejecting blood at a reduced rate
B. Increasing left ventricular pressure
C. Opening the mitral valve
D. Rapidly filling the left ventricle
E. Slowly filling the left ventricle

66. In the figure shown, the left ventricular pressure–volume loop of a patient is shown when healthy (solid line) and after chronic manifestation of a disease (dashed line). Which of the following diseases most likely caused the shift from the solid to the dashed line in this patient?

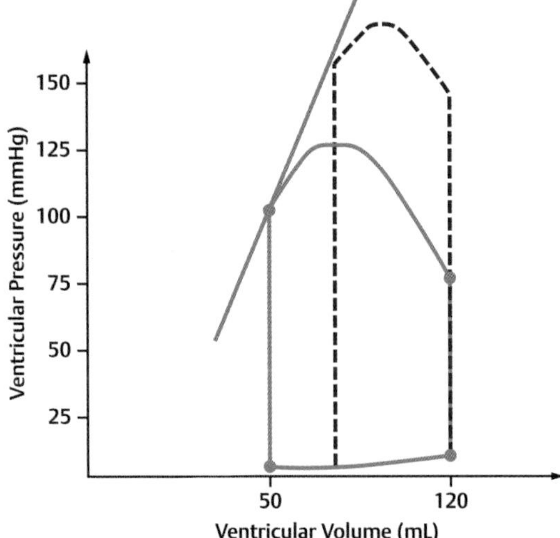

A. Aortic valve regurgitation
B. Left heart failure
C. Mitral valve stenosis
D. Pulmonary hypertension
E. Systemic hypertension

67. The image shown is a left ventricular pressure–volume loop. Which of the following points (M, N, O, P) correctly describe when diastole begins, when systole begins, when the aortic valve opens, when the mitral valve opens, and when the mitral valve closes, respectively?

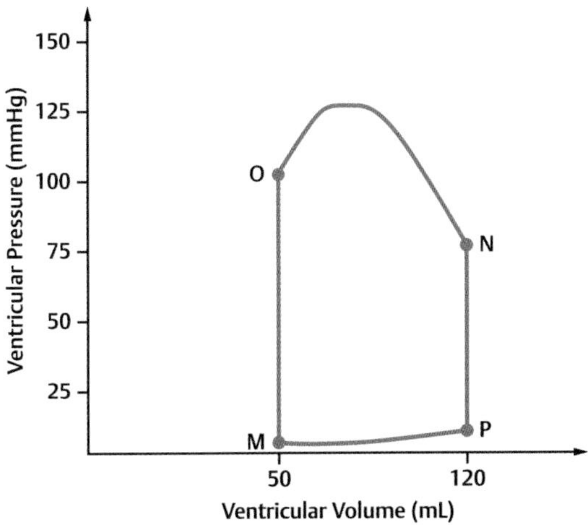

	Diastole begins	Systole begins	Aortic valve opens	Mitral valve opens	Mitral valve closes
A.	O	P	N	M	P
B.	M	N	P	M	N
C.	P	M	P	O	M
D.	O	P	P	M	P
E.	M	P	N	O	N
F.	P	N	N	O	P

68. The figure shown is a left ventricular pressure–volume loop. What are the patient's approximate mean arterial pressure (mm Hg), stroke volume (mL), and ejection fraction (%)?

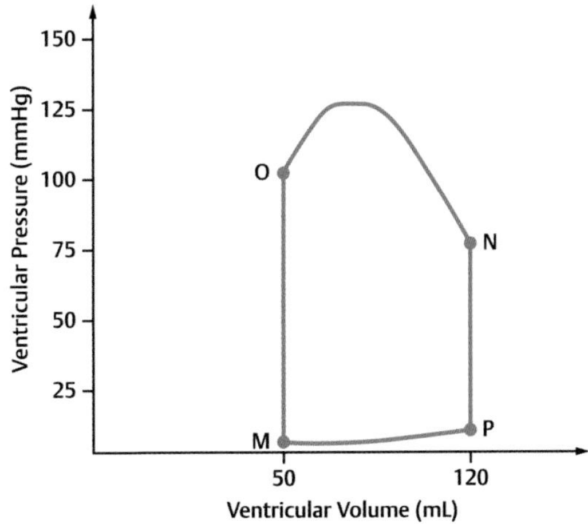

	Mean arterial pressure (mm Hg)	Stroke volume (mL)	Ejection fraction (%)
A.	100	120	42
B.	92	120	42
C.	100	120	58
D.	92	70	58
E.	92	70	42
F.	100	70	58

69. The figure shown is a left ventricular pressure–volume loop for a person at rest. What effect would aerobic exercise have on the maximal left ventricular (LV) afterload and slope of the end systolic pressure–volume relationship (ESPVR) line?

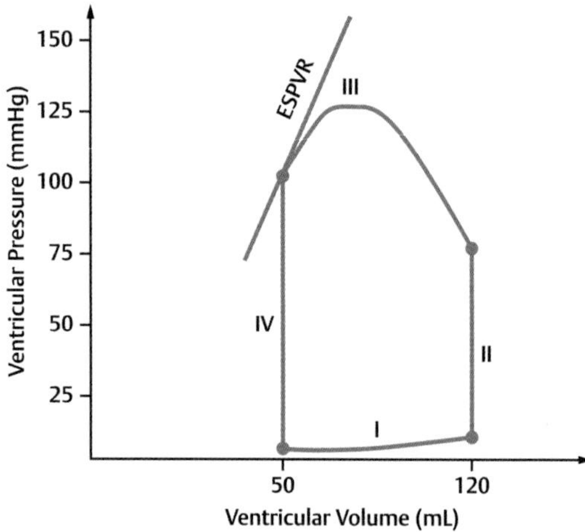

	Maximal LV afterload	Slope of ESPVR line
A.	↑	↑
B.	↓	↓
C.	↑	↔
D.	↓	↔
E.	↑	↓
F.	↓	↑

70. A 68-year-old woman presents to the emergency department with episodes of syncope. On auscultation, a diastolic murmur is heard at the apex of the heart. Her arterial blood pressure is 90/60 mm Hg. Which of the following valve pathologies best explains these findings?

A. Aortic valve regurgitation
B. Aortic valve stenosis
C. Mitral valve prolapse
D. Mitral valve regurgitation
E. Mitral valve stenosis

71. In the image the left ventricular pressure–volume loop drawn with the solid line was recorded in a healthy patient at rest (normal). Compared to the normal pressure–volume loop, what cardiovascular parameter is reduced in the pressure–volume loop drawn with the dashed line?

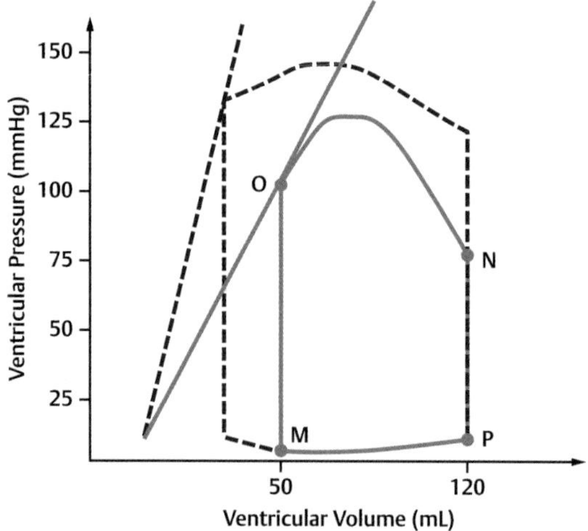

A. Afterload
B. Arterial systolic blood pressure
C. Cardiac contractility
D. End diastolic volume
E. End systolic volume
F. Stroke volume

72. An 88-year-old man with a history of atherosclerosis presents to the emergency department complaining of shortness of breath. His aortic pulse pressure curve is shown. What are this patient's approximate mean arterial pressure in mm Hg and pulse pressure in mm Hg?

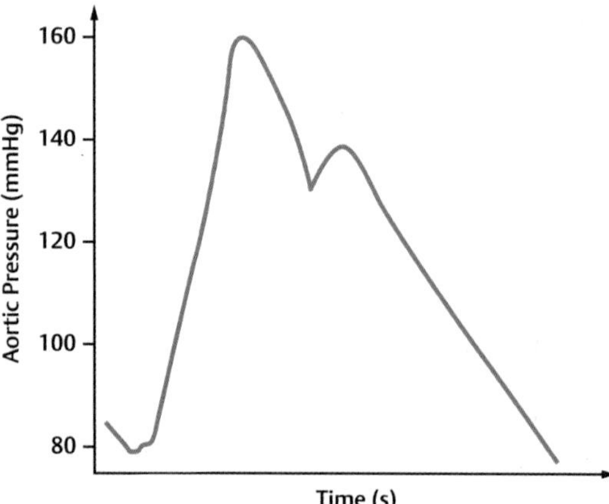

A. 120; 160
B. 107; 160
C. 120; 80
D. 107; 80
E. 120; 120
F. 107; 120

Questions 73 to 75

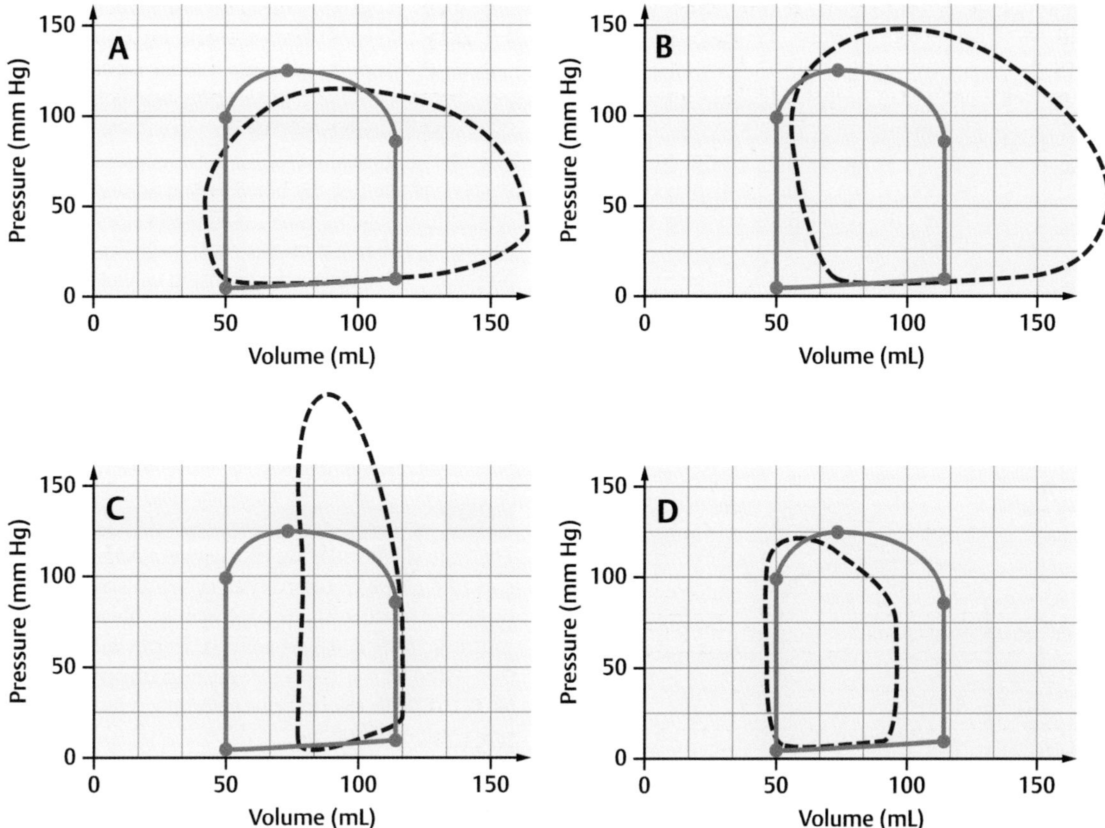

73. In the image, the black dotted line in each of the four panels shows the left ventricular pressure–volume loop of a person with a valvular heart defect compared to healthy (red lines). Which of the panels represents mitral valve stenosis? (Do not consider cardiac and systemic compensatory body mechanisms such as vasoconstriction, inotropy, and increase in blood volume.)

A. A
B. B
C. C
D. D

74. As part of a clinical trial with subjects who have been diagnosed with valvular heart defects, a 55-year-old woman presents with palpitations and chest pain. She has a high-pitched, blowing, holosystolic murmur. It is difficult to hear but most prominent at the apex. Her clinical trial portfolio most likely includes which panel of the left ventricular pressure–volume loops shown in the image?

A. A
B. B
C. C
D. D

75. A 40-year-old male, who is enrolled in the same clinical trial as in the previous question, is transferred for cardioelectrographic assessment. His portfolio reveals the left ventricular pressure–volume loop shown in panel C of the figure, and his chest echocardiogram indicates an enlarged heart. Which of the following are the most likely additional findings of this subject in regards to the mean QRS axis of his electrocardiogram (ECG) and his arterial blood pressure?

	Mean QRS axis of ECG (degrees)	Arterial blood pressure (mm Hg)
A.	–65	115/79
B.	–65	140/50
C.	+65	115/79
D.	+65	140/50
E.	+130	115/79
F.	+130	140/50

76. In order to study the exercise tolerance of patients with congestive heart failure (CHF), eight dogs were catheterized and heart failure was induced by rapid ventricular pacing. The image shows the average left ventricular pressure–volume loops of the dogs while standing on a stationary treadmill (solid black lines) and while running on the operating treadmill (red dotted lines). Panel A displays data from dogs without CHF, panel B shows data from dogs with CHF. The timings of their cardiac cycle phases were comparable. Which of the following is a correct conclusion for the exercise response of dogs with CHF in panel B, in comparison to the dogs without CHF in panel A?

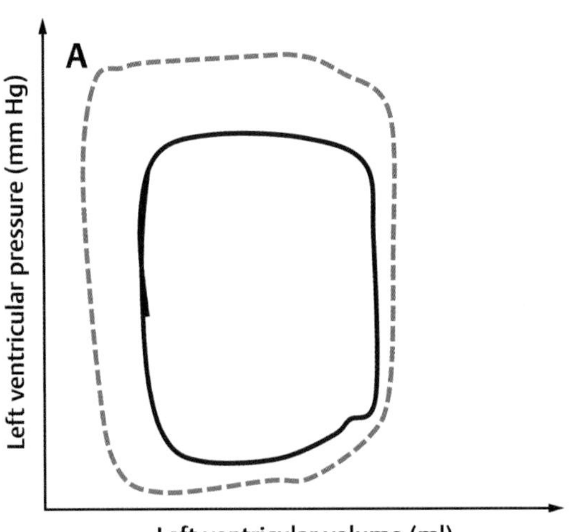

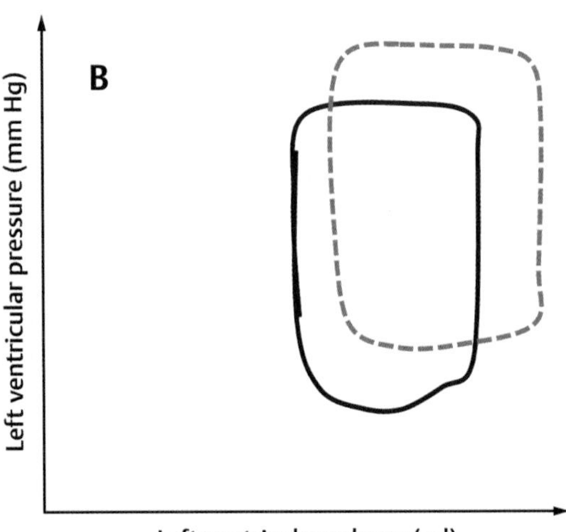

A. End-systolic volume is decreased.
B. Heart rate has not increased.
C. Rate of left ventricular relaxation is slower.
D. Sympathetic stimulation has not occurred.
E. The aortic valve does not close completely.

5.8 Answers and Explanations

54. Correct: Tricuspid (D)

Infective endocarditis (IE) is an infection caused by bacteria that enter the bloodstream and settle in the heart lining, a heart valve, or a blood vessel. IE can be caused by the injection of drugs, in this case heroin, and most often affects the tricuspid valve for reasons not well understood. In addition, the auscultation point of the murmur (lower left sternal border) is the tricuspid valve auscultation location. (**A, B, C, E**) While these valves can be affected by IE with drug use, they are not the most likely, and they do not have the correct auscultation points.

55. Correct: Mitral valve stenosis (B)

The region labeled X on the Wiggers diagram is the diastolic phase of the cardiac cycle, so any murmur produced during this phase would be a diastolic murmur. Mitral valve stenosis is the only condition listed that produces a murmur during diastole. (**A, C, D, E**) These conditions all produce systolic murmurs, not diastolic.

56. Correct: U (F)

The S3 heart sound is produced by conditions that have a chronically high preload, which produces eccentric hypertrophy of the ventricular chamber. When a large volume of blood rushes into an enlarged ventricular chamber, it produces the S3 heart sound. This occurs during the rapid ventricular filling phase of the cardiac cycle, which is point U. (**A**) This point is where an S4 heart sound would be heard, during atrial contraction. (**B**) This point is where the S1 heart sound is heard, as the mitral valve closes. (**C**) The aortic valve opens here, but no heart sounds are produced by this event. (**D**) This point is where the S2 heart sound is heard, as the aortic valve closes. (**E**) The mitral valve opens here, but no heart sounds are produced by this event. The S3 sound is not heard until after the mitral valve opens and blood is rushing into the enlarged ventricular chamber.

57. Correct: A (A)

The aortic valve opens when ventricular pressure becomes greater than aortic pressure, in order to allow blood to exit the left ventricle into the aorta. This is the case when the blue and the red lines intersect at point A before systole. In aortic valve stenosis, the valve fails to open all the way, resulting in much greater left ventricular pressure than aortic pressure during left ventricular ejection (difference between the peaks of the red and blue line). (**B, C**) At these points, the aortic valve is already open since aortic pressure rises as blood enters the aorta. (**D**) At this point the aortic valve closes. (**E**) This point is close to when the mitral valve opens, but for the exact place, left atrial pressure changes would need to be available.

58. Correct: Aortic valve regurgitation (A).

The aortic valve is located at the second right intercostal space. Regurgitation produces a diastolic murmur that reverberates to the aorta in the upper right sternal border. Amplification and noise reduction of an electronic stethoscope helps to hear the murmur. When chronic, it manifests with a high systolic pressure due to a high stroke volume in response to increased preload and with a high diastolic pressure due to increased afterload in response to vasoconstriction. (**B**, **C**, **F**, **G**) Aortic valve stenosis, mitral valve regurgitation, tricuspid valve regurgitation, and pulmonic valve regurgitation all produce systolic murmurs. (**D**, **E**, **H**) Auscultation is at the sites to where the sound waves of the malfunctioning valves reverberate. For mitral valve stenosis, pulmonic valve regurgitation, and tricuspid valve stenosis, these sites are the left lower midclavicular line, the upper left sternal border, and the lower left sternal border, respectively.

59. Correct: Bradycardia and increased CVP (B)

The patient's murmur and S2 split is consistent with pulmonary valve stenosis: The murmur is during systole and best heard in the pulmonic auscultation area. The normal S2 split during inspiration becomes wider, because it takes longer for the right ventricle to eject the blood through the stenotic valve and the pulmonary valve closure is delayed. This typically congenital heart disease may remain asymptomatic until adulthood, but can lead to arrhythmias. The patient's ECG shows a third-degree heart block with complete absence of atrioventricular conduction. Since none of the supraventricular impulses (P waves) are conducted to the ventricles and since ventricular rate (R waves) is about 40 bpm, the patient's ventricular heart rate is low (bradycardia), leading to dizziness and shortness of breath. The obstruction of blood flow from the right ventricle to the pulmonary artery during systole causes right ventricular hypertrophy. Forceful atrial contraction against the hypertrophied ventricle increases central venous pressure. (**A**, **C**, **D**, **E**, **F**) The patient is not tachycardic and does not have a decreased or normal central venous pressure.

60. Correct: Bulging of tricuspid valve toward the atrium (B)

The jugular venous pulse waveform correlates to pressure changes that occur in the right atrium during the cardiac cycle. The c-wave is produced by pressure changes associated with the isovolumetric contraction phase, which causes the tricuspid valve to bulge backwards into the right atrium and causes a slight increase in pressure in the right atrium, which is reflected backwards to the jugular vein. (**A**) Atrial contraction produces the a-wave on the jugular venous pulse waveform. (**C**) The slow filling phase of the ventricle occurs during the upstroke of the a-wave on the jugular venous pulse waveform. (**D**) The tricuspid valve opens at the peak of the v-wave on the jugular venous pulse waveform. (**E**) Rapid ejection of blood from the ventricle occurs during the downstroke of the v-wave.

61. Correct: Passive left atrial filling (C)

A Swan-Ganz catheter, when balloon inflated, provides pulmonary capillary wedge pressure (PCWP), which closely reflects left atrial pressure. PCWP fluctuates due to cardiac events of the left heart, similarly to how the venous pulse fluctuates due to cardiac events of the right heart. The "v" wave is generated by the passive filling of the left atrium before the opening of the mitral valve. Pathological conditions that affect atrial filling during systole, such as mitral regurgitation, cause a large "v" wave. (**A**) Left atrial contraction produces the "a" wave. (**B**, **E**) The bulging of the mitral valve into the left atrium during isovolumetric left ventricular contraction produces the "c" wave. For the PCWP curve, it is typically not very prominent. (**D**) The opening of the mitral valve and the rapid filling of the ventricle from the atrium represent the y-descent.

62. Correct: Prominent a-wave (C)

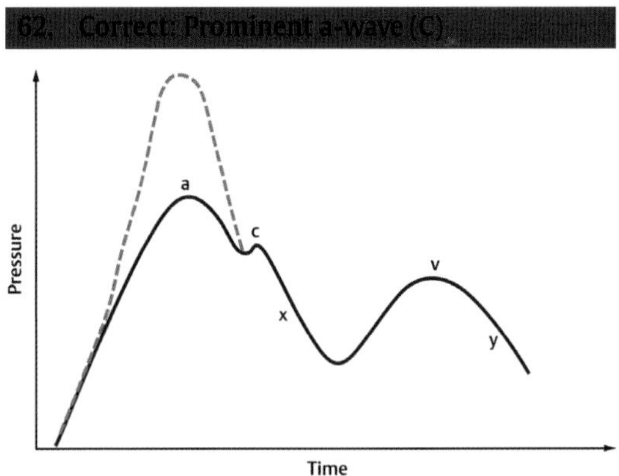

Anything that increases resistance to ventricular filling, including tricuspid valve stenosis, will produce a prominent a-wave. (**A**) An absent a-wave is seen in atrial fibrillation due to the irregularity of the heart rhythm, which prevents differentiation of atrial contraction and relaxation on the jugular venous pulse waveform. (**B**) A cannon a-wave is due to the contraction of the right atrium against a closed tricuspid valve, which results in the generation of a high atrial pressure. This is seen is complete heart blocks. (**D**) A prominent v-wave is caused by conditions that increase right atrial pressure during atrial diastole, such as tricuspid valve regurgitation. (**E**) A steep y-descent is produced by conditions that restrict adequate stretching of the cardiac wall, such as constrictive pericarditis; thus, when the tricuspid valve opens, the pressure in the right atrium decreases more rapidly.

63. Correct: 6 (F)

The phase labeled 6 is the rapid filling phase of the cardiac cycle, where 60–70% of the blood moves passively from the atria to the ventricles down a pressure gradient. (**A**) Phase 1 is the atrial contraction phase, where the final 10% of the blood is actively pumped from the atria to the ventricles. (**B**) Phase 2 is the isovolumetric contraction phase, and no blood is moving from the atria or ventricles during this phase. (**C**) Phase 3 is the rapid ejection phase, where most of the blood in the ventricle is forcefully ejected into the aorta. (**D**) Phase 4 is the slow ejection phase, where a small volume of blood in the ventricle is ejected into the aorta. (**E**) Phase 5 is the isovolumetric relaxation phase, and no blood is moving from the atria or ventricles during this phase. (**G**) Phase 7 is the slow filling phase (diastasis), where about 20% of the blood moves passively from the atria to the ventricles.

64. Correct: S4 (D)

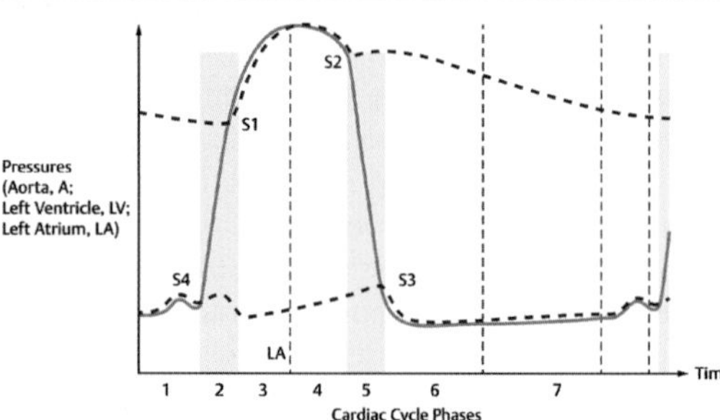

The carotid pulse is felt simultaneously with auscultation of the S1 heart sound. The heart sound that occurs just before S1 is the S4 heart sound, which is pathologic, caused from conditions that chronically increase cardiac afterload (e.g., hypertension). (**A, E**) The S1 and split S1 heart sounds are heard simultaneous to palpation of the carotid pulse. (**B, C**) S2 and S3 are heard after the carotid pulse is palpated.

65. Correct: Ejecting blood at a reduced rate (A)

The beginning of the T wave on the electrocardiogram (ECG) indicates that the ventricles repolarize and cardiomyocytes are no longer contracting. The aortic valve is still open and blood continues to be ejected into the aorta, but at a reduced rate compared to the rate right after the aortic valve has opened. Commotio cordis seems to involve potassium currents that are normally inhibited but occur when ATP decreases during cellular hypoxia. They alter normal cardiac action potential repolarization and lead to cardiac arrhythmias. (**B**) Left ventricular pressure increases during the isovolumetric contraction and the rapid ejection phases of the cardiac cycle, which coincide with the QRS complex and the S-T segment of the ECG. (**C, D, E**) The mitral valve opens at the lowest left ventricular pressure and allows the ventricle to fill with blood, initially at a rapid, then at a reduced rate. On the ECG, it is the time between the T wave and the P wave of the next cardiac cycle.

66. Correct: Systemic hypertension (E)

The left ventricular pressure–volume (PV) loop shown with the dashed line is demonstrating a high afterload on the left ventricle, which could be produced by systemic hypertension. The elevated maximum ventricular pressure and reduced stroke volume are key components of high afterload. (**A, B**) Aortic valve regurgitation and left heart failure would increase the end diastolic volume (EDV). (**C, D**) Mitral valve stenosis and pulmonary hypertension would reduce EDV and maximum ventricular pressure.

67. Correct: O, P, N, M, P (A)

Diastole begins at the start of the isovolumetric relaxation phase, which is point O. Systole begins at the start of the isovolumetric contraction phase, which is point P. The aortic valve opens at the end of the isovolumetric contraction phase, which is point N. The aortic valve opens at the end of the isovolumetric relaxation phase, which is point M. The mitral valve closes at the start of systole, which is the start of the isovolumetric contraction phase, at point P. (**B, C, D, E, F**) These answer choices have the wrong combination of answers.

68. Correct: 92, 70, 58 (D)

In the pressure–volume (PV) loop, the diastolic blood pressure (P_d) is approximated by the pressure at point N, and the systolic blood pressure (P_s) is estimated by the pressure at the peak of the PV loop. End systolic volume (ESV) is estimated by the volume at point M, and end diastolic volume (EDV) is estimated by the volume at point P. In the given PV loop,

Mean arterial pressure = $P_d + (1/3)(P_s - P_d) = 75 + (1/3)(125 - 75) = 75 + (1/3)(50) = 75{+}17 = 92$ mm Hg.

Stroke volume = EDV – ESV = 120 mL – 50 mL = 70 mL.

Ejection fraction = (SV/EDV) 100 = (70/120) 100 = 58%

69. Correct: ↑, ↑ (A)

With aerobic exercise, cardiac output increases, which increases systolic blood pressure, and thus afterload. In addition, cardiac contractility increases due to increased sympathetic innervation of the heart, thus increasing the slope of the ESPVR line. (**B, C, D, E, F**) These choices have wrong combinations of answers.

70. Correct: Mitral valve stenosis (E)

Mitral valve stenosis is the most likely cause of the symptoms because it produces a diastolic murmur, is heard best at the apex of the heart, and produces a low systolic and diastolic blood pressure due to a small ejection volume. (**A**) Aortic regurgitation produces a diastolic murmur, but it is heard best at the upper right sternal border, and it would produce a high systolic pressure (due to a large ejection volume) and a low diastolic pressure (due to the regurgitation of blood back into the ventricle). (**B, C, D**) Aortic stenosis, mitral regurgitation, and mitral prolapse are eliminated because they produce systolic, not diastolic, murmurs.

71. Correct: End systolic volume (E)

The only parameter that is reduced, compared to normal, is the left ventricular end systolic volume, which is represented by point M on the normal loop. (**A**) Left ventricular afterload is elevated in the dashed loop, as indicated by the increase in the height of the loop. (**B**) Systolic blood pressure is elevated in the dashed loop, as indicated by the increase in the height of the loop. (**C**) Cardiac contractility is increased in the dashed loop, as indicated by the increase in the slope of the end systolic pressure–volume relationship line. (**D**) Left ventricular end diastolic volume does not change in the two loops, as indicated by point P. (**F**) Stroke volume increases in the dashed loop, as indicated by the width of the loop, relative to normal.

72. Correct: 107; 80 (D)

The diastolic blood pressure (P_d) is approximated by the pressure at the base of the curve, and the systolic blood pressure (P_s) is estimated by the pressure at the peak of the curve.

Pulse Pressure (PP) = $P_s - P_d$ = 160 – 80 mm Hg = 80 mm Hg.

Mean arterial pressure (MAP) = P_d + 1/3(PP) = 80 + 1/3(80) = 80 + 27 = 107 mm Hg.

73. Correct: D (D)

Mitral valve stenosis impairs left ventricular filling, so there is a decrease in preload. This leads to a decrease in stroke volume (SV) and a fall in cardiac output and aortic pressure. This reduction in afterload enables the end-systolic volume (ESV) to decrease slightly, but not enough to overcome the decline in end-diastolic volume (EDV). (**A, B**) Panel A represents mitral valve regurgitation, and panel B shows aortic valve regurgitation. The backflow of blood through leaky valves does not allow true isovolumetric contraction and relaxation, as present in these panels. (**C**) Panel C shows aortic stenosis, which presents with an increase in ventricular afterload, a decrease in SV, and an increase in ESV. SV decreases because the velocity of fiber shortening is decreased by the increased afterload. The excess residual volume added to the incoming venous return causes the EDV to increase. This activates the Frank-Starling mechanism, but the compensation is not enough to overcome the increased outflow resistance.

74. Correct: A (A)

Panel A shows the left ventricular volume pressure loop of mitral valve regurgitation. It presents with a holosystolic heart murmur, since the mitral valve is unable to contain the blood within the ventricle for the entire systolic period. During auscultation, it is best heard at the “mitral area,” or apex, with radiation into the axilla. (**B, D**) Panel B shows aortic valve regurgitation, and panel D shows mitral valve stenosis, both leading to diastolic (not systolic) murmurs. (**C**) Panel C shows aortic stenosis, which presents with a mid-systolic, crescendo-decrescendo murmur. During auscultation, it is best heard over the “aortic area,” or right second intercostal space, with radiation to the right neck.

75. Correct: –65, 115/79 (A)

The subject of the clinical trial has a stenotic aortic valve leading to the characteristic left ventricular pressure–volume loop shown in panel C of the figure. To eject blood, ventricular pressure must rise to a greater than normal level during isovolumetric contraction. The cardiac muscle fibers adapt to this increased work by hypertrophy, so that the mean QRS axis of the man’s ECG shows a left axis deviation of –65°. Moreover, his aortic systolic blood pressure and pulse pressure will be decreased, which makes A the best choice. (**B**) An ECG leftward axis shift, systolic hypertension, and a wide pulse pressure are present in aortic valve regurgitation (not aortic valve stenosis). (**C, D**) A mean electrical axis of 65° falls into the normal range between –30° to +90°, seen in healthy (not hypertrophied) hearts. (**E, F**) A mean electrical axis greater than +90° is termed a right axis deviation, which occurs due to hypertrophy of the right (not the left) side of the heart.

76. Correct: Rate of left ventricular relaxation is slower. (C)

For the dogs with congestive heart failure (CHF), one can see that the rate of left ventricular relaxation is slower, since at the end of isovolumetric relaxation, the ventricular pressure does not decrease to the level present for the CHF dogs at rest. Considering a fixed isovolumetric relaxation time (comparable timing of the cardiac cycles), this is significantly different from the exercise response of dogs without CHF, where the end-systolic pressure of exercising dogs is lower compared to resting dogs. (**A**) End-systolic volume (ESV) is increased (not decreased) in CHF dogs in response to exercise. This is different in healthy dogs, in which exercise-induced sympathetic stimulation results in a faster rate of relaxation and decreased ESV so that there is more time for refilling. (**B**) Volume–pressure loops do not provide direct information about heart rate. Nevertheless, the increased pressure at the end of isovolumetric contraction in CHF dogs points to sympathetic stimulation, which increases heart rate. (**D**) Sympathetic stimulation has occurred, since for all dogs, including CHF dogs, there is a significant increase in peak myocardial tension in response to exercise. (**E**) Ventricular relaxation remains isovolumetric, which would not be the case with a regurgitant aortic valve.

5.9 Questions

77. The image shows a group of Starling curves plotting cardiac stroke work versus left ventricular end diastolic volume. If a patient is currently at the steady-state operating point 1, what change in cardiac contractility and preload must occur to shift toward point 2?

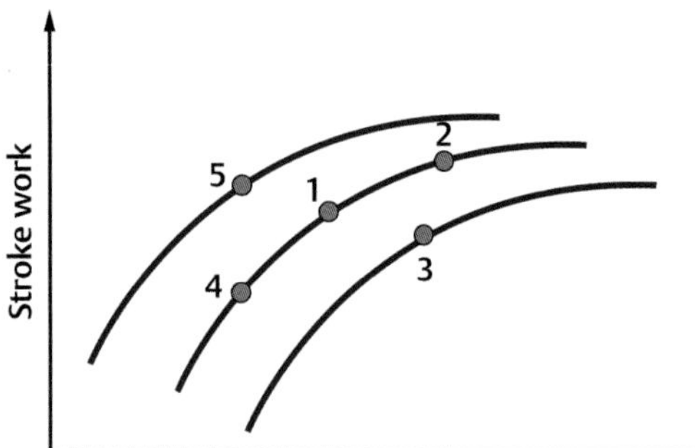

	Contractility	Preload
A.	↓	↑
B.	↓	↓
C.	↑	↑
D.	↑	↓
E.	↔	↑
F.	↔	↓

78. A 21-year-old female college student is running a 5 km (~3.1 miles) race. She is relatively new to running and has trained minimally for the race. Compared to her resting values, how will her left ventricular contractility, end systolic volume, and end diastolic volume change while she is running?

	Left ventricular contractility	Left ventricular end systolic volume	Left ventricular end diastolic volume
A.	↑	↓	↓
B.	↑	↑	↑
C.	↑	↓	↑
D.	↓	↑	↓
E.	↓	↓	↑
F.	↓	↑	↑

79. In a healthy person, the heartbeat immediately following an increase in cardiac preload will exhibit which of the following changes?

A. Decreased diastolic arterial blood pressure
B. Increased pulse pressure
C. Decreased stroke volume
D. Decreased systolic arterial blood pressure
E. Increased peripheral arteriolar resistance

80. A 22-year-old woman occasionally faints. Her resting blood pressure is 120/75 mm Hg, and 95/60 mm Hg after standing up. Her resting heart rate is 95 beats per minute and 115 beats per minute after standing up. Which of the following physiologic cardiovascular changes most likely causes her abnormal response to the postural change?

A. Decrease in blood volume
B. Decrease in left ventricular afterload
C. Decrease in cardiac contractility
D. Decrease in venous compliance
E. Increase in venous return

81. A healthy 5-year-old girl experienced a mild nosebleed, which threw her in a frantic state of anxiety. Which of the following sets of cardiovascular changes would be observed during the incident, relative to normal?

	Mean circulatory filling pressure	Heart rate	Cardiac output
A.	↑	↑	↑
B.	↑	↑	↓
C.	↑	↓	↓
D.	↓	↓	↓
E.	↓	↑	↑
F.	↓	↓	↑

82. A patient is undergoing a stent placement in the left anterior descending coronary artery, and the following data are collected during the procedure.

Heart rate = 65 beats/min
Mean arterial blood pressure = 90 mm Hg
Oxygen consumption = 250 mL oxygen/min
Pulmonary artery oxygen content = 0.19 mL oxygen/mL blood
Pulmonary vein oxygen content = 0.14 mL oxygen/mL blood

What is the patient's cardiac output (L/min) during the procedure?

A. 3
B. 5
C. 10
D. 15
E. 20

83. As part of a supervised research study at the university hospital, a healthy normovolemic woman with an estimated blood volume of 5 liters is voluntarily donating 1.2 liters (about two and a half pints) of blood by venipuncture. The resultant effect on her mean systemic pressure could also be produced by which of the following?

A. Administration of a positive inotropic agent
B. Decrease in contractility
C. Decrease in total peripheral resistance
D. Excessive NaCl intake
E. Increase in venous compliance

84. A physician sees two different patients. Patient 1 has pheochromocytoma and Patient 2 has untreated right heart failure. On the cardiac function curves shown, if the star indicates the normal operating point for a healthy person, at what points will the two patients be operating?

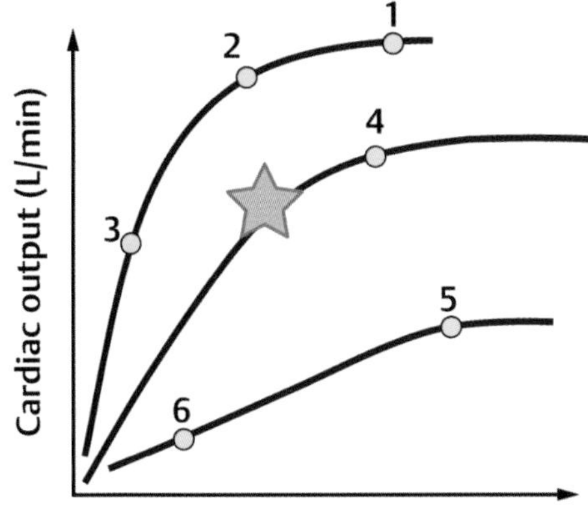

	Patient 1	Patient 2
A.	1	3
B.	1	5
C.	1	6
D.	2	3
E.	2	5
F.	2	6
G.	3	3
H.	3	5
I.	3	6
J.	4	3
K.	4	5
L.	4	6

85. In which of the following scenarios do both central venous pressure and venous return decrease?

A. Inhaling compared to exhaling
B. Late compared to early pregnancy
C. Sustained increase in intrapleural pressure
D. Suddenly standing up compared to lying
E. Walking compared to standing

86. A patient with dehydration has the steady-state operating point labeled B on the cardiac-vascular function curves shown in the figure. The patient's normal operating point is at point A. Administration of a drug producing which of the following changes would help to return the patient's cardiac function back to normal (i.e., from point B to point A)?

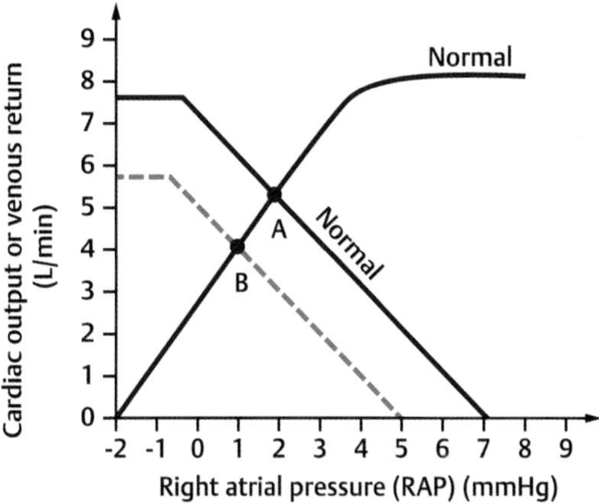

A. Decreased cardiac contractility
B. Decreased venous compliance
C. Increased arteriole tone
D. Increased cardiac contractility
E. Increased venous compliance

87. A patient has a cardiac output of 5 L/minute and a right atrial pressure of 2 mm Hg. His mean systemic filling pressure is 7 mm Hg. Maximum cardiac output in this individual without any cardiac or vascular changes before venous collapse is 7.5 L/minute. An intervention is given and results in a mean systemic filling pressure of 8 mm Hg; cardiac output of 6 L/minute; and right atrial pressure of 2.5 mm Hg. The patient has most likely received which of the following interventions, considering only the effect of the intervention, and not any resulting compensation?

A. A β_1 adrenergic receptor agonist
B. An α_1 adrenergic receptor blocker
C. An IV infusion of 2.5 pints of normal saline
D. A nitric oxide vasodilator drug
E. A therapeutic dose of a cardiac glycoside

88. On the following diagram, point X represents the resting state of a 55-year-old woman with intact reflexes, as determined by her cardiac function curve (orange) and her vascular function curve (purple). Which of the following best explains the change in her cardiovascular status from Point X to point Y?

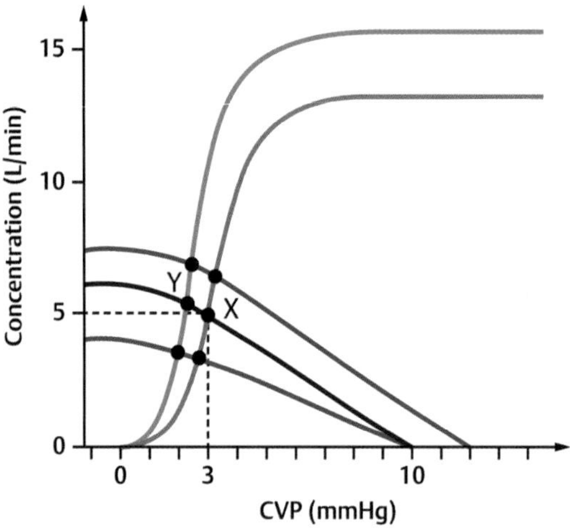

A. She began exercising.
B. She was in severe pain due to peripheral artery occlusive disease.
C. She suddenly stood up.
D. She was given a blood transfusion.
E. She was given a positive inotropic drug.

89. A 63-year-old woman read about atypical presentation of heart failure in women and requests a thorough checkup. Her history reveals that for months she has felt tired, weak, and without energy. She describes having fibromyalgia and heartburn for years. She was diagnosed with type II diabetes 2 years ago. Electrocardiography of inferior leads II, III and aVF show no S-T segment elevation, but distinct Q waves. Extensive cardiovascular assessment reveals high right atrial pressure and low cardiac output (point X), as compared to values from a checkup 10 years ago (point Y). Left ventricular volume-pressure assessment reveals loop X, overlaid with loop Y from the 10-year-old checkup. Which of the following cardiovascular parameters is currently most likely decreased in this patient?

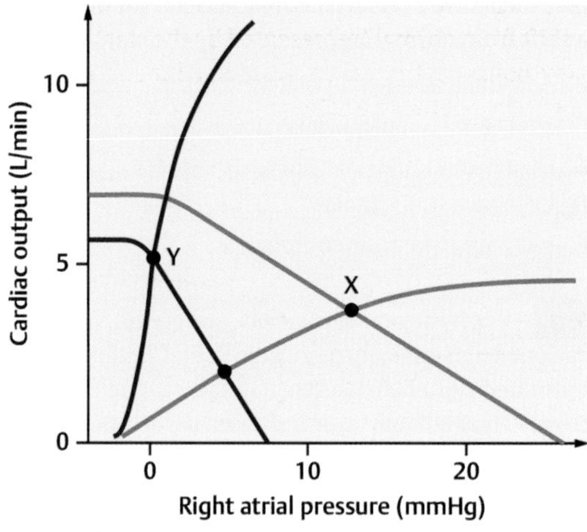

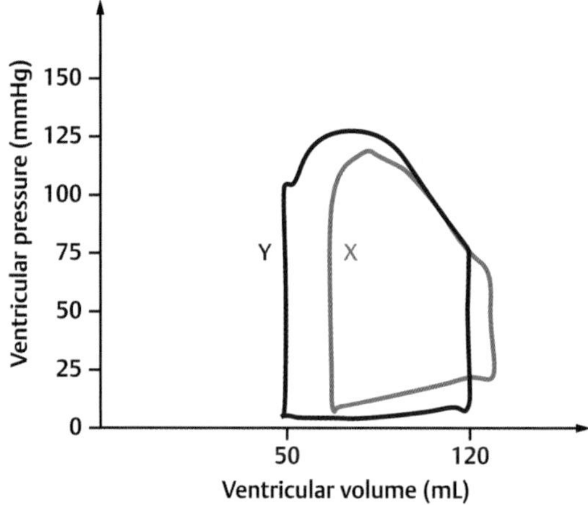

A. Blood volume
B. End-systolic volume
C. Preload
D. Systemic vascular resistance
E. Venous compliance

90. An herbal supplement advertised to enhance weight loss was found to increase cardiac contractility and decrease arteriolar tone. This supplement was taken by a healthy person with a normal cardiac output (CO), venous return (VR), and right atrial pressure (RAP). The effect of this supplement caused a shift from normal (represented by the star) to what new point on the cardiac-vascular function curve? (Assume no other cardiovascular changes occur.)

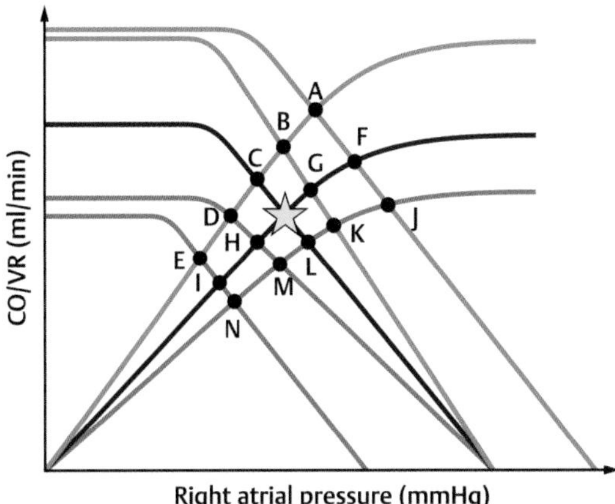

A. A
B. B
C. C
D. D
E. E
F. F
G. G
H. H
I. I
J. J

91. The vascular function curves of six different people (labeled A–F) are shown in comparison to a given cardiac function curve in green. The vascular function curve B in purple is from a healthy resting person. Which person has the lowest resistance to venous return?

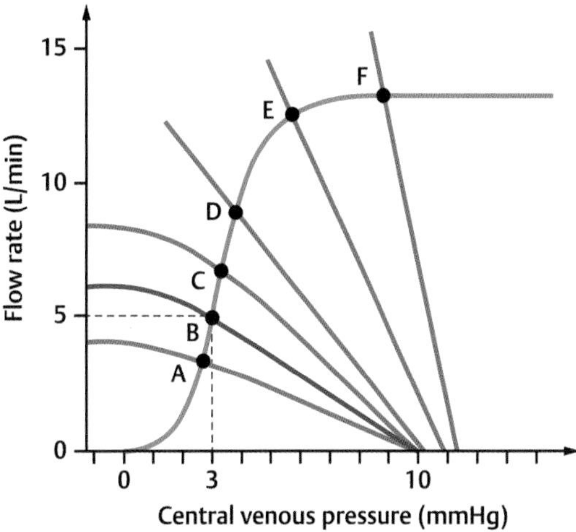

A. A
B. C
C. D
D. E
E. F

92. A 30-year-old woman presents 1 week following a surgical procedure with a blood pressure of 80/60 mm Hg, a pulse rate of 120 beats per minute, and a low central venous pressure. Based on her medical history and physical examination, she is determined to have distributive shock. Which of the following conditions is this patient most likely suffering from?

A. Cardiac tamponade
B. Hemorrhage
C. Myocardial infarction
D. Pulmonary embolism
E. Sepsis

93. Two patients in the emergency department are diagnosed with shock. One is suffering from anaphylactic shock from a bee sting, and the other is suffering from obstructive shock from cardiac tamponade. What is expected for each patients' central venous pressures (CVP) when compared to healthy?

	Patient with anaphylactic shock	Patient with obstructive shock
A.	↑	↑
B.	↑	↓
C.	↑	↔
D.	↓	↑
E.	↓	↓
F.	↓	↔

94. A 23-year-old healthy woman runs two miles at a moderate pace. Based on the exercise-induced changes that occur while running, which left ventricular pressure–volume loop most likely represent the woman's status during her run? (Dashed line represents the "normal" left ventricular pressure–volume loop at rest.)

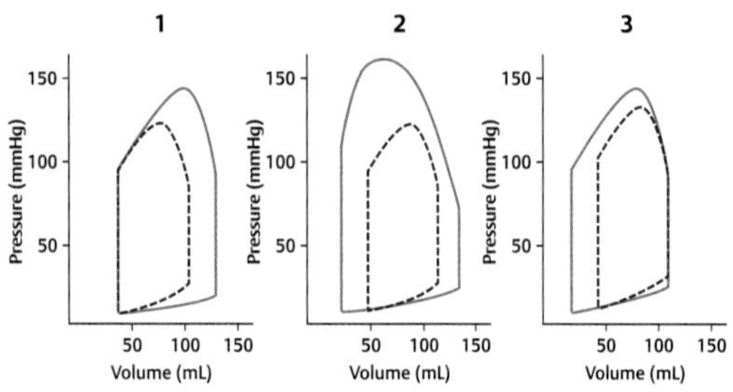

A. 1
B. 2
C. 3

95. A 33-year-old man is roller skating with his kids. Which of the following changes to ventricular preload is expected during this period of exercise?

A. Increase in right ventricular preload
B. Decrease in right ventricular preload
C. Increase in left ventricular preload
D. Decrease in left ventricular preload
E. Increase in right and left ventricular preload
F. Decrease in right and left ventricular preload

96. A 72-year-old man is hospitalized following a massive myocardial infarction. His blood pressure is 90/50 mm Hg, pulse is 125 beats per minute, and respiratory rate is 23 breaths per minute. Physical exam reveals weak distal pulses; cool, clammy skin; and crackles in both lungs. Shock is diagnosed. Which type of shock is most associated with these signs and symptoms?

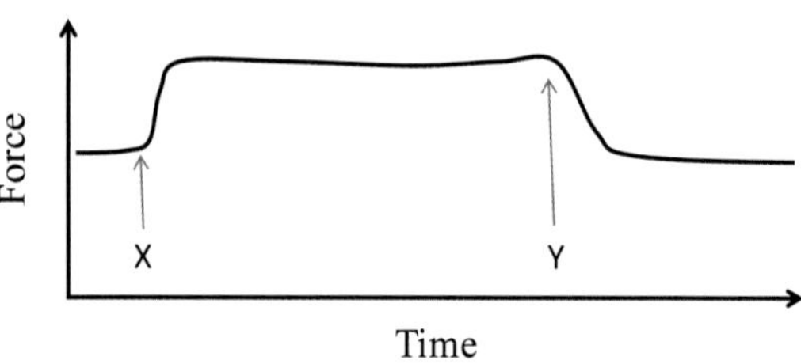

A. Cardiogenic
B. Distributive
C. Hypovolemic
D. Neurogenic
E. Obstructive

97. A 47-year-old woman is transported to the emergency department after fainting at a baseball game. She is conscious but feels dizzy, cold, and clammy. Her blood pressure is 82/55 mm Hg, pulse is 120 beats per minute, and respiratory rate is 21 breaths per minute. Body temperature is normal. She admits to chronic constipation for several months and seeing blood in her feces. Physical exam reveals profuse bleeding from the anus, and shock is diagnosed. Which type of shock is most associated with these signs and symptoms?

A. Cardiogenic
B. Distributive
C. Hypovolemic
D. Neurogenic
E. Obstructive

98. A 38-year-old woman came to the emergency department complaining of left-sided flank pain for 2 days. She was noted to have had vomiting and headache for the past 24 hours. Her blood pressure is 79/50 mm Hg, pulse is 115 beats per minute, respiratory rate is 18 breaths per minute, and temperature is 102.6°F. The patient is admitted to the ICU and given IV fluids, but her blood pressure does not respond. Which type of shock is most associated with these signs and symptoms?

A. Cardiogenic
B. Distributive
C. Hypovolemic
D. Neurogenic
E. Obstructive

99. A 42-year-old woman presents to the emergency department with a cough and weakness for 3 days. She has smoked 1 pack of cigarettes per day for 20 years. She takes medication for a hypothyroid condition, hypertension, and oral contraceptives. Physical examination reveals tachycardia, tachypnea, and jugular venous distention. Her blood pressure is 100/70 mm Hg. Which type of shock is most associated with these signs and symptoms?

A. Cardiogenic
B. Distributive
C. Hypovolemic
D. Neurogenic
E. Obstructive

5.10 Answers and Explanations

77. Correct: ↔, ↑ (E)

Points 1 and 2 are on the same Starling curve, so no change in contractility occurs when shifting from 1 to 2. An increase in contractility would shift up to point 5, and a decrease in contractility would shift down to point 3. To shift up the Starling curve from point 1 to 2, the cardiac preload must increase, thus increasing left ventricular end diastolic volume. A decrease in preload would cause the shift to point 4. (**A**, **B**, **C**, **D**, **F**) These answer choices have the wrong combination of answers.

78. Correct: ↑, ↓, ↑ (C)

During periods of increased physical activity, the sympathetic innervation to the heart is increased and parasympathetic innervation is decreased. The increase in sympathetic innervation will increase left ventricular contractility, which will in turn reduce the left ventricular end systolic volume by contracting more forcefully and ejecting a greater volume of blood. The left ventricular end diastolic volume will increase due to reduced vascular compliance, which drives some of the venous reservoir to the heart. This increases venous return, end diastolic volume, and ultimately cardiac output. (**A**, **B**, **D**, **E**, **F**) These answer choices have the wrong combinations of answers.

79. Correct: Increased pulse pressure (B)

Pulse pressure is increased since the Frank-Starling law of the heart dictates that in response to increased preload there is an increase in stroke volume, which then leads to a higher systolic arterial blood pressure on the next beat. Any time thereafter, it is not so easy to predict, since changes in arterial blood pressure will activate autonomic cardiovascular control, and especially, any change in parasympathetic control will be evident in a few heartbeats. (**A**) Diastolic arterial blood pressure is mainly a function of heart rate and peripheral arteriolar resistance, not of preload. (**C**, **D**) Stroke volume and systolic arterial blood pressure are increased, as explained in answer B. (**E**) Change in arteriolar resistance is a function of the sympathetic nervous system, which acts too slowly to affect the next heartbeat.

80. Correct: Decrease in blood volume (A)

When blood pools in the lower extremities after standing up, decreased preload causes low stroke volume, which is compensated for with elevated heart rate to maintain cardiac output. This normal compensatory body response is overwhelmed in the presence of hypovolemia, such as caused by low blood volume. (**B**) A physiologic decrease in left ventricular afterload will not cause orthostatic hypotension in a young person. It will increase stroke volume due to increased velocity of fiber shortening and decrease end-diastolic volume. The Frank-Starling mechanism and the baroreceptor-induced heart rate response will normalize cardiac output. (**C**) A decrease in cardiac contractility due to decreased sympathetic activity would also decrease heart rate. A decrease in cardiac contractility due to decreased afterload (Anrep effect) is unlikely, as explained in B. (**D**) A decrease in venous compliance redistributes blood from the unstressed volume to the stressed volume, which causes an increase in blood pressure and a decrease in heart rate (**E**) An increase in venous return increases cardiac output through the Frank-Starling mechanism and does not explain an abnormal response to gravitational changes.

81. Correct: ↑, ↑, ↑ (A)

Extreme anxiety leads to sympathetic activation. As a consequence, mean circulatory filling pressure increases due to a decrease in venous compliance that shifts blood to the arteries or stressed volume of the cardiovascular system. This effect outweighs the small decrease in mean circulatory filling pressure due to the minor hemorrhage. Heart rate increases, because norepinephrine and epinephrine activate β_1 adrenergic receptors in the sinoatrial node of the heart. Cardiac output increases, because sympathetic activation has a positive inotropic effect, which leads to increased stroke volume, and together with increased heart rate, to increased cardiac output. (**B**, **C**, **D**, **E**, **F**) These choices have one or more wrong consequences of exercise- or severe stress–induced sympathetic activation.

82. Correct: 5 (B)

Use the Fick principle to solve for cardiac output: cardiac output (CO) = oxygen consumption/(arterial oxygen content – venous oxygen content)

CO = 250 mL/min/(0.19 mL oxygen/mL blood – 0.14 mL oxygen/mL blood) = 250 mL/min/ (0.05 mL oxygen/mL blood) = 5000 mL/min = 5 L/min.

(**A, C, D, E**) These answer choices do not contain the correct response.

83. Correct: Increase in venous compliance (E)

The mean systemic pressure (MSP) is the pressure of the cardiovascular system that the blood exerts upon the walls of blood vessels when there is no venous return. It is affected by the volume of blood (donating blood decreases MSP) and by the "tightness" of the blood vessels (increase in venous compliance decreases MSP). With increased venous compliance, blood shifts to the veins, which hold it there without any significant pressure increase, while the blood that is removed from the arteries significantly decreases their pressure. In the clinical vignette, the blood loss is large since a small loss would be counterbalanced in a healthy person by a decrease in venous compliance, so that overall MSP would be minimally affected. (**A, B**) Positive or negative changes in contractility, also called inotropy, alter heart function but have no effect on vascular function and MSP. (**C**) Total peripheral resistance is primarily determined by the resistance of the arterioles. It affects how easily blood flows from the arterial to the venous side, but not how full the circulatory system is. In other words, MSP is not affected. (**D**) Excessive intake of NaCl would cause hyperosmotic volume expansion and increase MSP.

84. Correct: 2, 5 (E)

Patient 1 has pheochromocytoma, a tumor that arises from the adrenal medulla and causes elevated levels of circulating epinephrine. This will increase sympathetic activity, including β_1 adrenergic receptor activity of the heart. This increase in β_1 receptor activity increases cardiac contractility (among other things), which shifts the cardiac function curve upward to point 2. Patient 2 has untreated right heart failure, which is shown by a downward shift on the cardiac function curve, since the heart cannot contract as forcefully as usual. In this case, the right atrial pressure would be elevated, since the right heart is not effectively pumping blood, so the patient is operating at point 5. (**A, B , C, D, F, G, H, I, J, K, L**) These answer choices do not include the correct combination of responses.

85. Correct: Suddenly standing up compared to lying (D)

Central venous pressure (CVP) and venous return (VR) decrease when a person moves from supine to standing position, since large amounts of blood pool in the veins due to gravity and the high capacitance of the veins. Decreased VR decreases cardiac output and mean arterial pressure, and the pressure gradient through the entire circulation system is decreased. (**A**) During respiratory inhalation, CVP decreases and VR increases in response to an increased venous pressure gradient. (**B, C**) During late pregnancy and with sustained increased intrapleural pressure (such as during a Valsalva maneuver), CVP increases due to external vena cava compression and VR decreases. (**E**) The rhythmical contraction of the limb muscles (the so-called muscle pump) increase CVP and VR by propelling blood toward the heart.

86. Correct: Decreased venous compliance (B)

Point B is on a different vascular function curve than point A, so either blood volume or vascular compliance must change to shift the intersection point from B to A. Since intersection point B is at a lower venous return (VR) and lower right atrial pressure (RAP), an increase in blood volume or a decrease in venous compliance will shift the curve upward toward point A. (**A, D**) Points A and B are on the same cardiac function curve, so there is no difference in cardiac contractility. (**C**) The downward shift of point B is not due to a change in arteriole tone because the vascular function curves have different *x*-axis intercepts, which indicate mean systemic filling pressures (MSFP). A change in arteriole tone alters the curve, but the MSFP remains unchanged. (**E**) An increase in venous compliance will shift the vascular function curve downward, not upward.

87. Correct: An IV infusion of 2.5 pints of normal saline (C)

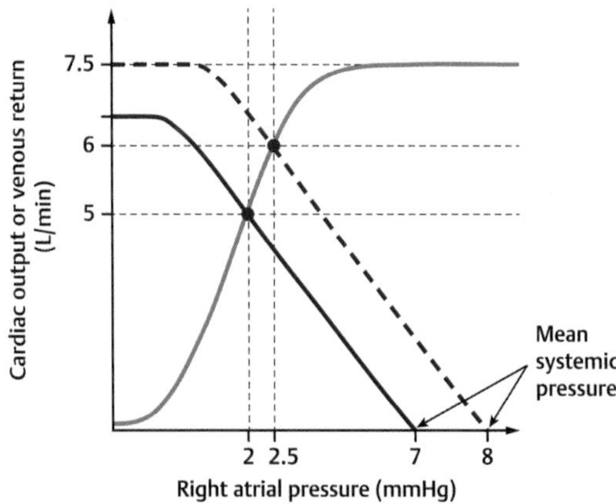

The image shows that the cardiovascular parameter changes can be explained by a parallel shift of the blue vascular function curve to the right (from solid to dotted line). This happens when blood volume increases, such as by intravascular fluid expansion, and mean systemic pressure (MSP) increases. In the new steady state, right atrial pressure and cardiac output are increased. (**A, E**) Both a β_1 adrenergic receptor agonist (e.g., dobutamine) and a cardiac glycoside (e.g., digitalis) increase contractility. There would be no change in MSP. (**B**) Blocking α_1 adrenergic receptors (e.g., terazosin) would cause vasodilation and a decrease in total peripheral resistance (TPR), but no change in MSP. (**D**) A nitric oxide vasodilator drug decreases TPR, which does not cause a change in MSP. It additionally dilates veins and increases their compliance, which leads to decreased (not increased) MSP.

88. Correct: She was given a positive inotropic drug. (E)

Positive inotropy affects only the cardiac function curve without altering the venous function curve, as is the case here. As a result of increased contractility and increased stroke volume, more blood is ejected on each beat, so that at equilibrium cardiac output (y-axis) is increased and end-diastolic volume is decreased (x-axis). (**A**) During exercise, total peripheral resistance (TPR) initially increases, followed by a decrease with time and increasing intensity. A change in TPR affects both the cardiac and venous function curves. (**B**) A peripheral artery blockage that causes severe pain due to diminished blood flow indicates increased TPR and would alter both the cardiac and venous function curves. (**C**) When suddenly standing up, contractility and TPR increase and venous compliance decreases, affecting both the cardiac and venous compliance curves. (**D**) A blood transfusion would affect the venous curve and shift X to the right.

89. Correct: Venous compliance (E)

The woman's venous compliance is decreased as part of a partially compensated left ventricular failure, most likely due to old inferior wall myocardial infarction (distinct Q waves, no S-T segment elevation in inferior wall leads). Silent infarcts or infarcts mistaken as fibromyalgia or heartburn are more prevalent in older people with diabetes mellitus. Point X of both figures indicate a failing heart (decreased contractility) with reduced stroke volume/cardiac output (causing her tiredness). As compensation, the woman's venous compliance decreased, shifting the vascular function curve to the right. (**A**, **C**) Another compensatory response is an increase in blood volume, further shifting the vascular function curve to the right and increasing preload in the left ventricular pressure–volume loop. (**B**) End-systolic volume is increased (not decreased) since the heart is overstretched and cannot cope with the increased preload. (**D**) Systemic vascular resistance is increased (not decreased), as evident from the decreased slope of the vascular function curve.

90. Correct: B (B)

When starting from the star on the cardiac-vascular function curve, an increase in cardiac contractility will shift the cardiac function curve upward to a new intersection point (point C). From there, a decrease in arteriole tone will shift the vascular function curve to the right to intersection point B, but the mean systemic filling pressures (MSFP; x-axis intercept) of the new curve remains unchanged. (**A**, **E**, **F**, **I**, **J**) These choices have a different MSFP, which indicate a change in blood volume or venous compliance. These are not affected by the herbal supplement based on the given information. (**C**) This choice does not show a shift of the vascular function curve, which must shift for a change in arteriolar tone. (**G**, **H**) These choices do not include a shift of the cardiac function curve, which would be the case for a change in contractility. (**D**) An increase (not a decrease) in arteriolar tone would shift the vascular function curve to the left.

91. Correct: F (E)

The slope of the vascular function curve is determined by total peripheral resistance (TPR). Decreased TPR rotates the venous return curve clockwise, so that for a given central venous pressure (CVP), venous return is increased. One can also express resistance as pressure difference divided by flow rate ($R = \Delta P/Q$), which shows that the lowest resistance is given at a small ΔP and/or at a large Q. For venous resistance, ΔP represents the difference between mean systemic pressure and central venous pressure at the steady-state operating point, and Q represents venous return. (**A**, **B**, **C**, **D**) These curves all have a lower slope, indicating a higher resistance to venous return.

92. Correct: Sepsis (E)

Sepsis is a systemic infection in which systemic vasodilation occurs, causing blood to be distributed in the peripheral vessels, and blood pressure to drop dangerously low. This is one example of distributive shock. (**A**) Cardiac tamponade is a compression of the heart by fluid accumulation in the pericardial sac. This can result in obstructive shock. (**B**) Hemorrhage is blood loss, which can lead to hypovolemic shock. (**C**) Myocardial infarction can damage the heart muscle tissue and lead to cardiogenic shock. (**D**) Pulmonary embolism (blood clots in pulmonary vasculature) can obstruct blood flow to the left heart and cause obstructive shock.

93. Correct: ↓, ↑ (D)

Anaphylactic shock is a distributive shock, causing a drop in blood pressure due to systemic vasodilation and blood distribution to the peripheral vessels. Due to this peripheral blood distribution, the central venous pressure will be low. Cardiac tamponade is a compression of the heart by fluid accumulation in the pericardial sac. This compression prevents proper filling of the heart and causes blood to back up in the venous system. This results in an elevated central venous pressure. (**A**, **B**, **C**, **E**) These answer choices do not contain the correct combination of responses.

94. Correct: 2 (B)

The second pressure–volume (PV) loop shows both an increase in end diastolic volume (EDV) and a decrease in end systolic volume (ESV), which is representative of the changes seen during exercise. The increase in EDV is due to an increase in venous return, primarily from the reduced venous compliance, which displaces the venous reservoir to the heart. The decrease in ESV is primarily due to the increase in cardiac contractility, with increases the force of contraction and ejects more blood from the heart. (**A**) The first loop shows only an increase in EDV. (**C**) The third loop shows only a decrease in ESV.

95. Correct: Increase in right and left ventricular preload (E)

During exercise, venous compliance is decreased, which increases venous return. This increase in venous return increases the preload (end diastolic volume) of both the right and left ventricles, since they are arranged in series. (**A**, **C**) These answers are both correct, but they are not the best choice, since both right and left ventricular preload increases. (**B**, **D**, **F**) Preload increases, not decreases, during exercise.

96. Correct: Cardiogenic (A)

Cardiogenic shock is caused by a failure of the heart to pump correctly, either due to damage to the heart muscle through myocardial infarction or through cardiac valve problems, congestive heart failure, or dysrhythmia. The reduced cardiac output causes the patient's hypotension, elevated pulse, weak distal pulses, and cool, clammy skin. The backup of blood into the lung causes the crackles (edema) and elevated respiratory rate. (**B**) Distributive shock is caused by an abnormal distribution of blood to tissues and organs and includes septic, anaphylactic, and neurogenic causes. (**C**) Hypovolemic shock is the most common type and is caused by insufficient circulating volume, typically from hemorrhage, although severe vomiting and diarrhea are also potential causes. Typical symptoms include a rapid, weak pulse due to decreased blood flow combined with tachycardia; cool, clammy skin; and rapid and shallow breathing. (**D**) Neurogenic shock arises due to damage to the central nervous system, which impairs cardiac function by reducing heart rate and reducing the blood vessel tone, resulting in severe hypotension. (**E**) Obstructive shock is caused by an obstruction of blood flow to the heart. This typically occurs due to a reduction in venous return but may also be caused by blockage of the aorta.

97. Correct: Hypovolemic (C)

Hypovolemic shock is caused by insufficient circulating volume, typically from hemorrhage, although severe vomiting and diarrhea are also potential causes. Typical symptoms include a rapid, weak pulse due to decreased blood flow combined with tachycardia; cool, clammy skin; and rapid and shallow breathing. (**A**) Cardiogenic shock is caused by a failure of the heart to pump correctly, either due to damage to the heart muscle through myocardial infarction or through cardiac valve problems, congestive heart failure, or dysrhythmia. (**B**) Distributive shock is caused by an abnormal distribution of blood to tissues and organs and includes septic, anaphylactic, and neurogenic causes. (**D**) Neurogenic shock arises due to damage to the central nervous system, which impairs cardiac function by reducing heart rate and loosening the blood vessel tone, resulting in severe hypotension. (**E**) Obstructive shock is caused by an obstruction of blood flow to the heart. This typically occurs due to a reduction in venous return, but it may also be caused by blockage of the aorta.

98. Correct: Distributive (B)

Distributive shock is caused by an abnormal distribution of blood to tissues and organs and includes septic, anaphylactic, and neurogenic causes. This patient has septic shock, most likely from a urinary tract or kidney infection. Her high temperature and unresponsiveness to IV fluids are the two major indicators. (**A**) Cardiogenic shock is caused by a failure of the heart to pump correctly, either due to damage to the heart muscle through myocardial infarction or through cardiac valve problems, congestive heart failure, or dysrhythmia. (**C**) Hypovolemic shock is caused by insufficient circulating volume, typically from hemorrhage, although severe vomiting and diarrhea are also potential causes. Typical symptoms include a rapid, weak pulse due to decreased blood flow combined with tachycardia; cool, clammy skin; and rapid and shallow breathing. (**D**) Neurogenic shock arises due to damage to the central nervous system, which impairs cardiac function by reducing heart rate and loosening the blood vessel tone, resulting in severe hypotension. (**E**) Obstructive shock is caused by an obstruction of blood flow to the heart. This typically occurs due to a reduction in venous return but may also be caused by blockage of the aorta.

99. Correct: Obstructive (E)

Obstructive shock is a form of shock associated with physical obstruction of the great vessels or the heart itself. Pulmonary embolism and cardiac tamponade are the most common causes of obstructive shock. This patient likely has a pulmonary embolism, based on her history of smoking, age, and use of oral contraceptives. In addition, distended jugular veins are seen only in cardiogenic and obstructive shocks, but she has no signs of pump failure, so cardiogenic can be excluded. (**A**) Cardiogenic shock is caused by a failure of the heart to pump correctly, either due to damage to the heart muscle through myocardial infarction or through cardiac valve problems, congestive heart failure, or dysrhythmia. (**B**) Distributive shock is caused by an abnormal distribution of blood to tissues and organs and includes septic, anaphylactic, and neurogenic causes. (**C**) Hypovolemic shock is caused by insufficient circulating volume, typically from hemorrhage, although severe vomiting and diarrhea are also potential causes. Typical symptoms include a rapid, weak pulse due to decreased blood flow combined with tachycardia; cool, clammy skin; and rapid and shallow breathing. (**D**) Neurogenic shock arises due to damage to the central nervous system, which impairs cardiac function by reducing heart rate and loosening the blood vessel tone, resulting in severe hypotension.

5.11 Questions

100. Stimulation of which of the following receptors will directly increase vascular smooth muscle tone?

A. Angiotensin II (AT_1)
B. β_1 adrenergic (β_1)
C. β_2 adrenergic (β_2)
D. Histamine-2 (H_2)
E. Muscarinic-2 (M_2)

101. A 63-year-old obese woman is treated for hypertension with a drug that antagonizes both α- and β-adrenergic receptors. What direct effect will this drug have on total peripheral resistance and cardiac inotropy?

	Total peripheral resistance	Cardiac inotropy
A.	↓	↓
B.	↓	↑
C.	↓	↔
D.	↑	↓
E.	↑	↑
F.	↑	↔

102. The tracing shows the force generation in isolated arterial smooth muscle when two vasoactive agents, X and Y, are given at the indicated times. X and Y most likely represent which of the following pharmacologic agents?

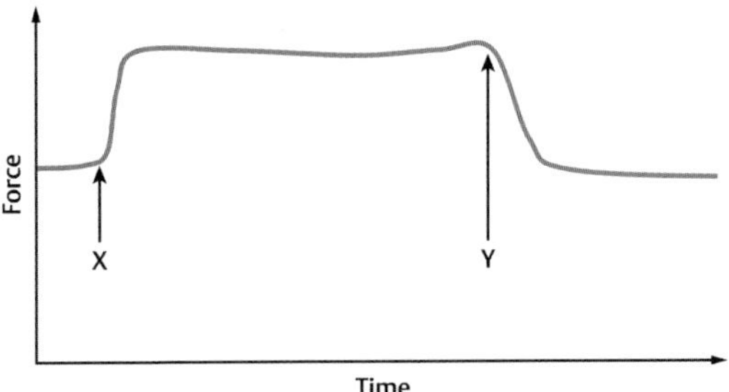

	Agent X	Agent Y
A.	α1 adrenergic agonist	Calcium channel antagonist
B.	Atrial natriuretic peptide	β1 receptor antagonist
C.	β2 receptor agonist	Angiotensin II
D.	Histamine	Serotonin
E.	Nitric oxide	Norepinephrine

103. When blood pressure is measured with a sphygmomanometer, blood flow through the brachial artery is temporarily increased above normal immediately following deflation of the blood pressure cuff around the arm. Which of the following correctly describes this change in blood flow, and what are the primary local metabolites responsible for the change in flow?

	Increased blood flow phenomenon	Primary local metabolites
A.	Active hyperemia	Carbon dioxide and hydrogen
B.	Active hyperemia	Adenosine and potassium
C.	Active hyperemia	Calcium and magnesium
D.	Reactive hyperemia	Carbon dioxide and hydrogen
E.	Reactive hyperemia	Adenosine and potassium
F.	Reactive hyperemia	Calcium and magnesium

104. In an experimental procedure, blood flow to the leg muscles of a mouse is measured at rest and again during exercise. During exercise, blood flow to the leg muscles triples compared to rest. What is the primary cause of this increase in blood flow?

A. Decreased plasma carbon dioxide levels
B. Decreased β_2 sympathetic activity
C. Increased plasma oxygen levels
D. Increased metabolite production in the legs
E. Increased parasympathetic activity

105. A 33-year-old woman with no known health concerns is exercising about three times per week. Her resting heart rate is 60 beats per minute, her resting blood pressure 122/78 mm Hg. By the end of 1 hour of submaximal exercise, her myocardial oxygen consumption has doubled, compared to rest. Which of the following best describes her coronary blood flow (mL/min) and coronary oxygen extraction (%) at that time?

	Coronary blood flow	Coronary oxygen extraction
A.	Less than double increase	Less than double increase
B.	About double	Little or no change
C.	Small decrease	More than double
D.	Small increase	About double
E.	More than double	Small decrease

106. A lean 75-year-old woman is being evaluated for burning muscle pain in her left leg during brisk walking. She reports no discomfort in her right leg. Ultrasound analysis reveals that the blood flows in her left and right calf muscles are similar at rest. Blood flow is increased twofold on the left side and fivefold on the right side when she walks on a treadmill. Which of the following is the most reasonable explanation of her symptoms?

A. A sedentary lifestyle made her peripheral vasculature stiffer.
B. Her heart is no longer able to sustain brisk walking exercise.
C. She suffers from generalized microvascular disease.
D. There is an increased vascular resistance in her left leg vasculature.
E. Vasculature of her right leg is inappropriately dilated during walking.

107. A medical student is studying fluid exchange in the skeletal muscle capillaries of a laboratory animal. He determines that fluid is being forced out of the capillaries with a net filtration pressure of 8 mm Hg, and he obtains the following laboratory values:

Capillary hydrostatic pressure = 22 mm Hg
Capillary colloid osmotic pressure = 17 mm Hg
Interstitial hydrostatic pressure = 7 mm Hg

Which of the following is the interstitial colloid osmotic pressure in mm Hg?

A. −9
B. −6
C. +6
D. +8
E. +10

108. A patient with right heart failure presents with shortness of breath. Tests reveal right ventricular hypertrophy, a systolic murmur, and pitting leg edema. There is no indication of left ventricular failure. Which of the following hemodynamic changes is expected in the pulmonary capillaries?

A. Decreased pulmonary capillary hydrostatic fluid pressure
B. Decreased pulmonary interstitial colloid osmotic pressure
C. Decreased pulmonary capillary filtration coefficient
D. Increased pulmonary interstitial hydrostatic fluid pressure
E. Increased pulmonary capillary colloid osmotic pressure

109. A 58-year-old woman presents with gradual weight loss, but an increase in belt size, over the past three years. The history assessment reveals that she has consumed substantial amounts of alcohol for years. Physical exam reveals an arterial blood pressure of 120/85 mm Hg, a positive abdominal fluid wave, and a bumpy and irregular liver on palpation. Which of the following changes in hydrostatic pressure is the reason for the patient's ascites?

A. It is abnormally high in the gastric artery.
B. It is abnormally high in the hepatic artery.
C. It is abnormally high in the splanchnic capillaries.
D. It is higher in the hepatic veins than in the portal vein.
E. It is higher in the hepatic veins than in the splenic vein.

110. A patient presents with peripheral edema in his lower right leg following a surgical procedure in that region. Which of the following changes to capillary hydrostatic pressure and interstitial hydrostatic pressure are expected in the patient's lower right leg?

	Capillary hydrostatic pressure	Interstitial hydrostatic pressure
A.	↓	↑
B.	↓	↓
C.	↑	↑
D.	↑	↓
E.	↔	↑
F.	↔	↓

111. A 50-year-old male patient with liver cancer is in advanced-stage hepatic failure. What effect will this have on his capillary colloid osmotic pressure, his interstitial hydrostatic pressure, and the net filtration in his systemic capillaries?

	Capillary colloid osmotic pressure	Interstitial hydrostatic pressure	Net filtration
A.	↑	↑	↑
B.	↑	↓	↓
C.	↑	↔	↑
D.	↓	↑	↓
E.	↓	↑	↑
F.	↓	↔	↓

112. In a healthy subject, which of the following is a correct statement in regards to lymph?

A. Lymph nodes clear it from lymphocytes.
B. In the digestive system, it may be rich in fat.
C. It may contain erythrocytes and platelets.
D. Production is decreased with a low-protein diet.
E. The spleen serves as the lymph "heart."

113. A 64-year-old man with a history of mitral valve stenosis presents to his general physician with complaints of difficulty breathing. If the patient is diagnosed with left heart failure due to chronic mitral valve stenosis, which of the following cardiac findings will most likely be present?

A. Decreased heart rate
B. Decreased jugular venous pulse
C. Increased mean arterial pressure
D. Peripheral edema
E. Pulmonary edema

114. During a brisk walk, the mechanism of autoregulation limits increases in perfusion to which of the following tissues/organs?

A. Kidney
B. Liver
C. Lungs
D. Skin
E. Spleen

115. A 23-year-old male had a snack 45 minutes ago and now lies relaxed on a bed in a room with a temperature of 72°F. He solves a crossword puzzle that lies on a tray in front of him. Under these conditions, which of his following organs has the lowest oxygen consumption in milliliters of oxygen per minute per 100 grams of tissue (mL O_2/min/100 g tissue)?

A. Brain
B. Heart
C. Kidney
D. Liver
E. Skeletal muscle

116. A mother informs the pediatrician that she wants to hold down her daughter during venipuncture since the girl is extremely fearful of needles. When the girl sees the venipuncture needle and becomes anxious, which of the following circulatory beds will respond with the largest percent decrease in blood flow compared to prestimulation?

A. Cerebral
B. Coronary
C. Cutaneous
D. Pulmonary
E. Skeletal muscle

117. The figure shows the brachial artery pulse pressure during one cardiac cycle. At which of the following times (labeled A–E) is left ventricular coronary blood flow highest?

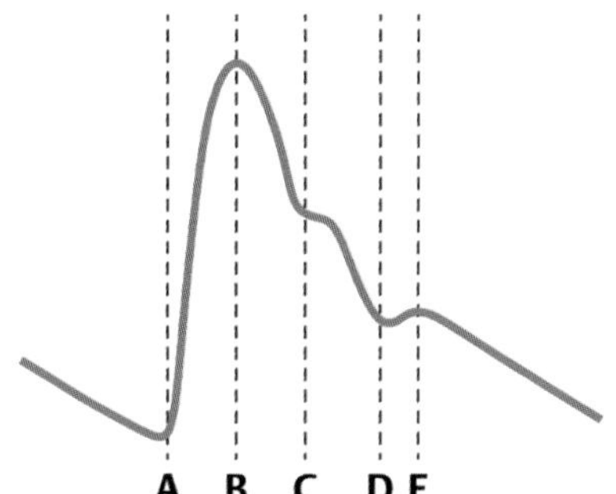

A. A
B. B
C. C
D. D
E. E

118. A patient with primary Raynaud's syndrome, a disorder that leads to extreme vasoconstriction in response to cold or stress, is preparing for a ski trip. Her past history shows that her attacks are resistant to behavioral therapy. From the following list, which pharmacological recommendation makes the most sense?

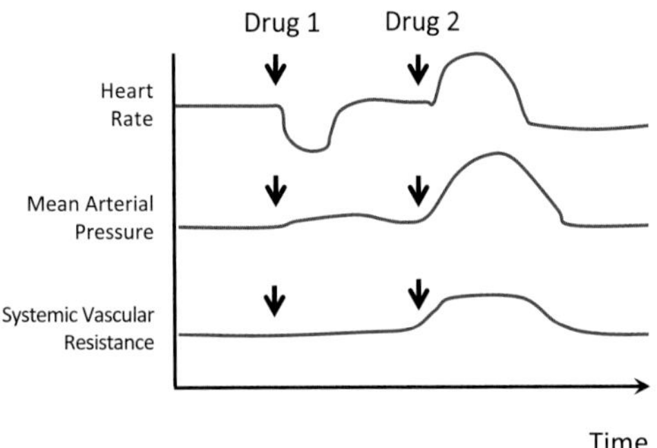

A. A nicotine patch
B. Arginine vasopressin analogues
C. Calcium channel blocker
D. Endothelin receptor agonist
E. Over-the-counter allergy medicine

119. In a healthy resting person, in which of the following circulatory beds is the arteriovenous oxygen difference independent of increased blood flow?
A. Cutaneous circulation
B. Hepatic circulation
C. Mesenteric circulation
D. Pancreatic circulation
E. Pulmonary circulation
F. Renal circulation
G. Skeletal muscle circulation
H. Splenic circulation

5.12 Answers and Explanations

100. Correct: Angiotensin II (AT1) (A)

Angiotensin II receptors are located in multiple organs, including blood vessels. They are activated by the circulating angiotensin II and stimulate vasoconstriction via G-protein receptor activation, thus increasing vascular tone. (**B**) β_1 receptors are primarily found in the heart and kidney. Their activation increases heart rate, cardiac contractility, and cardiac conduction velocity and the release of renin. (**C**) β_2 receptors are found in a multitude of tissues, and they generally cause smooth muscle cell relaxation (not contraction), particularly in the respiratory bronchi and blood vessels. (**D**) Histamine-2 receptors are located in various tissues and activated by local histamine release. They stimulate smooth muscle cell relaxation, not contraction. (**E**) Muscarinic-2 receptors are primarily located in the heart. Upon stimulation, they reduce heart rate and atrial contractility.

101. Correct: ↓, ↓ (A)

Antagonizing α-adrenergic receptors will decrease total peripheral resistance by reducing vascular tone. Antagonizing β-adrenergic receptors will decrease cardiac inotropy by reducing calcium availability in the cardiomyocytes. (**B, C, D, E, F**) These answer choices do not include the correct combination of responses.

102. Correct: α_1 adrenergic agonist, calcium channel antagonist (A)

Vasoactive agent X is a vasoconstrictor (increases arterial smooth muscle force), and vasoactive agent Y is a vasodilator (decreases arterial smooth muscle force). Hence, choice A is correct in that an α_1 adrenergic agonist causes vasoconstriction, and a calcium channel blocker causes vasodilation. (**B**) Atrial natriuretic peptide is a vasodilator, and a β_1 receptor antagonist has no direct effect on vascular smooth muscle. (**C**) A β_2 receptor agonist leads to vasodilation in skeletal muscle vasculature, and angiotensin II is a vasoconstrictor. (**D**) Histamine is a vasodilator, and serotonin is a vasoconstrictor. (**E**) Nitric oxide causes vasodilation, and norepinephrine causes vasoconstriction.

103. Correct: Reactive hyperemia, adenosine and potassium (E)

Blood pressure measurement via sphygmomanometry involves a temporary occlusion of blood flow through the brachial artery, which leads to reactive hyperemia. The occlusion causes metabolites to accumulate in the vessel downstream of the occlusion, and the metabolites cause vasodilation of the blood vessel. Once the occlusion is removed, the increased radius of the vessel allows a temporary increase in blood flow until the excess metabolites are washed away. The most powerful metabolites for vasodilation in skeletal muscle tissue are adenosine and potassium. (**A, B, C, D, F**) These answer choices do not include the correct combination of responses.

104. Correct: Increased metabolite production in the legs (D)

Exercise-induced increase in blood flow to skeletal muscle tissue is an example of active hyperemia, the increase in blood flow for a given tissue with increased demand. It is produced by an increase in metabolite production in response to the increase in activity. The metabolites have a vasodilatory effect on the vascular smooth muscle cells, which reduces vascular resistance and increases blood flow. (**A**) Elevated, not decreased, plasma carbon dioxide concentration promotes vascular dilation. (**B**) Increased, not decreased, β_2 receptor activity causes vasodilation in skeletal muscle vasculature. (**C**) Decreased plasma oxygen concentration, not increased, promotes vascular dilation. (**E**) The parasympathetic nervous system, except for a few special regions of the body, does not directly affect vascular resistance and will not increase blood flow to the extremities.

105. Correct: About double, little or no change (B)

In response to a doubling of oxygen consumption, coronary blood flow approximately doubled. In a healthy and fit person (evidenced by low resting heart rate and wide pulse pressure), increased oxygen demand of the heart is met by proportionally increasing blood flow, since oxygen extraction from blood is already close to optimal at rest. The relationship between blood flow and energy demand serves the heart well, since it is limited to oxidative metabolism and needs to perform continually, so there is no time to pay back any incurred oxygen debt. (**A, C, D, E**) These answers are not consistent with the principle that in the coronary arteries, vasculature flow is tightly coupled to oxygen demand.

106. Correct: There is an increased vascular resistance in her left leg vasculature. (D)

The woman presents with typical signs of peripheral artery disease, in which narrowed arteries due to plaque buildup increase her left leg vascular resistance and compromise the expected increase in blood flow during exercise. (**A**) While a sedentary lifestyle can accelerate the age-dependent increase in blood vessel stiffness, there is some additional impairment on the left that is not present on the right leg. (**B, C, E**) The normal response of increased blood flow with increased oxygen demand in her right leg vasculature indicates that her heart and body support exercise.

107. Correct: +10 (E)

Net filtration pressure (NFP) = (capillary hydrostatic pressure + interstitial colloid osmotic pressure) − (capillary colloid osmotic pressure + interstitial hydrostatic pressure). With the given values, interstitial colloid osmotic pressure equals 10 mm Hg, based on the following:

$$8 = (22 + X) - (17 + 7) = 22 + X - 24 = X - 2. \text{ When solved: } X = 8 + 2 = 10$$

108. Correct: Decreased pulmonary capillary hydrostatic fluid pressure (A)

The capillary hydrostatic fluid pressure is determined by the volume of blood in the capillaries. If the right heart is failing, then it cannot effectively pump blood to the lung; thus, the volume of blood in the lung capillaries will decrease and reduce the pulmonary capillary fluid pressure. (**B**) The pulmonary interstitial colloid osmotic pressure is produced by proteins in the interstitial space. This value will not be altered unless the vessel walls are damaged or inflamed, which can increase filtration of proteins. (**C**) The capillary filtration coefficient depends on the area of the capillary walls and their permeability to water. Ischemia such as potentially present for a patient with heart failure could increase it, but not decrease it. (**D**) The pulmonary interstitial fluid pressure is produced by fluid in the interstitial space. This increases if capillary blood volume increases or capillary colloid osmotic pressure decreases, which is not occurring in this patient. (**E**) The pulmonary plasma colloid osmotic pressure is produced by proteins in the plasma. This increases if protein concentration in the plasma is increased, which is not occurring in this patient.

109. Correct: It is abnormally high in the splanchnic capillaries. (C)

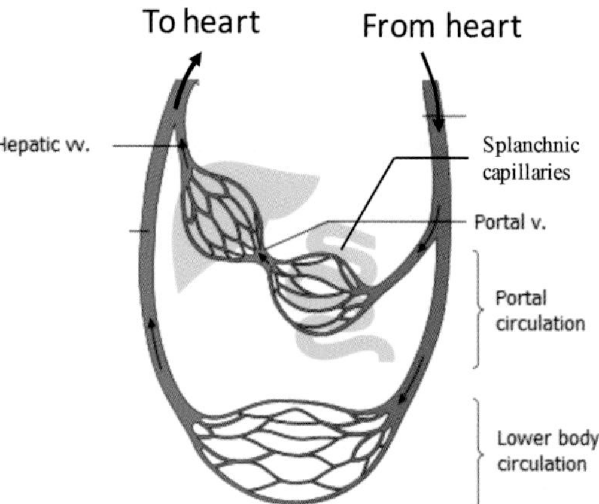

The hydrostatic pressure in the splanchnic capillaries (includes gastric, small intestinal, colonic, pancreatic, and splenic capillaries) is abnormally high due to hypertension of the portal vein in response to the increased intrahepatic resistance of a cirrhotic liver (irregular and bumpy appearance). When the splanchnic capillary hydrostatic pressure exceeds its capillary oncotic pressure, fluid moves into the abdominal cavity (positive abdominal fluid wave). (A, B) The hepatic and gastric artery pressures (not shown in the figure) are similar to the aortic pressure, which is normal. (**D**) The hepatic venous pressure has to be lower than the pressure in the portal vein; otherwise there would be no hepatic flood flow. (**E**) The splenic vein drains into the portal vein, so the same explanation applies as in D.

110. Correct: ↑, ↑ (C)

Surgical procedures can disrupt the lymphatic vessels in the region and affect fluid clearance from the interstitial space. If the excess interstitial fluid is not carried away by the lymph vessels, then it accumulates in the interstitial space and increases interstitial hydrostatic pressure (edema). The increased interstitial hydrostatic pressure promotes reabsorption of fluid back into the vessel and increases capillary hydrostatic pressure as well. (**A, B, D, E, F**) These choices do not include the correct combination of answers.

111. Correct: ↓, ↑, ↑ (E)

Since the liver synthesizes many of the plasma proteins, liver failure results in decreased plasma proteins and thus a decreased capillary colloid osmotic pressure. Since the concentration of proteins in the plasma plays an important role in the reabsorption of fluid from the interstitial space, low capillary colloid osmotic pressure will result in fluid accumulation in the interstitial space and increased interstitial hydrostatic pressure. Collectively, this will produce more filtration than reabsorption; thus, net filtration increases. (**A, B, C, D, F**) These choices do not include the correct combination of answers.

112. Correct: In the digestive system, it may be rich in fat. (B)

The lymph vessels of the digestive systems are rich in fat after a meal. The vessels, called lacteals, take up fats that have been released inside chylomicrons from small intestinal cells. (**A**) The function of lymph nodes is not to destroy but rather to activate the immune system and produce more lymphocytes, so that efferent lymphatic vessels carry lymphocytes to other nodes or to veins. (**C**) Lymph does not contain erythrocytes and platelets, because they are not present in the interstitial fluid that forms the lymph and that is carried one-way to the left subclavian vein. (**D**) Lymph production may be increased with an extremely low-protein diet, since a decrease in plasma oncotic pressure would cause more interstitial fluid and hence, lymph production. (**E**) The spleen does not act as a pump for lymph flow as the heart acts as a pump for blood flow. Lymph flow is mainly maintained by intrinsic smooth muscle and extrinsic skeletal muscle contraction.

113. Correct: Pulmonary edema (E)

In left heart failure, the left heart cannot effectively pump blood, which causes a backup of fluid in the lungs and commonly presents with pulmonary edema. (**A**) Patients with left heart failure have a small stroke volume due to reduced contractile force, and thus a reduced cardiac output. The heart partially compensates for this by increasing (not decreasing) heart rate. (**B**) Jugular venous pulse (JVP) will not be affected by left heart failure, unless it also leads to right heart failure, in which case JVP will increase due to the backup of blood from the right heart (not decrease). (**C**) Left heart failure reduces cardiac output, which reduces mean arterial pressure. (**D**) Peripheral edema results from right heart failure, not left heart failure.

114. Correct: Kidney (A)

While most systems of the body show some degree of autoregulation, it is most clearly observed in the kidneys, heart, and brain. Perfusion of these organs is essential for life, and autoregulation allows the body to divert blood flow where it is most needed. In the kidneys, autoregulation serves a second function in that it allows appropriate reabsorption of tubular biomolecules at a wide blood pressure range. (**B**, **C**, **D**, **E**) These organs have autoregulation, but to a much lesser degree than the kidneys.

115. Correct: Skeletal muscle (E)

Skeletal muscle at rest (note that the man is not even holding the puzzle) has the lowest oxygen consumption, of about 1 mL O_2/min/100 g tissue. (**A**) Compared to resting skeletal muscle, the oxygen consumption of the brain at rest is about threefold. It is most likely even higher for the man since he is solving a crossword puzzle. (**B**, **C**) Compared to resting skeletal muscle, the oxygen consumption at rest is about eightfold for the heart and about fivefold for the kidney, respectively. (**D**) Oxygen consumption of the liver is always higher than the normalized consumption by resting skeletal muscle. For the man, it is even higher due to the presence of dietary products 45 minutes after eating.

116. Correct: Cutaneous (C)

With no ambient temperature change, blood will be redirected during a fight-or-flight response (triggered by extreme fear) from the skin to vital organs that are needed for fighting and running. (**A**, **B**) Cerebral and coronary circulation beds are among the least sensitive systems in the body to the sympathetic constrictor action of norepinephrine/epinephrine, and their blood flow will not change. (**D**, **E**) Sympathetic activation redirects blood to the lung and skeletal muscle in anticipation of increased oxygen demand during times of high physiological stress.

117. Correct: C (C)

Point C (the dichrotic notch or incisura) is caused by a brief retrograde blood flow when the aortic valve closes and marks the end of systole and the beginning of diastole. During systole, coronary blood vessels are compressed, and blood flow is reduced. Immediately thereafter, reactive hyperemia occurs, with increased blood flow to repay the oxygen debt that was incurred during the compression. This is the time with highest coronary blood flow. (**A**, **B**) These time points mark rapid ejection during systole with reduced coronary blood flow. (**D**, **E**) These time points are in mid to late diastole, during which coronary blood flow continually declines from its highest point. Point E is an accentuated pressure point in diastole attributed to the delayed arrival of the reflected wave from the lower body.

118. Correct: Calcium channel blocker (C)

Calcium channel blockers (especially the class of dihydropyridines) are potent vasodilators by inhibiting L-type calcium channels on vascular smooth muscle, with little effect on cardiac contractility or conduction. (**A**, **B**, **D**, **E**) Nicotine, arginine-vasopressin, endothelin, and H_1-antihistamines as part of over-the-counter allergy medicine are all known to cause vasoconstriction and are hence not recommended for patients with Raynaud's disease.

119. Correct: Renal circulation (F)

Renal oxygen consumption is proportional to the sodium transport from the tubular fluid into the peritubular capillaries, which is coupled to the reabsorption of most other solutes in the renal cortex. An increase in renal blood flow, for instance by increased systemic blood pressure, increases glomerular filtration rate and concomitantly the quantity of solute to be reabsorbed in order to avoid excessive loss in urine. Hence, as blood flow increases, the arteriovenous oxygen difference remains constant. (**A**, **B**, **C**, **D**, **E**, **G**, **H**) In these circulatory beds, an increase in blood flow is accompanied by a decrease in arteriovenous oxygen difference, since oxygen extraction can be optimized with increased tissue oxygen demand.

5.13 Questions

120. A 53-year-old male presents with a hematocrit of 69%. He was diagnosed 3 years ago with renal abnormalities. The patient's systolic and diastolic arterial pressures are each increased by 15 mm Hg compared to his pre–kidney disease values. His hands and feet are cool, but there is no evidence of edema or cardiovascular problems at rest. Cardiac enzymes are within normal range. The man's arterial blood pressure at rest is increased because of an increase in which of the following parameters?

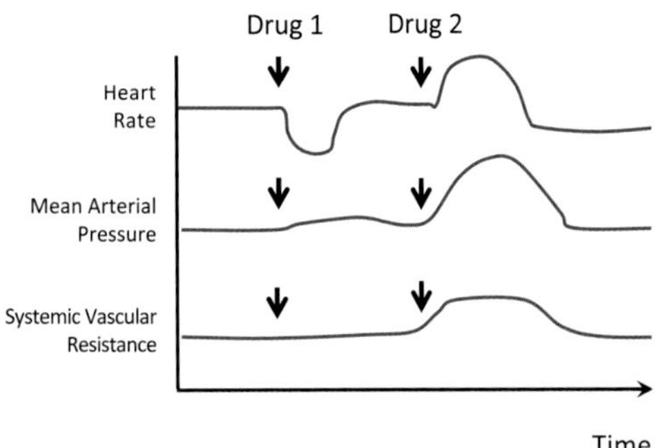

A. Arteriolar compliance
B. Blood density
C. Laminar blood flow
D. Total blood flow
E. Vascular resistance

121. An advanced martial art self-defense technique is pressure point fighting. One maneuver is to knock the opponent unconscious by striking at the neck and increasing stimulation of the carotid sinus baroreceptors. Which of the following is the most likely cardiovascular response to this technique in the targeted person?

A. Negative chronotropy
B. Negative inotropy
C. Positive chronotropy
D. Positive inotropy
E. Vasoconstriction

122. A 30-year-old woman experiencing tachycardia begins to massage the carotid region of her neck, which quickly reduces her heart rate. Which of the following mechanisms is responsible for this phenomenon?

A. Decreased activity of the cardioinhibitory center
B. Decreased afferent firing from baroreceptors to the nucleus tractus solitarii
C. Increased activity of the vasomotor center
D. Increased afferent firing from baroreceptors to the nucleus tractus solitarii
E. Decreased venous compliance

123. A 20-year-old college student was brought to an urgent care clinic with a severe headache. Her friends reported that she drank several liters of water in the previous hour as part of a game to see who could drink the most without urinating. The physician suspected overhydration, also called water intoxication. As part of the body's compensatory reflex against elevated blood pressure from overhydration, the activity of which component of the baroreceptor reflex is most likely to be decreased in this patient?

A. Cardioinhibitory center
B. High-pressure baroreceptors
C. Nucleus tractus solitarii (NTS)
D. Parasympathetic output to the heart
E. Vasomotor center

124. An anesthetized patient receives drug 1, which causes an acute bronchospasm, in response to which drug 2 is given. The relative changes in the patient's heart rate, mean arterial pressure, and systemic vascular resistance in response to the pharmacological interventions are shown in the image. Which of the following are most likely drug 1 and drug 2?

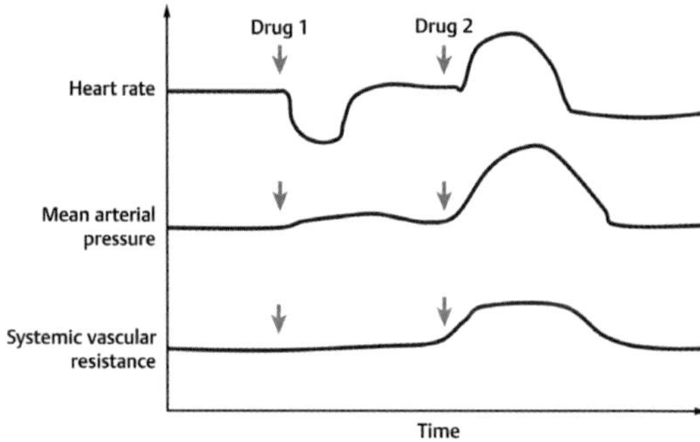

	Drug 1	Drug 2
A.	ACE inhibitor	Vagal stimulator
B.	α_1 receptor blocker	β_1 receptor blocker
C.	β_1 receptor blocker	Negative dromotropic drug
D.	Calcium channel blocker	Positive chronotropic drug
E.	Parasympathetic M_2 agonist	Epinephrine

125. A 17-year-old girl with orthostatic hypotension presents with complaints of multiple syncopal episodes over the past month when standing up. To prevent syncope, which of the following changes to cardiac output, arterial resistance, and venous compliance occur as part of the normal baroreceptor reflex in a healthy person when standing up?

	Cardiac output	Arterial resistance	Venous compliance
A.	↑	↑	↑
B.	↑	↓	↓
C.	↑	↑	↓
D.	↓	↑	↑
E.	↓	↓	↑
F.	↓	↓	↓

126. The solid line on the graph shows the profile of the mean blood pressure in the vasculature in a person at rest. Which of the following drug/drug categories will most likely cause the solid line to shift to the dashed line?

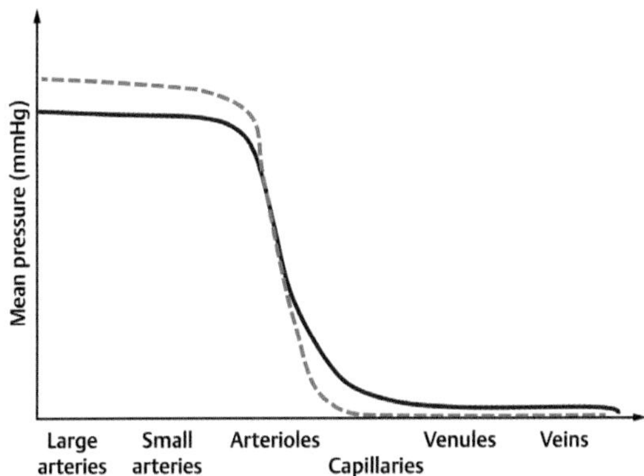

A. Arteriolar constrictor
B. Atropine
C. β_1 blocker
D. β_2 agonist
E. Venoconstrictor

127. When the Valsalva maneuver is used as a cardiac function test, the patient is asked to exhale forcibly against a closed glottis. The testing physician monitors the normal physiological body response to continued strain about 10–25 seconds after the beginning of the test. A rise in which of the following is monitored?

A. Arterial compliance
B. Cardiac contractility
C. Central venous pressure
D. Heart rate
E. Stroke volume

128. Six months after a heart transplant, the cardiac parameters of a 21-year-old man show normal cardiac output, pulmonary capillary wedge pressure, pulmonary artery pressure, ejection fraction, contractility, and blood pressure. However, there is no sign of reinnervation of the transplanted heart. Which of the following is expected for the man's heart rate when he starts to run as part of cardiac rehabilitation?

A. No change
B. Decrease
C. Increase, but slower than normal
D. Increase, but faster than normal
E. Unpredictable

129. The pharmacologic class of "neutral endopeptidase inhibitors" inhibits the degradation of vasoactive peptides. The body responds to the drug with a reduction in water and sodium, as well as vasodilation, thereby reducing blood pressure. Which of the following is a normal biological substrate of neutral endopeptidase?

A. Adenosine diphosphate (ADP)
B. Antidiuretic hormone (ADH)
C. Arginine (ARG)
D. Arginine vasopressin (AVP)
E. Atrial natriuretic peptide (ANP)

130. A 16-year-old boy involved in a knife fight is transported to the emergency department. A severed artery in his forearm was bleeding profusely but is now controlled. His blood pressure is 100/70 mm Hg. Which of the following cardiovascular parameters will be lower during compensation for hemorrhage than before the hemorrhage?

A. Arterial baroreceptor nerve activity
B. Arterial resistance
C. Capillary fluid reabsorption
D. Total peripheral resistance
E. Ventricular contractility

131. When comparing a healthy 70-year-old man to a healthy 20-year-old man, which of the following cardiac measurements will be decreased due to age?

A. Arterial intimal thickness
B. Early diastolic filling rate
C. Mean arterial blood pressure
D. Myocardial oxygen consumption
E. Myocardial wall stress

132. An 83-year-old man in overall good health presents with a blood pressure of 148/70 mm Hg. His medical records show a blood pressure of 121/80 mm Hg at age 42. Which of the following changes to the aortic pressure wave velocities contribute to the blood pressure changes in this patient?

	Forward wave velocity	Reflected wave velocity
A.	↓	↓
B.	↑	↑
C.	↓	↑
D.	↑	↔
E.	↔	↑

133. The following are the stroke volumes (in milliliters) and heart rates (in beats per minute), at rest and at maximal exercise, for 20-year-old twin brothers with similar stature. One is a nonathlete, and the other is a marathon runner.

		Stroke volume (mL)	Heart rate (bpm)
At rest	Nonathlete	75	75
	Marathon runner	105	50
Maximal exercise	Nonathlete	110	195
	Marathon runner	162	X

Which of the following is most likely the heart rate of the marathon runner at maximal exercise (indicated as *X* in the table)?

A. 300
B. 250
C. 200
D. 150
E. 100

Questions 134 to 136

A 55-year-old man is recovering from open heart surgery. Drainage chest tubes are in place to remove postoperative pus, blood, and other fluids. His wife visits him at the hospital bed the day after the surgery and notices that no fluids are draining from the tubes. Before she leaves, she tells the nurse that her husband seems restless and confused. The nurse alerts a rapid response team to assemble in order to assess and discuss the patient's status. It is summarized by the team as follows:

Complaint: Intermittent unstable angina
CNS: Glasgow coma scale: 12/15
Skin: Cold skin, mottled extremities
Capillary refill time: Prolonged
Heart Rate: Tachycardia
Heart sounds: Muffled
ECG: Tachycardia
CVP: Elevated
Respirations: Tachypnea
SpO_2: Hypoxia
Lung sounds: Clear
Urine output: Very low

134. Which of the following do you expect regarding the patient's blood pressure?

A. Normal blood pressure
B. Normal pulse pressure
C. Severe hypertension
D. Severe hypotension
E. Wide pulse pressure

135. Which of the following is the cause of the patient's red or purple patches of mottled skin?

A. Blood buildup due to constricted blood vessels
B. Blood buildup due to ruptured blood vessels
C. Blood stasis due to vasodilated blood vessels
D. Discoloration due to hemoglobin leaking into skin
E. Fluid buildup due to nondraining chest tubes

136. On further examination of the patient, a pulsus paradoxus is noted, which is the exaggerated response of the normal decrease in systolic blood pressure during inspiration. Which of the following results from inspiration and ultimately leads to the transient decrease in systolic arterial blood pressure during inspiration?

A. Filling of left heart is increased.
B. Left ventricular transmural pressure is decreased.
C. Pulmonary venous return is increased.
D. Right ventricular transmural pressure is decreased.
E. Systemic venous return is increased.

137. Hypovolemic shock, cardiogenic shock, and distributive shock due to sepsis have which of the following abnormally low features in common?

A. Arterial blood pressure
B. Central venous pressure
C. Contractility
D. Oxygen delivery to tissues
E. Systemic vascular resistance

138. As part of antihypertensive therapy, nitrates decrease preload and afterload, which leads to increased heart rate and contractility due to body reflexes. Nitrates are often prescribed in combination with β-blockers, which increase preload and decrease afterload, heart rate, and contractility. Considering this information, a decrease in which of the following is the main strategy for the use of a combination of β-blockers and nitrates as antihypertensive therapy?

A. End-diastolic volume
B. Contractility at given preload
C. Resting heart rate
D. Total blood volume
E. Work of the heart

139. Mr. Jones mixed his medication up with his wife's and accidentally took an α-antagonist drug, which decreased his mean arterial pressure temporarily. As a result of the decreased mean arterial pressure, compensation will occur. Which of the following compensatory changes to sympathetic and parasympathetic innervation of the heart, and cardiac output, are expected?

	Sympathetic innervation of the heart	Parasympathetic innervation of the heart	Cardiac output
A.	↑	↓	↑
B.	↑	↑	↑
C.	↑	↓	↓
D.	↓	↑	↓
E.	↓	↓	↓
F.	↓	↑	↑

5.14 Answers and Explanations

120. Correct: Vascular resistance (E)

Polycythemia (hematocrit of 69%) significantly increases blood viscosity and, hence, vascular resistance. With such progressive increase in afterload, the heart needs to work harder continuously to maintain normal cardiac output. The increased systolic pressure is likely due to a higher blood volume and the increased diastolic pressure due to an increased total peripheral resistance and higher heart rate. (**A**) An increase in arteriolar compliance (i.e., less stiff vessels) does not lead to an increase in blood pressure. (**B**) Blood density is proportional to the total protein concentration of blood and hence increased in polycythemia. However, blood density has no effect on resistance, the cause of the increased blood pressure. (**C**) The increased blood pressure is unrelated to whether blood flow is laminar or turbulent. (**D**) Total blood flow seems maintained (as indicated by cardiac enzymes in the normal range and the lack of cardiovascular problems) and not increased (as indicated by cold hands and feet).

121. Correct: Negative chronotropy (A)

Activation of the carotid sinus baroreceptors activates parasympathetic activity, which decreases heart rate within a few beats. If this happens suddenly without any physiological need, the sudden decrease in blood pressure can cause unconsciousness. Carotid sinus massage uses the same principle for the clinical purpose of lowering dangerously high heart rate. (**B**) The parasympathetic has no major negative inotropic effect. (**C, D, E**) Positive chronotropy, positive inotropy, and vasoconstriction are all sympathetic-mediated cardiovascular responses, which are inhibited by baroreceptor activation.

122. Correct: Increased afferent firing from baroreceptors to the nucleus tractus solitarii (D)

Carotid massage mechanically stimulates the baroreceptors in the carotid sinus and increases their activity (mimics high blood pressure). This increases afferent nerve firing from baroreceptors to the nucleus tractus solitarii, causing an increase in parasympathetic output to the heart and a decrease in sympathetic output to the heart and vessels. Among other things, this results in a decrease in heart rate. (**A, C, E**) Mechanical stimulation of the baroreceptors will mimic the effect of high blood pressure, which increases cardioinhibitory center activity, decreases vasomotor center activity, and increases venous compliance. (**B**) Mechanical stimulation increases, not decreases, afferent firing from baroreceptors.

123. Correct: Vasomotor center (E)

After drinking several liters of water, the patient's blood volume is increased and her mean arterial pressure (MAP) is elevated. As a result of the increased MAP, the baroreceptor reflex activity will increase, and the activity of the control center (nucleus tractus solitarii [NTS]) in the medulla will increase. This will decrease the activity of the vasomotor center, thus reducing sympathetic output to the heart. (**A**, **D**) The increased MAP will increase the activity to the cardioinhibitory center in the medulla, which will increase parasympathetic output to the heart. (**B**) Baroreceptor activity will increase as blood volume increases, since baroreceptors are activated by increased stretch. (**C**) NTS activity is directly related to baroreceptor activity, so as baroreceptor activity increases, NTS activity increases.

124. Correct: Parasympathetic M2 agonist, epinephrine (E)

Stimulation of the parasympathetic by M_2 muscarinic receptor agonists can be a cause of bronchospasms in anesthetized patients. It decreases heart rate (HR) and atrial contractility, which will not (or only minimally) affect mean arterial blood pressure (MAP) and systemic vascular resistance (SVR). Treating bronchospasm in an anesthetized patient is difficult, and epinephrine might be given, especially when a specific β_2 agonist is not available. The sympathetic activation increases HR, contractility, and vascular smooth muscle, resulting in increased MAP and SVR, as seen in the tracings. (**A**) An angiotensin-converting enzyme (ACE) inhibitor would affect MAP, and a vagal stimulator would not change MAP and SVR. (**B**) An α_1 receptor blocker would alter SVR, and a β_1 receptor blocker would not increase MAP. (**C**) A β_1 receptor blocker would affect MAP, and a negative dromotropic drug would not increase SVR. (**D**) A calcium channel blocker would cause vasodilation and decrease SVR, while a positive chronotropic drug would not increase SVR.

125. Correct: ↑, ↑, ↓ (C)

Upon standing up from a sitting position, the central venous pressure immediately drops as blood pools in the lower extremities. This triggers a decrease in baroreceptor activity due to the low blood volume and pressure in the thorax, which increases sympathetic output to the heart and vessels and decreases parasympathetic output to the heart. The increased sympathetic output increases arterial resistance, decreases venous compliance, and increases heart rate and contractility (stroke volume). The decreased parasympathetic output increases heart rate. The increase in heart rate and stroke volume increase the cardiac output. (**A**, **B**, **D**, **E**, **F**) These choices do not include the correct combination of answers.

126. Correct: Arteriolar constrictor (A)

Arteriolar vasoconstriction would increase mean pressure in upstream vessels such as large and small arteries and exacerbate the pressure decrease in the arterioles. Based on the equation $\Delta P = Q \times R$, an increase in resistance (R) due to vasoconstriction increases driving pressure (ΔP) at constant total blood flow (Q). (**B**) Atropine counters the actions of the parasympathetic system, which has no direct effect on vascular smooth muscle. It may cause vasodilation through indirect actions. (**C**) β_1 receptors are mainly located in the heart and kidneys, and blocking their actions has no direct effect on vascular smooth muscle. Indirectly, it may lead to vasodilation. (**D**) Vascular smooth muscle has β_2 receptors and their activation leads to arteriolar dilation. (**E**) Venoconstrictor drugs primarily decrease compliance of small veins, which consequently increases the volume and pressure of large veins, neither of which is seen in the graph.

127. Correct: Heart rate (D)

The increased strain of the Valsalva maneuver increases intrathoracic pressure, which primarily squeezes compliant venous vessels. Increased central venous pressure decreases venous return, which in turn decreases systolic and hence mean arterial pressure. In response, the baroreceptor reflex increases sympathetic outflow, resulting in increased heart rate during continued strain (phase II) of the maneuver. In modern cardiovascular medicine, the Valsalva maneuver is used as bedside tool for preliminary office examinations, when heart rate can be simply obtained. (**A**, **B**, **C**, **E**) Changes in arterial compliance contractility, central venous pressure, and stroke volume require sophisticated instruments and are not used to monitor a Valsalva body response.

128. Correct: Increase, but slower than normal (C)

The heart is expected to respond to exercise with increasing heart rate due to sympathetic nervous system activation and β_1 receptor activation from circulating catecholamines of the adrenal medulla. The response to hormones will take significantly longer compared to the fast response of direct nervous stimulation. Similarly, the time until the heart rate returns to normal after exercise will be significantly longer due to the slow decline of the circulating hormones. Resting heart rate is typically faster than normal due to the loss of parasympathetic inhibition. (**A**, **B**, **D**, **E**) The change in heart rate is a predictably slow increase.

129. Correct: Atrial natriuretic peptide (ANP) (E)

ANP, or atrial natriuretic peptide, is a biological substrate of neutral endopeptidase, which breaks peptide bonds that join amino acids together within the molecule. Hence, neutral endopeptidase inhibitors increase the lifetime of ANP, extending its normal biological response as counterregulator of the renin-angiotensin system. This leads to decreased water and sodium retention and decreased blood pressure. (**A**) ADP, or adenosine diphosphate, is not a peptide. While ADP can locally act as vasodilator, it is not a systemic blood pressure regulator and has no direct effect on body water and sodium. (**B, D**) Antidiuretic hormone and arginine vasopressin are two names for the same substance. This substance has two primary actions: (1) it increases water and sodium retention, thereby increasing blood pressure; and (2), it acts as a vasoconstrictor, hence elevating blood pressure. (**C**) ARG, or arginine, is an amino acid and by itself not affected by endopeptidase. As a substrate of nitric oxide synthase, it may have blood pressure–lowering effects.

130. Correct: Arterial baroreceptor nerve activity (A)

The blood loss will result in a decreased mean arterial pressure (MAP), which will reduce the baroreceptor stretch and thus reduce the activity of the baroreceptors. (**B, D**) Arterial resistance and venous tone, the major contributors to total peripheral resistance, will be increased by the baroreceptor reflex in order to increase MAP. (**C**) Capillary fluid reabsorption will increase because capillary hydrostatic pressure is reduced, thus changing the balance of the Starling forces to favor reabsorption in order to increase MAP. (**D**) Ventricular contractility will be increased to increase cardiac output in order to increase MAP.

131. Correct: Early diastolic filling rate (B).

The rate of early diastolic filling declines markedly with increasing age in normal subjects. Dying myocytes are replaced with fibroblasts, and remaining myocytes undergo hypertrophy. Such structural changes result in decreased ventricular compliance and negatively affect diastolic relaxation, which is further impacted by the prolongation of systolic contraction in response to increased afterload. (**A**) Arterial intimal thickness is most likely increased due to decreased venous compliance and increased arterial plaque buildup. (**C**) Mean arterial blood pressure increases with age due to decreased blood vessel and heart compliance, increased total peripheral resistance, changes in blood volume and composition, and other factors. (**D**) Myocardial oxygen consumption is most likely increased due to increased resistance to ejection of blood from the left ventricle. (**E**) Myocardial wall stress is most likely increased due to increased afterload, slightly offset by left ventricular hypertrophy.

132. Correct: ↑, ↑ (B)

At age 83, the man will have less compliant (stiffer) blood vessels due to age-related histological changes. Both the aortic forward pressure wave (down the pressure gradient along the cardiovascular circuitry) and the reflected pressure wave (reflected at arterial branching) travel faster in a stiffer vessel with less recoil. This is due to the inefficient conversion of pressure energy into elastic energy and vice versa. The consequence is that the two waves combine during systole (increasing systolic pressure) and not during diastole as is the case in younger people. This "lack of pressure increase" in the elderly slightly decreases their diastolic pressure. (**A, C, D, E**) These combinations of aortic pressure wave velocity changes are incorrect.

133. Correct: 200 (C)

During aerobic exercise training, there is an adaptive increase in stroke volume; however, the maximum heart rate (mainly dependent on hereditary factors and age) cannot be changed. Hence, with identical age, similar stature, and comparable resting cardiac output (in both men about 5.5 liters per minute), the maximum heart rates of the trained and untrained twin brothers will be similar. The increase in cardiac output (from about 21 liters per minute in the nonathlete to about 32 liters per minute in the marathon runner) is due to the increased stroke volume. (**A, B, D, E**) The maximal heart rate will not be significantly higher or lower in the two brothers.

134. Correct: Severe hypotension (D)

The patient most likely is experiencing obstructive shock, probably due to cardiac tamponade. Postoperatively, thrombi may form inside the chest tubes and cause fluid buildup in the pericardial sac. This diagnosis is supported by bedside clinical signs of poor tissue perfusion (such as cool and mottled skin, altered mentation, long capillary refill) and further backed by signs such as tachycardia, oliguria, low oxygen saturation, and elevated central venous pressure. Obstructive shock leads to severe hypotension, since the pericardial fluid accumulation reduces cardiac output. The obstruction causes decreased venous return, which leads to decreased stroke volume and decreased blood pressure (BP). (**A**) The clear signs of tissue underperfusion make the possibility of normal BP highly unlikely. (**B, E**) A normal or wide pulse pressure is unlikely. A small pulse pressure is likely, since decreased stroke volume leads to a lower systolic BP, while tachycardia and increased total peripheral resistance (cold skin) lead to a higher diastolic BP. (**C**) The history and physical examination do not provide information on end-organ damage as seen in a hypertensive crisis, nor do they point towards chronic hypertension, malignant hypertension, or pharmacological hypertension.

135. Correct: Blood buildup due to constricted blood vessels (A)

Irregular or patchy skin discoloration can have many causes, but in this case the cause is the severe vasoconstriction response of a patient in cardiogenic shock. Blood cannot be properly distributed and builds up in certain areas close to the skin's surface. (**B**, **D**) Rupture of blood vessels and/or release of hemoglobin would discolor the skin; however, this is not the case in this cardiac shock patient. (**C**) Severe vasodilation (such as for septic shock) can cause mottled skin due to underperfused skin areas, but this is not the case for this patient. (**E**) Postsurgery fluid buildup that is not drained leads to edema, but not to mottling by itself.

136. Correct: Systemic venous return is increased. (E)

During inspiration, intrathoracic pressure becomes more negative compared to atmospheric pressure. This opens up the thoracic vena cava, the right atrium, and the right ventricle, leading to increased systemic venous return due to a larger pressure gradient between the abdominal vena cava and the right atrium. (**A**) On the left side of the heart, filling is decreased (not increased as on the right side). This is because the low intrathoracic pressure also opens the compliant pulmonary vasculature. Blood is pooled there and the flow to the left heart is reduced. Low preload leads to a decreased stroke volume and the observed decrease in systolic blood pressure. In cardiac tamponade, the pressures in all chambers have equalized so that the overfilled right ventricle bulges into the underfilled left ventricle, further decreasing preload and exaggerating the respiratory effect (pulsus paradoxus). (**B**, **D**) The transmural pressures on the left and the right sides of the heart are increased (not decreased), because the intrathoracic pressure falls more than the pressures inside the heart chambers. This increase has to be taken into account to assess the hemodynamics of patients with cardiac tamponade, but it is typically neglected for healthy people. (**C**) Pulmonary venous return is decreased (not increased) due to the pooling of blood in the pulmonary vasculature as explained for A.

137. Correct: Oxygen delivery to tissues (D)

All types of shock have in common that there is abnormally low oxygen delivery to tissues to a point at which tissue perfusion is inadequate to meet the cellular metabolic needs. (**A**) Arterial blood pressure is not abnormally low; rather, it is maintained in early-stage hypovolemic shock, when the decrease in blood volume is compensated by sympathetic action, leading to tachycardia, increased conduction velocity, increased contractility, and vasoconstriction. (**B**) Central venous pressure is abnormally high (not low) in cardiogenic shock, where the decrease in cardiac output leads to fluid backup and distended jugular veins. (**C**) Contractility is high (not low) in hypovolemia. (**E**) Systemic vascular resistance is high (not low) in hypovolemia and cardiogenic shock due to sympathetic action.

138. Correct: Work of the heart (E)

Nitrate decreases blood pressure by vasodilation, and β-blockers decrease blood pressure through decreased stroke volume and heart rate. This decrease in afterload substantially diminishes heart work. (**A**) There is no substantial net effect on end-diastolic volume, since nitrates decrease and β-blockers increase preload. (**B**) There is no substantial net effect on the heart's ability to contract at a given preload, since nitrates increase and β-blockers decrease contractility. (**C**) Nitrates increase and β-blockers decrease heart rate, so that the net effect is unpredictable without information on the dosage or specific type of drug. (**D**) Nitrates and β-blockers have no direct effect on total blood volume.

139. Correct: ↑, ↓, ↑ (A)

As a result of the decrease in mean arterial pressure (MAP), the baroreceptor reflex activity will decrease, and the activity of the control center (nucleus tractus solitarii) in the medulla will decrease. This will decrease activity to the cardioinhibitory center in the medulla, which will decrease parasympathetic output to the heart, thus increasing heart rate. Concurrently, activity of the vasomotor center will be increased, and sympathetic output to the heart will increase, thus increasing heart rate and contractility (stroke volume), and reducing venous compliance (venous return). The increase of heart rate and stroke volume will increase cardiac output. (**B**, **C**, **D**, **E**, **F**) These choices do not contain the correct combination of answers.

Chapter 6

Respiratory System

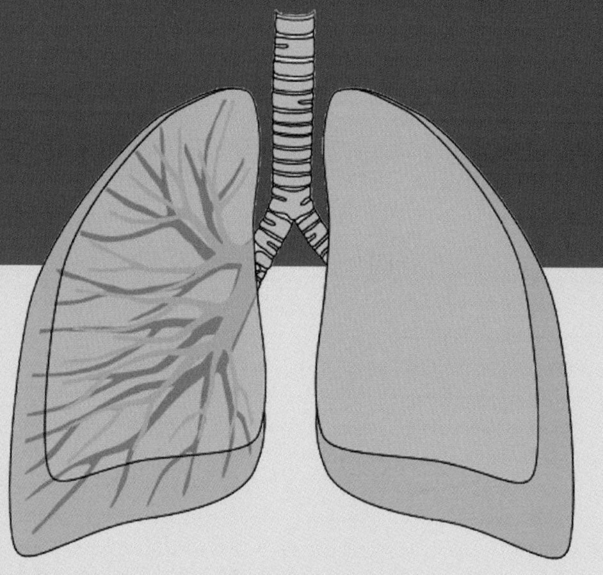

LEARNING OBJECTIVES

- Discuss the gas laws of the pulmonary system, describe the different lung volumes and how they are measured, and understand the mechanics of the lung.
- Discuss the factors that affect airway resistance, and describe how pulmonary function is assessed using spirometry and flow-volume loops.
- Discuss the factors that affect metabolic rate, alveolar ventilation, and gas exchange in normal and pathological conditions.
- Discuss the factors that affect pulmonary circulation and blood gas transport.
- Describe the mechanisms of arterial hypoxemia and discuss the different mechanisms for control of breathing.

6.1 Questions

Easy	Medium	Hard

1. Two alveoli of different sizes are connected to a common airway. If the surface tension is the same in both alveoli, the pressure produced by the surface tension will be higher in which alveolus, and in which direction will air flow between the two alveoli?

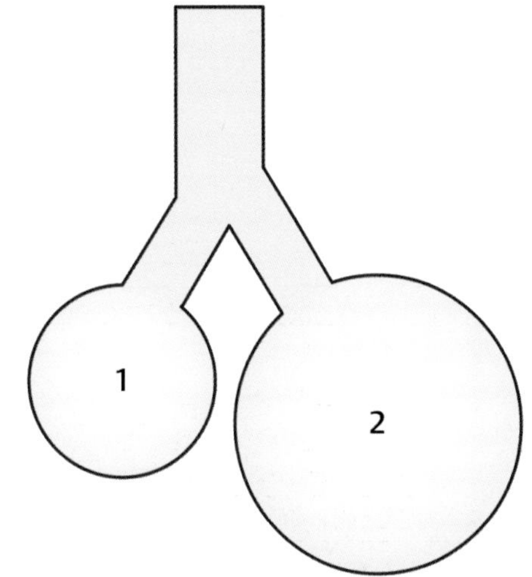

	Alveolar pressure	Direction of air flow
A	Higher pressure in alveolus 1	From alveolus 1 to 2
B	Higher pressure in alveolus 1	From alveolus 2 to 1
C	Higher pressure in alveolus 1	No net air movement
D	Higher pressure in alveolus 2	From alveolus 1 to 2
E	Higher pressure in alveolus 2	From alveolus 2 to 1
F	Higher pressure in alveolus 2	No net air movement

2. Which of the following lung volumes or capacities cannot be directly measured using spirometry?

A. Expiratory reserve volume
B. Inspiratory reserve volume
C. Tidal volume
D. Total lung capacity
E. Vital capacity

3. A healthy patient is connected to a 1.5-liter bag containing 9% helium and rapidly rebreathes over 10 seconds until the helium concentration in the bag and lungs is the same. If the final helium concentration is 3% and the subject is at functional residual capacity (FRC) when he is connected to the bag, what is his FRC (in liters)?

A. 2.0
B. 2.5
C. 3.0
D. 3.5
E. 4.0

4. As a person takes a deep breath, the compliance of the respiratory system changes with lung volume. At which lung volume or capacity does the respiratory system have the greatest compliance?

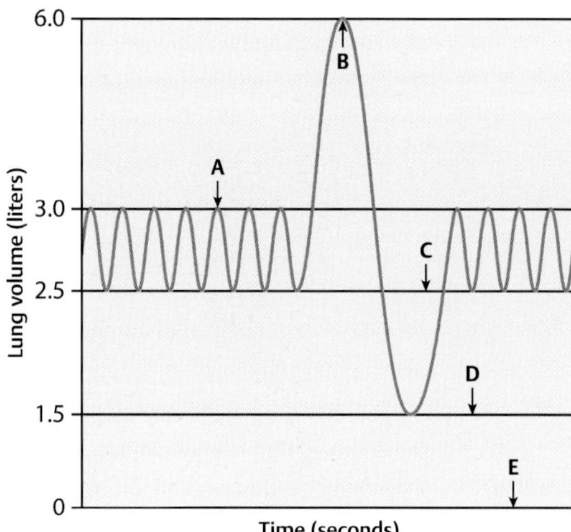

A. A
B. B
C. C
D. D
E. E

5. A 28-year-old woman is diagnosed with myasthenia gravis. She is referred to a pulmonologist for a pulmonary function test. Spirometry reveals that her pulmonary volumes are normal. Based on her spirometry, at which of the following lung volumes will the expiratory muscles have the greatest force?

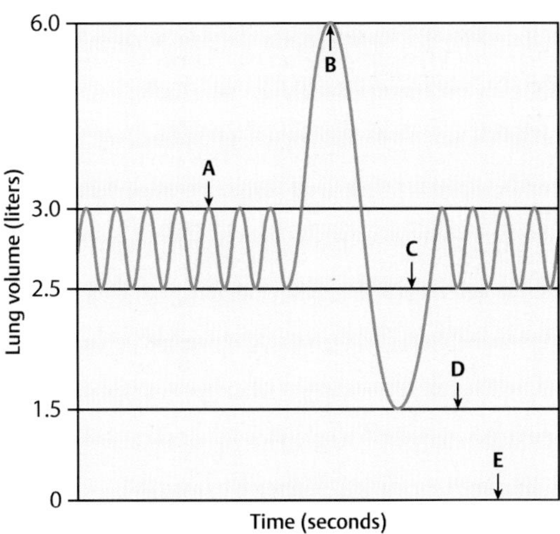

A. A
B. B
C. C
D. D
E. E

6. 35-year-old man presents to his primary care physician for a routine annual exam. His only complaint is of seasonal allergies. He weighs 70 kg and does not smoke cigarettes or drink alcohol. His heart rate is 71 beats per minute, respiratory rate is 16 breaths per minute, and blood pressure is 117/75 mm Hg. What is a typical tidal volume, vital capacity, and residual volume in a healthy adult such as this man (in mL)?

	Tidal volume	Vital capacity	Residual volume
A	300	3,500	1,500
B	300	5,500	1,200
C	300	6,500	500
D	500	3,500	500
E	500	5,500	1,200
F	500	6,500	1,200
G	1,200	3,500	500
H	1,200	5,500	1,500
I	1,200	6,500	1,500

7. In a lab experiment, mice were exposed to hypoxic conditions long enough to induce hypoxic alveolar epithelial damage. Which of the following types of cells are responsible for repairing damaged alveolar epithelial cells?

A. Type I alveolar epithelial cells
B. Type II alveolar epithelial cells
C. Alveolar macrophages
D. Clara cells
E. Goblet cells

8. A 27-year-old pregnant woman is rushed to the emergency department following a car accident and delivers a premature baby girl by cesarean section at 30 weeks of gestation. The baby is 3 pounds 4 ounces. The newborn is tachypneic and dyspneic. Which of the following changes to alveolar surface tension and lung compliance are expected in this newborn, compared to a healthy newborn?

	Alveolar surface tension	Lung compliance
A	↑	↑
B	↑	↓
C	↑	↔
D	↓	↑
E	↓	↓
F	↓	↔

9. A 71-year-old woman presents with complaints of dyspnea on exertion and a chronic cough for 18 months. She has an 80-pack-per-year smoking history. On exam, she has a "barrel-like" chest and breathes through "pursed lips." If this patient inhales 2.5 liters of room air and holds her breath, and her lung transmural pressure increases from 5 cm H_2O at the beginning of inspiration to 10 cm H_2O while she holds her breath, what is her lung compliance (in L/cm H_2O)?

A. 0.1
B. 0.2
C. 0.3
D. 0.4
E. 0.5

10. Inspiration and expiration are associated with changes in intrapleural pressure (P_{ip}). During which of the following modes of respiration can P_{ip} become positive (greater than atmospheric pressure)?

A. Breath holding at functional residual capacity
B. Forced expiration of a large volume (3 L)
C. Forced inspiration of a large volume (3 L)
D. Normal expiration
E. Normal inspiration

11. A 24-year-old man in a car accident sustains a puncture wound to the right side of the chest wall. Auscultation reveals absence of breath sounds on the right side and chest X-ray confirms a unilateral complete pneumothorax. Which of the following changes to lung volume and thoracic volume is expected in this patient?

	Lung volume	Thoracic volume
A	↑	↑
B	↑	↓
C	↑	↔
D	↓	↑
E	↓	↓
F	↓	↔

12. In the spirometry trace shown, which label correctly identifies the inspiratory reserve volume and which label correctly identifies the expiratory reserve volume?

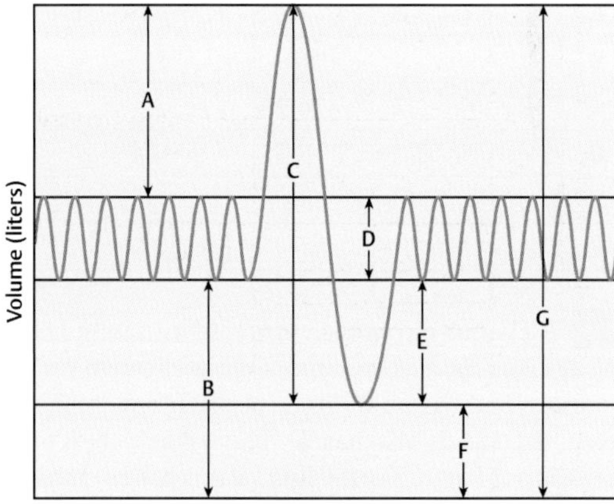

	Inspiratory reserve volume	Expiratory reserve volume
A	A	B
B	A	C
C	A	E
D	B	A
E	B	C
F	B	E
G	C	B
H	C	F
I	C	E

6.2 Answers and Explanations

Easy | Medium | Hard

1. Correct: Higher pressure in alveolus 1, From alveolus 1 to 2 (A)

The relationship between pressure in the alveolus and surface tension is demonstrated by Laplace's law: Tension = (Pressure × Radius)/2. If this equation is written to solve for pressure, Pressure = (2 × Tension)/Radius), then it is evident that the alveolus with the smaller radius (alveolus 1) will have the higher pressure. That pressure gradient will drive air from the smaller alveolus to the larger alveolus. (**B**, **C**, **D**, **E**, **F**) These options include one or more incorrect answers.

2. Correct: Total lung capacity (D)

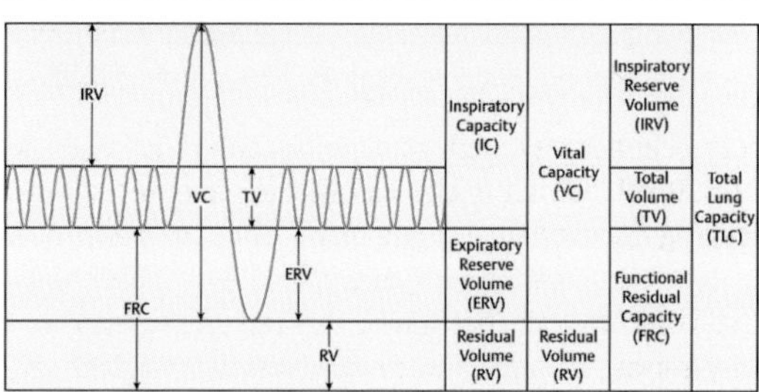

The total lung capacity (TLC) is a measurement of the total volume of air the lung can hold. It is the sum of the residual volume (RV), expiratory reserve volume (ERV), tidal volume (TV), and inspiratory reserve volume (IRV). Each of these volumes can be measured directly, except RV (the volume of air left in the lung after a maximal exhalation, which must be determined by other methods (inert gas dilution method). (**A**) Expiratory reserve volume (ERV), which is the additional amount of air that can be exhaled after a normal exhalation, can be measured directly. (**B**) Inspiratory reserve volume (IRV), which is the additional amount of air that can be inhaled after a normal inhalation, can be measured directly. (**C**) Tidal volume (TV), which is the amount of air that is inspired and expired during normal breathing, can be measured directly. (**E**) Vital capacity (VC), which is the maximum amount of air that can be inhaled or exhaled during a respiratory cycle, can be measured directly.

3. Correct: 3.0 (C)

The helium dilution method can be used to measure functional residual capacity because helium is almost insoluble in the blood. Since no helium is lost, the concentration before equilibration ($C_1 \times V_1$) equals the amount after equilibration [$C_2 \times (V_1 + V_2)$]. From this, $V_2 = V_1(C_1 - C_2)/C_2$.

$$V_2 = V_1(C_1 - C_2)/C_2$$
$$V_2 = 1.5L(9\% - 3\%)/3\%$$
$$V_2 = 1.5L(6\%)/3\%$$
$$V_2 = 9\ L\%/3\%$$
$$V_2 = 3.0\ L$$

4. Correct: C (C)

The respiratory system has its greatest compliance at functional residual capacity (FRC), which is the resting volume of the respiratory system. At FRC, the lung and chest wall are recoiling in opposite directions towards their resting volumes (lungs inward, chest wall outward). (**A**) This is the volume at the end of a tidal volume inspiration. (**B**) This is total lung capacity. (**D**) This is residual volume. (**E**) This is a lung volume of zero liters, which is not possible in a living person.

5. Correct: B (B)

The expiratory muscles have their greatest force at total lung capacity (TLC), which is approximately 6 liters in the typical person. This is because the chest is farthest above its relaxation volume (residual volume), and the expiratory muscles are at their optimal length, which is the best position to generate maximal tension. (**A, C, D, E**) These volumes do not represent TLC.

6. Correct: 500, 5,500, 1,200 (E)

A typical healthy adult male will have a tidal volume of 500 mL, which is the volume of air entering and leaving the lungs in a single respiratory cycle at rest. A typical vital capacity is 5,500 mL, which is the maximal volume of air that can be expired after a maximal inspiration. A typical residual volume is 1,200 mL, which is the volume of air that remains in the lungs after a maximal expiration. This volume of air cannot be expired from the lungs. (**A, B, C, D, F, G, H, I**) These do not contain the correct combination of answers.

7. Correct: Type II alveolar epithelial cells (B)

Type II alveolar cells cover a small fraction of the alveolar surface area (5%). Their major functions are the secretion of surfactant, which decreases the surface tension, and induction of cellular divisions to produce more Type I cells. (**A**) Type I alveolar cells cover approximately 90–95% of the alveolar surface and are involved in the process of gas exchange between the alveoli and the blood. (**C**) Alveolar macrophages clear the air spaces of infectious, toxic, or allergic particles that have evaded the mechanical defenses of the respiratory tract. (**D**) Clara cells secrete a lipoprotein with properties similar to surfactant to prevent airway collapse. (**E**) Goblet cells secrete mucus to trap debris that has been inhaled.

8. Correct: ↑, ↓ (B)

This newborn has surfactant insufficiency due to premature birth. Surfactant is a lipoprotein with a hydrophilic and hydrophobic end that is produced by type II pneumocytes to reduce the surface tension in the alveoli. Type II pneumocytes begin to appear at approximately 21 weeks of gestation and surfactant production begins between 25 and 32 weeks of gestation. A decrease of surfactant causes alveolar surface tension to increase and pulmonary compliance to decrease, which causes the smaller alveoli to collapse (atelectasis). (**A, C**) A decrease in surfactant levels will increase the alveolar surface tension and decrease lung compliance. (**D, E, F**) Low levels of surfactant cause alveolar surface tension to increase, not decrease.

9. Correct: 0.5 (E)

Lung compliance is a measure of lung dispensability. A normal value in adults is 0.1–0.2 L/cm H_2O, but this patient has a history that indicates emphysema, which causes a high lung compliance due to the poor elastic recoil. Compliance is calculated by the following formula:

Compliance (**C**) = Change in volume (ΔV)/Change in transmural pressure difference (ΔP).
$C = \Delta V/\Delta P = 2.5\ L/5\ cm\ H_2O = 0.5\ L/cm\ H_2O$.

(**A, B, C, D**) These answers do not contain the correct answer.

10. Correct: Forced expiration of a large volume (3 L) (B)

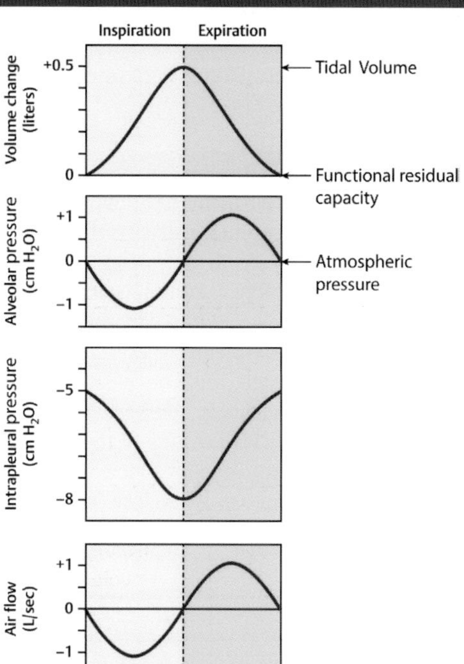

During forced expiration (i.e., during exercise), expiration can be active. The abdominal muscles contract to push the diaphragm up, and the internal intercostal muscles contract to pull the ribs downward and inward. This increases the intrapleural pressure above atmospheric pressure, and thus causes a proportionate increase in alveolar pressure. As a result, the lung transmural pressure difference and lung volume remain briefly unaffected, but as soon as increased alveolar pressure (at unchanged mouth pressure) drives the exhalation of alveolar gas, both lung transmural pressure difference and lung volume are continually decreasing toward end of expiration. (**A**) At functional residual capacity (FRC), the lungs have an inward recoiling force whereas the chest wall has an outward recoiling force. These opposing forces are equal and generate a negative pressure within the intrapleural space (roughly –6 cm H_2O or –4.6 mm Hg), which causes a positive lung transmural pressure difference that maintains the lungs inflated at functional residual capacity. (**C, E**) During inspiration (normal or forced), the inspiratory muscles actively expand the thoracic cavity, which in turn decreases the pleural pressure further to more negative values (–8 or –10 cm H_2O). This decrease in pleural pressure is transmitted into a negative alveolar pressure that leads to air flow from outside into the lungs. As a result, lung volume is increasing, which is associated with a larger lung transmural pressure difference (more negative pleural pressure) and a greater lung recoil force, which is counterbalanced in this condition by the force of inspiratory muscles. (**D**) In expiration, as soon as inspiratory muscles are relaxing, the recoil forces of both lung (high at the end of inspiration) and chest wall are no longer counterbalanced by the force of inspiratory muscles, and the higher inward-directed recoil force of the lung produces a positive alveolar pressure that drives the air out of the lung. As a result, the volumes of both the lung and thoracic cavity decrease continually until their opposing recoil forces become equal at FRC, with a resultant less negative intrapleural pressure.

11. Correct: ↓, ↑ (D)

The lung and thorax normally have opposing recoil forces at functional residual capacity that create a subatmospheric pressure in the pleural space. The pneumothorax consists of a communication through the chest wall between the atmosphere and pleural space. As air enters the pleural space, the lung and chest wall are separated, and the pleural pressure becomes equal to atmospheric pressure. This separation of lung and chest wall results in the chest wall recoiling outward (thoracic volume increases) and the lung recoiling inward towards collapse (lung volume decreases). (**A, B, C, E**) These answers do not represent the volume changes for a complete pneumothorax.

12. Correct: A, E (C)

The inspiratory reserve volume, which is the volume of air that can be inhaled after a tidal inhalation, is indicated by point A; the expiratory reserve volume, which is the volume of air that can be exhaled after a tidal exhalation, is indicated by point E. (**A, B, D, E, F, G, H, I**) Interval B is the functional residual capacity, which includes the expiratory reserve volume and the residual volume. Interval C is the vital capacity, which is the volume of air that can be maximally exhaled after a maximal inspiration. Interval D is the tidal volume, which is the volume of air moving in or out of the lungs during normal respiration. Interval E is the expiratory reserve volume, which is the additional volume of air that can be exhaled after a normal exhalation. Interval F is the residual volume, which is the volume of air remaining in the lung after a maximal exhalation. Interval G is the total lung capacity, which is the largest volume of the air that lung can occupy.

6.3 Questions

13. A 49-year-old man presents with a dry cough and progressively worsening dyspnea over 10 weeks. Physical exam reveals clubbed digits, and fine inspiratory crackles are heard on auscultation. A lung function test is ordered, and all lung volumes are reduced, but the FEV_1:FVC ratio (forced expiratory volume in 1 second to forced vital capacity) is unchanged or slightly higher than normal. Based on the likely diagnosis, which curve or line on the figure most likely represents the expected changes reflecting the lung compliance of this patient?

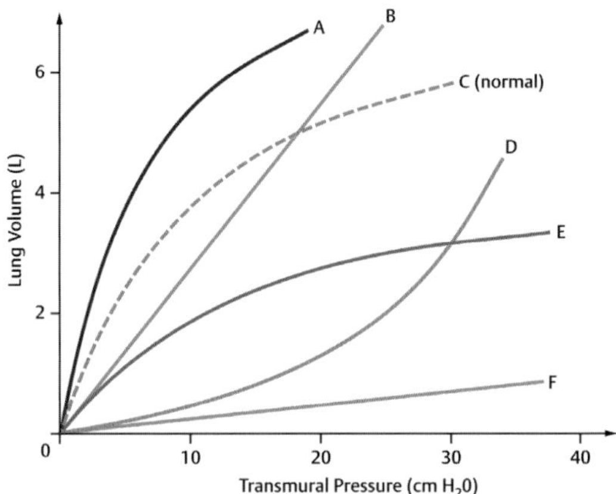

A. A
B. B
C. C
D. D
E. E

14. A 68-year-old woman presents with complaints of dyspnea on exertion and a chronic cough for 2 years. She has a 60-pack-per-year smoking history. On exam, she is thin with a "barrel-like" chest and breathes through "pursed lips." A lung function test reveals a decreased forced vital capacity (FVC), decreased forced expiratory volume in 1 second (FEV_1), and decreased FEV_1/FVC ratio. Based on the most likely diagnosis, which curve or line on the figure most likely represents the expected changes reflecting the lung compliance of this patient?

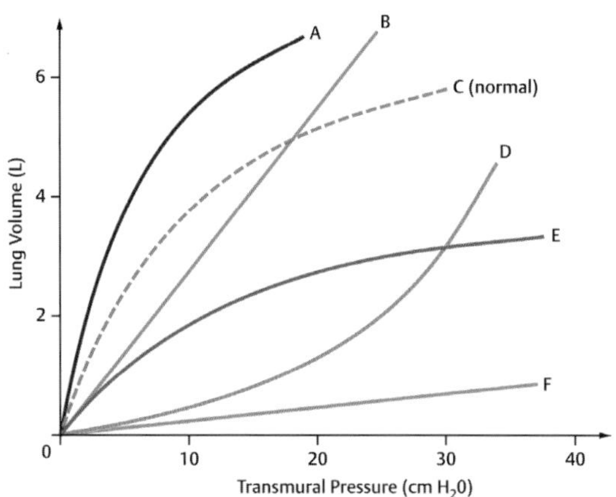

A. A
B. B
C. C
D. D
E. E
F. F

15. A 14-year-old boy presents to the urgent care facility with shortness of breath and wheezing after playing soccer for 30 minutes. Physical exam reveals a heart rate of 130 bpm, respiratory rate of 27/min, and blood pressure of 135/75 mm Hg. He is noted to be using accessory muscles for respiration. Wheezing on expiration is noted upon auscultation. Based on the most likely diagnosis, which combination of changes in total lung capacity (TLC), residual volume (RV), and functional residual capacity (FRC) are expected in this patient?

	TLC	RV	FRC
A	↑	↑	↑
B	↑	↑	↓
C	↑	↓	↔
D	↓	↑	↑
E	↓	↓	↓
F	↓	↓	↔
G	↔	↑	↑
H	↔	↓	↓

16. A 66-year-old man presents with a persistent and worsening cough for 7 months. He is a nonsmoker and worked in construction for 43 years before retiring last year. On questioning, he admits that he frequently worked with asbestos without protection in the early part of his career. Based on the most likely diagnosis, which combination of changes in total lung capacity (TLC), residual volume (RV), and functional residual capacity (FRC) are expected in this patient?

	TLC	RV	FRC
A	↑	↑	↑
B	↑	↑	↓
C	↑	↓	↔
D	↓	↑	↑
E	↓	↓	↓
F	↓	↓	↔
G	↔	↑	↑
H	↔	↓	↓

17. A healthy 22-year-old college student undergoes an experimental pulmonary function test. His flow-volume loop is shown. The generation of which part of the loop is dependent on the individual's effort during expiration?

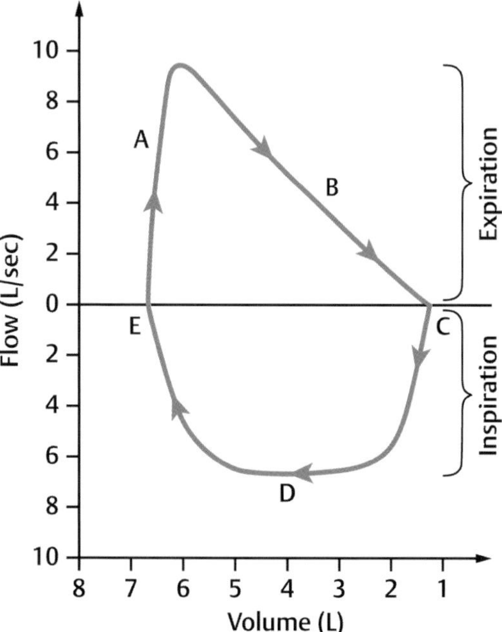

A. A
B. B
C. C
D. D
E. E

18. A healthy 22-year-old college student participates in an experimental pulmonary function test. His flow-volume loop is shown. Which point on the loop indicates his total lung capacity?

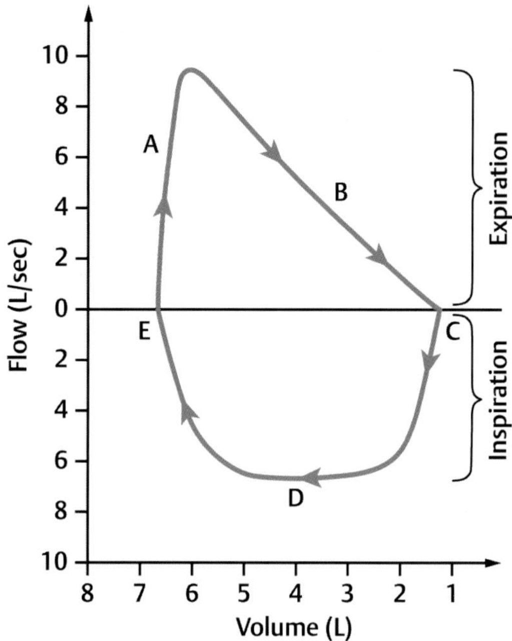

A. A
B. B
C. C
D. D
E. E

19. A healthy 39-year-old woman sees her primary care physician with complaints of dysphagia and dyspnea. Palpitation reveals an enlarged thyroid. A thyroid ultrasound is ordered, and a large goiter is confirmed. If the patient were asked to undergo a pulmonary function test, which of the following flow-volume loops would be expected?

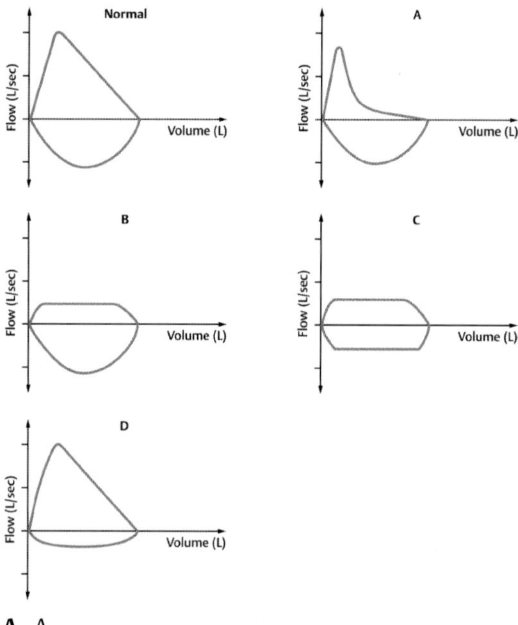

A. A
B. B
C. C
D. D

20. The spirometric measurement of lung volumes of a patient are shown in the figure. At which lung volume indicated by letters (A-E) will the airway resistance be the highest?

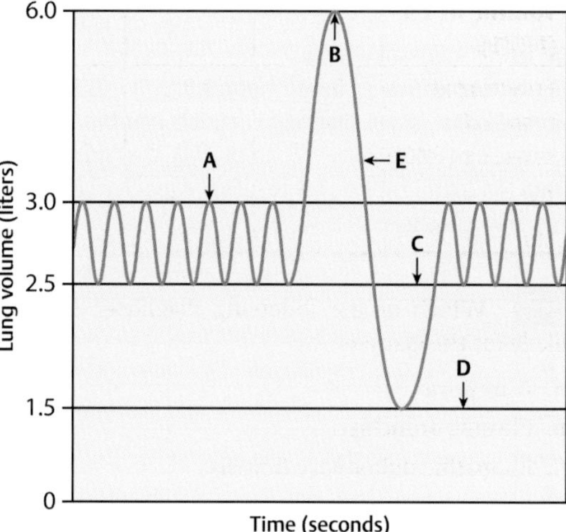

A. A
B. B
C. C
D. D
E. E

21. The schematic shown is a representation of the respiratory system that is enclosed by the intrapleural cavity. Which point on the figure represents the equal pressure point (EPP) during a forced exhalation in a healthy individual?

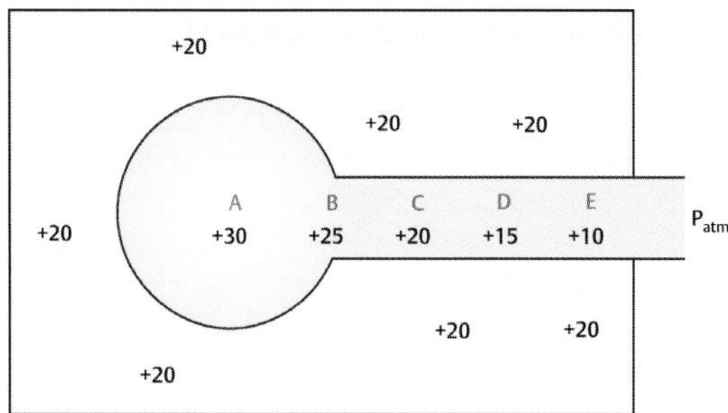

A. A

B. B

C. C

D. D

E. E

Questions 22 to 23

A 51-year-old male presents with a chronic cough with sputum and progressively increasing dyspnea for two weeks. He has been a 2-pack-per-day smoker for the past 30 years. A pulmonary function test is administered before and after the administration of isoproterenol, and the results are shown:

	Before isoproterenol	After isoproterenol	Reference range
Forced vital capacity (FVC)	4.1 L	4.2 L	4.5 L
Forced expiratory volume in 1 s (FEV1)	1.4 L	1.4 L	3.6 L
Functional residual capacity (FRC)	3.4 L	3.3 L	3.0 L
Total lung capacity (TLC)	7.0 L	7.0 L	6.0 L

22. Which of the following diagnoses is most likely for this patient?

A. Asbestosis

B. Chronic bronchitis

C. Idiopathic pulmonary fibrosis

D. Interstitial lung disease

E. Pulmonary embolism

23. Why is the patient's total lung capacity increased above normal, while the forced vital capacity remains normal?

A. Increased expiratory reserve volume

B. Increased functional residual capacity

C. Increased inspiratory capacity

D. Increased inspiratory reserve volume

E. Increased residual volume

24. Two climbers reach the summit of Mt. Everest (29,029 feet above sea level) at the same time. One climber is breathing 60% supplemental oxygen at the summit, and the other is not using supplemental oxygen. If the barometric pressure is 760 mm Hg at sea level and 250 mm Hg at the peak, what is the approximate inspired P_{O_2} for each climber (in mm Hg)?

	Inspired P_{O_2} with supplemental oxygen	Inspired P_{O_2} without supplemental oxygen
A	89.3	42.6
B	89.3	61.4
C	121.8	42.6
D	121.8	61.4
E	147.0	42.6
F	147.0	61.4

6.4 Answers and Explanations

13. Correct: E (E)

This patient's presentation indicates pulmonary fibrosis, which causes a decrease in lung compliance, as indicated by curve E on the graph. The decrease in compliance makes pulmonary fibrosis a restrictive lung disease. Pulmonary fibrosis involves gradual exchange of normal lung parenchyma for fibrotic (scar) tissue, causing an irreversible decrease in oxygen diffusion capacity. This disease causes dry cough, worsening dyspnea, and clubbing. The fine inspiratory crackles are due to opening of collapsed alveoli. Both the FEV1 and FVC are reduced, and the FEV1/FVC ratio is unchanged or higher than normal. (**A**) This curve represents an increase in compliance, as seen with conditions such as emphysema, in which there is a loss in elastic recoil of the lungs. (**B, F**) These options are incorrect because compliance curves are not linear. (**C**) The patient's presentation indicates pulmonary fibrosis, which is not consistent with normal lung compliance. (**D**) Lung compliance does not increase with increasing transmural pressures.

14. Correct: A (A)

This patient's presentation indicates emphysema, which results in an increase in lung compliance, as indicated by curve A on the graph. The increase in compliance makes emphysema an obstructive lung disease. The emphysematic lungs show loss of alveolar walls and enlargement of the air spaces distal to terminal bronchi. The small airways are narrowed and have atrophied walls. Reduction of the lung recoil force is the cause of closure of the small airways during forced expiration (air trapping). The patient has a "barrel chest" because the increase in compliance causes the ribs to recoil outwards, resulting in widening of the thoracic cavity. Also, she breathes through "pursed lips" to increase the pressure in the small airways to keep them open longer. Finally, the FEV_1 and FVC are both reduced, but the FEV_1 is reduced more, so the FEV_1/FVC ratio is reduced. (**B**, **F**) These options are incorrect because compliance curves are not linear. (**C**) The patient's presentation indicates emphysema, which is not consistent with normal lung compliance. (**D**) Lung compliance does not increase with increasing transmural pressures. (**E**) This compliance curve indicates decrease in lung compliance, such as with pulmonary fibrosis.

15. Correct: ↑, ↑, ↑ (A)

The patient most likely has an acute exacerbation of asthma, an obstructive lung disease, which increases resistance to airflow. In this condition, airway inflammation, bronchoconstriction, and mucus production obstruct airflow, causing wheezing (especially on expiration) and shortness of breath. The airway obstruction reduces the proper emptying of the lung volume and thus increases residual volume. Since RV makes up part of the functional residual capacity (FRC) and total lung capacity (TLC), these volumes are increased as well. (**B, C, D, E, F, G, H**) These options include one or more incorrect changes in lung volumes.

16. Correct: ↓, ↓, ↓ (E)

The patient most likely has pulmonary fibrosis from asbestos exposure, which thickens alveolar walls and reduces compliance of the lungs, leading to reduced lung volumes. The result is a lower expiratory reserve volume (ERV) and residual volume (RV), which decreases FRC (FRC = ERV + RV). Together these contribute to the reduced TLC. (**A, B, C, D, F, G, H**) These options include one or more incorrect changes in lung volumes.

17. Correct: A (A)

At high lung volumes, airflow increases with increasing effort and is therefore effort-dependent. This occurs because alveolar elastic recoil pressure is high and positive intrapleural pressures cannot be attained at such high lung volumes with the airway wide open. (**B**) These regions of the flow-volume loop are effort independent because there is less alveolar elastic recoil pressure, and thus less airway traction and a smaller pressure gradient. (**C**, **D**, **E**) These regions of the flow-volume loop are produced during inspiration.

18. Correct: E (E)

This point represents the total lung capacity (TLC). It is found at the end of maximal inspiration, before expiration begins. (**A**, **B**) These points are part of the expiratory phase and are at lung volumes that are greater than residual volume (RV) but less than TLC. (**C**) This point represents the RV of the lung, which is the volume of air remaining in the lung after a maximal expiration. (**D**) This point is part of the inspiratory phase, before TLC is achieved.

19. Correct: C (C)

The patient has a fixed upper airway obstruction from a large thyroid goiter, which produces the flow-volume loop shown in C. Flow limitation occurs during both the inspiratory and expiratory phases due to the continuous presence of the obstruction. (**A**) An obstructive lung disease, such as emphysema, will produce the flow-volume loop shown in A. The air in the large airways usually can be expired without problems, but with obstructive lung disease the smaller airways are partially blocked, so exhalation from these regions will be slower. This will result in a lower flow and concave shape of the flow-volume curve. (**B**) A variable intrathoracic upper airway obstruction, such as a lower trachea tumor, will produce the flow-volume loop shown in B. The key finding is flow limitation during the expiratory phase. This occurs during expiration when the tumor is pushed into the trachea, causing partial obstruction. (**D**) A variable extrathoracic upper airway obstruction, such as vocal cord paralysis, will produce the flow-volume loop shown in D. The key finding is flow limitation during the inspiratory phase. The obstruction is pushed outwards by the force of the expiration, then sucked into the trachea with partial obstruction during inspiration.

20. Correct: D (D)

Point D represents the residual volume of the lung, which is the amount of air left in the lung after a forced expiration. Since lower lung volumes have higher airway resistance, the residual volume (point D) will have the highest resistance. This is due to bronchi and bronchioles residing within the lung tissue surrounded by alveoli. At low lung volumes, the inward directed recoil force of alveoli is less, which leads to less expansion of airways and increases airway resistance. As lung volumes increase, the airways stretch to a greater diameter and have a reduced resistance. (**A, B, C, E**) These volumes do not represent residual volume.

21. Correct: C (C)

The equal pressure point (EPP) is the point at which pressure inside the airway equals pressure outside (intrapleural pressure). Proximal to the EPP (toward the alveoli), transairway pressure is positive, and therefore the airways are not compressed and remain open with a low resistance. Distal to the EPP (toward the mouth), the transairway pressure becomes negative, resulting in a compression of the airways, which produces a higher airway resistance and a tendency for airway collapse. This is opposed by cartilaginous support in larger airways. (**A**, **B**) These points have an airway pressure that is greater than (not equal to) the intrapleural pressure. (**D**, **E**) These points have an airway pressure that is less than (not equal to) the intrapleural pressure.

22. Correct: Chronic bronchitis (B)

This patient has a low FEV_1/FVC, which indicates an obstructive disease. In obstructive lung disease, the FEV_1 is reduced because of increased airway resistance produced by the obstruction, which reduces flow at the same pressure difference. Bronchitis is the only obstructive disease listed as a choice, and it fits his presentation (dyspnea and cough with sputum), so it is the best answer. His condition is chronic because it was not improved much with bronchodilator use. (**A**, **C**, **D**) These choices are all characterized as restrictive diseases and can be eliminated because the total lung capacity is normal (this would be reduced in a patient with restrictive disease), and the FEV_1/FVC is low (this would be normal or slightly increased in a patient with restrictive disease due to the proportional decrease in FEV_1 and FVC). Asbestosis, a chronic inflammatory condition of the lung parenchyma that results from inhalation of asbestos dust, is a type of interstitial lung disease. Idiopathic pulmonary fibrosis is fibrosis of an unknown origin. (**E**) This patient does not exhibit the classic signs of pulmonary embolism, such as acute onset of dyspnea and chest pain; therefore, pulmonary embolism is unlikely.

23. Correct: Increased residual volume (E)

This patient has an obstructive lung disease (indicated by the low FEV_1/FVC ratio). This causes an increased residual volume (RV) due to gas trapping on expiration. Since the total lung capacity (TLC) is equal to vital capacity (VC) plus residual volume (RV), if the VC is normal, then the RV must increase to increase TLC. (**A**, **B**, **C**, **D**) An increase in expiratory reserve volume, functional residual capacity, inspiratory capacity, and inspiratory reserve volume would all increase VC, which is not seen in this patient.

24. Correct: 121.8, 42.6 (C)

Inspired P_{O_2} is the P_{O_2} of the air in the trachea and airways during inhalation. To calculate this, the water vaper pressure (P_{H_2O}), barometric pressure (P_B), and fraction of inspired O_2 (F_{IO_2}) are needed.

Climber without O_2: Inspired $P_{O_2} = (P_B - P_{H_2O}) \times F_{IO_2} = (250 \text{ mm Hg} - 47 \text{ mm Hg}) \times 0.21 = 42.6 \text{ mm Hg}$

Climber with O_2: Inspired $P_{O_2} = (P_B - P_{H_2O}) \times F_{IO_2} = (250 \text{ mm Hg} - 47 \text{ mm Hg}) \times 0.60 = 121.8 \text{ mm Hg}$

(**A**, **B**, **D**, **E**, **F**) These choices do not include the correct combination of answers.

6.5 Questions

25. An 80-year-old female presents to the emergency department with dyspnea that worsens when lying down, cough producing a frothy sputum, and anxiety. The patient has a history of myocardial infarction 2 years prior with a subsequent coronary artery bypass. On exam, she is tachypneic and tachycardic. Blood pressure is 100/82 mm Hg, and inspiratory crackles are heard bilaterally in the lower lung fields. A chest X-ray reveals pulmonary edema, and left heart failure is diagnosed. Which of the following additional findings is most likely present in this patient?

A. Decreased pulmonary artery pressure
B. Decreased pulmonary lymph flow
C. Increased pulmonary venous pressure
D. Increased vital capacity
E. Normal arterial oxygen partial pressure

26. A 20-year-old male college student participates in a pulmonary study in his physiology lab. He is healthy and in good physical shape. He is asked to run on a treadmill for 20 minutes at a moderate pace, during which time his arterial P_{CO_2} is measured. What is his predicted arterial P_{CO_2} (in mm Hg)?

A. 10
B. 20
C. 40
D. 60
E. 80

27. A 17-year-old boy presents to the urgent care facility with shortness of breath and wheezing after jogging for 1 mile. Physical exam reveals a heart rate of 110 and respiratory rate of 27. He is using accessory muscles for respiration, and wheezing is noted on expiration. If his tidal volume is 300 mL, what is his alveolar ventilation (in mL/min)?

A. 2,450
B. 4,050
C. 4,600
D. 5,200
E. 8,900

28. Five healthy men participating in a pulmonary function study are each asked to modify their tidal volume and respiration rate for 2 minutes. The following data were measured in each man during this time:

	Tidal volume (mL)	Respiration rate (breaths per minute)
Volunteer 1	300	25
Volunteer 2	500	15
Volunteer 3	1,000	10
Volunteer 4	1,500	5
Volunteer 5	2,000	3

Which volunteer has the lowest alveolar ventilation (mL/min)?

A. Volunteer 1
B. Volunteer 2
C. Volunteer 3
D. Volunteer 4
E. Volunteer 5

29. The arterial P_{O_2} and arterial P_{CO_2} from five patients in the intensive care unit are shown.

	Arterial P_{O_2} (mm Hg)	Arterial P_{CO_2} (mm Hg)
Patient 1	100	40
Patient 2	80	33
Patient 3	105	42
Patient 4	80	40
Patient 5	70	50

Which patient is most likely hypoventilating?

A. Patient 1
B. Patient 2
C. Patient 3
D. Patient 4
E. Patient 5

30. Which of the following combinations of alveolar ventilation and pulmonary perfusion will produce the highest arterial P_{O_2}?

	Alveolar ventilation	Pulmonary perfusion
A	Normal	Increased
B	Normal	Decreased
C	Decreased	Increased
D	Decreased	Decreased
E	Increased	Increased
F	Increased	Decreased

31. A patient has signs of arterial hypoxemia. According to Fick's law of diffusion, an increase in which of the following factors will cause a decrease in the oxygen diffusion rate from the alveoli to the capillaries?

A. Oxygen partial pressure difference (ΔC)
B. Alveolar surface area
C. Krogh diffusion constant (K)
D. Distance of diffusion (ΔX)
E. Body temperature

32. A patient has a respiratory exchange ratio (R) and respiratory quotient (RQ) of 1.0. His P_{IO_2} and P_{ACO_2} are normal. What does this R value indicate about the macronutrient being primarily metabolized by this patient, and what effect will it have on the patient's alveolar P_{O_2}?

	Macronutrient being primarily metabolized	Effect on alveolar P_{O_2}
A	Carbohydrates	Increase above normal
B	Carbohydrates	Decrease below normal
C	Fats	Increase above normal
D	Fats	Decrease below normal
E	Proteins	Increase above normal
F	Proteins	Decrease below normal

6.6 Answers and Explanations

25. Correct: Increased pulmonary venous pressure (C)

As a result of the left heart failure, fluid backs up into the lungs and increases pulmonary venous and capillary pressures. This leads to increased filtration and edema formation. (**A**) Pulmonary artery pressure will be increased in this patient as fluid backs up toward the right heart. (**B**) Pulmonary lymph flow will increase as filtration increases. Once filtration exceeds lymph flow, edema forms. (**D**) Edema interferes with lung inflation and would probably cause a decrease in vital capacity. (**E**) Edema interferes with gas exchange, possibly causing a decrease in arterial oxygen partial pressure.

26. Correct: 40 (C)

In moderate exercise, both CO_2 production and alveolar ventilation are increasing proportionally. This proportional increase in CO_2 production and ventilation allow the arterial P_{CO_2} to be maintained at its normal value, which is 40 mm Hg. (**A, B, D, E**) These values are not correct.

27. Correct: 4,050 (B)

Ventilation is the movement of air between the environment and the lungs via inhalation and exhalation. Approximately 150 mL of each inspiration does not contribute to the alveolar ventilation because it does not clear the respiratory dead space, so no gas exchange occurs with that air.

Alveolar ventilation = (tidal volume – dead space volume) × respiratory rate

$V_A = (V_T - V_{DS})f = (300 - 150)27 = 4{,}050$ mL.

(A, C, D, E) These answers do not contain the correct alveolar ventilation.

28. Correct: Volunteer 1 (A)

Alveolar ventilation is the volume of gas that reaches the alveoli per unit time. Approximately 150 mL of each tidal volume does not reach the alveoli (dead space volume), so no gas exchange occurs within that air. Alveolar ventilation = (Tidal volume – Dead space volume) × respiratory frequency.

$V_A = (V_T - V_{DS}) \times f$.

(**A**) Volunteer 1 $V_A = (300 - 150) \times 25 = 3{,}750$ mL/min.
(**B**) Volunteer 2 $V_A = (500 - 150) \times 15 = 5{,}250$ mL/min.
(**C**) Volunteer 3 $V_A = (1{,}000 - 150) \times 10 = 8{,}500$ mL/min.
(**D**) Volunteer 4 $V_A = (1{,}500 - 150) \times 5 = 6{,}750$ mL/min.
(**E**) Volunteer 5 $V_A = (2{,}000 - 150) \times 3 = 5{,}550$ mL/min.

29. Correct: Patient 5 (E)

With hypoventilation, alveolar ventilation decreases, which leads to a decrease in P_{AO_2} (below 80 mm Hg) because ventilation is reduced, and an increase in P_{ACO_2} (above 45 mm Hg) because CO_2 is retained. (**A**, **C**, **D**, **E**) These answers do not represent the correct values for hypoventilation.

30. Correct: Increased, decreased (F)

The ventilation-perfusion ($\dot{V}/\dot{Q}$) ratio has a direct effect on arterial P_{O_2} and arterial P_{CO_2}. An increase in the $\dot{V}/\dot{Q}$ ratio, caused by an increase in ventilation or a decrease in perfusion, will result in an increase in arterial P_{O_2} and decrease in arterial P_{CO_2}. When the $\dot{V}/\dot{Q}$ ratio is increased, this means ventilation is in excess of the metabolic needs being met by perfusion, so we blow off CO_2 and increase and arterial P_{O_2}. (**A**, **C**) These will decrease the $\dot{V}/\dot{Q}$ ratio and decrease arterial P_{O_2}. (**B**) This will increase the $\dot{V}/\dot{Q}$ ratio and increase arterial P_{O_2}, but not as much as choice F. (**D**, **E**) If these changes are proportional, then $\dot{V}/\dot{Q}$ ratio and arterial P_{O_2} will be maintained.

31. Correct: Distance of diffusion (ΔX) (D)

Fick's law of diffusion [$J = (KD/\Delta X) \times A(\Delta C)$] describes the variables that affect the rate of solute diffusion across a biological membrane. Based on this equation, only ΔX (the distance of diffusion) is inversely related to the rate of diffusion, so an increase in ΔX will produce a decrease in the oxygen diffusion rate. (**A**) Oxygen partial pressure difference (ΔC) is proportional to the rate of diffusion. (**B**) Surface area is proportional to the rate of diffusion. (**C**) Krogh diffusion constant, which is solubility (α) × diffusion coefficient (D), is proportional to the rate of diffusion. K, which is the solubility of a solute to a lipid membrane, is proportional to the rate of diffusion. (**E**) The diffusion coefficient (D), which takes body temperature into account, is proportional to the rate of diffusion.

32. Correct: Carbohydrates, effect on alveolar P_{O_2} (A)

The ratio of CO_2 output to O_2 uptake is called the respiratory quotient (RQ) in the tissues and respiratory exchange ratio (R) in the lungs. When carbohydrates are metabolized, the RQ and R = 1.0, which is what we see in this patient. If we assume normal values for P_{IO_2} and P_{ACO_2} in the alveolar gas equation, $P_{AO_2} = P_{IO_2} - (P_{ACO_2}/R)$, then an R of 1 will yield a P_{O_2} of 107 mm Hg, which is increased above normal. $P_{AO_2} = P_{IO_2} - (P_{ACO_2}/R) = 147 - (40/1) = 107$ mm Hg.

(**B**) The alveolar P_{O_2} is increased, not decreased, as explained for option A.

(**C**, **D**) When fats are metabolized, the RQ and R = 0.7. This will yield a P_{O_2} of 90 mm Hg, which is lower than a P_{O_2} for an average R. $P_{AO_2} = P_{IO_2} - (P_{ACO_2}/R) = 147 - (40/.7) = 90$ mm Hg.

(**E**, **F**) When proteins are metabolized, the RQ and R = 0.8. This will yield a P_{O_2} of 97 mm Hg, which is normal. $P_{AO_2} = P_{IO_2} - (P_{ACO_2}/R) = 147 - (40/0.8) = 97$ mm Hg.

6.7 Questions

33. A 16-year-old male is rushed to the emergency department following a heroin overdose. Physical exam reveals a respiratory rate of 9 breaths per minute, blood pressure of 98/62 mm Hg, and an irregular pulse. He is afebrile. Which of the following oxygen-hemoglobin dissociation curves is predicted for this patient?

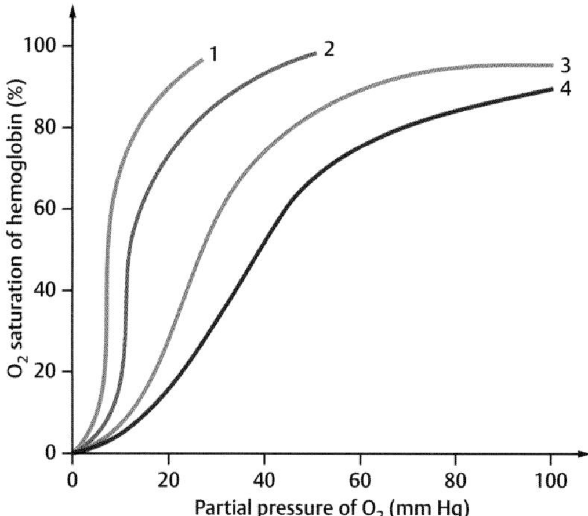

A. 1
B. 2
C. 3
D. 4

34. A healthy person participating in a lab experiment takes a deep breath. As lung volume increases toward total lung capacity, which of the following changes occurs to alveolar and extra-alveolar vascular resistance?

	Alveolar vascular resistance	Extra-alveolar vascular resistance
1	↑	↑
2	↑	↓
3	↑	↔
4	↓	↑
5	↓	↓
6	↓	↔

A. 1
B. 2
C. 3
D. 4
E. 5
F. 6

35. During exercise, pulmonary vascular resistance (PVR) is reduced. Which of the following pulmonary changes most likely contributes to this decrease in PVR?

A. Constriction of open capillaries
B. Decrease in pulmonary artery pressure
C. Decrease in pulmonary venous pressure
D. Recruitment of closed capillaries

36. In a healthy individual standing upright, what is the relationship between pulmonary artery pressure (Pa), alveolar pressure (PA), and pulmonary vein pressure (Pv) that is responsible for the low perfusion of Zone 1 of the lung?

A. Pa > PA > Pv
B. Pa > Pv > PA
C. PV > PA > Pa
D. PA > Pa > Pv

37. In a lab experiment, a healthy adult male is running on a treadmill while oxygen uptake, cardiac output, and arterial oxygen content are measured simultaneously. The measurements are:

Oxygen uptake: 1.2 L/min
Cardiac output: 16 L/min
Arterial oxygen content: 0.25 L of O_2/L of blood

Based on these data, what is the man's mixed venous oxygen content during exercise (in mL O_2/L of blood)?
A. 50
B. 75
C. 100
D. 150
E. 175

38. A teenage girl is found in a closed garage with her car running, with a suicide note on the seat. It is unknown how long she was exposed to carbon monoxide (CO), but she is breathing on her own and her skin color is cherry red. Which of the following findings is expected to be decreased is this girl?

A. Alveolar P_{O_2}
B. Arterial O_2 concentration
C. Arterial P_{CO_2}
D. Arterial P_{O_2}
E. Hemoglobin-oxygen affinity

39. A 26-year-old woman presents to the urgent care facility with rapid and shallow breathing for 1 hour. She describes having an anxiety attack and cannot catch her breath, and complains of dizziness and tingling in her hands and feet. Her heart rate and blood pressure are slightly elevated, and body temperature is normal. Which of the following changes is expected in this patient?

A. A left shift of the O_2 dissociation curve
B. A right shift of the O_2 dissociation curve
C. An increase in plasma HCO_3^-
D. A decrease in arterial P_{O_2}
E. An increase in arterial P_{CO_2}

40. Which of the following best describes the blood flow, vascular resistance, and arteriolar compliance for the pulmonary circulatory system, relative to the systemic circulatory system?

	Blood flow	Vascular resistance	Arteriolar compliance
A	Higher	Higher	Lower
B	Higher	Lower	Higher
C	Lower	Higher	Lower
D	Lower	Lower	Higher
E	Same	Higher	Lower
F	Same	Lower	Higher

41. A 62-year-old man with a history of chronic obstructive pulmonary disease (COPD) presents to the emergency room with a 3-day history of worsening shortness of breath. His oxygen saturation is 86% on room air. He has labored breathing and speaks only in short sentences. An arterial blood gas (ABG) shows the following: pH = 7.17, P_{CO_2} = 55, P_{O_2} = 62, HCO_3 = 19.4. The patient is mechanically ventilated using positive end-expiratory pressure (PEEP) and begins to show signs of right heart failure (cor pulmonale) over the next few days, most likely due to elevated pulmonary vascular resistance (PVR). Which of the following is the most likely cause of the patient's elevated PVR?

A. Alveolar hyperoxia due to ventilation
B. Alveolar hypocapnia due to ventilation
C. High blood viscosity due to polycythemia
D. Mechanical ventilation at high lung volumes
E. Systemic hypertension

42. Regional differences in ventilation and perfusion of the normal upright lung affect gas tensions in the pulmonary blood. Which of the following best describes the gas tensions (P_{O_2} and P_{CO_2}) in the alveolar capillaries at the apex or base of the lung in a healthy individual standing upright?

	Apex	Base
A	Lowest P_{O_2}	Highest P_{O_2}
B	Highest P_{O_2}	Lowest P_{O_2}
C	Lowest P_{O_2}	Lowest P_{O_2}
D	Lowest P_{CO_2}	Highest P_{O_2}
E	Highest P_{CO_2}	Lowest P_{O_2}
F	Highest P_{CO_2}	Highest P_{O_2}

43. A patient sees a cardiologist with complaints of chest tightness during exercise. A treadmill stress test is ordered. While walking at a brisk pace, the patient's cardiac output is 6000 mL/min and his arterial saturation decreases from 97% to 86%. Assuming a pulmonary capillary volume of 180 mL, what is the approximate pulmonary capillary transit time in this patient (in seconds)?

A. 0.30
B. 0.50
C. 0.75
D. 1.00
E. 1.80

6.8 Answers and Explanations

33. Correct: 4 (D)

Heroin overdose causes depression of the respiratory center, leading to hypoventilation. With hypoventilation, CO_2 is retained leading to hypercapnia (↑ P_{CO_2}) and respiratory acidosis (↓ pH). The increase in P_{CO_2} and resulting drop in pH shifts the oxygen-hemoglobin dissociation curve to the right. Other factors that can cause a rightward shift include an increase in 2,3-diphosphoglycerate (2,3-DPG) levels and an increase in body temperature. (**A**, **B**) A leftward shift of the oxygen-hemoglobin dissociation curve indicates an increased affinity of hemoglobin for oxygen and is produced by a decrease in P_{CO_2} and increase in blood pH, a decrease in 2,3-diphosphoglycerate (2,3-DPG) levels, or a decrease in body temperature. The patient is not experiencing any of these changes. (**C**) This is the normal oxygen-dissociation curve of a healthy person.

34. Correct: ↑, ↓ (B)

Alveolar capillaries are located in the alveolar walls, so as lung volume increases, these capillaries are mechanically stretched and compressed, increasing pulmonary vascular resistance and decreasing blood flow. Extra-alveolar vessels are located in the parenchymal tissue of the lung, so as lung volume increases and the lung recoils inward, this tissue is pulled apart and these vessels are pulled open, thus reducing pulmonary vascular resistance and increasing blood flow. (**A, C, D, E, F**) These do not contain the correct combination of answers.

35. Correct: Recruitment of closed capillaries (D)

During exercise, the increase in pulmonary blood flow and perfusion causes a transient increase in pulmonary artery pressure (PaP). This increase in PaP initiates pulmonary capillary recruitment and distension, thus increasing total capillary area in the lung, and decreasing pulmonary vascular resistance. (**A**) Constriction of open capillaries would increase, not decrease, pulmonary vascular resistance (PVR). (**B**) An increase in PaP, not decrease, stimulates capillary recruitment and decreases PVR. (**C**) The increased pulmonary blood flow during exercise would increase the venous pressure if the total diameter of the veins is not increased by other means (mediators). Therefore, a decrease in pressure is unlikely.

36. Correct: Pa > Pa > Pv (D)

Zone 1 is the apex of the lung and has low perfusion due to the effects of gravity on blood flow. In zone 1, the alveolar pressure (P_A) is greater than the arterial (Pa) and venous (Pv) pressures, causing compression of the alveolar capillaries, which increases alveolar capillary resistance and prevents perfusion of this region of the lung. (**A, B, C**) These choices are ordered incorrectly.

37. Correct: 175 (E)

Mixed venous oxygen content can be calculated using the Fick equation:

Cardiac output (CO) = Oxygen uptake ($\dot{V}O_2$) / [Arterial O_2 content (CaO_2) – Mixed venous O_2 content (CvO_2)]
But the equation must be rewritten to solve for CvO_2.
$CvO_2 = C_a - (\dot{V}O_2/CO)$
CvO_2 = 0.25 L of O_2/L of blood – (1.2 L/min)/(16 L/min)
CvO_2 = 0.25 L of O_2/L of blood – 0.075
CvO_2 = 0.175 L of O_2/L of blood or 175 mL O_2/L of blood

(**A**, **B**, **C**, **D**) These answer do not contain the correct calculations.

38. Correct: Arterial O_2 concentration (B)

The arterial O_2 concentration decreases because hemoglobin has 200 times more affinity for carbon monoxide (CO) than for oxygen, thus decreasing overall oxygen binding to hemoglobin and decreasing overall arterial O_2 concentration. (**A**, **D**) Alveolar and arterial PO_2 are normal in patients with CO poisoning, because arterial PO_2 is equilibrated at and determined by alveolar PO_2 and is independent of hemoglobin. The alveolar fraction of CO in a living person suffering from CO poisoning is too low to be able to produce any significant change in alveolar O_2 fraction and thus in alveolar PO_2. (**C**) Arterial PCO_2 levels are unaffected by CO poisoning. (**E**) The hemoglobin structure undergoes a conformational change when CO is bound at one of the four heme sites, resulting in an increase in the affinity of the remaining heme groups for oxygen.

39. Correct: A left shift of the O_2 dissociation curve (A)

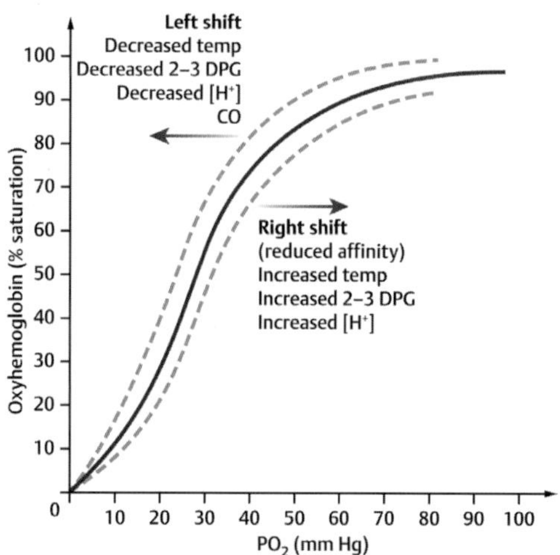

The patient is hyperventilating due to an anxiety attack, leading to a decrease in arterial PCO_2 (hypocapnia) and elevation in blood pH (alkalosis), which causes a left shift of the O_2 dissociation curve. (**B**) This patient does not have any of the changes that produce a right shift (increased body temperature, 2-3-DPG, or [H^+]). (**C**) Since carbon dioxide is carried as HCO_3^- in the blood, the loss of carbon dioxide will drive bicarbonate to combine with hydrogen ions to form more carbon dioxide, and bicarbonate levels will be more or less below normal, depending on the level of hyperventilation. (**D**) Arterial PO_2 increases with hyperventilation, unless the stimulus of hyperventilation in hypoxia, which is not the case in this patient. (**E**) Arterial PCO_2 decreases with hyperventilation because the higher alveolar ventilation induced by rapid shallow breathing blows off more CO_2.

40. Correct: Same, lower, higher (F)

The blood flow is the same for both circulations, since they are linked in series (the left ventricle cardiac output is about 1–2% higher due to normal shunts in the heart and lung). The vascular resistance of the pulmonary vasculature is lower than that of the systemic vessels as seen from the ratio of driving pressure to flow: Resistance (R) = driving pressure (ΔP)/flow (**F**) (pulmonary vascular resistance is about 9 times less than systemic vascular resistance). The pulmonary arterioles have high compliance, relative to the systemic arteries, due to their histological makeup.
(**A**, **B**, **C**, **D**, **E**) These choices contain the wrong combination of answers.

41. Correct: Mechanical ventilation at high lung volumes (D)

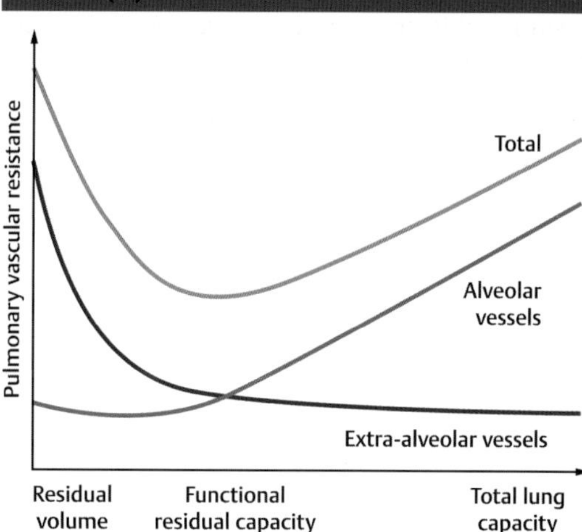

Lung volume is an important determinant of pulmonary vascular resistance (PVR). PVR is minimum at functional residual capacity (FRC), and PRV increases as lung volumes increase or decrease from FRC. At low lung volumes, the extra-alveolar vessels are compressed due to reduced retraction force of the lung tissue on these vessels as a result of smaller lung recoil force, which increases total PVR. At high lung volumes, the intra-alveolar capillaries are compressed by the expanded alveoli, as these vessels are located just within the wall of neighboring alveoli, which increases total PVR. This effect at high lung volumes is important to remember for patients on a PEEP ventilation since high PVR causes increased afterload for the right ventricle and can lead to right heart failure. (**A**) Alveolar hyperoxia causes cell damage through increased production of reactive oxygen species, but it is not a stimulus for vasoconstriction; therefore. it would not be responsible for the increased PVR. (**B**) Alveolar hypocapnea (low CO_2) may cause some pulmonary vessel dilation, which reduces PVR. (**C**) High blood viscosity may increase vascular resistance, but this patient's history does not indicate polycythemia. (**E**) Systemic hypertension is not an indicator for cor pulmonale, which is abnormal enlargement of the right side of the heart as a result of disease of the lungs or pulmonary vessels.

42. Correct: Lowest P_{O_2}, lowest P_{O_2} (C)

In regions with high $\dot{V}/\dot{Q}$ ratios, such as the apex of the lung, ventilation occurs in excess of perfusion and contributes to alveolar dead space. Due to this, alveolar gas tensions approach those of inspired air (alveolar P_{O_2} is highest in this region and alveolar P_{CO_2} is lowest). In regions with low $\dot{V}/\dot{Q}$ ratios, such as the base of the lung, ventilation is less than perfusion, which contributes to physiological shunting, and alveolar gas tensions approach those of mixed venous blood (alveolar P_{O_2} is lowest in this region and alveolar P_{CO_2} is highest). (**A, B, D, E, F**) These do not include the correct combination of answers.

43. Correct: 1.80 (E)

Gas transfer can be limited by the length of time blood stays in capillaries. Since flow is defined as volume/time, this "transit time" can be calculated using the equation: Time = volume/flow. While running on the treadmill, this patient's cardiac output is 6,000 mL/min (100 mL/second). Given that his pulmonary capillaries have a volume of 180mL, the transit time is 180 mL/(100 mL/sec) = 1.8 seconds.
(**A, B, C, D**) These answers do not have the correct calculated value.

6.9 Questions

44. A 55-year-old female passenger on a commercial airline flight is experiencing severe dyspnea. On questioning, she reports a history of deep vein thrombosis. The plane makes an emergency landing and the passenger is taken to the nearest emergency department by ambulance. Arterial blood gas (ABG) labs on room air are as follows:

PaO2 = 72 mm Hg
PaCO2 = 30 mm Hg
PIO2 = 150 mm Hg
pH = 7.49
Respiratory exchange ratio = 0.8

What is the patient's A – a difference?

A. 14.0 mm Hg
B. 26.5 mm Hg
C. 40.5 mm Hg
D. 70.0 mm Hg
E. 110.0 mm Hg

45. Three patients in the intensive care unit have arterial blood gas (ABG) labs ordered. The results are as follows:

	PaO_2 (mm Hg)	$PaCO_2$ (mm Hg)
Patient 1	40	45
Patient 2	135	20
Patient 3	100	40

Based on these data, which patient most likely has a mucus plug in a small airway, and which has a pulmonary embolus?

	Mucus plug in airway	Pulmonary embolus
A	Patient 1	Patient 2
B	Patient 1	Patient 3
C	Patient 2	Patient 1
D	Patient 2	Patient 3
E	Patient 3	Patient 1
F	Patient 3	Patient 2

46. A 26-year-old farm worker presents to the emergency department with diarrhea, vomiting, bradycardia, diaphoresis, and severe respiratory distress. History reveals an acute exposure to malathion, an organophosphate, while working in the fields 4 hours prior. Which of the following is responsible for his severe respiratory distress?

A. Decreased airflow velocity
B. Decreased surfactant production
C. Increased airway diameter
D. Increased sympathetic stimulation
E. Increased parasympathetic stimulation

47. A 21-year-old female with a history of heroin use is brought to the emergency department in an unconscious state by her mother. A heroin overdose is suspected. Her breathing is slow and erratic. Exam reveals a respiratory rate of 7 and heart rate of 55. Her pulse is irregular. An arterial blood gas is performed on arrival, before she is intubated. What change to the patient's pH, P_{CO_2}, and P_{O_2} is most likely to be measured?

	pH	P_{CO_2}	P_{O_2}
A	↑	↑	↑
B	↑	↑	↓
C	↑	↓	↔
D	↑	↓	↓
E	↓	↑	↓
F	↓	↑	↔
G	↓	↓	↓
H	↓	↓	↔

48. A 30-year-old man begins a climbing expedition on Mount Kilimanjaro. The climber lives at sea level and is unacclimated to high altitude. He reaches the first base camp at 9,000 ft above sea level on the first day, where he meets a guide who resides at the base camp, to escort him on the rest of his climb. Which of the following physiologic parameters would be expected to be increased in the climber and guide on the day the climber arrived at base camp?

	Climber	Guide
A	Blood pH	Hemoglobin concentration
B	Blood pH	Po_2
C	Blood pH	Blood pH
D	Hemoglobin concentration	Hemoglobin concentration
E	Hemoglobin concentration	Po_2
F	Hemoglobin concentration	Blood pH
G	Po_2	Hemoglobin concentration
H	Po_2	Po_2
I	Po_2	Blood pH

49. A 16-year-old girl with a head injury from a car accident was brought to the emergency department by ambulance. On exam, she had a respiratory rate of 8 breaths per minute, and a prolonged duration of inhalation was noted. Damage to which of the following groups of neurons in the brainstem is most likely responsible for this abnormal respiration?

A. Dorsal respiratory group
B. Nucleus tractus solitarii
C. Pneumotaxic center
D. Vasomotor center
E. Ventral respiratory group

50. Which of the following receptors is activated by irritants in the lungs, and what is the effect of the receptor activation?

	Receptor	Effect of receptor activation
A	Slowly adapting stretch receptor	Induces cough reflex
B	Slowly adapting stretch receptor	Induces rapid, shallow breathing
C	Rapidly adapting stretch receptor	Induces cough reflex
D	Rapidly adapting stretch receptor	Terminates inspiration
E	J-receptor	Induces cough reflex
F	J-receptor	Terminates inspiration

51. A 26-month-old girl becomes cyanotic and faints after holding her breath for 40 seconds during a temper tantrum. She regains consciousness 30 seconds later and calms down. What effect does the breath holding have on the girl's alveolar Po_2 and alveolar Pco_2 during the episode?

	Alveolar Po_2	Alveolar Pco_2
A	↑	↑
B	↑	↓
C	↑	↔
D	↓	↑
E	↓	↓
F	↓	↔
G	↔	↑
H	↔	↓
I	↔	↔

52. A 36-year-old woman presents with shortness of breath. She has a history of blood clots and is currently not taking any medication for prevention. If she has a pulmonary embolism, what physiological change will most likely be present?

A. Decreased heart rate
B. Decreased respiratory rate
C. Hypoventilation
D. Increased alveolar dead space
E. Increased left ventricular preload

53. A 4-year-old girl presents with dyspnea after swallowing a marble. On arrival, her arterial Po_2 is 70 mm Hg on room air. She is given pure oxygen (100% 02) for 10 minutes, and her arterial Po_2 increases to 120 mm Hg. Which of the following clinical findings is expected in this patient?

A. Pulmonary vasodilation
B. Decreased Pco_2
C. Increased blood pH
D. Pulmonary right-to-left shunt

54. A 21-year-old collegiate football player was involved in a helmet-to-helmet collision during a game. He collapsed after the play and was rushed to the emergency department. On admission, he was cyanotic with no visible respiration. He was intubated and placed on mechanical ventilation. At what level was the spinal cord most likely damaged?

A. C1
B. C5
C. C7
D. T8
E. T10

6.10 Answers and Explanations

44. Correct: 40.5 mm Hg (C)

To determine the A – a difference (PAO2 – PaO2), one must first solve for the partial pressure of O2 at the alveolar membrane (PAO2).

Patient's PAO2 = PIO2 – (PaCO2/R) = 150 – (30/0.8) = 150 – 37.5 = 112.5 mm Hg

Note: R = respiratory exchange ratio = 0.8.

The patient's A – a difference = PAO2 – PaO2 = 112.5 – 72 = 40.5 mm Hg.

The patient's predicted A – a difference is 14 mm Hg (2.5 + 0.21 × 55 years). The calculated value (40.5 mm Hg) is 26.5 mm Hg higher than predicted. The combination of suspected pulmonary embolism and increased A – a difference indicates a $\dot{V}A/\dot{Q}$ mismatch, suggesting impaired O2 uptake by the lungs. This occurs because the vascular obstruction reduces or blocks blood flow to the lungs, and thus prevents adequate perfusion. (**A, B, D, E**) These values are not correct.

45. Correct: Patient 1, Patient 2 (A)

In a patient with an airway obstruction (patient 1), as seen with a mucus plug in the lung, alveolar gas equilibrates with mixed venous blood at a $Paco_2$ of 45 mm Hg and PaO_2 of 40 mm Hg. Since blood leaving the area of obstruction has no opportunity to exchange O_2 or Co_2, it remains unchanged as it flows past the alveoli. In a patient with a vascular obstruction (patient 2), as seen with a pulmonary embolus, alveolar gas composition remains unchanged in the affected region of the lung following inspiration (PIo_2 = 150 mm Hg; $PIco_2$ = 0) because there is no blood perfusion to that region, and thus no gas exchange. This will lower the mixed $Paco_2$ and raise the mixed Pao_2, relative to normal. (**B, C, D**) These choices contain the wrong combination of answers. (**E, F**) Patient 3 has normal values for $Paco_2$ and Pao_2.

46. Correct: Increased parasympathetic stimulation (E)

Organophosphates block acetylcholinesterase activity, leading to an increase in acetylcholine, which enhances all parasympathetic activity. In the airway, parasympathetic stimulation causes bronchoconstriction via activation of muscarinic-3 (M3) cholinergic receptors, which increases airway resistance, leading to respiratory distress. (**A**) A decrease in airflow velocity will reduce turbulence, which lowers airway resistance and lessens respiratory distress. (**B**) A decrease in surfactant production is not linked to organophosphate poisoning or parasympathetic stimulation. (**C**) An increase in airway diameter will decrease airway resistance and lessen respiratory distress. (**D**) Sympathetic stimulation causes dilation of the airways via activation of β2 adrenergic receptors, which decreases airway resistance and lessens respiratory distress.

47. Correct: ↓, ↑, ↓ (E)

Heroin overdose causes depression of the respiratory center, leading to hypoventilation. With hypoventilation, Co_2 is retained, leading to hypercapnia (↑ Pco_2) and respiratory acidosis (↓ pH), and Po_2 is reduced, leading to hypoxia (↓ Po_2). Since this is acute, the kidneys have not yet compensated. (**A, B, C, D, F, G, H**) These options include one or more incorrect changes.

48. Correct: Blood pH, hemoglobin concentration (A)

The climber is acclimated to sea level. At high altitude, the atmospheric pressure is reduced relative to sea level, which means ambient air Po_2 is reduced, and thus alveolar and arterial Po_2 will also be reduced. The low arterial Po_2 will reduce hemoglobin saturation, which will stimulate the peripheral chemoreceptors, causing an increase in alveolar ventilation (at high altitude, low Po_2, rather than high Pco_2, is the primary stimulus for chemoreceptors). The result is hyperventilation, which will decrease Pco_2 and subsequently increase blood pH acutely, until renal compensation occurs. The guide is acclimated to high altitude. At high altitude, chronically low arterial Po_2 activates transcription factors that upregulate erythropoietin production, thus leading to an increase in hemoglobin concentration over time. The guide's blood pH will be in the normal range due to renal compensation. (**B, C, D, E, F, G, H, I**) These contain an incorrect combination of answers.

49. Correct: Pneumotaxic center (C)

The pneumotaxic center sends inhibitory signals to the inspiratory center of the medulla and controls the "switch-off" of inspiration, which directly affect inspiratory time. Decreased signals increase the duration of inspiration and tidal volume and decrease the respiratory rate. (**A, B**) The dorsal respiratory group (DRG), which is located in the nucleus tractus solitarii, is composed mainly of inspiratory neurons located bilaterally in the medulla. It controls the normal basic rhythm of breathing (along with the pre-Botzinger complex) by triggering inspiratory impulses to the motor nerves of the diaphragm and external intercostal muscles. (**D**) The vasomotor center is primarily involved in blood pressure homeostasis. (**E**) The ventral respiratory group (VRG) contains both inspiratory and expiratory neurons located bilaterally in the medulla. They are active primarily in exercise and stress. The VRG sends impulses to multiple muscle groups of respiration.

50. Correct: Rapidly adapting stretch receptor, induces cough reflex (C)

Rapidly adapting stretch receptors are the primary afferent nerve fibers that evoke the cough reflex and can be activated by airway smooth muscle constriction, mucus accumulation, mechanical irritation, and chemical stimuli, such as spices. (**A**, **B**) Slowly adapting stretch receptors are responsible for eliciting the reflexes evoked by moderate lung inflation. They play a role in terminating large inspirations and expirations and controlling breathing pattern, airway smooth muscle tone, systemic vascular resistance, and heart rate. (**D**) Rapidly adapting stretch receptors initiate the cough reflex, not terminate inspiration. (**E**, **F**) J-receptors respond to events such as pulmonary edema or pulmonary embolus and produce a rapid, shallow breathing.

51. Correct: ↓, ↑ (D)

Voluntary apnea (breath holding) causes alveolar Po_2 to decrease and alveolar Pco_2 to increase, due to lack of respiration. These alterations cause similar changes in the arterial Po_2 and Pco_2. The decreased arterial Po_2 directly stimulates peripheral chemoreceptors, and the increased Pco_2 indirectly stimulates central chemoreceptors. (**A**, **B**, **C**, **E**, **F**, **G**, **H**, **I**) These do not contain the correct combination of answers.

52. Correct: Increased alveolar dead space (D)

A pulmonary embolism blocks blood flow to the affected alveolar region. Although the alveoli of this region are ventilated with air, they are not perfused with blood (alveolar dead space ventilation). (**A**, **E**) A pulmonary embolism will reduce blood flow to the left ventricle (LV), thus decreasing LV preload and cardiac output. As compensation, heart rate will increase, leading to tachycardia. (**B**) Tachypnea, not bradypnea (reduced respiratory rate), is typically seen with pulmonary embolism. (**C**) Hyperventilation, not hypoventilation, is typically seen with pulmonary embolism.

53. Correct: Pulmonary right-to-left shunt (D)

If arterial pressure of O_2 (Pao_2) does not increase after administration of pure oxygen at 100% for 5 to 10 minutes, then a pulmonary shunt is present. Following administration of pure O_2 the estimated alveolar Po_2 will be:

$PAO_2 = PIO_2 - PACO_2/R = [FIO2\ (PB - PH2O)] - PACO_2/R = [1 \times (760 - 47) - 40/0.8 = 713 - 50 = 663$ mm Hg.

The arterial Po_2 is assumed to be roughly equal to alveolar Po_2 (within 10 mm Hg). Therefore, the arterial Po_2 is expected to rise to 663 mm Hg during pure O_2 breathing, but it does not come even close to this value. This means that a significant volume of venous blood bypasses the alveolar gas exchange surface and mixes with a fraction of oxygenated blood coming from normally perfused lung areas. This venous "right-to-left shunt" reduces the Po_2 of mixed blood, which is arterial blood. Therefore, the arterial Po_2 remains low, and far below alveolar Po_2. (**A**) The blocked airway will produce a hypoxic vasoconstriction in the lung. This is unique to the lung, since other tissues produce hypoxic vasodilation. (**B**, **C**) The blockade of some airways may reduce alveolar ventilation and cause an increase (not a decrease) in Pco_2 and a decrease in pH.

54. Correct: C1 (A)

Damage at the level of C1 is above the brachial plexus and phrenic nerve and would paralyze the upper extremities and diaphragm, requiring a ventilator for respiration. (**B**) Damage at the level of C5 would cause upper extremity paralysis, but the diaphragm would maintain partial function, so respiration could occur without a ventilator. (**C**) Damage at the level of C7 would cause paralysis of the lower extremities, abdominal muscles, and intercostal muscles, because the nerves that innervate these regions are below C7, but the nerves that innervate the diaphragm are above C7, so mechanical ventilation would not be required. (**D**, **E**) Damage at the level of T8 or T10 would have no effect on the upper body. Partial paralysis of the lower body and legs would be present, and breathing would be normal.

Chapter 7

Renal and Urinary Systems

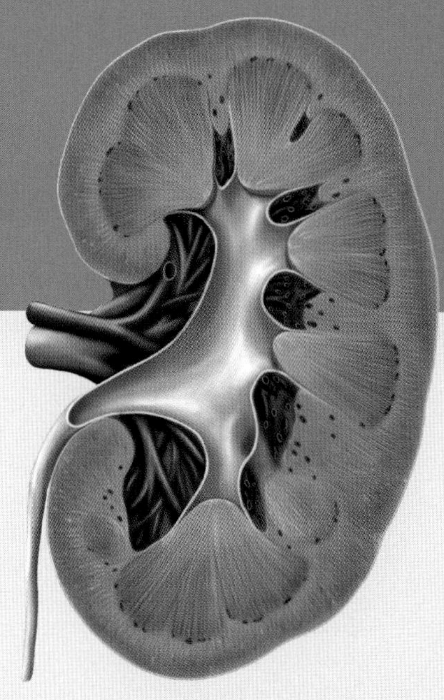

LEARNING OBJECTIVES

- Understand the relationship between the renal structure and function in regards to blood flow, glomerular filtration, and renal clearance. Be able to apply this knowledge to common physiologic and pathophysiologic situations, as well as the concepts for treatment.
- Describe renal reabsorption and secretion of common substances with distinguishing the site and mechanism of action, as well as their regulation by hormones and common pharmaceuticals categories. Describe clinical syndromes related to defects in specific renal transporters.
- Describe urine formation and micturition and understand the role of the urine composition for diagnosis of pathologies and clearance of toxic substances. Understand the role of the kidneys for acid-base homeostasis.
- Describe body fluids and predict the changes in extracellular/intracellular volume and osmolality, plasma protein concentration, and hematocrit caused by volume contraction and expansion. Discuss the body's balances of major electrolytes and the role of the kidneys to maintain water and salt homeostasis.
- Discuss how the kidneys handle special substances, such as erythropoietin, vitamin D, prostaglandins, renin, atrial natriuretic peptide (ANP), kinins, and endothelin.
- Recognize the signs and symptoms of acute and chronic renal injury, and describe the underlying physiologic processes that produce them.

7.1 Questions

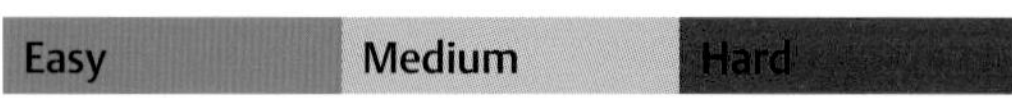

1. A 58-year-old female, who recently received a coronary artery bypass graft, presents with granular casts in her urine and a progressively increasing serum creatinine concentration. Amongst other tests, a renal biopsy is obtained. The pathologist in particular investigates which of the following nephron segments, since they are particularly susceptible to ischemia?

A. Proximal convoluted tubule
B. Proximal straight tubule
C. Descending loop of Henle
D. Ascending loop of Henle
E. Distal convoluted tubule
F. Collecting duct

2. Which of the following best describes the function of the renal structure indicated by the red arrows the image?

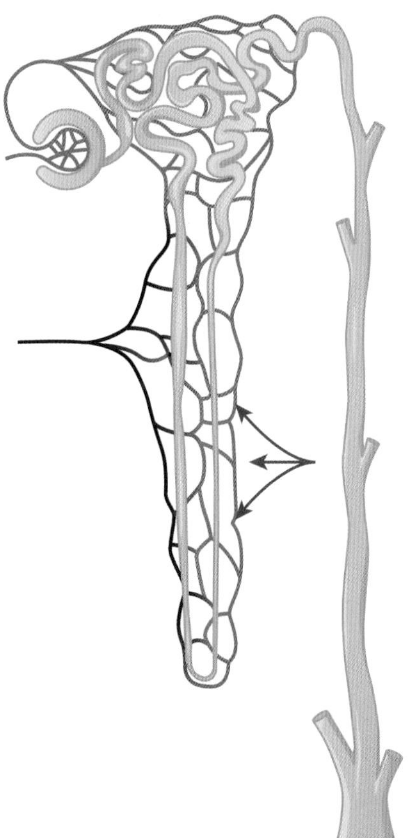

A. Accelerate blood flow around the loops of Henle
B. Delivers nutrients and oxygen to the cortical nephrons
C. Maintains corticopapillary gradient of juxtamedullary nephrons
D. Transports filtrate from the glomerulus
E. Transports blood to the afferent arteriole

3. Researchers discuss an improved renal imaging tool that provides functional information on the type of nephron that is outlined in the blue box in the image. Which of the following is a main function of the tubular structure?

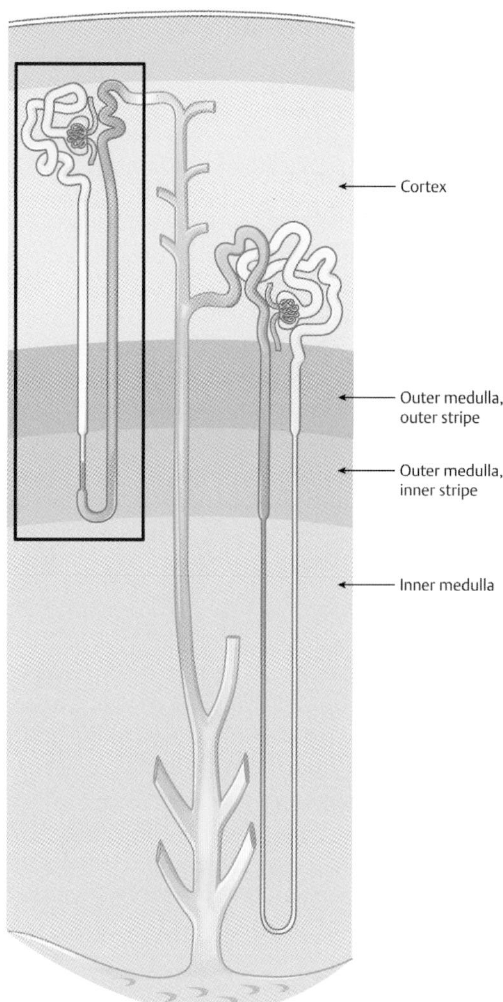

A. Bulk reabsorption of solutes
B. Erythropoietin production
C. Formation of the corticopapillary gradient
D. Urine-concentrating mechanisms
E. Urine-diluting mechanisms

4. A newborn has been diagnosed with a loss-of-function mutation of the *NPHS1* gene, which encodes for nephrin. Abnormal nephrin leads to the absence of glomerular slit diaphragms of glomerular podocytes. Considering this information, which of the following characteristic would most likely be present in this baby without treatment?

A. Bright yellow urine
B. Generalized edema
C. High urine output
D. Normal birth weight
E. Normal immune response

5. A patient presents with a twofold-elevated serum creatinine level compared to baseline for 12 hours. In order to prevent worsening azotemia, the patient's glomerular filtration rate must be increased. Which of the following is an appropriate manipulation?

A. Constricting renal afferent arteriole
B. Dilating renal afferent arteriole
C. Dilating renal efferent arteriole
D. Increasing glomerular capillary colloid oncotic pressure
E. Increasing hydrostatic pressure in Bowman's space

6. A 45-year-old woman donates a healthy kidney to her sister. In regards to creatinine, which of the following is expected to be decreased in the donor after full recovery from the operation?

A. Clearance
B. Plasma concentration
C. Production
D. Renal excretion
E. Storage

7. A 35-year-old woman suffers from acute liver failure due to liver cancer. She is jaundiced and edematous. Which of the following Starling forces in the kidney are likely to be primarily and secondarily affected by her condition?

	Primary change in glomerular capillary	Secondary change in Bowman's space
A.	↑ Hydrostatic pressure	↑ Hydrostatic pressure
B.	↑ Hydrostatic pressure	↑ Oncotic pressure
C.	↑ Hydrostatic pressure	↓ Oncotic pressure
D.	↓ Oncotic pressure	↑ Hydrostatic pressure
E.	↓ Oncotic pressure	↓ Hydrostatic pressure
F.	↓ Oncotic pressure	↑ Oncotic pressure

8. In a laboratory experiment, renal efferent arterioles are stimulated to constrict, and then the glomerular Starling forces are measured. The values are reported as follows:

Glomerular capillary hydrostatic pressure = 65 mm Hg
Glomerular capillary oncotic pressure = 28 mm Hg
Bowman's space hydrostatic pressure = 20 mm Hg
Bowman's space oncotic pressure = 0 mm Hg
Based on these data, what is the glomerular net filtration pressure (in mm Hg)?

A. −17
B. −8
C. 0
D. 8
E. 17

9. A patient presents with severe renal artery stenosis. When an angiotensin-converting enzyme (ACE) inhibitor is administered, the patient has to be carefully monitored for which of the following?

A. Increased renal resistance to blood flow
B. Increased protein excretion in the urine
C. Increased systemic blood pressure
D. Reduced renal tubule potassium reabsorption
E. Reduced glomerular filtration rate

10. In an experiment, the renal vein of a rat was cannulated, and para-aminohippurate (PAH) was infused. Following a sufficient period of equilibration, plasma PAH concentration was 0.2 mg/mL and urinary concentration was 100 mg/ml. Urinary flow was 1 mL/min. Inulin clearance was found to be 100 mL/min. The fraction of filtered plasma at the glomerulus is which of the following?

A. 0.1
B. 0.2
C. 0.3
D. 0.4
E. 0.5

11. Using the following table and assuming that renal perfusion pressure remains constant, which of the following combined changes in afferent and efferent arteriolar resistance would result in an immediate increase in renal plasma flow and glomerular filtration rate?

	Afferent arteriolar resistance	Efferent arteriolar resistance
A.	↑	↑
B.	↑	↓
C.	↑	↔
D	↓	↓
E.	↓	↔

A. A
B. B
C. C
D. D
E. E

12. A 29-year-old man presents with diarrhea. Physical examination reveals a palpated blood pressure of 100 and a heart rate of 120. Neck veins are flat, and there is poor skin turgor. Three months ago, a baseline serum creatinine was 0.8 mg/dL. Current serum creatinine concentration is unchanged. Which of the following correctly describes the man's status in regards to the synthesis of the following renal vasoactive compounds?

A. Decrease of histamine
B. Decrease of prostaglandin E_2
C. Decrease of prostaglandin I_2
D. Increase of angiotensin II
E. Increase of endothelin

13. A 55-year-old man presents to the emergency room complaining of burning epigastric pain, a 2-hour history of vomiting blood, and feeling faint. His vital signs are: ear temperature 97.8°F, pulse 109 bpm, blood pressure 90/63 mm Hg, and respiratory rate 30 breaths/min. His skin is pale, extremities are cold, and mucous membranes are dry. His condition affects the kidney in which of the following ways as compared to a healthy individual?

	Glomerular filtration rate	Renal blood flow	Filtration fraction	Renin release juxtaglomerular cells	Renal PGE_2 and PGI_2* synthesis
A.	↓	↓	↓	↓	↓
B.	↓	↓	↓	↓	↑
C.	↓	↓	↓	↑	↑
D	↓	↓	↓	↑	↓
E.	↓	↓	↑	↑	↑
F.	↑	↑	↓	↑	↑
G	↑	↓	↑	↑	↑

*PGE_2: prostaglandin E_2, PGI_2: prostaglandin I_2

14. The image below is used to explain the kidneys' ability for tubuloglomerular feedback in response to increased renal arterial pressure. Which of the sites labeled 1–4 are correctly identified as the sites where a change is sensed and the site(s) primarily respond(s) to the change?

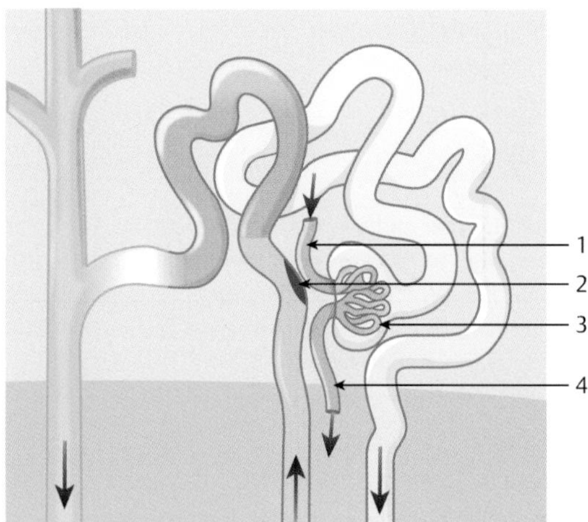

	Sensor site	Response site(s)
A.	1	1
B.	1	2
C.	2	1
D.	1	3
E.	2	4
F.	1	1, 3 and 4

15. A healthy 25-year-old man with a resting blood pressure of 120/80 mm Hg is running on a treadmill, which increases his blood pressure to 140/100 mm Hg. Which of the following is the most likely change in the diameters of his renal afferent and efferent arterioles when exercising?

A. Constriction of afferent and dilation of efferent arterioles
B. Constriction of both afferent and efferent arterioles
C. Constriction of efferent arterioles only
D. Constriction of afferent arterioles only
E. Dilation of afferent and constriction of efferent arterioles

16. A 40-year-old woman experiencing an acute hypertensive event has a renal mean arterial pressure that is fluctuating between 120 and 150 mm Hg. The resulting renal blood flow (RBF) and glomerular filtration rate (GFR) are shown on the graph. Which of the following physiological mechanisms is most responsible for this patient's minimal change in RPF and GFR, despite the large changes in renal arterial pressure?

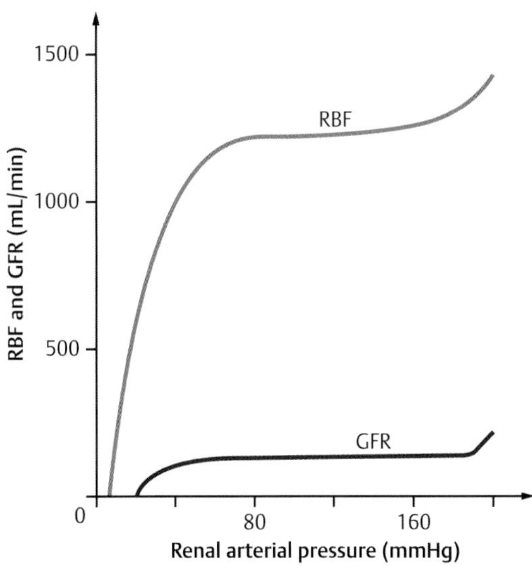

A. Autoregulation of renal arteriolar diameter
B. Release of aldosterone from the adrenal cortex
C. Release of epinephrine from the adrenal medulla
D. Reactive hyperemia of the renal arterioles
E. Sympathetic-mediated vasoconstriction of renal arterioles

17. The physician uses the image of the renal glomerular filtration apparatus in the image to explain to a patient his proteinuria. Which layer (labeled A–C) is the primary barrier that normally inhibits the passage of serum albumin from the glomerular capillaries into Bowman's space?

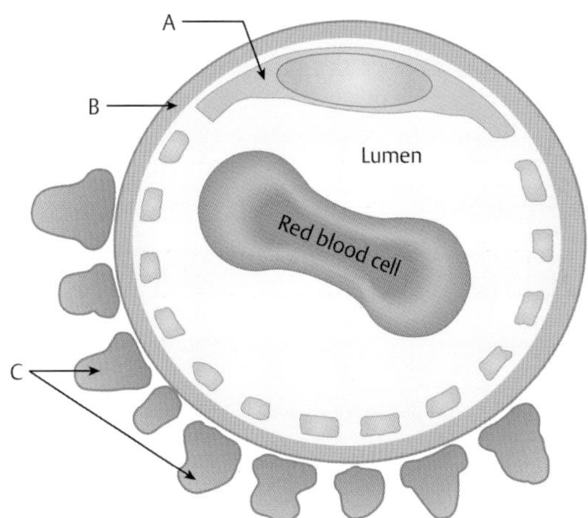

A. A only
B. B only
C. C only
D. A & B both contribute equally
E. A & C both contribute equally
F. A, B & C all contribute equally

18. The following graph shows the relative filtration rate for various dextrans (polysaccharides) that have different molecular radii and are differently charged. Which layer of the renal glomerular filtration barrier is most responsible for the change in the relative glomerular filtration rate of cationic dextran (blue line) relative to neutral dextran (red line)?

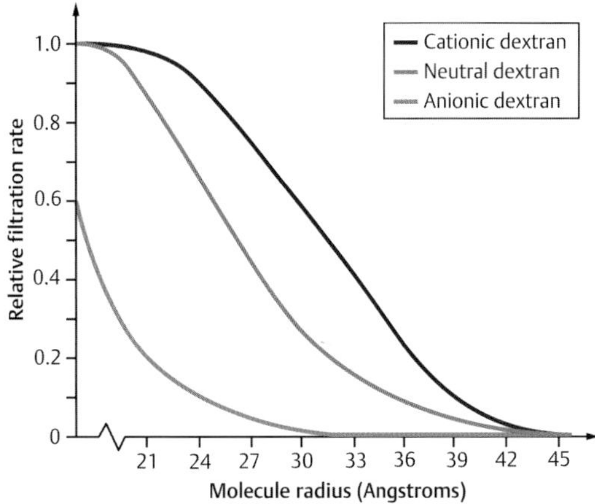

A. Basement membrane only
B. Basement membrane and podocytes
C. Capillary endothelium only
D. Capillary endothelium and basement membrane
E. Capillary endothelium and podocytes
F. Podocytes only

19. A 7-year-old boy presents to his primary care physician with mild edema in his hands and feet, slightly elevated blood pressure, and cola-colored, foamy urine. An image of his urine sample is shown in the image. His mother reports that he has complained of a sore throat a few times over the past 2 weeks but otherwise has been healthy until last night, when she noticed the swelling and unusual urine. Which of the following change of the glomerulus best describes the presence of foamy urine in this patient?

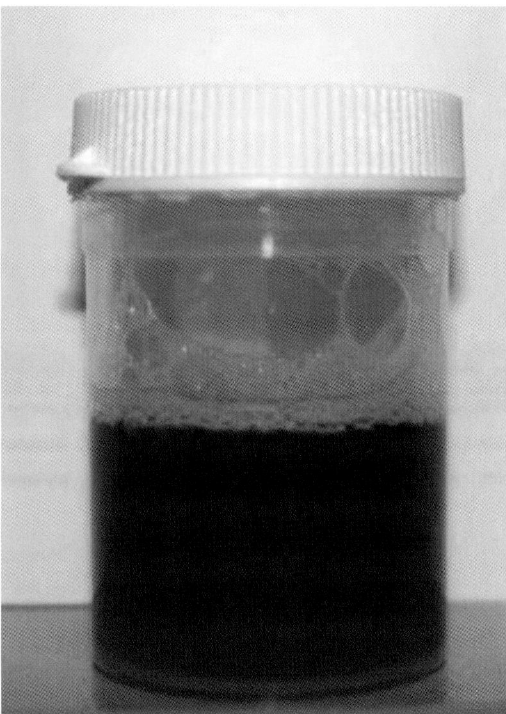

A. Inflammation of the basement membrane
B. Inflammation of the epithelial layer
C. Inflammation of the podocytes
D. Sclerosis of the basement membrane
E. Sclerosis of the epithelial layer
F. Sclerosis of the podocytes

20. A 71-year-old woman with a recent history of urinary tract infections presents with pain on her side and back, justifying renal function tests. As part of it, which of the following is tested by the creatinine clearance test?

A. The amount of creatinine being filtered per minute
B. The amount of creatinine being secreted per minute
C. The amount of creatinine being reabsorbed per minute
D. The volume of urine being cleared of creatinine per minute
E. The volume of plasma being cleared of creatinine per minute

21. An 11-year-old boy presents with polydipsia, polyuria, fatigue, and headache, so a series of renal function tests are ordered. Which of the following test results would be an abnormal finding?

A. Creatinine clearance of 130 mL/min
B. Glucose clearance of 10 mL/min
C. Inulin clearance of 120 mL/min
D. PAH clearance of 600 mL/min
E. Plasma creatinine concentration of 0.5 mg/dL

22. As part of a two-day clinical study, the following data are collected from a young adult:

	Day 1	Day 2
Plasma inulin (mg/mL)	0.006	0.006
Plasma urea (μmol/mL)	6.5	6.5
Plasma glucose (mg/dL)	100	400
Urine inulin (mg/mL)	0.2	0.1
Urine urea (μmol/mL)	250	150
Urine glucose (mg/dL)	1	1
Urine flow (mL/min)	2	4

Which of the following changes occurred on day 2?

	Glomerular filtration rate	Urea excretion	Urea clearance	Glucose excretion	Glucose clearance
A	↔	↓	↑	↑	↓
B	↔	↑	↑	↑	↓
C	↓	↓	↑	↑	↑
D	↓	↑	↓	↓	↔
E	↑	↓	↓	↓	↔

23. Assuming constant glomerular filtration rate, plasma volume, and urine flow rate, the renal clearance of which of the following substances will increase when its plasma concentration is significantly increased?

A. Creatinine
B. Inulin
C. Mannitol
D. Phosphate
E. Urea

24. A 75-year-old woman is treated for urinary infection with an antibiotic. She weighs 320 pounds. The antibiotic is completely eliminated in urine. Its dosage must be adjusted by 1% for every 1% change from the normal glomerular filtration rate, which is 100 mL/min for a woman of her age and weight. Two weeks ago, the patient underwent a creatinine clearance test, in which her serum creatinine was 5 mg/dL and urine creatinine was 50 mg/dL. One liter of urine was collected within 200 minutes. What is the most appropriate antibiotic dosage (in % of normal) for this patient?

A. 10

B. 20

C. 50

D. 80

E. 100

25. A 50-year-old patient with chronic hypertension is diagnosed with renal artery stenosis. As part of the differential diagnosis, creatinine clearance and the plasma/blood concentrations of creatinine and urea nitrogen were obtained. Which of the following changes from his normal healthy values best characterize the current patient's status?

	Creatinine clearance	Plasma creatinine concentration	Blood urea nitrogen (BUN)
A	↓	↑	↓
B	↓	↑	↑
C	↑	↑	↑
D	↓	↓	↓
E	↓	↓	↑
F	↑	↓	↓

26. Substance X is filtered by renal tubules but is not secreted or reabsorbed. Substance X is infused into a volunteer until a steady-state plasma level of 0.1 mg/mL is achieved. The subject then empties his bladder and waits 2 hours, at which time he urinates again. The volume of urine in the second specimen is 120 mL, and the concentration of substance X is 8 mg/mL. What is the clearance of this substance in mL/min, and which parameter (glomerular filtration rate, GFR, or renal plasma flow, RPF) is the clearance measuring?

	Clearance of X (mL/min)	Measured parameter
A.	30	GFR
B.	30	RPF
C.	80	GFR
D.	80	RPF
E.	100	GFR
F.	100	RPF

27. A healthy 80-year-old man and a healthy 21-year-old man of the same race and similar height, weight, diet, and hydration status both produce 1.5 liters of urine within a day. However, the older man has a serum creatinine concentration of 2 mg/dL, while the younger man has a serum creatinine concentration of 1 mg/dL. Relative to the younger man's glomerular filtration rate, what percentage of glomerular filtration rate would be expected in the older man?

A. 2

B. 10

C. 50

D. 100

E. 200

28. A 35-year-old woman presents at the emergency department with flank pain and painful urination. Her ear temperature is 100.6°F (38.1°C) and blood pressure is 115/75 mm Hg. Ultrasound reveals a bilateral hydronephrosis, and blood tests reveal a plasma creatinine level of 3.1 mg/dL. Which of the following is the most likely cause of her hydronephrosis and elevated plasma creatinine level?

A. Adrenal medulla tumor

B. Blocked urethra

C. Hyperalbuminemia

D. Hypovolemia

E. Renal artery stenosis

29. In a healthy person with a normal balanced diet, which of the following substances has the greatest fraction excreted in the urine compared to plasma?

A. Creatinine

B. Glucose

C. Inulin

D. Para-aminohippurate

E. Urea

30. The glomerular filtration rate of a person is 100 mL/min. The plasma concentration of drug X is 2 mg/mL; the urine concentration of drug X is 50 mg/mL; and the urine flow rate is 1 mL/min. Drug X is a small molecule that is not bound to plasma proteins. Which of the following can be concluded about drug X in regards to renal tubules?

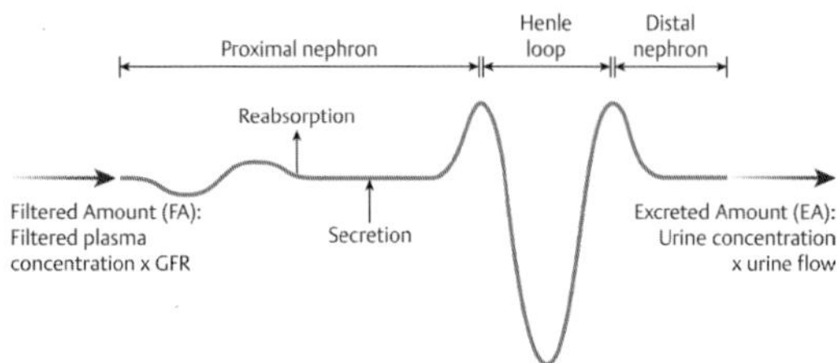

A. It is neither secreted nor reabsorbed by tubules.
B. The tubules reabsorbed 50 mg/min of it.
C. The tubules reabsorbed 150 mg/min of it.
E. The tubules secreted 50 mg/min of it.
D. The tubules secreted 150 mg/min of it.

31. The following measurements are from a renal clearance study on a young adult woman.

Plasma inulin concentration:	1 mg/mL
Urine inulin concentration:	50 mg/mL
Urine flow rate:	2 mL/min
Plasma concentration of substance Y	0.02 mg/mL
Urine concentration of substance Y	5.00 mg/mL

If substance Y is a small molecule, of which 50% is bound to plasma protein, which of the following actions of the kidney tubules is correct?

A. Reabsorbed 1 mg/min
B. Reabsorbed 8 mg/min
C. Reabsorbed 9 mg/min
D. Secreted 1 mg/min
E. Secreted 8 mg/min
F. Secreted 9 mg/min

32. A 28-year old patient is discovered to have a solitary kidney during preparation for a knee surgery. He has been asymptomatic in regards to kidney function. When compared with a person with two functional kidneys and similar diet and stature, which of the following would be expected for the patient with one kidney compared to the person with two kidneys?

A. Elevated glomerular filtration rate
B. Higher plasma creatinine concentration
C. Low blood pressure
D. Peripheral edema
E. Twofold higher sodium clearance

33. As part of a continuing medical education training session on the advances of diabetes mellitus treatment, the following renal titration curve for glucose is shown for a patient. Which of the following is the patient's renal threshold for glucose?

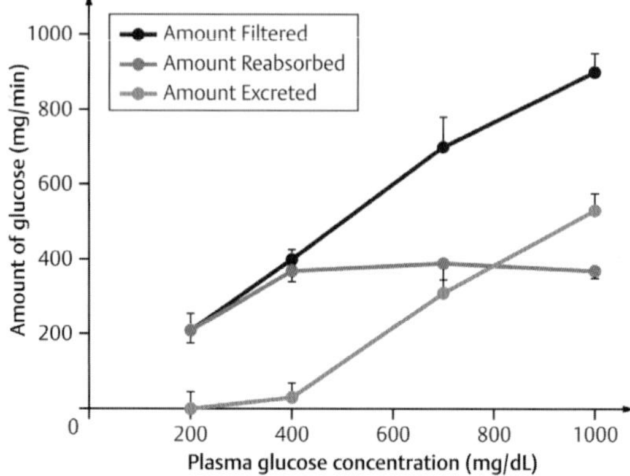

A. 200 mg/dL
B. 200 mg/min
C. 400 mg/dL
D. 400 mg/min
E. 800 mg/dL
F. 800 mg/min

34. The following graph is a glucose titration curve showing changes in glucose transport in the proximal tubule relative to glucose plasma concentration. Which of the following changes to plasma glucose concentration, glucose transport, or nephron diversity would create a greater "splay"?

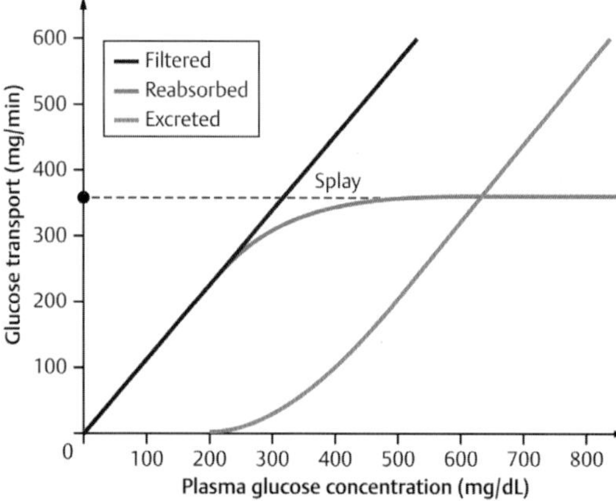

A. Glucose concentration, decreased
B. Glucose concentration, increased
C. Glucose transport, decreased
D. Glucose transport, increased
E. Nephron diversity, decreased
F. Nephron diversity, increased

35. To help with the diagnosis of hyponatremic and hypernatremic disorders, the physician frequently orders a free-water clearance and an osmolar clearance test. Which of the following parameters can be determined from the sum of the two clearances?

A. Creatinine clearance
B. Inulin clearance
C. Renal plasma flow rate
D. Urea clearance
E. Urine flow rate

Questions 36 to 38

A 28-year-old man of average height is brought to the emergency department after being lost in the woods for three days while hiking. When found, he is given plenty of fluids to drink and he is thoroughly checked out. It seems that there are no major injuries, except that he was dehydrated. The following test results were obtained from this patient:

Plasma concentration inulin	P_{inulin}	= 2.5 mg/mL
Plasma osmolarity	$P_{osmolarity}$	= 315 mOsm/L
Plasma concentration sodium	P_{Na+}	= 36 mg/mL
Urine concentration inulin	U_{inulin}	= 24 mg/mL
Urine osmolarity	$U_{osmolarity}$	= 350 mOsm/L
Urine concentration sodium	U_{Na+}	= 3.5 mg/mL
Urine flow	$\dot{V}$	= 10 mL/min

36. What is the patient's approximate glomerular filtration rate in milliliters per minute (mL/min)?

A. 6
B. 42
C. 60
D. 96
E. 120

37. What is the patient's approximate free water clearance in milliliter per minute (mL/min)?

A. −11.1
B. −1.1
C. 0.0
D. +1.1
E. +11.1

38. What does the patient's free water clearance value indicate when comparing his urine to his plasma?

A. It contains more glucose.
B. It contains more proteins.
C. It is hyperosmotic.
D. It is hypoosmotic.
E. It is isoosmotic.

7.2 Answers and Explanations

Easy | Medium | Hard

1. Correct: Proximal convoluted tubule (A)

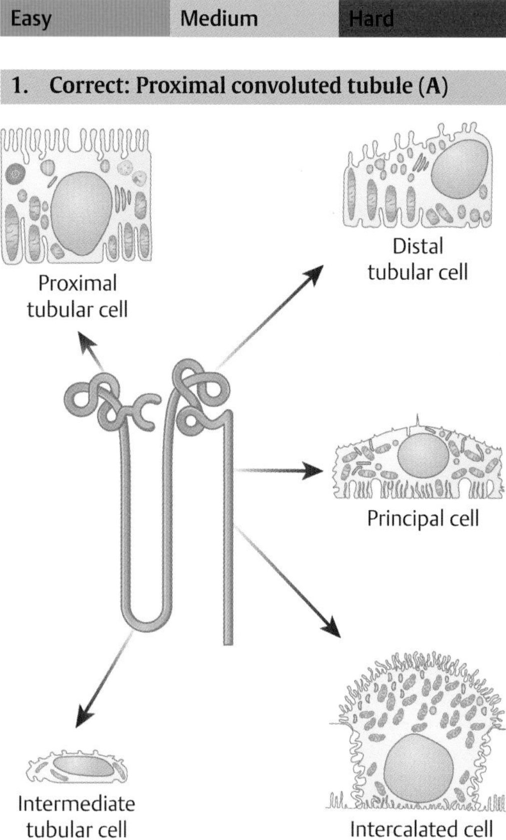

The epithelial cells of the proximal convoluted tubule have a brush border of microvilli, which can be seen in a microscopic preparation (image). In this first segment of the nephron, nutrients and most other solutes are reabsorbed into peritubular capillaries while organic wastes are secreted into the tubular lumen. This requires an enormous number of cellular transporters, which are accommodated by an increased apical surface area. The high energy demand makes those cells especially susceptible to ischemia. In all other segments of the nephron, there is quantitatively less transport. (**B**) In the late proximal tubule, including the straight part, there is mainly reabsorption of NaCl. (**C, D**) The main function of the loop of Henle is to reabsorb water without solute in the descending part and solute without water in the ascending part. (**E, F**) In the early distal nephron, including the convoluted tubule, the main function is reabsorption of NaCl without water, while in the late distal convoluted tubule and the collecting duct, water and NaCl are reabsorbed.

2. Correct: Maintains corticopapillary gradient of juxtamedullary nephrons (C)

The arrows point to the vasa recta, blood vessels that branch off the efferent arterioles of the juxtamedullary nephrons (deep nephrons that extend into the medulla), then enter the medulla and surround the loops of Henle. They deliver nutrients and oxygen to the juxtamedullary nephrons and help to maintain the corticopapillary gradient. (**A**) Vasa recta carry blood at a very slow (not fast) rate to avoid washout of the interstitial corticopapillary osmotic gradient. (**B**) Vasa recta are a series of straight capillaries in the medulla that lie parallel to the loop of Henle of juxtamedullary nephrons, not cortical nephrons. (**D**) These are blood vessels, not renal tubules, so they do not transport filtrate. (**E**) These vessels transport blood from the efferent arterioles to the medulla of the kidney, not to the afferent arterioles.

3. Correct: Bulk reabsorption of solutes (A)

From the one million nephrons per kidney, about seven of eight are cortical nephrons (the structure in the blue box). They primarily function to reabsorb and secrete solutes in the kidney. (**B**) Erythropoietin-producing cells in the healthy kidney are interstitial cells close to peritubular capillaries in the cortex and outer medulla. (**C, D, E**) Cortical nephrons are short in length and extend only slightly into the renal medulla, so they have little impact on the formation of the corticopapillary gradient or urine-diluting and concentrating mechanisms.

4. Correct: Has generalized edema (B)

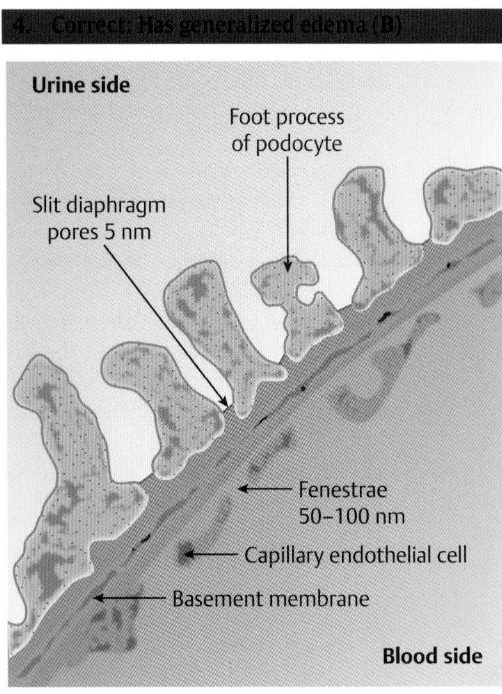

The baby has generalized edema due to urinary loss of albumin and other proteins, which leads to decreased serum oncotic pressure, the main force that normally keeps water inside blood vessels. Mutations in genes that encode podocyte proteins, such as nephrin, disrupt the normal glomerular architecture, in which podocytes form foot processes and slits, the latter being covered by a membrane called slit diaphragm (image). This organization is critical to retain proteins on the blood side of the glomerular filtration barrier; disruption leads to proteins passing to the urine side (image). The described condition is called congenital nephrotic syndrome of the Finnish type. (**A**) The presence of proteins in urine make it foamy and cloudy, not bright yellow colored. (**C**) Since fluids leave the bloodstream, urine output is low (not high), and the baby could suffer acute kidney failure. (**D**) As a result of hypoproteinemia, the nutritional status and the birth weight is low, not normal. Hypothyroidism (due to the loss of thyroxine-binding protein) and poor appetite contribute to poor growth. (**E**) The loss of immunoglobulins in urine does not leave enough antibodies that help fight body infections, and there is no normal immune response.

5. Correct: Dilating renal afferent arteriole (B)

Dilating the afferent arteriole increases hydrostatic glomerular capillary pressure (P_{GC}). This increases the force that drives plasma from the capillary into the capsule and increases glomerular filtration rate (GFR). (**A, C**) Constricting the afferent arteriole or dilating the efferent arteriole decreases P_{GC} and thus decreases GFR. (**D**) Increasing the glomerular capillary colloid oncotic pressure will draw fluid from Bowman's capsule into the capillary, hence decrease GFR. (**E**) Increasing hydrostatic pressure in Bowman's space, such as seen in postrenal failure, opposes filtration and decreases GFR.

6. Correct: Clearance (A)

Creatinine clearance is an estimate of glomerular filtration rate (GFR), which is decreased after the donation of a kidney due to the decreased total number of functioning nephrons. (**B, D**) Plasma creatinine concentration is expected to increase (not decrease) until steady state has been reached, so that the rate of creatinine production is equal to the rate of excretion. In other words, a person with decreased GFR also excretes all creatinine that is produced, but at the expense of a higher plasma creatinine concentration. (**C**) Creatinine production is unchanged (not decreased), since it is proportional to a person's muscle mass and the clinical vignette does not provide any indication of change. (**E**) Creatinine is not stored, and when produced, it is excreted by the kidney. It is a spontaneous byproduct of the reaction between creatine and phosphocreatine, catalyzed by creatine kinase.

7. Correct: ↓ Oncotic pressure, ↑ hydrostatic pressure (D)

Liver failure will reduce the amount of plasma proteins produced by the liver, which will reduce the glomerular capillary oncotic pressure (primary change). This reduction in glomerular capillary oncotic pressure will reduce the reabsorption of fluid from the nephron back into the glomerulus, thus increasing Bowman's space hydrostatic pressure (secondary change). (**A, B, C**) The glomerular hydrostatic pressure will be decreased due to the reduced protein production, which leads to a systemic reduction in capillary hydrostatic pressure; however, this is not the primary change that occurs. (**E, F**) Reduced glomerular capillary oncotic pressure is the primary change (see explanation above), but the hydrostatic pressure in Bowman's space will be increased, and the oncotic pressure it not affected since no proteins are filtered.

8. Correct: 17 (E)

Net filtration pressure (NFP) is calculated as follows:

$NFP = (P_{GC} - P_{BS}) - (\pi_{GC} - \pi_{BS}) = (65 - 20) - (28 - 0) = 45 - 28 = 17$ mm Hg

P_{GC} = glomerular capillary hydrostatic pressure

P_{BS} = Bowman's space hydrostatic pressure

π_{GC} = glomerular capillary oncotic pressure

π_{BS} = Bowman's space oncotic pressure

Under normal conditions, the net filtration pressure always favors filtration. This is further augmented with a constricted efferent arteriole and a consequently higher P_{GC}, so that the numeric value of NFP will definitely have a positive sign. (**A, B, C, D**) All other answers are incorrect.

9. Correct: Reduced glomerular filtration rate (E)

A patient with renal artery stenosis has reduced blood flow to the kidneys and, thus, reduced glomerular filtration rate (GFR). Administration of an ACE inhibitor might reduce systemic blood pressure and thus reduce driving pressure to the kidneys below the limits of autoregulation. This might further reduce GFR and can lead to acute renal failure. Moreover, the body's compensation to maintain GFR in these patients includes an increase in efferent arteriolar resistance, partly mediated by angiotensin II (AngII). Blunting this effect by an ACE inhibitor can aggravate the situation. While patients still receive ACE inhibitors, they need to be carefully monitored for the possibility of acute renal failure. (**A**) An ACE inhibitor, and hence a decrease in AngII, would dilate the afferent arterioles and decrease renal resistance to blood flow. In this case the renal stenosis might prevent the vessel from dilating, though. (**B**) Administration of an ACE inhibitor will have no effect on protein excretion in the urine. (**C**) A decrease in AngII will decrease (not increase) systemic blood pressure. (**D**) A decrease in AngII will have no effect on potassium reabsorption in the renal tubules.

10. Correct: 0.2 (B)

The fraction of filtered plasma at the glomerulus, or filtration fraction (FF), equals glomerular filtration rate (GFR) divided by renal plasma flow (RPF), or inulin clearance divided by para-aminohippurate (PAH) clearance. Inulin clearance is given as 100 mL/min. PAH clearance can be calculated as 500 mL/min, when PAH urine concentration (100 mg/mL) is multiplied by urine flow (1 mL/min) and divided by PAH plasma concentration (0.2 mg/mL). GFR of 100 mL/min divided by RPF of 500 mL/min equals 0.2. (A, C, D, E) These are incorrect results.

11. Correct: ↓, ↔ (E)

If afferent arteriolar resistance is decreased (i.e., arteriole is dilated), renal plasma flow (RPF) increases. In order for glomerular filtration rate (GFR) to increase, the efferent arteriolar resistance must be maintained. This will produce an increased volume in the glomerulus and increase glomerular hydrostatic pressure (P_{GC}), which will increase GFR. (**A, B, C**) These choices are incorrect because in order to increase RPF, the afferent arteriole must dilate, i.e., decrease resistance. (**D**) This choice is incorrect because if both afferent and efferent arteriolar resistances are decreased (i.e., both vessels are dilated), then RPF would increase, but GFR would remain constant since there would be no increase in outflow resistance to increase the glomerular blood volume, and thus P_{GC} and GFR.

12. Correct: Increase of angiotensin II (D)

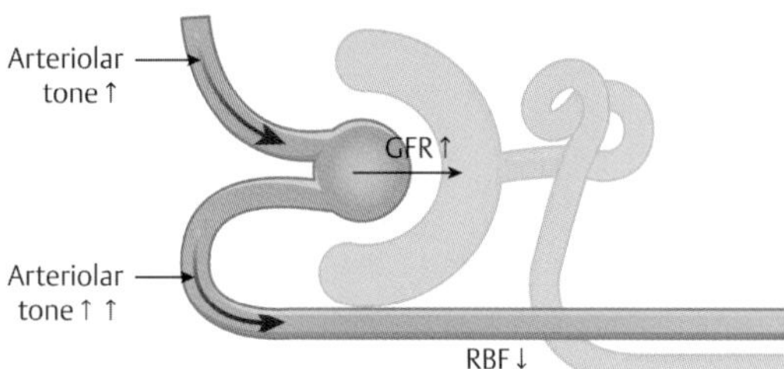

Angiotensin II (AngII) synthesis is increased in response to increased renin, which has been produced in the patient due to volume contraction (flat neck veins, poor skin turgor, low systolic blood pressure) as a complication of diarrhea. While renal perfusion could be compromised, glomerular filtration rate (GFR) appears to be maintained (stable creatinine). AngII will have contributed to it, since it is a potent vasoconstrictor, especially of the efferent arteriole. This raises hydrostatic glomerular pressure and hence maintains GFR (image). (**A**) Histamine synthesis induces vasodilation, in the kidney most likely via stimulation of renin and nitric oxide release. Like many other renal vasoactive substances, its role is not well understood; however, a decrease would not contribute to maintaining GFR. (**B, C**) Renal prostaglandin E_2 and I_2 are vasodilators, and an increase (not a decrease) may have been involved in renal blood flow autoregulation. (**E**) Renal endothelin is an extremely powerful vasoconstrictor. It is released in an extreme prerenal condition, which is not the case in the patient with a systolic blood pressure of 100, in order to decrease renal blood flow further and maintain coronary and cerebral perfusion.

13. Correct: ↓, ↓, ↑, ↑, ↑ (E)

The patient presents with signs of sympathetic nervous system (SNS) stimulation (increased pulse and respiratory rate, pale skin, and cold extremities), most likely due to a gastrointestinal bleed (epigastric pain, vomiting blood, feeling faint, low blood pressure, dry mucous membranes). The SNS has been activated by the low mean arterial blood pressure of 72 and acts on α_1 receptors of renal arteriolar smooth muscles. As a result, resistance increases in afferent and somewhat less in efferent arterioles. Afferent arteriolar constriction leads to decreased glomerular capillary hydrostatic pressure (P_{GC}), hence decreased glomerular filtration rate (GFR). This decrease is somewhat offset by an increase in P_{GC} as a result of efferent arteriolar constriction. On the other hand, simultaneous constriction of both arterioles results in a profound decrease in renal plasma flow (RPF). A small decrease in GFR and a large decrease in RPF increases filtration fraction (FF). Increased FF leads to high colloid osmotic pressure in peritubular capillaries, which favors reabsorption of fluid and Na^+. Additionally, the SNS acts on β_1 receptors of renal juxtaglomerular cells that release renin. The renin–angiotensin–aldosterone-system further supports Na^+ reabsorption. Last, SNS activation leads to renal prostaglandin PGE_2 and PGI_2 synthesis and local vasodilation in order to offset the otherwise excessive sympathetic renal vasoconstriction. In summary, sympathetic stimulation redirects blood flow to more vital organs such as heart and brain, while maintaining renal perfusion as best as possible and reducing urinary Na^+ excretion. (**A, B, C, D, F**) All other choices have one or more changes in the wrong direction.

14. Correct: 2, 1 (C)

The tubuloglomerular feedback mechanism is an intrinsic negative feedback response between the distal tubule and the glomerulus, which has evolved to protect against fluctuations in solute excretion by maintaining renal blood flow and glomerular filtration rate (GFR) within a narrow range. In the case of increased renal arterial pressure, GFR is increased and an increased tubular sodium load is sensed by macula densa cells at the beginning of the distal convoluted tubule (2: sensor site). It triggers vasoconstriction of the renal afferent arteriole (1: response site) to decrease GFR. (**A, B, D, E**) These are incorrect, since the feedback loop exists between the sensing distal nephron and the responding afferent arteriole. (**F**) The glomerular response mechanism is complex and indeed involves to a minor extent efferent vasodilation (site 4) and capillary modulation (site 3), but the change in renal artery pressure is sensed by macula densa cells as increased sodium chloride load (not by afferent arterioles).

15. Correct: Constriction of afferent and dilation of efferent arterioles (A)

The man's increase in blood pressure when running indicates an increase in cardiac output. Increased systemic blood flow increases his renal arterial blood flow (RBF) and consequently glomerular filtration rate (GRF). However, when a mean arterial blood pressure (MAP) between 80 and 180 mm Hg is present (the man's running MAP is 113 mm Hg), renal autoregulatory mechanisms are active to overwrite the systemic influence and locally maintain RBF, GFR, and solute excretion relatively constant. One mechanism of such renal autoregulation is tubuloglomerular feedback. When GFR temporarily increases, more NaCl is transported into macula densa cells via Na–K–2Cl cotransporters, which causes more water absorption. This causes the macula densa cells to swell, which causes a stretch-activated nonselective anion channel to open, and ATP escapes, and is converted to adenosine. Adenosine constricts the afferent arteriole via A_1 receptors and dilates (to a lesser degree) efferent arterioles via A_2 receptors. (**B, C, D, E**) These are incorrect because they do not accurately describe the effect of increased GFR on the diameter of the renal afferent and efferent arterioles.

16. Correct: Autoregulation of renal arteriolar diameter (A)

Regulation of renal blood flow (RBF) is important for maintaining glomerular filtration rate (GFR) despite changes in mean arterial blood pressure between 80 and 180 mm Hg. Autoregulation utilizes both the myogenic reflex and tubuloglomerular feedback mechanisms, both affecting renal arteriolar diameter. (**B**) Aldosterone would be released from the adrenal cortex in response to hypotension, not hypertension. (**C, E**) The release of epinephrine by the sympathetic nervous system potently vasoconstricts the renal vasculature and overrides the autoregulatory system. Override of renal autoregulation happens at more marked decreases in blood pressure than present in the patient. (**D**) Reactive hyperemia is the temporary increase in blood flow that would follow the brief occlusion of renal arterioles, which has not occurred in this patient.

17. Correct: B only (B)

Label B is the basement membrane, which contains anionic proteoglycan clusters that deter large, negatively charged proteins such as albumin. (**A**) Label A is the capillary endothelium layer, which primarily prevents the filtration of blood cells. (**C**) Label C points to podocytes, which form slits covered by slit diaphragms that further prevent the filtration of medium-sized proteins such as albumin. However, since most albumin has already been screened by the basement membrane, the podocytes are not the primary barrier, nor do they contribute equally to the glomerular barrier for protein filtration. (**D–F**) Each of these choices contain answer A and/or C, which makes them incorrect.

18. Correct: Basement membrane and podocytes (B)

The basement membrane and podocyte layers both have negative charges; thus they deter negatively charged (anionic) substances and attract positively charged (cationic) substances. Therefore, cationic dextrans have a greater relative filtration rate across the glomerulus than neutral dextrans do. (**A, C, D, E, F**) Each of these answer choices is incorrect because they do not include both correct answers.

19. Correct: Inflammation of the podocytes (C)

Glomerulonephritis may develop a week or two after recovery from a strep throat infection. To fight the infection, the body produces extra antibodies, which may eventually settle in the glomeruli, causing inflammation and increased permeability of the podocytes. This allows protein filtration and causes foamy urine. The cola-colored urine stems from the presence of hematuria. (**A, B**) There may also be inflammation in other layers of the glomerulus, but the inflammation of the podocytes allows the excess protein filtration that causes foaminess. (**D, E, F**) Sclerosis of the glomerular layers occurs more commonly as a consequence of chronic renal diseases such as lupus erythematosus or diabetes mellitus, not in acute cases like poststreptococcal glomerulonephritis.

20. Correct: The volume of plasma being cleared of creatinine per minute (E)

Renal clearance is the kidneys' ability to clear a given substance (in this case creatinine) completely from a given volume of plasma per unit time (in this case per minute) as it passes through the renal vasculature. Creatinine clearance is used clinically to estimate glomerular filtration rate. (**A, B, C**) The amount of creatinine (the product of creatinine concentration and flow rate) being filtered, secreted, or reabsorbed does not define renal clearance. (**D**) Renal clearance is the volume of plasma cleared of a substance per unit time, not the volume of urine cleared of the substance.

21. Correct: Glucose clearance of 10 ml/min (B)

Glucose is normally completely reabsorbed in the renal proximal tubule, so any clearance of glucose would be considered abnormal. Without memorizing values, one should understand whether and to which extend the listed substances are normally expected in urine due to the function of the kidneys. (**A, C**) Creatinine clearance can be used as a rough estimate of glomerular filtration rate (GFR), while inulin clearance is equivalent to the GFR. Average normal GFR between 2 and 12 years is 127 mL/min/1.73 m^2, with a range between 89 and 165. Hence, the boy's value is normal. (**D**) PAH clearance can be used as an estimate of renal plasma flow (RPF). Normal RPF is 600 mL/min, so the boy's PAH clearance would be considered normal. (**E**) Plasma creatinine levels can be used to calculate estimated GFR. Normal plasma creatinine concentrations in children are 0.0 to 0.7 mg/ dL, indicating that the boy's value is normal. High serum values due to lack of clearance indicate abnormal GFR.

22. Correct: ↔, ↑, ↑, ↑, ↓ (B)

Glomerular filtration rate (GFR), defined by inulin clearance, is unchanged: Day 1: 0.2 × 2/0.006; Day 2: 0.1 × 4/0.006. Urea excretion, or urea urine concentration times urine flow, is increased: Day 1: 250 × 2 = 500; Day 2: 150 × 4 = 600. Urea clearance, or urea excretion divided by urea plasma concentration, is increased: Day 1: 500/6.5; Day 2: 600/6.5. Glucose excretion, or glucose urine concentration times urine flow, is increased: Day 1: 1 × 2; Day 2: 1 × 4. Glucose clearance, or glucose excretion divided by glucose plasma concentration, is decreased: Day 1: 2/100 = 0.02; Day 2: 4/400 = 0.01. (**A, C, D, E**) All other choices have one or more incorrect changes.

23. Correct: Phosphate (D)

At constant glomerular filtration rate (GFR), constant urine flow, and no change in extracellular fluid volume, the clearance of a substance is increased when the substance's urine concentration is higher than its plasma concentration. This is the case when the plasma concentration exceeds the renal threshold for reabsorption, such as in the case of phosphate, which has a low threshold and appears in urine at a plasma level only slightly above normal. (**A, B, C**) Creatinine, inulin, and mannitol are freely filtered and not (or negligibly) reabsorbed or secreted, so their clearances will not change with increasing plasma concentration. (**E**) Urea is reabsorbed or secreted in the nephron by simple and facilitated diffusion, which means that the transport rate is determined (at a given permeability and constant flow rates), by the concentration difference between tubular fluid and blood, not by a saturatable transport process. Practically speaking, for a healthy, normally hydrated person, increased plasma urea concentration will lead to increased urea urine concentration but no change in clearance.

24. Correct: 50 (C)

To compare the patient's glomerular filtration rate (GFR) with a normal GFR of 100 mL/min, her creatinine clearance has to be calculated. For that, one has to first convert the units to mg, mL, and min. A urine creatinine concentration of 50 mg/dL converts to 0.5 mg/mL. A plasma creatinine concentration of 5 mg/ dL converts to 0.05 mg/mL. One liter of urine converts to 1000 mL. When collected in 200 minutes, it converts to a urine flow of 5 mL/min. Hence, creatinine clearance = (0.5 × 5)/0.05 = 50 mL/min. This is 50% of normal GFR, so that the antibiotic dosage should be 50% of normal. (**A, B, D, E**) These are incorrect dosages for a patient with a half-normal GFR.

25. Correct: ↓, ↑, ↑ (B)

Renal artery stenosis reduces renal blood flow (RBF) and glomerular filtration rate (GFR). When GFR is reduced, less plasma creatinine is filtered and excreted in the urine, so creatinine clearance decreases. This test is useful with a decline of GFR up to 50% of normal. Since the body's creatinine production is typically constant, when GFR decreases, plasma creatinine concentration increases after some time to a new steady-state concentration (column 2). Moreover, when RBF is reduced, less urea will be filtered and excreted, so the plasma concentration of urea (BUN) increases as well. While single test values per se are of limited use, the changes of the values in a particular individual throughout chronic disease (adjusting for potential weight or diet changes) are clinically useful for monitoring GFR and hence renal function. (**A, C, D, E, F**) Each of these choices has an incorrect sequence of answer choices.

26. Correct: 80, GFR (C)

The clearance of substance X:

= (Urine concentration)(Urine flow)/(Plasma concentration)
= (8 mg/mL)(120 mL/2 hr)(hr/60 min)/(0.1 mg/mL)
= (8 mg/mL)(1 mL/min)/(0.1 mg/mL)
= (8 mg/min)/(0.1 mg/mL)
= 80 mL/min

Since substance X is filtered but not secreted or reabsorbed, this quantity measures glomerular filtration rate (GFR). To measure renal plasma flow, a substance is needed that is filtered and secreted, so that it is completely excreted in urine during one passage through the kidney. (**A, B, D, E, F**) All other answers are incorrect.

27. Correct: 50 (C)

Steady state for creatinine:

Produced = Filtered = Excreted
Produced (↔) = Serum Concentration (↑) ´ GFR (↓) = Excreted (↔)

Double serum creatinine indicates half, or 50 percent, of the glomerular filtration rate (GFR), as shown in the image. In healthy people, creatinine is relatively constantly produced in the body as a metabolic byproduct of muscle creatine. The two men have a similar muscle mass (affected by race and body mass index) and a similar diet (creatine is present in meat and available as supplements), so that their creatinine production is similar. Since creatinine is eliminated from serum by glomerular filtration and since it appears in urine unchanged (a small addition to the tubular fluid is typically neglected), urinary creatinine clearance estimates the rate by which urinary blood ultrafiltrate is produced, or GFR. In the steady state, there is always a constant plasma concentration of creatinine because the production is equal to its urinary excretion (see image above). Since the older man produces and excretes the same amount of creatinine as the young man, and since his plasma concentration is double, the amount of filtered fluid per time has to be the reciprocal, or half. (**A, B, D, E**) All other percentages are incorrect because the filtered load of creatinine in both men are similar, so that a higher serum creatinine concentration can be the case only if GFR is lower by the same proportion.

28. Correct: Blocked urethra (B)

Hydronephrosis is the swelling of the kidney(s) from a buildup of urine due to a blockage or obstruction. This patient is in acute renal failure due to the obstructed urethra, which elevates Bowman space hydrostatic pressure. This reduces glomerular filtration rate (GFR) and results in elevated plasma creatinine. (**A**) A functional adrenal medulla tumor that releases epinephrine would lead to an elevated (not normal) blood pressure. (**C**) Hyperalbuminemia would reduce GFR by reducing glomerular filtration and therefore would not cause hydronephrosis. (**D**) Hypovolemia would lower blood pressure and GFR, so that the woman's normal blood pressure and hydronephrosis make this choice unlikely. (**E**) Renal artery stenosis would lead to a reduced GFR and no hydronephrosis.

29. Correct: Para-aminohippurate (D)

The ratio of urine to plasma concentration for para-aminohippurate (PAH) is about 585, compared to a ratio of 1 for a substance with the same plasma and urine concentration. The reason for the extensive increase in concentration is the fact that PAH is both filtered and secreted. In fact, it is so rapidly secreted by the proximal tubule that the PAH plasma concentration is nearly completely removed while flowing through the kidney and excreted in urine, which makes it a clinical estimate for renal plasma flow. (**A, C**) The urine-to-plasma ratio for creatinine and inulin are indeed high, since both become concentrated when 99% of water is reabsorbed while they remain in the tubular fluid, and in the case of creatinine a small amount is even secreted. However, the ratio is about 125 for inulin and 140 for creatinine, which is lower compared to PAH. (**B**) Glucose is completely reabsorbed in the proximal tubule, so its urine-to-plasma ratio is close to zero. (**E**) Urea also becomes concentrated in urine in order to function as a waste product for nitrogen. However, a significant amount of urea is reabsorbed to contribute to the corticopapillary osmotic gradient, so the urine-to-plasma ratio is lower than that of PAH.

30. Correct: The tubules reabsorbed 150 mg/min of it. (C)

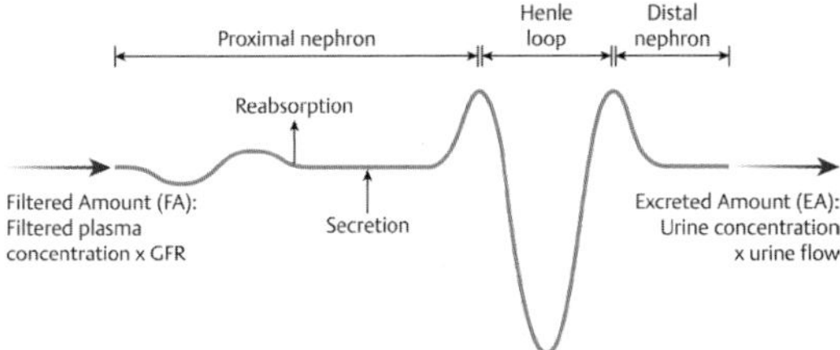

The filtered amount (image, FA) of drug X can be calculated as plasma concentration times glomerular filtration rate, or 2 mg/mL × 100 mL/min = 200 mg/min. The excreted amount (image, EA) of drug X can be calculated as urine concentration times urine flow, or 50 mg/mL × 1 mL/ min = 50 mg/min. Since the filtered amount exceeds the excreted amount, 200 – 50 = 150 mg/min of drug X have been reabsorbed. (**A, B, D, E**) These choices are incorrect.

31. Correct: Secreted 9 mg/min (F)

The amount of secreted or reabsorbed substance Y per unit time can be determined by comparing its filtered amount with the excreted amount (see image answer 30 above). The filtered amount of Y per time (FA) equals 50% of the plasma concentration of Y, multiplied by GFR, or 0.01 mg/mL × GFR. GFR can be determined as 100 mL/min, since it equals inulin clearance: urine concentration of inulin, multiplied by urine flow, divided by plasma concentration of inulin, or 50 mg/mL × 2 mL/min/1 mg/mL = 100 mL/min. This determines FA as 0.01 mg/mL × 100 mL/min = 1 mg/min. The excreted amount of Y per time (EA) equals urine concentration of Y, multiplied by urine flow, or 5 mg/mL × 2 mL/min = 10 mg/min. Since EA exceeds FA, 9 mg/min of substance Y were secreted. (**A, B, C**) A substance is reabsorbed when EA is less than FA. (D. E) Substance Y is indeed secreted, but by a different amount.

32. Correct: Higher plasma creatinine concentration (B)

Plasma creatinine concentration would be elevated in the patient with one kidney because if glomerular filtration rate (GFR) is reduced, then the total creatinine filtered per minute is reduced, leaving more in the plasma. (**A**) The patient with one functional kidney would have a lower GFR than the person with two functional kidneys. However, one kidney functionally adapts to the renal plasma flow and increases renal filtration in every single nephron, so that GFR is significantly larger than 50% of that for the person with two kidneys. (**C, D**) Plasma sodium concentration would be normal with one functional kidney; therefore, neither hypotension nor edema would be expected. (**E**) Sodium clearance would be decreased because GFR is reduced.

33. Correct: 200 mg/dL (A)

The renal threshold for glucose is the plasma concentration of glucose above which glucose appears in the urine. At 200 mg/dL and above (image), tubular glucose reabsorption can no longer keep up with filtered glucose loads, so filtered glucose appears in the urine. (**B, D, F**) The units of mg/min indicate a flow rate (i.e., passage per unit time), not a concentration. (**C**) At the plasma concentration of 400 mg/dL, all glucose carriers are saturated, which means that transport maximum, or T_m, has been reached. (**E**) At plasma concentrations above 800 mg/dL, all glucose is still filtered, but more of it is lost in urine than reabsorbed.

34. Correct: Nephron diversity, increased (F)

"Splay" refers to the difference between the renal threshold and saturation of transporters (T_m) for a specific substance. Splay occurs primarily due to heterogeneity of nephrons, which produces variability in the T_m of nephrons. This means some nephrons are saturated before others and begin excreting glucose before other nephrons hit their T_m. For this reason, an increase in nephron diversity will likely increase the observed splay. (**A, B**) Changes in plasma glucose concentration will affect the amount of filtered glucose, but if the nephrons are the same, then this will only impact how much glucose is reabsorbed and/or excreted, not the splay. (**C, D**) Changing the glucose transport will raise or lower the transport maximum but not the splay, which is created by the variation in transport maxima among nephrons. (**E**) Decreased nephron diversity will reduce the variation in nephron transport maxima and reduce the splay.

35. Correct: Urine flow rate (E)

Urine flow rate can be calculated be adding the free water clearance and the osmolar clearance. This is best conceptualized by understanding that the produced urine can be artificially separated into an amount of solute-free water and an amount of osmotically active particles, in order to describe the kidney's ability to produce concentrated or diluted urine. Since the cardiovascular and renal systems are flow systems, it is best expressed by comparing plasma and urine concentrations over time, or clearances. Understanding a patient's kidney function in regards to water and solute reabsorption is critical for the correct diagnosis of diseases with abnormal plasma tonicity. (**A, B, D**) Clearance of a substance is calculated by urine concentration times urine flow, divided by plasma concentration. (**C**) Renal plasma flow rate is the renal blood flow minus the hematocrit.

36. Correct: 96 (D)

Glomerular filtration rate is estimated best by calculating the clearance of inulin. The following equation is used to calculate inulin clearance (C_{inulin}):

$$
\begin{aligned}
C_{inulin} &= (U_{inulin})(\dot{V})/(P_{inulin}) \\
&= (24\ mg/mL)(10\ mL/min)/(2.5\ mg/mL) \\
&= 96\ mL/min
\end{aligned}
$$

A GFR above 90 mL/min/1.73 m^2 indicates normal kidney function. (**A, B, C, E**) All other answers are incorrect.

37. Correct: -1.1 (B)

Free water clearance (CH_2O) is the difference between urine flow (V̇) and the osmolar clearance ($U_{osmolarity} \times \dot{V}/P_{osmolarity}$):

$CH_2O = \dot{V} - (U_{osmolarity} \times \dot{V}/P_{osmolarity})$
$CH_2O = 10$ mL/min – (350 mOsm/L × 10 mL/min/315 mOsm/L)

One can see that a slightly larger number is subtracted from 10, so that CH_2O is slightly negative (exactly –1.1 mL/min)
(**A, C, D, E**) All other answers are incorrect.

38. Correct: It is hyperosmotic. (C)

The urine is hyperosmotic relative to the plasma. Free water clearance values less than zero imply that the kidney is conserving water, as would be the case in a dehydrated person who unexpectedly hiked for three days in the woods. (**A, B**) The patient is dehydrated, which will not increase the amount of proteins or glucose in the urine. (**D**) Free water clearance measures the excretion of solute-free water, relative to normal, so it can be used as an indicator of how the body is regulating water. Values greater than zero imply that the kidney is producing dilute (hypoosmotic) urine relative to the plasma, through the excretion of solute-free water. (**E**) A free water clearance of zero means the kidney is producing isoosmotic urine relative to plasma.

7.3 Questions

39. The physician is asked whether it is true that drinking too much soda causes hyperphosphatemia. She quickly recalls a few facts about renal tubular phosphate handling. Which of the following is true?

A. All of the filtered phosphate is reabsorbed.
B. More phosphate is excreted than is filtered.
C. More phosphate is reabsorbed than is filtered.
D. Phosphate that is not reabsorbed can buffer H^+ ions.
E. The renal threshold of phosphate is rarely exceeded.

40. A 53-year-old woman presents with cloudy urine. Her past history includes the induction of hypogonadism to treat an estrogen-dependent disorder. To minimize bone loss, she received intermittent doses of a hormone analogue. At which of the following nephron segments did the drug act to cause the abnormal urine?

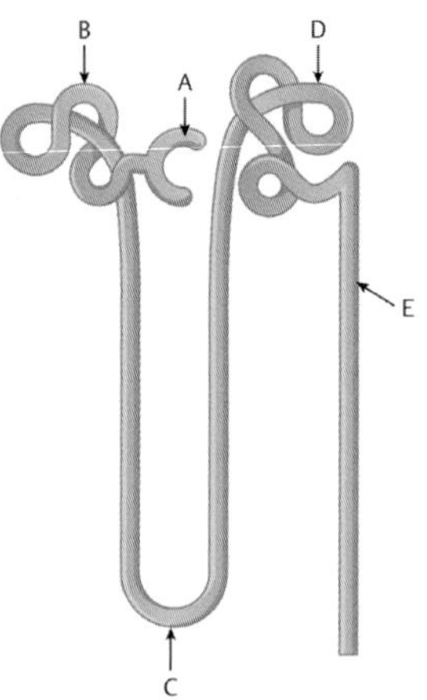

A. A
B. B
C. C
D. D
E. E

41. A patient with advanced type 2 diabetes mellitus and stage 2 chronic kidney disease is referred to the dietitian to discuss protein supplementation. In which of the following form does the kidney handle the reabsorption of amino acids, peptides, and small proteins?

	Amino acids	Peptides	Small proteins
A.	Na^+ cotransport	H^+ cotransport	Endocytosis
B.	Na^+ cotransport	H^+ cotransport	Not reabsorbed
C.	Na^+ cotransport	Endocytosis	Na^+ cotransport
D.	H^+ cotransport	Na^+ cotransport	Endocytosis
E.	H^+ cotransport	Na^+ cotransport	Not reabsorbed
F.	H^+ cotransport	Endocytosis	Na^+ cotransport

42. A 45-year-old man recently moved to a different state. At his first routine doctor's visit, he mentions that about 10 years ago he had been diagnosed with glucosuria, but he is not affected by it. He eats a normal diet and denies diarrhea or being abnormally thirsty. His current lab values show that his urine is indeed positive for glucose, but otherwise unremarkable. His fasting glucose level is 80 mg/dL; his hemoglobin A1C is 4.5%; and the result of his 2-hour oral glucose tolerance test is 130 mg/dL. The patient's presentation is typical for a loss-of-function gene mutation that encodes for which of the following cellular transporters?

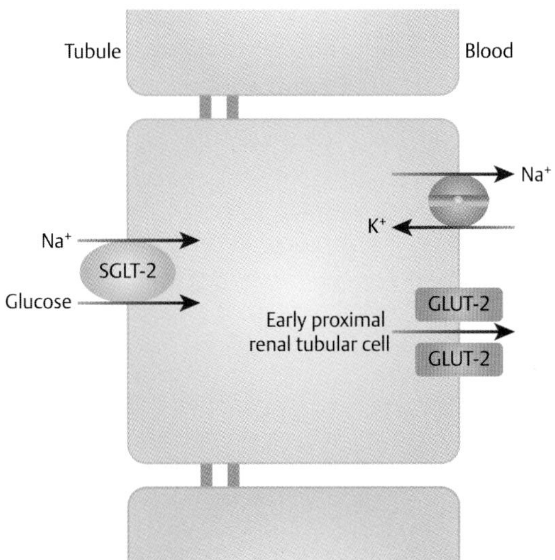

A. GLUT-3
B. GLUT-4
C. Na-K-ATPase
D. SGLT-1
E. SGLT-2

43. Due to a temporary problem with accessing the hospital patient records, the only available information for a patient is elevated urine phosphate. Based solely on this information, which of the following could have caused the phosphaturia?

A. Chronic renal failure
B. Fruit and vegetable diet
C. Mutation of Na^+-P_i cotransport
D. Pseudohypoparathyroidism
E. Surgical hypoparathyroidism

44. Fanconi's syndrome is a renal disease, either hereditary or acquired, that results from the impaired ability of renal proximal tubular transport. Based on this information, which of the following substances has the smallest increase in fractional urinary excretion in Fanconi's patients compared to normal?

A. Amino acids
B. Bicarbonate
C. Glucose
D. Magnesium
E. Phosphate
F. Small proteins

45. In animal experiments, the activity of renal organic anion transporters is investigated. Which of the following substances is used in the negative control experiment?

A. ACE inhibitor
B. Inulin
C. Loop diuretic
D. Para-aminohippurate
E. Penicillin
F. Salicylate

46. An adolescent female is delivered to the emergency department after a drug overdose suicide attempt. The patient history points toward aspirin ingestion more than 24 hours ago. This is supported by her clinical presentation, including dehydration and metabolic acidosis. Intravenous administration of which of the following pharmacologic agents would be indicated?

A. Ammonium chloride
B. Antidiuretic hormone
C. Loop diuretic
D. Sodium bicarbonate
E. Thiazide diuretic

Questions 47 to 48

The image below shows the tubular fluid/plasma (TF/P) ratio for several different substances that are freely filtered (labeled 1–8) along the length of the proximal tubule.

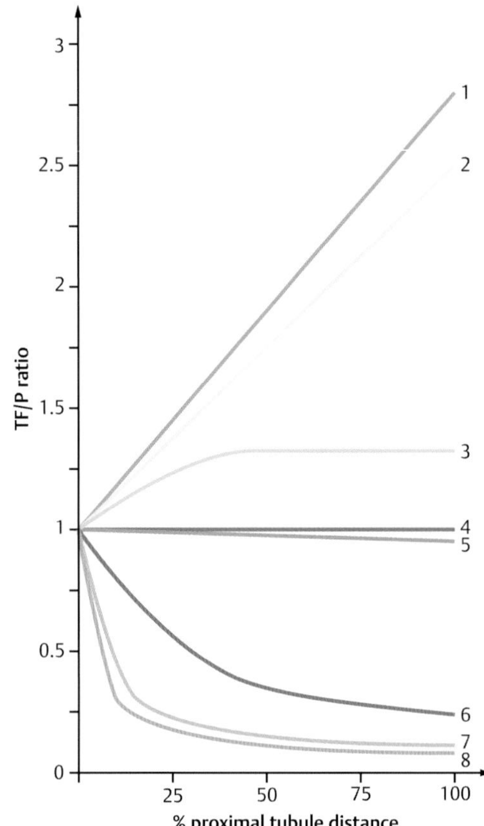

47. Which of the following best describes the proximal tubule reabsorption of the substance represented by line 3?

A. Not reabsorbed at all in the proximal tubule
B. Reabsorbed at a rate that is equal to water reabsorption
C. Reabsorbed at a rate that is faster than water reabsorption
D. Reabsorbed at a rate that is slower than water reabsorption
E. Reabsorbed completely in the proximal tubule

48. The clearance of which substance can be used to determine glomerular filtration rate?

A. 1
B. 2
C. 3
D. 4
E. 5
F. 6
G. 7
H. 8

49. As part of the efficacy test for a new diuretic drug, the following clearance measurements were made in a healthy human subject. What fraction (in percent) of filtered water did her renal tubules reabsorb?

Plasma inulin concentration 1 mg/mL
Urine inulin concentration 10 mg/mL
Urine flow rate 1 mL/min

A. 9
B. 10
C. 90
D. 99
E. 100

50. A patient experiences unexplained low blood clotting, and a problem in renal magnesium reabsorption is eventually considered. Under normal conditions, which segment of the renal tubule labeled on the image below (A–G) reabsorbs the largest percentage of the total filtered load of magnesium?

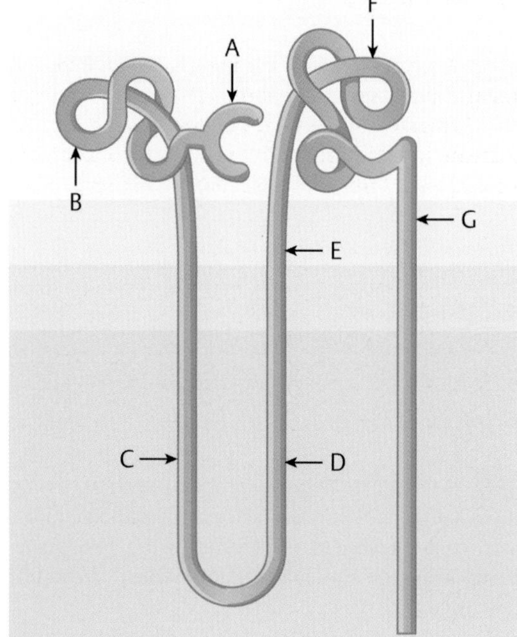

A. A
B. B
C. C
D. D
E. E
F. F
G. G

51. Decreased potassium secretion by the thick ascending limb of the loop of Henle will decrease which of the following tubular parameters at this site?

A. Ca^{2+} concentration
B. Fluid osmolality
C. H_2O reabsorption
D. Mg^{2+} concentration
E. Na^+ concentration

52. A side effect of an experimental cancer drug is the destruction of potassium channels on the apical membrane of the thick ascending limb of the loop of Henle. Which of the following electrolytes is the most likely one to become low in the serum of an otherwise healthy patient taking the drug?

A. Bicarbonate
B. Chloride
C. Magnesium
D. Phosphate
E. Potassium

53. A drug inhibits a common apical membrane renal tubular cell transporter at the nephron site that is marked in the image below by a red box. An increase in which of the following is the most likely consequence after administration of this drug?

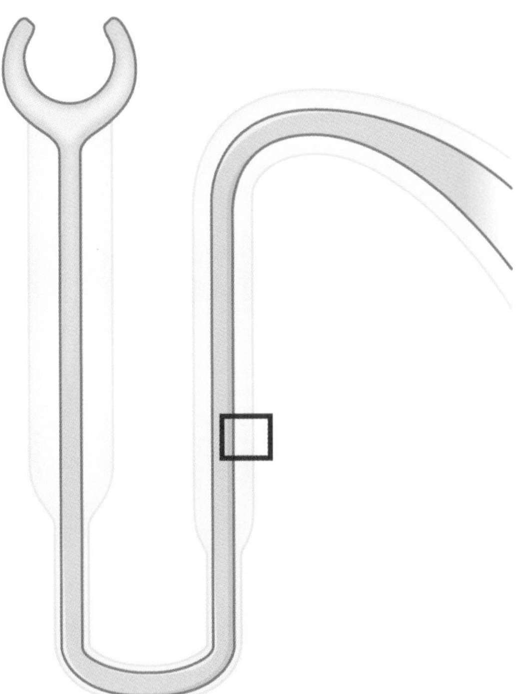

A. Glomerular capillary hydrostatic pressure
B. Glomerular filtration rate
C. Renal arterial hydrostatic pressure
D. Renal plasma flow
E. Urine potassium excretion

54. A 47-year-old woman with chronic hypertension is prescribed a diuretic drug that acts in the segment of the nephron labeled X on the image below. Which of the following drug category is part of the woman's treatment plan?

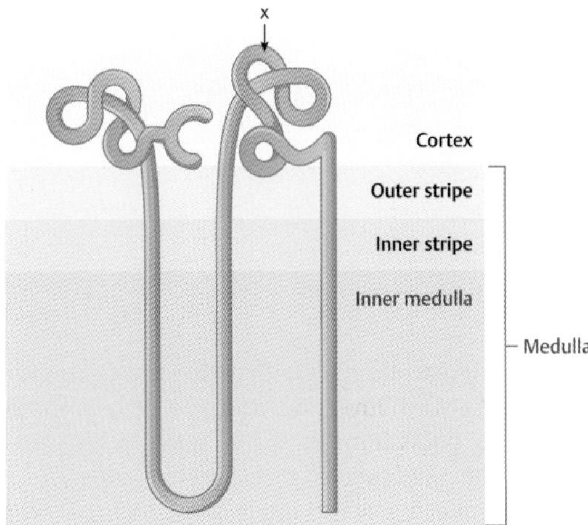

A. Antimineralocorticoid
B. Carbonic anhydrase inhibitor
C. Loop diuretic
D. Potassium-sparing diuretic
E. Sodium-chloride symport inhibitor

55. A 23-year-old man is in the intensive care unit with stage 4–5 renal failure. He was diagnosed with type 2 diabetes mellitus at the age of 12 and has been noncompliant with treatment and lifestyle choices for the past 5 years. He has peripheral and abdominal edema, headaches, anuria, and muscle cramps. His plasma is acidemic, and his glomerular filtration rate is 15 mL/min. The patient is ineligible for a transplant because of his unwillingness to comply with treatment, so he is currently on dialysis. Which of the following pharmaceutical treatments would be most useful in this patient?

A. Aldosterone antagonists
B. Calcium channel blockers
C. Carbonic anhydrase inhibitors
D. Epithelial sodium channel inhibitors
E. Loop diuretics

56. A 58-year old woman consults her chiropractor due to downward-radiating flank pain that she describes with an intensity of 8/10 on a verbal analogue scale. Her past history includes several calcium stones, and conventional abdominal radiography confirms a right ureteric calculus. After dealing with her pain and existing stone, which of the following drugs is most appropriate for this patient to lower the likelihood of new stone formation?

A. Carbonic anhydrase inhibitor
B. Loop diuretic
C. Osmotic diuretic
D. Potassium-sparing diuretic
E. Thiazide diuretic

57. A 71-year-old man with congestive heart failure is prescribed amiloride, a drug that belongs to the class of potassium-sparing diuretics. Which segment of the renal tubule labeled on the image (A–E) is directly affected by this drug?

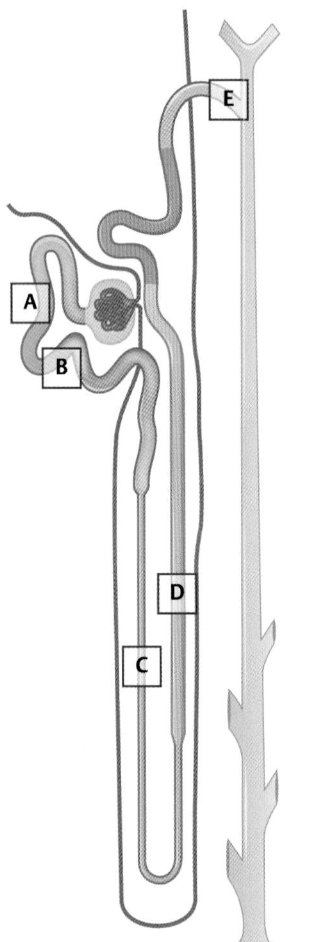

A. A
B. B
C. C
D. D
E. E

58. Colonic crypt cells were studied in order to see whether aldosterone and antidiuretic hormone (ADH) act in the gastrointestinal system the same way as they do in renal principal cells, where they act in which of the following ways?

	Action of aldosterone	Action of ADH
A.	Na+ reabsorption and K+ secretion	Water reabsorption
B.	Na+ reabsorption and K+ secretion	Water secretion
C.	K+ reabsorption and Na+ secretion	Water reabsorption
D.	K+ reabsorption and Na+ secretion	Water secretion
E.	Water reabsorption	Na+ reabsorption and K+ secretion
F.	Water reabsorption	K+ reabsorption and Na+ secretion

59. A 63-year-old patient reports that whenever he is outdoors on a very cold day, he has a strong urge to urinate and then produces a fairly large volume of urine that is light in color. This response is most likely mediated by the decrease of a hormone that normally acts at which of the following sites at the nephron?

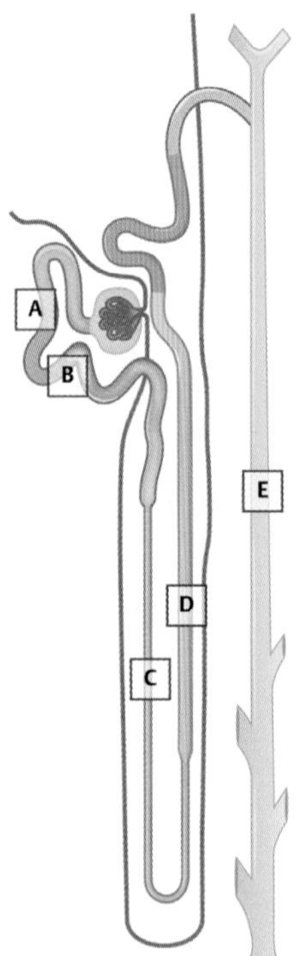

A. A
B. B
C. C
D. D
E. E

60. Five people are diagnosed with stage 3 chronic kidney disease that led to various symptoms. Which of the following persons is most likely to be the one with the lowest serum aldosterone level?

A. A nauseated person vomiting
B. A person with hyperkalemia
C. A person with congestive heart failure
D. A severely stressed person
E. A volume-overloaded person

61. The image below represents the renal tubular principal cell and shows membrane transport of Na^+ and K^+ (labeled A, B, and C), as well as binding of antidiuretic hormone (ADH) to its receptor (labeled D). After acting on the nuclear mineralocorticoid receptors, the effectors of aldosterone action in principal cells enhance which of the following?

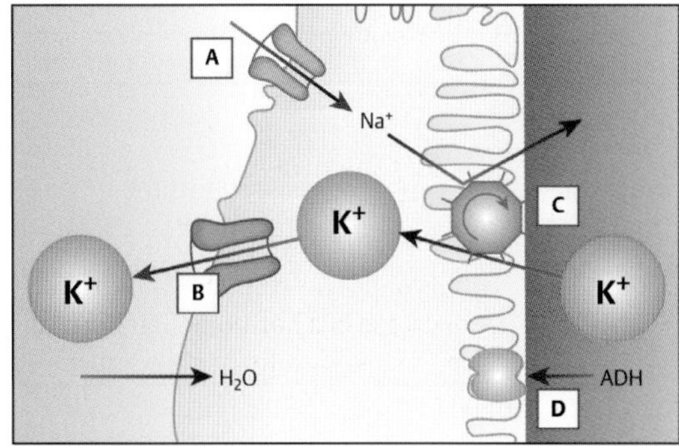

A. A only
B. B only
C. C only
D. D only
E. A and B only
F. A and D only
G. A, B, and C only
H. A, B, C, and D

62. A patient with congestive heart failure is managed over the first days with a loop diuretic in combination with a potassium-sparing diuretic. The rationale for giving the potassium-sparing diuretic is that the loop diuretic by itself produces hypokalemia. This hypokalemia is partly due to the serum increase of which of the following hormones?

A. Aldosterone
B. Atrial natriuretic peptide
C. Glucagon
D. Insulin
E. Parathyroid hormone

63. A 20-year-old marathon runner presents to the emergency department with muscle tenderness and weakness. Her urine is dark in color and positive for myoglobin, but no blood is present. Serum potassium, creatine kinase, and myoglobin are elevated. Which of the following indicates the normal body response of the adrenal glands and kidneys in this situation?

	Aldosterone	K^+ secretion by principal cells	Reabsorption of sodium
A.	↓	↓	↓
B.	↓	↓	↑
C.	↓	↑	↑
D.	↑	↑	↓
E.	↑	↑	↑

Questions 64 to 65

A 37-year-old female patient presents with fatigue and muscle weakness for several weeks, during which she gained about 7 pounds (about 3 kg) of weight. She is diagnosed with primary hyperaldosteronism resulting from an adrenal tumor.

64. Which of the following additional clinical findings would most likely be increased in this patient?

A. Angiotensin II
B. Blood pressure
C. Plasma $[K^+]$
D. Plasma $[Na^+]$
E. Plasma renin

65. Which of the following is expected in the patient in regards to her acid-base homeostasis?

A. Maintained homeostasis
B. Metabolic acidosis
C. Metabolic alkalosis
D. Respiratory acidosis
E. Respiratory alkalosis

66. A patient has a syncopal episode and is brought to the emergency department. The following clinical and laboratory data are collected over a 24-hour period:

Urine volume/24 hours	600 mL
Urine osmolarity	1,100 mOsm/L
Plasma osmolarity	280 mOsm/L
Plasma potassium	4.1 mmol/L

As a direct effect, a large increase in plasma of which of the following most likely produced these data?

A. Aldosterone
B. Angiotensin II
C. Antidiuretic hormone
D. Atrial natriuretic peptide
E. Renin

67. In which portion of the nephron (labeled **A–E** on the image) will the tubular fluid osmolality remain constant in the presence or absence of antidiuretic hormone?

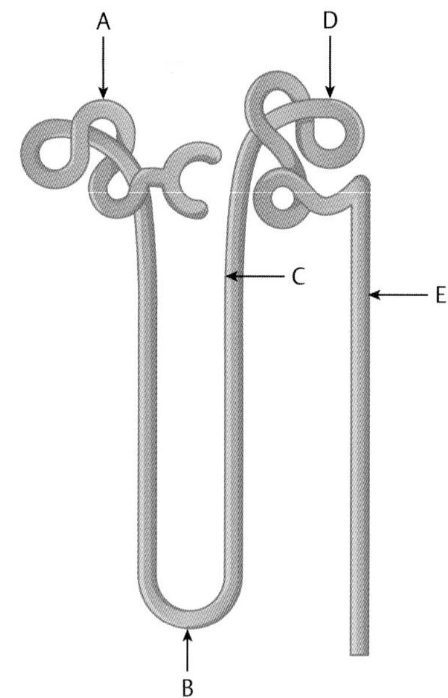

A. A
B. B
C. C
D. D
E. E

68. A 92-year old woman with a 15-year history of type 2 diabetes mellitus, atherosclerosis, and an enlarged heart sees her family physician with the complaint of severe fatigue and labored breathing. Evaluation shows generalized edema, hyponatremia, and increased antidiuretic hormone. A vasopressin receptor antagonist is administered. Which of the following best represents the expected physiological changes after administration of the drug as compared to her status beforehand?

	Urea permeability in outer medullary collecting ducts	Urea permeability in inner medullary collecting ducts	Water permeability in outer medullary collecting ducts	Water permeability in inner medullary collecting ducts	Free water clearance
A.	↓	↓	↓	↓	↓
B.	↔	↔	↓	↓	↓
C.	↔	↓	↓	↓	↓
D.	↔	↓	↓	↓	↑
E.	↑	↓	↔	↓	↑
F.	↑	↑	↔	↑	↑
G.	↑	↑	↑	↑	↑

69. As part of an experiment with healthy dogs, the experimental group is given diluted ethanol to drink, while the control group is given water only. After one week, *in vivo* micropunctures are used to measure the dogs' renal tubular fluid segment osmolalities. Assuming that a dog nephron is comparable to a human nephron, in the experimental group, what would be the trend in osmolality in the loop of Henle, the distal tubule, and urine compared to proximal tubule osmolality?

	Thin descending limb of the loop of Henle	Distal tubule	Urine
A.	Hypoosmotic	Hyperosmotic	Hyperosmotic
B.	Hyperosmotic	Hyperosmotic	Isoosmotic
C.	Hypoosmotic	Hypoosmotic	Isoosmotic
D.	Hyperosmotic	Isoosmotic	Hypoosmotic
E.	Hyperosmotic	Hypoosmotic	Hypoosmotic

70. A 43-year-old man with small-cell carcinoma of the lung is being evaluated for syndrome of inappropriate antidiuretic hormone (SIADH). Which of the following laboratory values for plasma sodium and plasma osmolality would be expected if the diagnosis is confirmed?

	Plasma Na^+ (mEq/L)	Plasma osmolality (mOsm/kg)
A.	160	310
B.	160	290
C.	160	250
D.	120	310
E.	120	290
F.	120	250

71. A 39-year-old man with a closed head injury resulting from a fall has a urine output of 5–7 L/day and the urine is hypoosmotic. Labs for plasma antidiuretic hormone (ADH) are ordered, and a water deprivation test is administered. The laboratory results reveal a low plasma ADH, and with no fluid intake for 6 hours, there is no change in the patient's urine output. What disease or condition do these test results indicate?

A. Central (neurogenic) diabetes insipidus
B. Nephrogenic diabetes insipidus
C. Osmotically induced diuresis
D. Primary (psychogenic) polydipsia
E. Syndrome of inappropriate antidiuretic hormone

72. Gitelman's syndrome has similar features to excess administration of a thiazide diuretic. Hence, it is best described by a mutation that inactivates which transporter or channel at which of the following places?

A. ENaC in the collecting duct
B. ENaC in the distal tubule
C. Na-Cl cotransporter in the early distal tubule
D. Na-Cl cotransporter in the late proximal tubule
E. Na-K-2Cl transporter in the loop of Henle

73. Patients with Liddle's syndrome respond to amiloride (a potassium-sparing diuretic) treatment but are insensitive to aldosterone receptor antagonists. Hence, which of the following is most likely an expected symptom of Liddle's syndrome?

A. Hyperaldosteronism
B. Hypokalemia
C. Hyponatremia
D. Hypotension
E. Metabolic acidosis

74. The primary defect of both Bartter's and Gitelman's syndrome is inhibition of renal sodium chloride reabsorption. The clinical manifestation is analogous to patients abusing a loop diuretic (mimicked by Bartter's syndrome) or a thiazide diuretic (mimicked by Gitelman's syndrome). Since the genetic tubular defects cannot be directly repaired, which of the following is part of adequate symptomatic treatment?

A. ACE inhibitor
B. Insulin and glucose
C. Low-magnesium diet
D. $NaHCO_3$ tablets
E. Synthetic cortisone

7.4 Answers and Explanations

39. Correct: Phosphate that is not reabsorbed can buffer H^+ ions. (D)

Phosphate excretion by the kidneys is controlled by an overflow mechanism. When the transport maximum for reabsorption of phosphate is exceeded, the remaining phosphate in the renal tubules is excreted in the urine and can buffer H^+ there. Hyperphosphatemia is rarely due to food. About 12 Coca-Cola 12-oz cans equal the dietary reference intake for phosphorus of 800 mg/d. (**A, C**) Since phosphorus is found in almost every food, generally more phosphate is filtered than reabsorbed, and not all of it is reabsorbed. (**B**) Most of the filtered phosphate is reabsorbed (about 85%), so no more is excreted than filtered. (**E**) The threshold for phosphate reabsorption is regularly exceeded under normal conditions.

40. Correct: B (B)

The woman received intermittent doses of parathyroid hormone (PTH) to avoid osteoporosis, which is likely to develop with low estrogen in a postmenopausal woman. PTH therapy to improve bone mass seems initially counterintuitive, since the physiologic result of increased PTH is bone resorption, but it can be understood by the true role of PTH to modulate the complex process of bone remodeling. In the kidneys, PTH acts in the proximal renal tubules at the sodium–phosphate cotransporter. The transporter is normally responsible for reabsorption of about 85% of filtered phosphate, and PTH regulates this transport by inhibiting it. This is to avoid $Ca_3(PO_4)_2$ precipitates in blood, since PTH increases renal calcium reabsorption. Hence, a PTH analogue drug can cause phosphaturia, which makes the patient's urine cloudy. Hypophosphatemia is typically asymptomatic if not extreme. (**A**) There are no transporters for solute reabsorption in Bowman's capsule. (**C, D, E**). Little or no phosphate reabsorption occurs beyond the proximal tubule.

41. Correct: Na^+ cotransport, H^+ cotransport, endocytosis (A)

Many oligopeptides are broken down in the proximal tubule by brush border peptidases to amino acids, which are primarily cotransported with sodium across the apical membrane. The peptides that are not broken down by peptidases can be cotransported across the apical membrane with hydrogen ions in the proximal tubule. Small proteins, such as myoglobin, can be reabsorbed across the apical membrane by receptor-mediated endocytosis. (**B, C, D, E, F**) These choices do not include the correct transport mechanisms for each substance.

42. Correct: SGLT-2 (E)

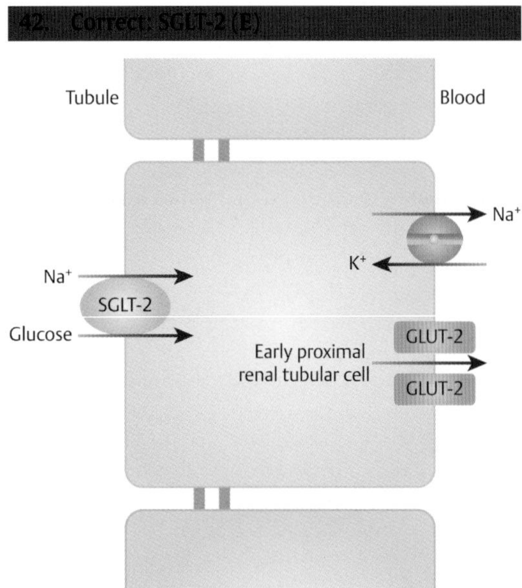

SGLT-2 is the high-capacity, low-affinity glucose transporter of the early proximal renal tubule (see image). When defective, it significantly impairs renal glucose reabsorption and leads to glucosuria. Patients with this rare disorder, called familial renal glucosuria, are not diabetic and are not symptomatic for hypoglycemia, due to ongoing gluconeogenesis. (**A**, **B**) GLUT-3 is the glucose transporter that is present in neurons and the placenta, while GLUT-4 is the insulin-sensitive transporter found in fat and muscle cells. GLUT-2 are the facilitated glucose transport channels at the basolateral membrane of renal proximal cells (see image). (**C**) A defect in Na-K-ATPase would lead to a wide variety of symptoms, since the pump-generated sodium gradient is necessary for reabsorption of many substances (not only glucose) in renal and gastrointestinal cells. (**D**) SGLT-1 mutations lead to glucosuria as well, since this low-capacity, high-affinity transporter is present in late proximal tubular cells. However, patients suffer from severe osmotic diarrhea and dehydration, because the transporter is also present in small-intestine cells, where it is responsible for absorption of glucose and galactose.

43. Correct: Mutation of Na^+-P_i cotransport (C)

The proximal tubule sodium-phosphate (Na^+-P_i) cotransporter is responsible for reabsorption of about 80% of filtered phosphate. A genetic defect leads to phosphaturia and contributes to calcium phosphate stone formation. (**A**) Chronic renal failure presents with hyperphosphatemia and hypophosphaturia due to a decreased filtered load of phosphorus. (**B**) Fruits and vegetables are low (not high) in phosphorus, a useful knowledge for patients with kidney problems. (**D**) Pseudohypoparathyroidism is a disorder, in which the Gs protein for parathyroid hormone (PTH) is defective. Since PTH normally inhibits phosphate reabsorption and favors phosphate excretion, defective PTH action leads to low (not high) urine phosphate. (**E**) Similarly, hypo-PTH caused by removal of the parathyroid gland results in low (not high) urine phosphate.

44. Correct: Magnesium (D)

The renal tubular reabsorption pattern for Mg^{2+} differs from other solutes in that about 30% of filtered load is reabsorbed in the proximal tubule, while about 65% is reabsorbed thereafter, with the majority in the thick ascending limb of the loop of Henle. Since Fanconi's syndrome affects proximal tubular transport, there is a relatively smaller increase of Mg^{2+} expected in urine compared to the other compounds. (**A, B, C, E, F**) In regards of filtered load, 100% of amino acids, 80% of HCO_3^-, 100% of glucose, 80% of inorganic phosphate, and 100% of small proteins are normally reabsorbed in the proximal tubule. Because other segments of the nephron cannot reabsorb these substances, the increase in their fractional excretion in Fanconi's patients is larger than for substances for which distal transporters are present.

45. Correct: Inulin (B)

Inulin is a good substance for the negative control experiment. It produces a negative result when studying the activity of renal organic anion transporters (OATs), since inulin is readily filtered but neither secreted nor reabsorbed in any appreciable amount along the nephron. This uncommon feature makes inulin clearance the ideal renal diagnostic for the glomerular filtration rate. (**A, C, D, E, F**). An ACE inhibitor (antihypertensive), a loop diuretic (e.g., furosemide), para-aminohippurate (diagnostic for renal plasma flow), penicillin (antimicrobial), and salicylate (NSAID) are all known substrates of OATs, which are present in the basolateral membrane of proximal tubular kidney cells. They play critical roles for the excretion of water-soluble, negatively charged molecules that are not freely filtered through the negatively charged glomerular filtration barrier.

46. Correct: Sodium bicarbonate (D)

Administration of sodium bicarbonate favors urinary excretion of the active ingredient of aspirin, salicylic acid, since at an alkaline pH it primarily exists in its base or charged form. In this form, it stays in the tubular fluid (charged molecules cannot diffuse through membranes) and can be eliminated from the body, supported by the increased urine flow rate. (**A**) Ammonium chloride will acidify the urine. At low pH, a weak acid such as salicylic acid primarily exists in its uncharged form, which diffuses back from the renal tubular fluid into blood. (**B**) Administering antidiuretic hormone will support both water and aspirin reabsorption into blood. (**C, E**) While a diuretic will increase urine flow rate and favor urinary excretion, it is not the treatment of choice. Loop diuretics and thiazide diuretics are counterproductive in an already dehydrated patient and will advance hypokalemia, which might exist as a result of the patient's metabolic acidosis.

47. Correct: Reabsorbed at a rate that is slower than water reabsorption (D)

Any lines that fall above a tubular fluid/plasma (TF/P) ratio of 1 represent a substance that is reabsorbed at a slower rate than water, which causes these substances to become concentrated in the proximal tubule. Thus, they are more concentrated in tubular fluid than in the plasma, and the TF/P ratio becomes greater than 1. Line 3 represents chloride, which fits this description. (**A, E**) Chloride (line 3) is reabsorbed in the proximal tubule, though not completely. (**B**) Substances that are reabsorbed at a rate equal to water will fall on the TF/P = 1 line, because they are present in the same concentration as in plasma. (**C**) Substances that are reabsorbed faster than water will fall below a TF/P ratio of 1, because they are less concentrated than in plasma.

48. Correct: 2 (B)

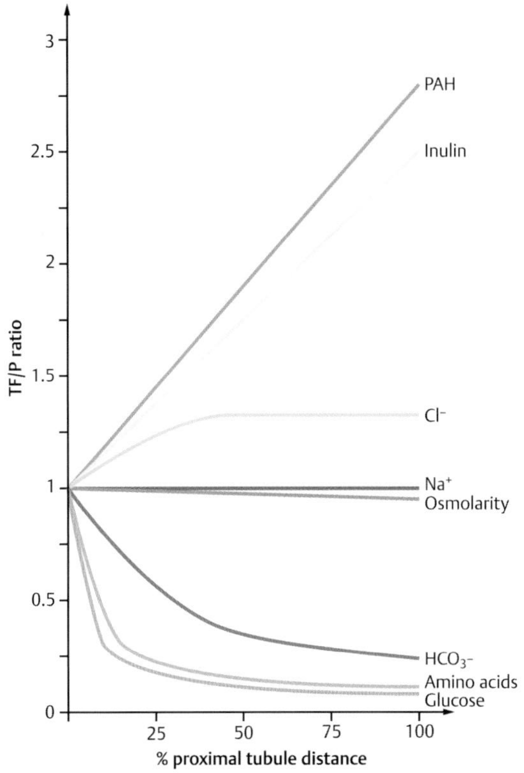

Inulin (image) is a freely filtered substance that is not secreted or reabsorbed. This line steeply increases along the length of the proximal tubule because water is being reabsorbed, but inulin is not. Therefore, inulin in tubular fluid (TF) is becoming more concentrated compared to plasma (P). By the end, TF concentration is about threefold, indicating that about 2/3 (67%) of the water has been reabsorbed. (**A**) Para-aminohippurate (PAH) is filtered (about 10–20%), secreted (about 80–90%), and not reabsorbed, so all PAH is excreted. This line steeply increases, because water is being reabsorbed, but PAH is not, therefore increasing its TF concentration. The slope of the line is even steeper than that of inulin because PAH is secreted, so the concentration of PAH is increasing more rapidly than inulin. (**C**) Chloride is freely filtered and in the early proximal tubule mainly reabsorbed in a paracellular manner, driven by the electrochemical Cl^- gradient. At the beginning, there is no gradient and reabsorption is slow, mainly driven by a lumen negative potential. The potential gradually becomes positive (opposing Cl^- reabsorption), but the TF_{Cl} concentration increases in comparison to P_{Cl} due to faster HCO_3^- than Cl^- reabsorption. The chemical gradient keeps Cl^- reabsorption going (curve levels off). In the late proximal tubule, transcellular pathways dominate. Overall, TF_{Cl}/P_{Cl} creates a characteristic curve. (**D, E**) The lines for Na^+ and fluid osmolarity are generally flat because Na^+ and water are being absorbed at approximately the same rate, thus their TF/P ratios do not change much. (**F, G, H**) The lines for bicarbonate, amino acids, and glucose all decrease below 1.0 because these substances are reabsorbed faster than water, thus reducing their relative concentrations along the length of the proximal tubule.

49. Correct: 90 (C)

Water reabsorption in the renal tubules can be calculated from the ratio between the inulin concentration of tubular fluid at the level of inner medullary collecting ducts (estimated by urine inulin concentration) and plasma inulin concentration, or $[TF/P]_{inulin}$. In the subject, this ratio is 10, indicating that inulin is tenfold concentrated and nine-tenths, or 90%, of the filtered water is not available in urine and has been reabsorbed. The following formula can also be used: $1 - 1/[TF/P]_{inulin}$, or $1 - 1/10 = 0.9$, or 90%. As long as the inulin concentration is in steady state, urine flow rate can be neglected. (**A, B, D, E**) These values are incorrect.

50. Correct: E (E)

Approximately 60–70% of the filtered load of Mg^{2+} is reabsorbed in the thick ascending loop of Henle. Serum Mg^{2+} competes with Ca^{2+} and has a complex interaction with coagulation proteins, so its net action on coagulation is still difficult to predict. For the patient, Mg^{2+} is considered, since the patient's blood clotting problem cannot be explained by more common causes. (**A, B**) Approximately 10–30% of the filtered load of Mg^{2+} is reabsorbed in the proximal tubule. (**C, D**) No Mg^{2+} is reabsorbed in the thin descending or ascending loop of Henle. (**F**) Virtually no Mg^{2+} is reabsorbed in the early distal tubule. (**G**) Approximately 5–10% of the filtered load of Mg^{2+} is reabsorbed in the late distal convoluted tubule/cortical collecting duct, and 5% is excreted in the urine.

51. Correct: H_2O reabsorption (C)

K^+ secretion drives several processes in the thick ascending loop of Henle (LOH), including the movement of water from the renal tubule to the interstitium. This will be reduced if K^+ secretion is reduced (continue reading for more details). (**A, D**) LOH K^+ secretion helps to create an electropositive filtrate, which drives the paracellular reabsorption of cations (Mg^{2+}, Ca^{2+}, Na^+, K^+). This increases the osmolality of the intracellular space, which promotes osmosis from the renal tubule to the interstitium. If K^+ secretion is reduced, then LOH reabsorption of Ca^{2+} and Mg^{2+} is reduced. (**B**) Since fewer cations are reabsorbed via the paracellular pathway, and less Na^+ and Cl^- is reabsorbed via the Na-K-2Cl cotransporter, the LOH fluid osmolality will be increased (not decreased). (**E**) K^+ is secreted into the renal tubule to promote the Na-K-2Cl cotransporter, which reabsorbs all three ions across the LOH apical membrane. If K^+ secretion is decreased, then Na^+ reabsorption will be decreased due to the reduced activity of the Na-K-2Cl cotransporter.

52. Correct: Magnesium (C)

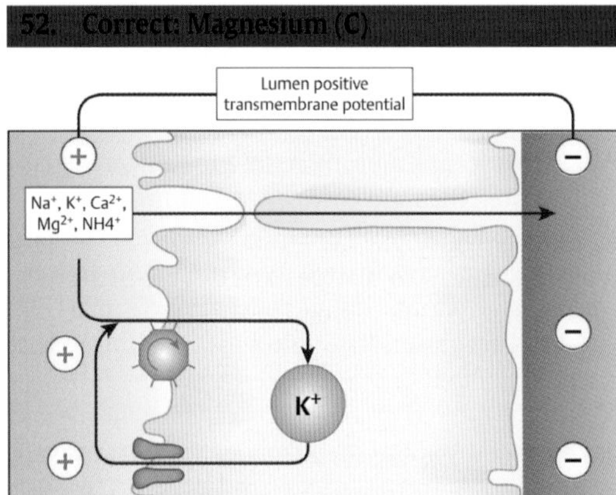

The K^+ channels on the apical membrane of the thick ascending limb of the loop of Henle allow recycling of some K^+ that has been absorbed by the Na-K-2Cl cotransporter (see image). Based on this recycling, a lumen-positive transmembrane potential develops, which drives movement of other positively charged ions out of the lumen into the cell. Since about 60% of filtered Mg^{2+} is reabsorbed by this process, loss of the transmembrane potential may lead to hypomagnesemia. (**A**) By far, the majority of HCO_3^- is reabsorbed in the proximal renal tubule, so that acidosis by loss of HCO_3^- is unlikely. (**B**) Renal Cl^- reabsorption generally follows Na^+ reabsorption. The presence of multiple downstream Na^+ transporters that can adjust for some variations upstream make NaCl imbalances not the best choice. (**D**) About 85% of filtered PO_4^{3-} is reabsorbed in the proximal tubule and the remainder is excreted, which makes phosphate imbalances unlikely. (**E**) Some K^+ reabsorption will be impaired by an impaired transmembrane potential; however, the distal tubule and the collecting ducts are responsible for the adjustments in K^+ excretion. They are well equipped to deal with large quantities of K^+, since this can frequently occur through food intake.

53. Correct: Urine potassium excretion (E)

The most common transporter at the apical membrane of renal tubular epithelial cells of the thick ascending limb of the loop of Henle (marked in the red box) are the Na-K-2Cl triporters. Hence, this question is asking about a drug like furosemide, which belongs to the class of loop diuretics that inhibit these transporters. Inhibition of the Na-K-2Cl triporters will decrease reabsorption of K+, as well as many other cations. This increases renal tubular flow to the extent that downstream K^+ equilibrium processes have not enough time to act, so that urine potassium excretion is increased. (**A, B, C, D**) A loop diuretic will decrease blood volume and thus decrease glomerular capillary hydrostatic pressure, glomerular filtration rate, renal arterial hydrostatic pressure, and renal plasma flow.

54. Correct: Sodium-chloride symport inhibitor (E)

A diuretic that acts in the distal convoluted tubule inhibits the sodium-chloride symporter and belongs to the class of thiazide diuretics. (**A**) A synthetic antimineralocorticoid (e.g., spironolactone) counteracts the normal actions of aldosterone in the distal tubule and collecting duct. It belongs to the class of potassium-sparing diuretics. (**B**) A diuretic that inhibits carbonic anhydrase (e.g., acetazolamide) acts in the proximal tubule. By inhibiting carbonic anhydrase, bicarbonate, sodium, and chloride are excreted, along with excess water. (**C**) A loop diuretic (e.g., furosemide) inhibits Na-K-2Cl- triporters in the thick ascending limb of the loop of Henle. (**D**) Potassium-sparing diuretics either compete with aldosterone (see **A**) or inhibit epithelial sodium channels (ENaC) in the late distal tubule and collecting duct (e.g., amiloride).

55. Correct: Loop diuretics (E)

Loop diuretics are the preferred drug to treat stage 4–5 renal failure because they allow for volume contraction (edema, headaches, anuria) while addressing the hyperkalemia (muscle cramps) and acidosis (plasma is acidemic), or at least not augmenting it. (**A, D**) Aldosterone antagonists and epithelial sodium channel inhibitors both are potassium-sparing diuretics. They are usually contraindicated, as they may aggravate the H^+ and K^+ retention. (**B**) Calcium channel blockers will not help with volume contraction, and they can stimulate aldosterone production, which is detrimental, as explained. (**C**) Carbonic anhydrase inhibitors will have little effect since they are typically mild diuretics. Moreover, since bicarbonate is already low, they can exacerbate the acidemia.

56. Correct: Thiazide diuretic (E)

Thiazide diuretics decrease urinary calcium excretion and hence the likelihood of stone formation by two mechanisms: First, volume depletion leads to a compensatory rise in proximal Na^+ and Ca^{2+} reabsorption. Second, the inhibition of the Na-Cl cotransporter leads to membrane hyperpolarization of the early distal tubular epithelial cell, and this negativity increases the driving force for Ca^{2+} reabsorption. Moreover, a tendency toward positive calcium balance might be beneficial, since a postmenopausal woman typically benefits from an increase in bone mineralization. (**A**) Inhibition of carbon anhydrase leads to no significant change of urinary Ca^{2+}, since the main renal role of the enzyme is for HCO_3^- and Na^+ reabsorption in the proximal tubule. The excess tubular fluid that results from the inhibition of this process is mainly reclaimed in the more distal tubular segments. (**B**) Loop diuretics increase Ca^{2+} excretion by inhibiting paracellular Ca^{2+} reabsorption in the thick ascending limb of the loop of Henle. There, reabsorption of up to 25% of filtered Ca^{2+} normally occurs when positive charges in the lumen drive cations such as Ca^{2+} toward the interstitial space. This lumen-positive electrochemical gradient has been created by the Na-K-2Cl transporter, so that its inhibition by loop diuretics leads to hypercalciuria. (**C**) Osmotic diuretics are nonreabsorbable substances that inhibit water and Na^+ reabsorption in the proximal tubule and the loop of Henle and concomitantly passive reabsorption of Ca^{2+}. (**D**) Potassium-sparing diuretics are the next best choice, since some have been shown to reduce urinary calcium excretion mildly, probably by a similar membrane-hyperpolarizing effect as described for choice E. However, the effect is much smaller and less understood than for thiazide diuretics, so these medications are not/rarely used clinically.

57. Correct: E (E)

Amiloride inhibits epithelial sodium channels (ENaC) in the late distal convoluted tubules, connecting tubules, and collecting ducts. This promotes the loss of sodium and water from the body without depleting potassium. (**A, B, C, D**) Amiloride works by directly blocking the ENaC, and these channels are not present in the proximal tubule or loop of Henle; therefore, amiloride has no direct effect on these sections of the tubule.

58. Correct: Na+ reabsorption and K+ secretion, water reabsorption (A)

In renal principal cells of the collecting duct, aldosterone increases the number of epithelial sodium channels (ENaC) on the apical plasma membrane, as well as the number and activity of Na-K-ATPases on the basolateral membrane. This stimulates Na^+ absorption across the apical membrane and Na^+ transport out of the cell in exchange for K^+. Most of the intracellular K^+ diffuses into the tubular lumen (secretion) based on its electrochemical gradient. Renal principal cells also are the pathway for water absorption, which is stimulated by antidiuretic hormone (ADH), which inserts aquaporin-2 channels in the luminal membrane. In colonic crypt cells, aldosterone has a similar physiological role; a physiological role of ADH is currently unlikely. (**B, C, D, E, F**) All other answers have an incorrect combination of actions.

59. Correct: E (E)

On a cold day, blood is redirected from the skin to the core of the body, so that the central (thoracic) blood volume increases. This stretches atrial cells and results in an increase of atrial natriuretic peptide and reflex inhibition of antidiuretic hormone (ADH) release. ADH normally acts at the principal cells of collecting ducts to increase water reabsorption. Without it, water diuresis ensues. Elderly men might be more susceptible to this effect, since the ADH effect may augment the urge for urination due to a benign enlargement of the prostate, a common occurrence with increasing age. (**A, B, C, D**) ADH does not act at the proximal tubule or loop of Henle.

60. Correct: A volume-overloaded person (E)

Due to the kidney's role in controlling blood pressure and electrolyte homeostasis, chronic kidney disease can lead to a wide variety of symptoms. A volume-overloaded person is expected to have low serum aldosterone, since aldosterone is released in response to low (not high) blood pressure and volume (via the renin-angiotensin-aldosterone system, RAAS). (**A**) Vomiting may lead to low extracellular fluid and low effective arterial blood volume, which stimulates the RAAS and hence aldosterone release. (**B**) Increased plasma K^+ concentration stimulates aldosterone release. (**C**) Congestive heart failure can lead to reduced effective circulating blood volume and hence secondary hyperaldosteronism. (**D**) Increased activity of the sympathetic nervous system due to severe stress will stimulate renin release and, via the RAAS aldosterone release.

61. Correct: A, B and C only (G)

The effectors of aldosterone action in principal cells are the luminal epithelial Na^+ channel (ENaC, labeled A), the luminal K^+ channel (labeled B) and the basolateral Na-K-ATPase (labeled C). Upregulation and/or enhanced activity of A, B, and C lead to reabsorption of Na^+ and H_2O and secretion of K^+. (**A, B, C, E**) These choices list correct but incomplete effector sites for aldosterone actions. (**D, F, H**) Aldosterone has no stimulatory effect on antidiuretic hormone binding to its receptor.

62. Correct: Aldosterone (A)

Congestive heart failure leads to generalized edema when blood backs up on the venous side of the circulation and increases capillary hydrostatic pressure so that fluid moves out of the capillaries into the interstitium. A decrease in the effective arterial blood volume (EABV) increases aldosterone release via the renin-angiotensin-aldosterone system. Aldosterone reabsorbs sodium in exchange for potassium, which leads to hypokalemia when excessive. A loop diuretic decreases intravascular volume and capillary pressure, allowing the edema fluid to move back from the interstitium to the blood vessels. However, the increased renal tubular flow rate leads to further potassium wasting. Hence, the rationale for a potassium-sparing diuretic, such as an aldosterone antagonist, is to blunt hyperaldosteronism and hypokalemia. (**B, C, E**) Atrial natriuretic peptide, glucagon, and parathyroid hormone are not released in response to decreased EABV, and elevated levels of these hormones do not produce hypokalemia. (**D**) While elevated serum insulin levels can produce hypokalemia, insulin is not released in response to decreased EABV.

63. Correct: ↑, ↑, ↑ (E)

The presence of myoglobin in serum and urine indicates excessive skeletal muscle tearing. Since skeletal muscle cells are the main storage site of K^+ in the body, a positive K^+ balance can be expected. High serum K^+ stimulates adrenal cortex cells to release aldosterone. Aldosterone increases the number and activity of Na-K-ATPases, which leads to increased K^+ concentrations inside renal tubular principal cells. Additionally, it increases the number of K^+ channels in the luminal membrane, thus effectively driving K^+ from the cell to the lumen. Last, aldosterone increases the number and activity of principal cell epithelial Na^+ channel, which increases Na^+ reabsorption. (**A, B, C, D**) These choices have one or more incorrect body responses to hyperkalemia.

64. Correct: Blood pressure (B)

In primary hyperaldosteronism, excess aldosterone initially induces more sodium and thus water reabsorption. After a few days (the patient's symptoms exist for weeks), a spontaneous diuresis, called aldosterone escape, occurs, which leads to a new homeostatic level between Na^+ intake and Na^+ excretion. The extracellular fluid volume becomes stable at a new, increased steady state (about 3 L of water retention). This makes hypertension the most common symptom of primary hyperaldosteronism, independent of the clinical subcategory. (A, E) Increased blood volume and hypertension decrease (not increase) renin release and subsequently angiotensin II. Suppressed renin is diagnostically important to distinguish primary from secondary hyperaldosteronism. (**C**) Aldosterone increases renal K^+ secretion in the late distal tubule and collecting duct, so plasma K^+ concentration will decrease (not increase). It could be normal due to the aldosterone escape effect just mentioned; however, the patient's muscle weakness indicates hypokalemia. (**D**) Aldosterone increases renal Na^+ reabsorption. However, after the aldosterone escape mechanism, a new steady state between Na^+ intake and excretion is reached, so that plasma Na^+ concentration is typically normal (and rarely increased).

65. Correct: Metabolic alkalosis (C)

Hyperaldosteronism causes increased urinary H^+ excretion due to a direct and indirect aldosterone effect. Aldosterone directly stimulates a luminal H^+ ATPase of α-intercalated cells. Aldosterone increases renal tubular potassium, and this indirectly stimulates luminal H^+-K^+ ATPases of α-intercalated cells, which reabsorb potassium in exchange for protons. Excess urinary H^+ loss decreases plasma H^+, and unmatched serum HCO_3^- causes metabolic alkalosis. (**A**) Muscle weakness in this patient points to hypokalemia. When muscle symptoms are present, the plasma $[K^+]$ is typically below 2.5 mEq/L, and such low levels are accompanied by metabolic alkalosis due to the transport processes of the distal renal tubule. (**B**) Renal H^+ wasting does not cause acidosis. (**D, E**) The kidney/adrenal gland as cause of the acid-base disturbance identifies it as metabolic (not respiratory).

66. Correct: Antidiuretic hormone (C)

The laboratory data indicate a small volume of concentrated urine (normal average 800–2000 mL/24 hours, with an osmolarity of 500–800 mOsm/L), and a low plasma osmolarity (normal > 285 mOsm/L). This could be directly produced by a large increase in antidiuretic hormone (ADH). ADH promotes water reabsorption in the distal nephron and leaves a smaller than normal volume of solute-free water for excretion. Syncope could be due to hyponatremia as a result of the inappropriate ADH release by the pituitary gland. (**A, B, E**) With a large increase of aldosterone (either directly or stimulated by renin or angiotensin II), hypokalemia is more likely than normokalemia. Low plasma osmolarity is not likely due to an aldosterone escape phenomenon. Overall, all three bioactive compounds would cause similar effects, and one could not distinguish the best answer. (**D**) Atrial natriuretic peptide is released in response to right atrial stretch due to high blood volume, which is not the case here.

67. Correct: A (A)

(**A**) Water and solute reabsorption in the proximal tubule is not impacted by antidiuretic hormone (ADH); it is simply bulk reabsorption, so fluid osmolality (in mOsm/kg) remains constant in the presence or absence of ADH. (**B, C, D**) Fluid osmolality in the loop of Henle and early distal tubule is indirectly impacted by ADH. ADH supports a large corticopapillary interstitial osmotic gradient, via the stimulatory effect of ADH on the Na-K-2Cl cotransporters and the ADH-mediated increase in reabsorption and secretion of urea. (**E**) The fluid osmolality of the collecting duct is directly impacted by the effects of ADH and its effect on water reabsorption.

68. Correct: ↔, ↓, ↓, ↓, ↓ (D)

Vasopressin, also called antidiuretic hormone (ADH), has three main effects in the kidneys: (1) It stimulates urea reabsorption exclusively in the inner medullary collecting duct in order to enhance urea recycling. Hence, administration of an antagonist does not impact urea permeability in outer medullary collecting ducts, but it decreases urea deposition in the inner medullary interstitial fluid. (2) ADH increases the water permeability of late distal tubules and all parts of collecting ducts. Hence, the drug leads to diminished back diffusion of solute-free water in these nephron segments and increased free water clearance. (3) ADH increases Na-K-2Cl cotransport in the ascending limb of the loop of Henle, and an inhibition of this effect results in a less hypertonic interstitium. The drug is indicated in this patient with advanced heart failure (enlarged heart, fatigue, edema), since the reduced effective arterial blood volume is erroneously recognized by hypovolemic hormones such as ADH (leading to hyponatremia). So, water diuresis (inhibition of V_2 receptors) and a decrease in afterload (inhibition of V_1 receptors) are helpful. (**A, B, C, E, F, G**). All other choices have one or more incorrect changes in response to vasopressin receptor antagonists.

69. Correct: Hyperosmotic, hypoosmotic, hypoosmotic (E)

Ethanol inhibits the pituitary secretion of antidiuretic hormone (ADH) by blocking voltage-gated calcium channels and thus vesicular exocytosis of the peptide hormone. Hence, the question asks about renal tubular osmotic fluid changes in the absence of ADH. Independent of ADH, the fluid in the thin descending limb of the loop of Henle is always hyperosmotic, since water is reabsorbed into the always hypertonic interstitial medullary fluid until equilibrium has been reached. Again, regardless of whether ADH is present or not, the beginning portion of the distal tubule is always hypoosmotic relative to the proximal tubule, because in the ascending limb of the loop of Henle solutes have been reabsorbed without water. From there on, the distal tubular fluid gradually becomes hyperosmotic in the presence of ADH on its way to make final urine. However, when ADH is inhibited, the filtrate remains hypoosmotic from distal tubule to urine. (**A, B, C, D**) The other choices have one or more incorrect statements.

70. Correct: 120, 250 (F)

In the presence of SIADH, the patient would exhibit hyponatremia and hypoosmolality. The key to understanding the pathophysiology of SIADH is the fact that the hyponatremia is the result of an excess of water rather than a deficiency of sodium. SIADH is defined by the hyponatremia and hypoosmolality resulting from inappropriate, continued secretion of ADH, despite normal or increased plasma volume, impairing normal urinary water excretion. (**A, B, C**) These choices are all incorrect because they exhibit hypernatremia (plasma sodium above 145mEq/L), not hyponatremia. (**D, E**) These choices are incorrect because they are not hypoosmotic (plasma osmolality below 275 mOsm/kg).

71. Correct: Central (neurogenic) diabetes insipidus (A)

Central diabetes insipidus (DI) in adults is usually due to damage to the pituitary gland or hypothalamus (patient had a head injury). This disrupts the normal production, storage, and /or release of antidiuretic hormone (ADH), leading to low plasma ADH, and thus large volumes of diluted urine (polyuria). (**B**) Nephrogenic DI occurs when there is a reduced response to ADH in the kidney tubules, but plasma ADH levels are not low. The defect may be due to an inherited disorder, chronic kidney disorder, or certain drugs, such as lithium or a tetracycline antibiotic. (**C**) Osmotically induced diuresis causes polyuria due to a high concentration of osmotically active substances in the renal tubules, which limit the reabsorption of water. With no fluid intake, an eventually low effective arterial blood volume would trigger ADH release. (**D**) Primary polydipsia causes excretion of large volumes of dilute urine due to excessive intake of fluids. The restriction of fluid would impact ADH secretion. (**E**) Syndrome of inappropriate antidiuretic hormone (SIADH) is due to continued secretion of ADH despite normal or increased plasma volume, which results in impaired water excretion. This results in elevated plasma ADH levels.

72. Correct: Na-Cl cotransporter in the early distal tubule (C)

The clinical manifestations of Gitelman's syndrome are analogous to those described in patients with chronic ingestion of a thiazide diuretic. Recent molecular studies indeed support that the majority of the patients have mutated, nonfunctioning Na-Cl cotransporters in the early distal tubule, the transporters that are specifically inhibited by thiazide diuretics. (**A, B, D, E**) The other renal tubular sodium transporters are not sensitive to thiazide diuretics and are not involved in Gitelman's syndrome.

73. Correct: Hypokalemia (B)

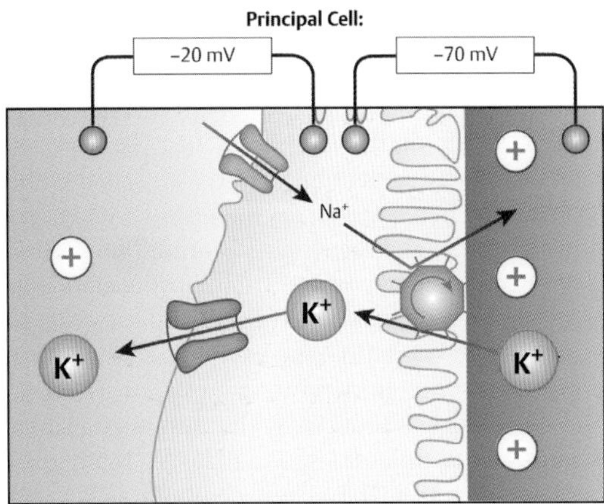

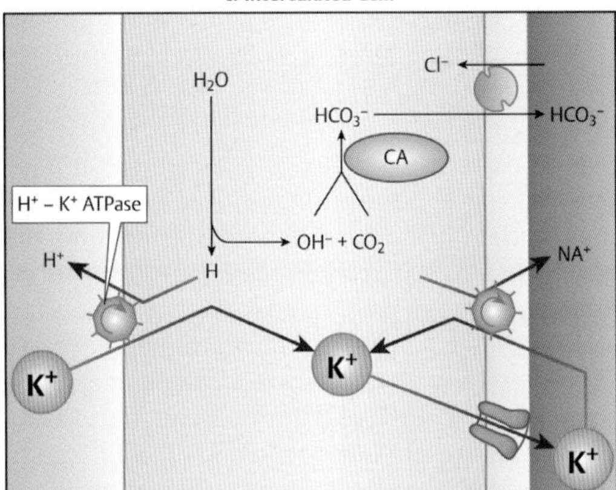

Liddle's patients have enhanced epithelial sodium channel (ENaC) activity, due to a dysregulated channel degradation. This leads to enhanced Na^+ reabsorption and enhanced K^+ secretion (resulting in hypokalemia) via two mechanisms: First, principal cells (image) reabsorb Na^+ through ENaC along its electrochemical gradient, which has been created by the basolateral Na-K-ATPase. The pump's activity raises intracellular K^+ concentration, which then favors K^+ secretion. Second, Na^+ reabsorption creates a transepithelial potential (lumen negative compared to the cells' basolateral side), which facilitates secretion of cations such as K^+. Amiloride directly blocks ENaC. Aldosterone receptor antagonists would avoid any further upregulation of ENaC but do not affect the chronically existing channels. (**A**) Although the symptoms of Liddle's syndrome are similar to hyperaldosteronism, serum aldosterone is low or normal, due to a low renin-angiotensin-aldosterone system in response to hypertension. (**C, D**) Enhanced ENaC activity increases tubular Na^+ reabsorption and leads to hypernatremia and hypertension (not hyponatremia and hypotension). (**E**) The lumen-negative transepithelial potential favors secretion of H^+, which can lead to unbuffered HCO_3^- in blood and metabolic alkalosis (not acidosis). Alkalosis is further supported by α-intercalated cells, which reabsorb luminal K^+ in exchange for H^+ secretion (image).

74. Correct: ACE inhibitor (A)

An angiotensin-converting enzyme (ACE) inhibitor is an adequate treatment to counteract the effects of secondary hyperaldosteronism. Aldosterone is inappropriately high since the inhibition of Na^+ reabsorption in the loop of Henle (Bartter's syndrome) or the early distal convoluted tubule (Gitelman's syndrome) overwhelms the Na^+ reabsorption capacity of the late distal convoluted tubule and collecting ducts and leads to salt wasting and volume depletion. The body's response is hyperactivity of the renin-angiotensin-aldosterone system, leading to hyperreninemia and hyperaldosteronism. (**B, D**) Administration of insulin and glucose (treatment for severe hyperkalemia) or $NaHCO_3$ tablets (treatment for severe metabolic acidosis) are counterproductive, because maximal Na^+ reabsorption in collecting ducts more likely leads to hypokalemia (due to K^+ secretion of principal cells) and metabolic alkalosis (due to H^+ secretion of α-intercalated cells). (**C**) A low-magnesium diet is not recommended since forms of both syndromes can lead to renal Mg^{2+} wasting and hypomagnesemia. (**E**) Although renal aldosterone receptors have a low affinity for natural cortisone (not to be confused with cortisol), a synthetic cortisone might still act as an aldosterone analogue, which is counterproductive for hyperaldosteronism.

7.5 Questions

75. A 32-year-old man suffers third-degree burns over 50% of his body following a car accident. At which point of his nephron (labeled A–E) will the tubular fluid be most concentrated?

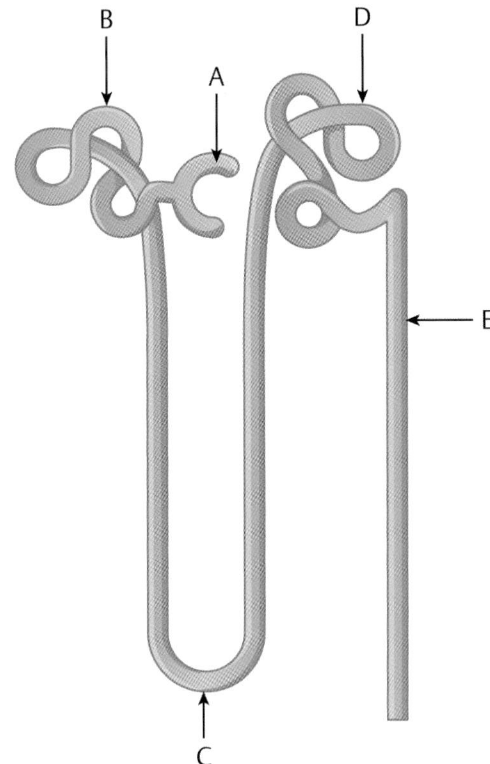

A. A
B. B
C. C
D. D
E. E

76. A 71-year-old man lives alone and reports that he gets up from bed several times a night to urinate. He was tested for his ability to concentrate urine maximally by a simple water deprivation test. It was found that his maximum urine osmolality was only 300 mOsm/kg at a time when his plasma antidiuretic hormone (ADH) levels were appropriately elevated. This indicated a problem with the renal interstitial osmotic gradient. Which of the following could account for his impaired ability to concentrate urine?

A. Diet high in steak and eggs
B. Eating a lot of potato chips
C. Elevated glomerular filtration rate
D. Increased UT-1 ubiquitination
E. Stimulated Na-K-2Cl transport

77. A 22-year-woman experiencing polydipsia and polyuria for the past 3 months sees her primary care physician. Her blood pressure and pulse are normal, but a brain scan reveals a lesion on the hypothalamus. A water deprivation test is ordered. The patient's plasma and urine osmolality are measured before the test, then again after a 4-hour water deprivation test. Following the water deprivation test, the patient receives a single injection of arginine vasopressin (AVP), and after a period of time, plasma and urine osmolality are measured again. The results of these three plasma and urine osmolality measurements are reported in the following table:

	Preliminary lab results	After water deprivation test	After first AVP injection
Plasma osmolality	310 mOsm/kg	330 mOsm/kg	290 mOsm/kg
Urine osmolality	240 mOsm/kg	240 mOsm/kg	600 mOsm/kg

Which of the following processes best explains the observed results?

A. Decreased corticopapillary gradient
B. Degenerated vasa recta
C. Increased countercurrent exchange
D. Increased countercurrent multiplication
E. Stimulated urea recycling

78. Which of the following patients in the hospital ward is the most likely to present with an impaired ability to maximally concentrate urine?

A. Patient being on a diet for phenylketonuria
B. Patient feeling cold due to overt hypothyroidism
C. Patient receiving carbonic anhydrase inhibitors
D. Patient presenting with gastrointestinal bleeding
E. Patient receiving high-dose corticosteroid therapy

79. A patient with food poisoning presents to the emergency department after 24 hours of vomiting and diarrhea. The patient is dehydrated, so intravenous therapy with normal saline is started. Which of the following correctly describes his renal function during this period of dehydration?

A. Blood volume leaving the vasa recta exceeds that entering them.
B. Free water clearance is zero to positive.
C. Inner medullary collecting ducts are impermeable to water.
D. Recycling of urea in the medulla is reduced compared to normal.
E. Water permeability in the ascending loop of Henle is increased.

80. A 9-year-old girl presents with frequent urination, bed wetting at night, and fever. On questioning, she also admits to back pain, but denies polyphagia or polydipsia. Her past history includes the diagnosis of sickle cell trait. Her complete genetic profile exists and does not show any other abnormalities. Her current history reveals stress due to the divorce of her parents. Her physical examination shows that normal values for the basic metabolic panel. Blood urea nitrogen and serum creatinine are at the high end of normal. Her renal function tests reveal that her maximum urine osmolality is 450 mOsm/kg. Her urine is somewhat cloudy. Which of the following is the most likely underlying mechanism for her nocturia and polyuria?

A. Defect of the collecting duct urea transporter
B. Defect of the vasa recta urea transporter
C. Erythrocyte sickling in medulla of vasa recta
D. Substantial increase in vasa recta blood flow
E. Uncontrolled diabetes mellitus type 1

81. After eating a meal that is very high in sodium (3,000 mg), plasma hyperosmolarity triggers which of the following change to the thirst response, antidiuretic hormone (ADH) secretion, and ultimately urine output?

	Thirst response	ADH secretion	Urine output
A.	↑	↑	↑
B.	↓	↑	↓
C.	↑	↑	↓
D.	↑	↓	↑
E.	↓	↓	↑
F.	↓	↓	↓

82. A clinical trial with healthy subjects aims to collect data in order to optimize an intervention. In a 27-year-old male subject, plasma osmolality, fractional excretion of sodium, and osmolar clearance remain unchanged after the intervention, compared to before the intervention. However, his urine osmolality decreased and his urine flow rate increased. The administration of which of the following is most likely tested?

A. A high-potassium drink
B. A new isotonic fluid
C. A new loop diuretic
D. A new thiazide diuretic
E. A V_2 receptor antagonist

83. In a healthy person with a normal balanced diet, which of the following substances is present in urine at the highest concentration?

A. Glucose
B. Magnesium
C. Sodium
D. Urea
E. Uric acid

84. As part of a micropuncture study of renal transport in rats, a fluid sample from a renal tubular segment was analyzed and showed an osmolality of 1,100 mOsm/kg and a pH of 4.8. If the results were extrapolated to a human nephron, from which segment of the renal nephron (labeled A–E in image) was the fluid most likely taken?

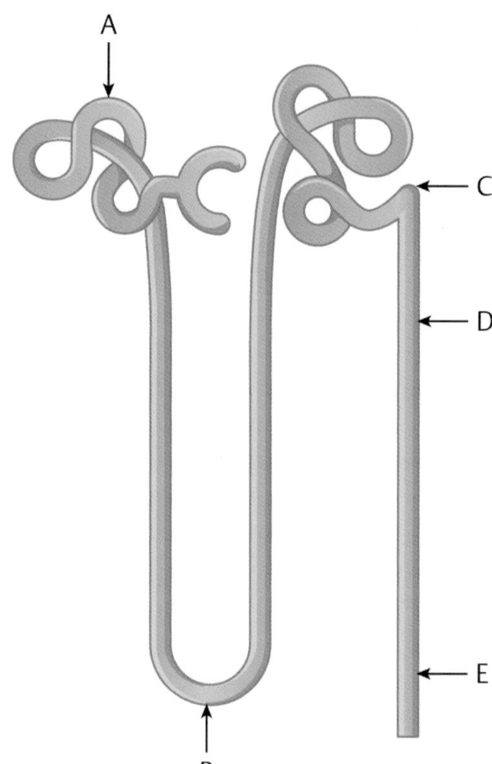

A. A
B. B
C. C
D. D
E. E

85. A 4-year-old girl is brought to the emergency department with signs of lower extremity and periorbital edema. After a series of blood tests and urinalysis, she is diagnosed with nephrotic syndrome due to minimal change disease (MCD). MCD disrupts glomerular anion production. Which of the following are the most likely results of her urinalysis?

	Proteinuria	Hematuria	Pyuria	Specific gravity of urine
A.	Present	Rare	Present	Elevated
B.	Present	Rare	Rare	Elevated
C.	Present	Present	Present	Normal
D.	Rare	Rare	Rare	Normal
E.	Rare	Present	Present	Elevated
F.	Rare	Present	Rare	Normal

86. At the beginning of an experimental study, the renal clearance of a substance was determined to be on average 100 mL/min on a balanced diet. The participants were asked to eat a high-meat diet for several days. When the clearance of the same substance was measured again, it had decreased to an average of 50 mL/min. The substance is most likely which of the following?

A. Ammonia (NH_3)
B. Insulin
C. Myoglobin
D. Weak acid drug
E. Weak base drug

87. A pharmaceutical sales representative is pitching a new drug that will lead to an increase in the rate of reabsorption of filtered bicarbonate by the proximal renal tubule. Which of the following is the most likely mechanism?

A. Decreasing arterial blood Pco_2
B. Decreasing glomerular filtration rate
C. Increasing pH inside the tubule cells
D. Inhibiting of carbonic anhydrase activity
E. Stimulating of the luminal Na^+/H^+ exchanger

88. A young, healthy woman obtained acetazolamide, a carbonic anhydrase inhibitor drug, from a friend at base camp of an 8,000-meter (26,247-feet) mountain. Now, several months later, back at sea level, she misuses the diuretic and takes it over weeks in the misguided hope to help her lose weight. Which of the following best characterizes the expected effects of the carbonic anhydrase inhibitor on renal excretion of the following ions?

	K^+	Ca^{2+}	HCO_3^-	H^+
A.	↑	↑	↑	↑
B.	↑	↑	↑	↓
C.	↑	↑	↓	↓
D.	↑	↓	↓	↓
E.	↔	↔	↔	↔
F.	↔	↔	↔	↑

89. A 17-year-old woman contracts the flu (influenza) and vomits excessively for two days. She becomes extremely weak and is taken to the emergency department by her mother. Her blood pressure is 90/70 mm Hg, pulse is 110 beats per minute, and respiratory rate is 9 breaths per minute. Blood tests reveal a blood pH of 7.51 and plasma bicarbonate of 35 mEq/L. Which is the correct combination of the patient's acid-base status and the increased hormone levels that contributed to it?

	Acid Base Status	Contributing hormones
A.	Metabolic alkalosis	Aldosterone and atrial natriuretic peptide
B.	Metabolic alkalosis	Aldosterone and vasopressin
C.	Metabolic alkalosis	Aldosterone and angiotensin II
D.	Metabolic alkalosis	Vasopressin and atrial natriuretic peptide
E.	Respiratory alkalosis	Aldosterone and atrial natriuretic peptide
F.	Respiratory alkalosis	Aldosterone and vasopressin
G.	Respiratory alkalosis	Aldosterone and angiotensin II
H.	Respiratory alkalosis	Vasopressin and atrial natriuretic peptide

90. A patient with episodic seizures is being treated with the carbonic anhydrase inhibitor acetazolamide, which is known to cause mild diuresis as a side effect. Which of the following renal changes would be expected when taking this drug?

A. Decreased bicarbonate excretion in urine

B. Decreased extracellular fluid H^+ concentration

C. Decreased number of protons in urine

D. Increased distal tubule fluid H^+ concentration

E. Increased proximal tubule bicarbonate reabsorption

91. A 23-year-old woman presents with sharp stomach pain. On questioning, she tells that for the past 3 weeks, she has been taking high-dose iron supplements three times a day since she read in a magazine about iron shortage in child-bearing women. Which of the following is the renal compensation for her developing acid-base problem?

A. Decreased Na^+/H^+ exchanger activity in proximal tubule cells

B. Decreased renal tubular synthesis of new bicarbonate

C. Increased synthesis and excretion of ammonium

D. Increased urinary excretion of bicarbonate

E. Increased urinary excretion of carbon dioxide

92. A drug has a side effect of inhibiting the conversion of glutamine to bicarbonate and ammonium in renal proximal tubular cells. If this drug were administered for some time to a patient with a healthy kidney, which of the following changes would you expect to occur in response to this side effect?

A. A decrease of K^+ in plasma

B. A decrease in plasma pH

C. An increase in plasma NH_4^+

D. An increase in urinary pH

E. Excess H^+ excretion by titratable acid

93. A 3-year-old girl is found dizzy and stumbling in the garage with an open bottle of antifreeze (ethylene glycol), and confirms that she drank it. The increase of which of the following in urine is most critical to eliminate her excess acid load?

A. Ammonium

B. Free hydrogen

C. Sulfate

D. Phosphate

E. Urea

94. The following measurements are from a 70-kg adult man. No health concerns are known.

Serum	
Bicarbonate:	24 mEq/L
Chloride:	100 mEq/L
Phosphorus:	2.0 mEq/L
Potassium:	4.2 mEq/L
Sodium:	142 mEq/L
Creatinine:	1.1 mg/dL
Urea:	25 mg/dL
Urine	
Protein:	Negative
Casts:	Negative
pH:	4.9
Chloride:	150 mEq/day
Potassium:	50 mEq/day
Sodium:	100 mEq/ day

Based on the available information, which of the following dietary recommendations would be appropriate for this person?

A. A low-carbohydrate diet

B. A low-fat diet

C. A low-nucleic-acid diet

D. A low-protein diet

E. A normal balanced diet

95. A woman with multiple sclerosis takes the muscle relaxant dantrolene, which blocks the ryanodine receptor. As an adverse side effect, she experiences urinary incontinence. Which of the following parts of the urinary system is most likely affected?

A. Detrusor muscle

B. External sphincter

C. Internal sphincter

D. Ureters

E. Urethra

96. A 51-year-old woman presents to her primary care physician with complaints of frequent and sudden urges to urinate. She reports several incidences of incontinence in the past month, but no fever, painful urination, or vaginal discharge is reported. She is diagnosed with overactive bladder. One treatment for overactive bladder syndrome involves the injection of botulinum toxin type A into the bladder to produce muscular relaxation. On the image of the bladder, into what structure would the botulinum toxin be injected to best treat the symptoms of overactive bladder?

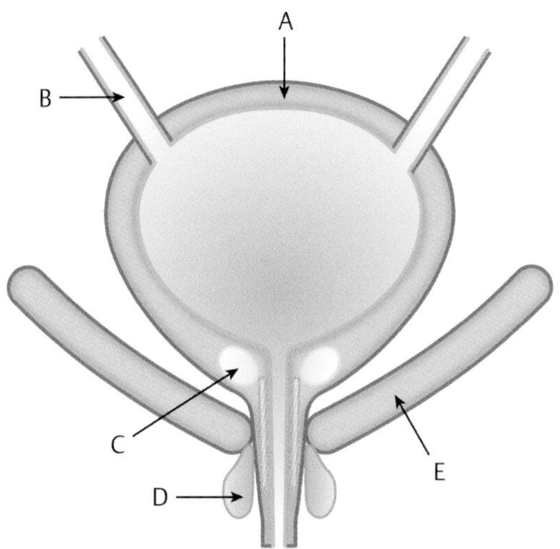

A. A
B. B
C. C
D. D
E. E

97. The image depicts the results of a cystometrogram that showed that the patient has a normal control of micturition. Which phase of the cystometrogram would have been most altered in the case of an overactive bladder?

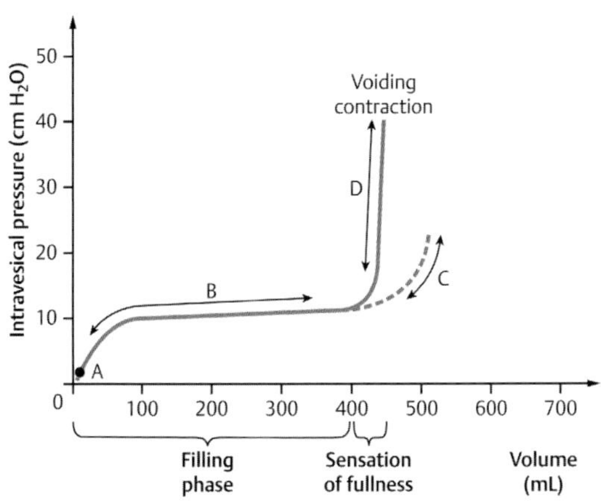

A. A
B. B
C. C
D. D

7.6 Answers and Explanations

75. Correct: C (C)

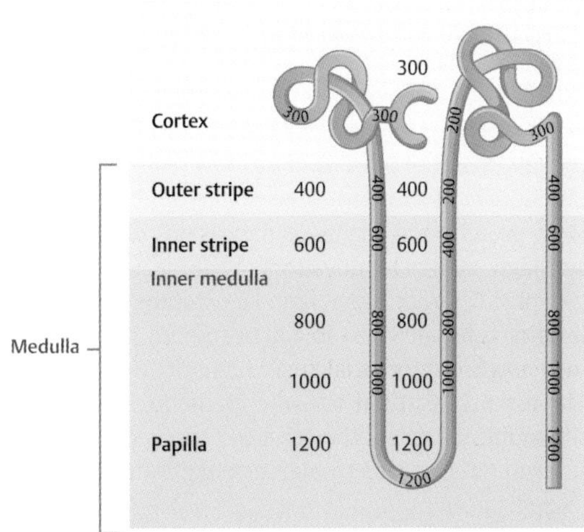

Severe burns increase capillary permeability. Fluids leak out of vessels, and the effective arterial blood volume decreases. In response, antidiuretic hormone (ADH) release is increased, which promotes urea reabsorption and recycling. The recycling of urea between the collecting duct, vasa recta, and loop of Henle (LOH) produces a corticopapillary gradient, which is greatest at the papillary tip of the LOH (see image). The gradient might not be as optimal as shown in the image, since renal capillary beds will be damaged as well. Nevertheless, the renal countercurrent multiplication mechanism will create an interstitial gradient that is higher in osmolality at the renal papilla compared to the renal cortex. There would be an equally concentrated tubular fluid at the inner medullary collecting duct (see image), but that position is not labeled on the nephron. (**A, B**) The osmolality of tubular fluid in Bowman's space and in the proximal tubule will be similar to plasma osmolality. (**D**) Fluid in the early part of the distal convoluted tubule will be hypoosmotic, independent of the patient's fluid status. (**E**) Osmolality along the collecting duct will increase and reach the highest concentration in the inner medullary part.

76. Correct: Increased UT-1 ubiquitination (D)

Ubiquitination, the tagging of the urea transport protein UT-1 with ubiquitin, marks the transporter for removal from the cell membrane and its intracellular destruction in lysosomes. UT-1 is the transporter in the medullary renal collecting ducts that allows urea to be deposited in the interstitial space by facilitated diffusion. If not present, a maximal corticopapillary osmotic gradient cannot be established, since urea contributes about half the osmoles during periods of urine concentration. The better the gradient, the more water can be reabsorbed, and the more concentrated urine can be produced. (A, B) High-protein and high-salt diets lead to high urea and high sodium loads, which can increase the renal interstitial osmotic gradient. (**C**) Elevated glomerular filtration rate leads to a high sodium load, which increase the interstitial renal osmotic gradient. (**E**) The renal interstitial osmotic gradient depends on the input of salt via the Na-K-2Cl transport, so that its stimulation leads to high osmolality in the renal interstitium.

77. Correct: Decreased corticopapillary gradient (A)

The results are consistent with a diagnosis of central diabetes insipidus, since arginine vasopressin (AVP) is not produced or released by the brain, even after water deprivation, but the kidneys respond by concentrating the urine after AVP is injected. A chronic lack of AVP will have decreased her corticopapillary gradient over time. Hence, the first injection only produces urine that equilibrates with a low medullary interstitial osmolality of 600 mOsm/kg. Further injections would eventually reconstitute a maximal medullary osmolality of 1,200 mOsm/kg, and she would again be able to produce a maximally concentrated urine of 1,200 mOsm/kg. (B) Degeneration of vasa recta is not a result of AVP deficiency. (C, D) AVP deficiency will have decreased (not increased) both countercurrent exchange and countercurrent multiplication, since water and urea reabsorption from the collecting duct are stimulated by AVP. (E) AVP deficiency will have decreased urea recycling, since it is AVP that stimulates the insertion of membrane urea transporters into the collecting duct.

78. Correct: Being on a diet for phenylketonuria (A)

The diet for patients with phenylketonuria is low in protein, which leads to low amounts of urea, the waste product of protein metabolism. A low urea concentration in the distal portion of the collecting ducts decreases the driving force for passive urea reabsorption into the medullary renal interstitium. This leads to a less than optimal corticopapillary osmotic gradient and an impaired ability to maximally concentrate urine. (**B**) Hyperthyroidism (not hypothyroidism) is known to increase the medullary blood flow in the vasa recta, which can lead to a washout of the interstitial osmotic gradient. (**C, E**) Gastrointestinal bleeding raises blood urea due to digestion and absorption of blood proteins, while high amounts of cortisol raise blood urea due to increased proteolysis. Urea can then be used in the kidneys as part of the urine concentration process. (**D**) Carbon anhydrase inhibitors inhibit Na^+ and H_2O reabsorption in the proximal tubule, which leads at the ascending limb of Henle to a higher solute load that can be used for creating an optimal renal interstitial osmotic gradient.

79. Correct: Blood volume leaving the vasa recta exceeds that entering them (A)

Vomiting and diarrhea leads to dehydration, and the body activates a number of mechanisms to conserve water. This means that water reabsorption in the renal tubule is increased, and the reabsorbed water is carried away from the renal tubules via the vasa recta and peritubular capillaries. Thus, blood volume leaving the vasa recta is greater than that entering. (**B**) A zero or positive free water clearance indicates that no or excess solute-free water is excreted in urine, which does not occur with dehydration, when a concentrated urine is produced. (**C**) Antidiuretic hormone (ADH) stimulates the insertion of aquaporin channels into the apical membrane of the renal collecting duct epithelial cells. This increases the cells' permeability to water and increases water reabsorption. (**D**) ADH stimulates urea recycling, which increases the corticopapillary gradient and thus increases water reabsorption. (**E**) In response to dehydration, antidiuretic hormone (ADH) increases water permeability in the collecting duct, not the ascending loop of Henle.

80. Correct: Erythrocyte sickling in medulla of vasa recta (C)

Slow blood flow and low oxygen tension make the medullary sites of vasa recta likely locations where erythrocytes sickle. Sickling is additionally promoted by the high blood osmolality, which pulls water out of passing erythrocytes and increases hemoglobin S concentration. Sickling causes microthrombotic infarctions and interferes with the function of the vasa recta as countercurrent exchanger in the inner medulla. This leads to less free water reabsorption and frequent urination with low-osmolality urine. In patients with sickle cell trait under stress, it can lead to renal papillary necrosis, causing fever and pain. (**A, B**) Genetic defects in the urea transporters of the renal nephron (UT-A) or the vasa recta (UT-B) could theoretically interfere with the process of countercurrent exchange and urea recycling and hence, impair the ability to maximally concentrate urine. However, symptoms of fever, back pain, and cloudy urine are inconsistent. Moreover, the girl's genetic profile would have shown these mutations.

Last, no major pathologies are currently linked with urea transporter dysfunction. (**D**) Increased vasa recta blood flow can wash out the renal interstitial osmotic gradient, but would not cause fever, pain or urea/creatinine backup. It is more likely that a decreased blood flow caused ischemia and necrosis, which impaired the function of ATP-dependent transporters. Decreased solute transport into the medullary interstitium led to the inability to maximally concentrate urine. (**E**) Diabetes mellitus type 1 is not likely, on the basis of her normal serum glucose level and acid-base status (glucose and bicarbonate are part of the basic metabolic panel). Additionally, the lack of polydipsia and polyphagia is uncharacteristic.

81. Correct: ↑, ↑, ↑ (A)

After a high-sodium meal, the plasma osmolality increases, which triggers the thirst response (leading to the intake of free water) and the release of antidiuretic hormone (ADH). Both promote volume expansion until plasma is isosmotic and the trigger subsides. The increase in effective arterial blood volume initiates several mechanisms that act at the kidneys (e.g., sympathetic nerve activity, atrial natriuretic peptide, renin-angiotensin-aldosterone system) to increase sodium and water excretion and return extracellular fluid volume and effective arterial blood volume back to normal. Hence, urine output increases. (**B, C, D, E, F**) These are incorrect because one or more changes is incorrect.

82. Correct: A V2-receptor antagonist (E)

A V_2 receptor antagonist inhibits the antidiuretic actions of vasopressin in the kidney, resulting in decreased water permeability of the collecting ducts. This results in urine with decreased osmolarity and increased urine flow rate. Due to the counterbalancing effects of osmolarity and flow rate, osmolar clearance ($C_{Osm} = U_{Osm} \times \dot{V}/P_{Osm}$) remains unchanged. In other words, in a healthy person, the capacity of the kidneys to excrete solutes is not affected. (**A**) High dietary potassium intake stimulates aldosterone release and, thus, increases renal Na^+ reabsorption. This would decrease fractional excretion of sodium (FENa). Urine flow would not be affected. (**B**) Isoosmotic volume expansion would increase atrial natriuretic peptide secretion, which would inhibit Na^+ reabsorption and increases FENa and C_{Osm}. (**C, D**) Diuretics (loop diuretic more than thiazide diuretic) would increase urine flow rate and, thus, increase FENa and C_{Osm}.

83. Correct: Urea (D)

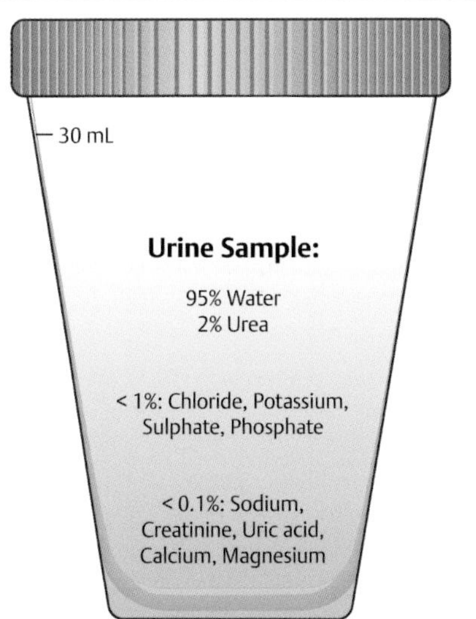

About 2% of urine is composed of urea. It is a waste product, created by the liver to eliminate nitrogen derived from protein catabolism. Urea is freely filtered, reabsorbed or secreted by simple or facilitated diffusion, and excreted in urine. The final excreted amount depends on antidiuretic hormone (ADH). In its absence, more urea is excreted due to a high urine flow rate. In its presence, urea becomes concentrated along the collecting ducts, which are impermeable to urea but permeable to water. Then, a high amount of urea is reabsorbed through an ADH-activated transporter in the inner medullary collecting duct in order to contribute to the water-drawing osmotic force of the interstitial fluid. On average, urea contributes about half of all solutes in urine (image). (**A**) In a healthy person on a balanced diet, there is no significant amount of glucose in urine. (**B**) Less than 0.01% of urine is composed of magnesium. (**C**) Less than 0.1% of urine is composed of sodium. (**E**) Less than 0.03% of urine is composed of uric acid, the byproduct of purine nucleotide catabolism.

84. Correct: E (E)

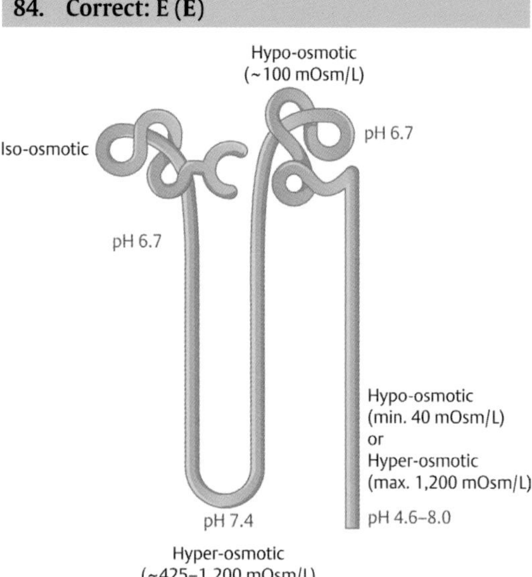

The high osmolality of 1,100 mOsm/kg and the low pH of 4.8 indicate that the renal fluid sample is from a segment beyond the distal nephron that passes through the inner renal medulla (image). There, an interstitial osmolality up to 1,200 mOsm/kg can exist under the influence of antidiuretic hormone, which increases the water permeability of the collecting duct so that intratubular fluid osmolality becomes equal with interstitial fluid osmolality. The pH is acidic since α-intercalated cells secrete protons, which are finally excreted in urine bound to ammonia, phosphate, and other buffers. (**A**) The proximal tubule fluid has an osmolality close to 300 mOsm/kg and a neutral pH due to isosmotic reabsorption. (**B**) The tip of the loop of Henle is hyperosmotic; however, the pH is close to neutral because of the increase in bicarbonate concentration due to water removal along the descending limb. (**C, D**) The cortical and outer medullary parts of the collecting duct are embedded in interstitial fluid with solute concentrations that create the low end of the interstitial corticopapillary osmotic gradient. Along the collecting duct, the pH gradually becomes acidic, but can only fall to a low level of 4.8, when maximal amounts of ammonia are added as buffers in the inner medullary collecting duct.

85. Correct: Present, rare, rare, elevated (B)

Minimal change disease (MCD) is a disorder in which T-cells release a cytokine that injures the glomerular epithelial foot processes. This disrupts the production of anions in the glomerulus, which allows the filtration of albumin into the nephron, leading to proteinuria and elevated specific gravity. Hematuria and pyuria are rarely seen in nephrotic syndromes. (**A, C, D, E, F**) These choices do not include the correct combination of answers.

86. Correct: Weak acid drug (D)

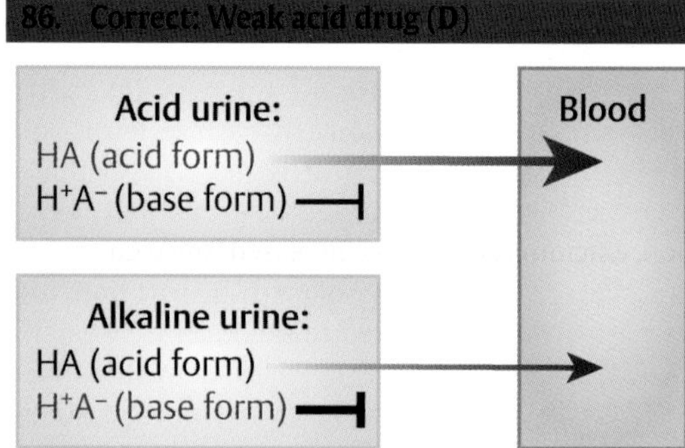

A high-meat diet produces acidic urine due to the metabolism of amino acids. When urine is acidic, weak acid drugs are more easily reabsorbed from tubular lumen by passive diffusion, since they predominate in their nonionized form (image). Consequently, their excretion (and clearance) decreases. (**A**) Ammonia is a weak base. At an acidic urine, its ionic form NH_4^+ predominates, which is trapped in urine so that clearance would increase (not decrease). (**B, C**) Filtered proteins and peptides, such as myoglobin and insulin, are not reabsorbed from the tubular lumen by passive diffusion, rather via endocytosis in the proximal tubule. Hence, clearance is not a direct function of urine pH. (**E**) With an acidic filtrate, a weak base drug is less extensively reabsorbed and its clearance would be increased (not decreased).

87. Correct: Stimulating of the luminal Na^+/H^+ exchanger (E)

Stimulation of the luminal Na^+/H^+ exchanger in the brush border of the proximal renal tubule will result in increased H^+ secretion and increased HCO_3^- reabsorption, since for every H^+ that is secreted, one HCO_3^- is returned to the systemic circulation (via H_2CO_3, in equilibrium with CO_2 and H_2O). (**A**) A decrease in arterial blood Pco_2 as primary disturbance will result in decreased H^+ secretion and decreased (not increased) reabsorption of filtered HCO_3^-. It is the renal compensation for respiratory alkalosis. (**B**) Decreasing glomerular filtration rate leads to less filtered and less (not more) reabsorbed HCO_3^-. (**C**) Increasing pH inside tubular cells (i.e., a decrease in H^+ concentration) will result in less H^+ secretion and hence decreased (not increased) HCO_3^- reabsorption. (**D**) Inhbiting carbonic anhydrase activity results in less renal HCO_3^- reabsorption, since the process of net reabsorption of HCO_3^- requires the enzyme's catalysis of the reaction between H_2CO_3 and CO_2 + H_2O.

88. Correct: ↑, ↑, ↑, ↓ (B)

In kidneys, carbonic anhydrase (CA) is abundant in proximal tubules, and the diuretic effect of CA inhibitor is mostly attributed to the inhibition of proximal Na^+ reabsorption by the Na^+-H^+ antiporter, which depends on the enzyme's activity. This inhibition of proximal Na^+ and H_2O reabsorption increases tubular fluid flow rate, which generally favors excretion of all electrolytes. However, due to the multiple tubular downstream transport processes, the excreted amount is less than predicted from the proximal process. Nevertheless, K^+ excretion is increased, because plasma volume contraction increases serum aldosterone, which stimulates renal principal cell K^+ secretion. Calcium excretion is increased, since Ca^{2+} is less soluble in alkaline urine. Urine is alkaline because proximal reabsorption of HCO_3^- requires H^+ secretion, which is inhibited by the diuretic. Hence, HCO_3^- excretion is increased and H^+ excretion is decreased. With long-term administration, a metabolic acidosis develops. The woman received the drug from high-altitude hikers. They use acetazolamide to avoid altitude-related respiratory alkalosis by increasing their urinary HCO_3^- excretion. (**A, C, D, E, F**) These include one or more incorrect choices.

89. Correct: Metabolic alkalosis, aldosterone and angiotensin II (C)

The combination of the alkaline pH and elevated serum bicarbonate indicates metabolic alkalosis. The excessive vomiting caused volume contraction, which activated the renin-angiotensin-aldosterone system (RAAS). Aldosterone stimulates the H^+-ATPase in the α-intercalated cells of the distal nephron, which in turn increases reabsorption of newly synthesized HCO_3^-. Angiotensin II stimulates Na^+-H^+ exchange in the proximal tubule. This leads to an increase in reabsorption of HCO_3^- that had been filtered by the glomerulus. Both proximal and distal processes increase plasma HCO_3^-. (**A, B, D**) Atrial natriuretic peptide is released in response to volume overload, which stretches the atrial wall. It opposes the RAAS and hence is downregulated in this woman. Vasopressin (or antidiuretic hormone, ADH) alters water permeability in the distal nephron but does not directly impact blood pH. (**E, F, G, H**) A respiratory alkalosis would present with decreased bicarbonate, compensating for low Pco_2 as the primary disturbance.

90. Correct: Decreased number of protons in urine (C)

Inhibition of carbonic anhydrase (CA) reduces the reabsorption of bicarbonate in the proximal tubule by indirectly inhibiting the renal proximal tubule Na^+-H^+ antiporter, which depends on the enzyme's activity. Bicarbonate reabsorption requires H^+ secretion. Thus, more bicarbonate is excreted in the urine, the urine pH increases, and a decreased number of protons is present. CA inhibitors act as mild diuretics due to the inhibition of proximal Na^+ and H_2O reabsorption, which increases tubular fluid flow rate. (**A**) Bicarbonate excretion in the urine is increased (not decreased) due to less reabsorption of bicarbonate in the renal tubule. (**B**) Bicarbonaturia will produce a metabolic acidosis due to decreased H^+ excretion. Hence, extracellular fluid H^+ concentration is increased (not decreased). (**D**) With an alkaline urine, the distal tubule fluid H^+ concentration is decreased (not increased). (**E**) Inhibition of CA will decrease (not increase) HCO_3^- reabsorption in the proximal tubule.

91. Correct: Increased synthesis and excretion of ammonium (C)

Iron overdose leads to metabolic acidosis as a result of mitochondrial toxicity and lactic acid buildup, as well as the reaction between ferric iron (Fe^{3+}) and water that leads to excess protons. The kidney responds to a chronic proton load by increasing intrarenal ammonium (NH_4^+) synthesis from glutamine metabolism. Increased NH_4^+ excretion is the most critical process for acid-base homeostasis in chronic metabolic acidosis. For each NH_4^+ excreted in urine, an HCO_3^- is released into the systemic circulation to restore buffer base reserves, so that ammonia excretion promotes acid excretion. (**A, B, D**) During acidemia, the kidneys recover all filtered HCO_3^- by maximal (not decreased) activation of the Na^+/H^+ exchanger; they synthesize more (not less) new HCO_3^-; and they decrease (not increase) urinary excretion of HCO_3^-. (**E**) The lungs (not the kidneys) increase CO_2 excretion.

92. Correct: A decrease in plasma pH (B)

A person on a typical Western diet produces about 1 mEq H^+ per kg body weight per day, which needs to be excreted to stay in acid-base balance. The renal process of ammoniagenesis contributes about 60–70%. It adds newly formed HCO_3^- to blood (the concomitantly added H_2O is negligible and CO_2 is eliminated by lungs), which is available there to buffer H^+. If this process were inhibited, excess acid would not be excreted and plasma pH would eventually decrease. (**A**) Excess H^+ is shifted into cells to be buffered by abundant intracellular buffers. This is often in exchange for K^+ leaving the cell, which leads to an increase (not decrease) of plasma K^+. (**C**) With inhibition of ammoniagenesis, NH_4^+ production would not increase. Additionally, NH_4^+ does not accumulate but rather is metabolized in the liver to urea. (**D**) With developing acidosis, more H^+ would be filtered and urine pH would decrease (not increase). However, urine pH would not fall beyond pH 4.5. The only way to get rid of more H^+ is to create more NH_4^+ buffer. (**E**) Titratable acid is not regulated by acid-base balance but rather depends on the amount of available buffer (mostly $H_2PO_4^-$). Hence, it cannot compensate for the missing NH_4^+ urinary buffers.

93. Correct: Ammonium (A)

Ethylene glycol is a neurotoxin, so the girl appears as if alcohol intoxicated for about the first 12 hours. During this time, the poison is metabolized and organic acids accumulate, leading to metabolic acidosis. Phosphate and ammonium are both buffers that bind and eliminate excess protons in the urine. Increased ammonium excretion is the best choice because the excretion rate of ammonium can be greatly increased in the face of a large acid load. Ammonium synthesis is stimulated by an increased H^+ concentration in the tubule filtrate. On the other hand, phosphate is not regulated to maintain acid-base balance as much as it is to maintain phosphorus homeostasis. (**B**) Urine has only a very small amount of free hydrogen ions, and the minimal urine pH of 4.5 cannot be lowered, because the concentration gradient becomes too great for proton transporters to overcome. Hence, increasing free H^+ is not the way to eliminate a large acid load. (**C**) Phosphate is a filtered buffer, and its excretion rate cannot be altered as easily as that of ammonium; therefore it is not the best choice here. (**D, E**) Increased sulfate and urea excretion are not used for urinary proton excretion.

94. Correct: A normal balanced diet (E)

The serum values do not show any electrolyte imbalance or signs of kidney damage (normal creatinine and urea). The low urinary pH indicates that the kidney excretes acidity. To address the question whether a change in diet is recommended to lower a potentially inappropriate amount of acid production, one has to understand conceptually how the kidney excretes daily produced nonvolatile acid, called Net Renal Acid Excretion (NAE). It is the sum of titratable acid and ammonia, minus bicarbonate. *Titratable acid* is urinary H^+ combined with buffers, mostly phosphates. The man's serum phosphorus level is within normal range, so his kidneys should have normal physiological amounts of urinary phosphate. *Ammonia* stands for urinary H^+ combined with NH_3 to NH_4^+. It can be estimated from the urine anion gap, UAG = Urine (Na + K – Cl). No gap or slightly positive values (in a Western diet, Na^+ and K^+ are typically higher than Cl^- ingestion) indicate normal ammonia production, as in the case of the man (100 + 50 – 150 = 0 mEq/day). *Bicarbonate* stands for urinary HCO_3^-. Normally, the kidneys completely reabsorb filtered HCO_3^-, so that any loss in urine is equivalent to an acidifying effect on the body and must be subtracted from the excreted acid load. In the case of the man, the low urinary pH does not indicate any significant amount of bicarbonate excretion. In summary, all given information indicates that the kidney normally deals with the produced acid load. A pH above 4.6, if not present for long times, is within normal range, so that a special diet is not indicated. (**A, B**) Carbohydrates and fats from diet do not contribute to acid-base stress as long as they are completely oxidized to CO_2 and H_2O. (**C**) Metabolism of phosphodiester bonds of nucleic acids produces phosphoric acid; however, a healthy kidney can easily deal with this acid load from a normal balanced diet. (**D**) Metabolism of proteins and amino acids produces sulfuric, hydrochloric, or phosphoric acid; however, a healthy kidney can easily deal with this acid load from normal diets.

95. Correct: External sphincter (B)

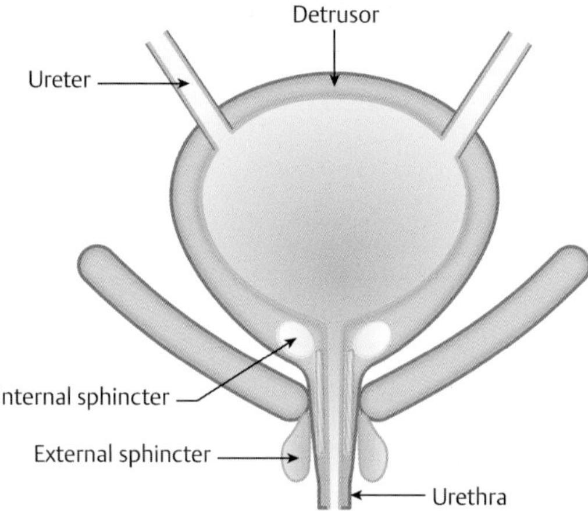

Multiple sclerosis is a demyelination disease that commonly presents with muscle spasms. Dantrolene decreases the intracellular calcium concentration of muscle fibers by binding to the ryanodine receptor; hence, it works primarily in skeletal muscle and minimally in smooth muscle. The external urethral sphincter is skeletal muscle and normally provides voluntary control of urination. Drug-induced relaxation of the external sphincter can cause urinary incontinence. (**A, C**) The internal sphincter and detrusor muscle are made of smooth muscle, which is under autonomic nervous system control. (**D, E**) The ureters and urethra are hollow tubes that carry urine but do not modulate its flow.

96. Correct: A (A)

This is the detrusor muscle, and sudden contraction of the detrusor muscle is the primary cause of overactive bladder, so injection of botulinum toxin (blocks acetylcholine neurotransmission) into that muscle will produce relaxation and ease the symptoms of overactive bladder for a few months. (**B**) This is the ureter, which simply carries urine from the kidney to the bladder. Relaxation of this structure would have no impact on the patient's symptoms. (**C, D**) These are the internal (**C**) and external (**D**) sphincters. Relaxation of these sphincters would promote uncontrolled urination, not prevent it. (**E**) This is the levator ani, which forms the floor of the pelvic cavity and supports the organs in the region.

97. Correct: B (B)

In a person with normal control of micturition, point A on the curve represents the empty bladder with a pressure of approximately zero. A small increase in volume causes the pressure to rise to about 10 cm H_2O, then a further increase of 300–400 mL can accumulate with very little change in pressure (phase B on the graph). Further distension of the bladder causes a rise in pressure and initiates the micturition reflex (phase D on the graph). Phase C indicates the voluntary suppression of the micturition reflex. Overactive bladder (OAB) is a condition that is characterized by sudden, involuntary contraction of the detrusor muscle in the wall of the urinary bladder, which results in a sudden and unstoppable need to urinate. This can occur at any point in phase B of the cystometrogram, thus cutting that phase short. (**A, C, D**) are not impacted by the sudden, involuntary contractions of the detrusor muscle.

7.7 Questions

98. At an international clinical conference, data are presented on the efficiency of magnesium chloride as oral tocolytic agent. A person in the audience asks how to translate a 3.0 mM $MgCl_2$ solution into milliequivalents per liter, and about the osmolarity of this solution in milliosmoles per liter. Which of the following is the correct answer, assuming an osmotic coefficient of 1.00?

	Mg^{2+} (mEq/L)	Cl^- (mEq/L)	Osmolarity (mOsm/L)
A.	3	3	3
B.	6	3	6
C.	3	6	6
D.	6	3	9
E.	6	6	9

99. An 11-year-old boy is admitted to the emergency department with a 3-day history of vomiting. The child is lethargic, has poor skin turgor, and a blood pressure of 80/60 mm Hg. One bag of normal saline (500 mL) is given intravenously. Approximately how much of the added fluid remains in the vascular compartment?

A. 50 mL
B. 125 mL
C. 250 mL
D. 400 mL
E. 500 mL

100. To determine the dialysis dose, a 65-kg, 24-year-old man is given 0.15 g of inulin intravenously. One hour later the plasma inulin concentration is 1.0 mg/100 mL. What is the approximate extracellular fluid volume (in liters) of this man?

A. 5
B. 10
C. 15
D. 20
E. 25

Questions 101 to 102

A computer animation shows the physiological body compartments of plasma, interstitial fluid, and intracellular fluid of a particular person, as seen in the image. When solutions are added to or removed from plasma, the program responds with fluid shifts between compartments in a comparable manner to a healthy person. Excretions and metabolic processes are neglected. After adequate time for diffusion to occur, the concentrations of the solutions are shown by the intensity of their colors.

101. Using the computer animation described, a user simulates an experiment on two different people with different fluid statuses. To each person, he adds 70 mL of Evans blue solution in 0.9% saline and analyzes the results after a given time has passed. For the first person, the color of the fluid compartment barely changes. For the second person, the fluid becomes dark blue. Which of the following can be concluded for the second person compared to the first person?

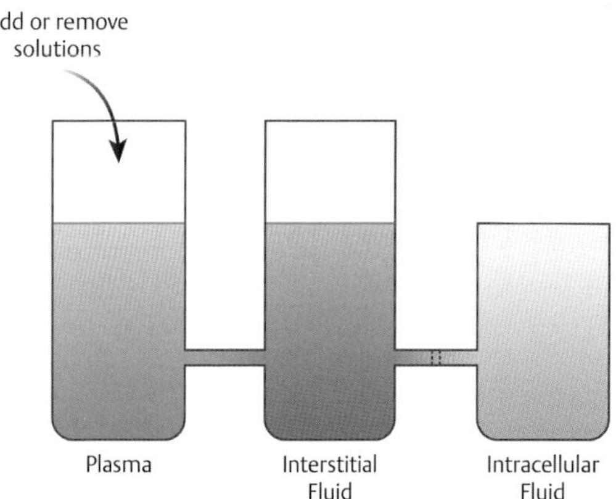

A. The plasma volume is larger.
B. The interstitial fluid volume is larger.
C. The intracellular fluid volume is larger.
D. The plasma volume is smaller.
E. The interstitial fluid volume is smaller.
F. The intracellular fluid volume is smaller.

102. Using the computer program as described, a known amount of mannitol solution is added, and the program responds by displaying the following volume and osmolality changes, as well as changes in plasma protein concentration:

ECF volume:	increase
ECF osmolality:	decrease
ICF volume:	increase
ICF osmolarity:	decrease
Plasma protein concentration:	decrease

Which of the following correctly describes the process that led to the indicated results?

A. Hypertonic volume contraction
B. Hypertonic volume expansion
C. Hypotonic volume contraction
D. Hypotonic volume expansion
E. Isotonic volume contraction
F. Isotonic volume expansion

103. 200 mCi of D_2O and 400 mg of mannitol are injected into a volunteer to determine the volumes of her fluid compartments. During the equilibration period, 20% of the D_2O and 10% of the mannitol are excreted in the urine. After equilibration, a plasma sample has a D_2O concentration of 3.5 mCi/L and a mannitol concentration of 25 mg/L. Based on these data, what are the woman's total body water, extracellular fluid volume, and intracellular fluid volumes?

	Total body water (L)	Extracellular fluid volume (L)	Intracellular fluid volume (L)
A.	41.3	14.4	31.3
B.	41.3	12.2	29.8
C.	41.3	12.2	29.8
D.	45.7	14.4	31.3
E.	45.7	14.4	29.8
F.	45.7	12.2	31.3

104. A patient with sickle cell disease needs to be rehydrated, and 1 liter of 0.25% sodium chloride is infused. After equilibration, which of the following box diagrams would most accurately represent changes to the patient's intracellular fluid (ICF), extracellular fluid (ECF), and plasma osmolarity, relative to normal?

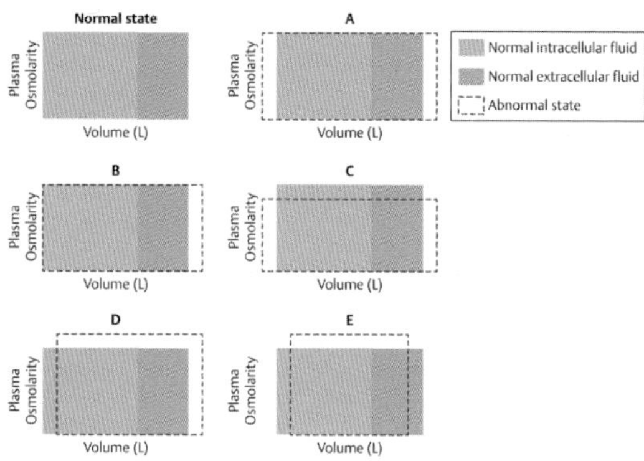

A. A
B. B
C. C
D. D
E. E

105. When 2.0 liters of each of the following clinical solutions are infused intravenously, which produces the greatest increase in extracellular fluid?

A. Dextrose in water, 5%
B. Lactated Ringer's solution
C. Sodium chloride, 0.45%
D. Sodium chloride, 0.9%
E. Sodium chloride, 3%

Questions 106 to 107

An 81-year-old woman with a history of recurrent kidney infections and acute renal failure presents in the emergency department with lower extremity edema, shortness of breath, lethargy, and confusion. She is diagnosed with stage 3 chronic kidney disease (CKD).

106. Given the patient's current condition, which of the following box diagrams would most accurately represent the changes to the patient's intracellular fluid (ICF), extracellular fluid (ECF), and plasma osmolarity, relative to normal?

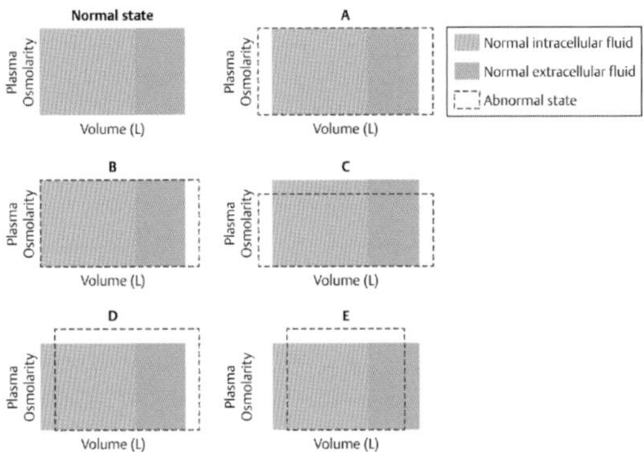

A. A

B. B

C. C

D. D

E. E

107. Which of the following symptoms would also be expected in this patient?

A. Hypokalemia

B. Hyponatremia

C. Hypophosphatemia

D. Hypotension

E. Uremia

108. In which of the following circumstances, in an otherwise unremarkable person in regards to health, can one most likely expect an increased hematocrit?

A. Being ill with syndrome of inappropriate antidiuretic hormone

B. Experiencing congestive heart failure

C. Having consumed pickled vegetables

D. Suffering from 21β-hydroxylase deficiency

E. Sweating during regular exercise

109. A 51-year-old woman presents to her primary care physician with complaints of frequent and sudden urges to urinate. She reports several incidences of incontinence in the past month, but no fever, painful urination, or vaginal discharge is reported. The history reveals that she eats a high-potassium diet. Which of the following mechanisms is responsible for the woman's urge incontinence?

A. Increased secretion of K^+ in the ascending loop of Henle

B. Increased secretion of K^+ in the collecting duct

C. Increased secretion of K^+ in the early distal tubule

D. Reduced reabsorption of K^+ in the proximal tubule

E. Reduced reabsorption of K^+ in the descending loop of Henle

110. The kidney of a large rodent is isolated and pump-perfused with hypernatremic plasma, containing 200 mEq/L of Na^+. Inulin clearance is 5 mL/min. Assuming the rodent nephron behaves like a human nephron, approximately how much Na^+ would be left in the tubular fluid (in mEq/min) at the end of the descending limb of the loop of Henle?

A. 0.13

B. 0.33

C. 0.43

D. 0.73

E. 1.00

111. Which of the following most likely leads to hypokalemia?

A. ACE inhibitors

B. β receptor blockers

C. Classic congenital adrenal hyperplasia

D. Excessive vomiting

E. Hypoaldosteronism

F. Traumatic rhabdomyolysis

112. A 58-year-old, 187-pound woman tells her primary care physician on a routine health check that for the last 3 months she eats a large bowl of miso soup (high-salt soybean paste soup) and a bag of chips daily. Her weight has not changed since her previous visit. Which of the following has been increased and explains her sodium balance?

A. Aldosterone

B. Angiotensin II

C. Glomerular hydrostatic pressure

D. Peritubular capillary oncotic pressure

E. Sympathetic activity

113. A patient presents with hematuria and sharp, stabbing back pain. His abdominal X-ray is shown.

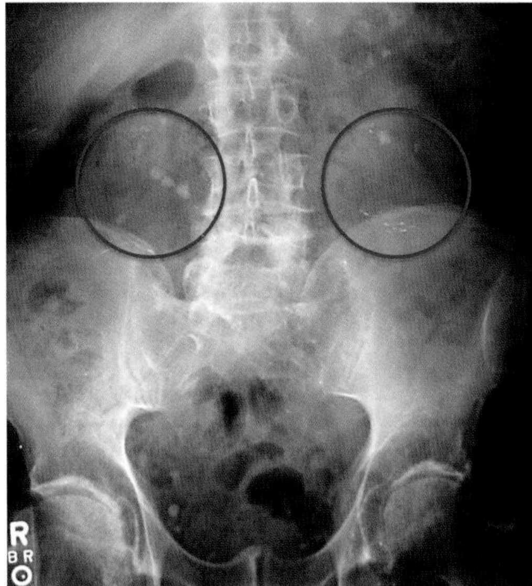

Based on the condition indicated in the X-ray image, which of the following hormones is the most likely one to be increased in this patient?

A. Aldosterone
B. Angiotensin II
C. Antidiuretic hormone
D. Parathyroid hormone
E. Renin

114. A 64-year-old woman with advanced metastatic cancer presents with hypercalciuria due to bone tumors. She is taking steroids. Which of the following would be a possible addition to her treatment plan?

A. A high-oxalate diet
B. A higher dose of steroids
C. A thiazide diuretic
D. A very-low-calcium diet
E. A vitamin D supplement

115. In a healthy person, which of the following changes to serum osmolarity and blood pressure result in the largest increase of serum antidiuretic hormone?

A. Decreased serum osmolarity and hypertension
B. Decreased serum osmolarity and hypotension
C. Increased serum osmolarity and hypertension
D. Increased serum osmolarity and hypotension
E. No change in osmolarity and hypertension
F. No change in osmolarity and hypotension

116. Which of the following is expected to happen after intravenous infusion of 0.5 liters of a 3% saline solution in a healthy adult male?

A. Decreased androgen synthesis
B. Decreased atrial natriuretic peptide synthesis
C. Increased aldosterone synthesis
D. Increased angiotensin synthesis
E. Increased antidiuretic hormone synthesis

117. An individual adjusted to a tropical climate loses 2 liters of fluid in sweat in a short period of time. Which of the following choices best describes the changes from normal that occur in the secretion of aldosterone, atrial natriuretic peptide (ANP), and antidiuretic hormone (ADH), as well as changes to urine osmolarity and Na^+ excretion?

	Aldosterone	ANP	ADH	Urine osmolarity	Na+ excretion
A.	↑	↑	↓	↓	↓
B.	↑	↓	↔	↔	↑
C.	↑	↓	↑	↑	↓
D.	↓	↑	↔	↑	↑
E.	↓	↓	↑	↔	↓
F.	↓	↑	↓	↓	↑

118. A group of college students has a contest to see who can drink 2 liters of water the fastest. They all finish the water in less than 10 minutes. Twenty minutes later, which of the following changes are most likely in the brainstem vasomotor (cardiac accelerator) center, the hypothalamic thirst center, and organum vasculosum of the lamina terminalis (OVLT)?

	Vasomotor center	Thirst center	OVLT activity
A	↑	↓	↑
B	↑	↑	↓
C	↑	↑	↑
D	↓	↓	↑
E	↓	↑	↓
F	↓	↓	↓

119. A tourist in Belize develops a severe case of diarrhea, with 8–10 L of watery stools per day. On examination, her mucous membranes are dry, her jugular veins are flat, she appears pale, and her skin is cool and clammy to the touch. Her blood pressure is 90/60 mm Hg while lying supine but drops to 60/40 mm Hg when standing upright. Her heart rate is 120 beats per minute. Respirations are deep and rapid at 26 breaths per minute. Which of the following renal characteristics would be expected to be increased in this person?

A. Collecting duct sodium channels
B. Blood flow through the vasa recta
C. Renal sodium excretion
D. Renal tubule flow rate
E. Renal urea excretion

120. A 31-year-old woman develops food poisoning. For 12 hours she has repeated vomiting and profuse diarrheal attacks and is unable to keep any fluid down. She is weak and dizzy on standing and is admitted to the hospital. Which of the following sets of pulse rate (pulse), blood pressure (BP), plasma and urine sodium (Na^+) concentration and urine osmolality would be expected in this patient?

	Supine		Standing		Plasma	Urine	
	Pulse (bpm)	BP (mm Hg)	Pulse (bpm)	PB (mm Hg)	Na^+ (mEq/L)	Na^+ (mEq/L/24 hr)	Osmolality (mOsm/kg H_2O)
A.	120	80/65	120	80/65	130	12	400
B.	100	120/80	100	120/80	150	140	900
C.	120	80/65	100	120/80	130	140	900
D.	100	120/80	120	80/65	130	12	900
E.	120	80/65	100	120/80	130	140	400
F.	100	120/80	120	80/65	150	12	400

121. An 8-year-old girl presents with muscle cramps and constipation. If it were due to a mild hypokalemia, which of the following is the most likely reason affecting the internal K^+ balance?

A. β-adrenergic antagonist
B. Insulin injection
C. Metabolic acidosis
D. Plasma hyperosmolarity
E. Renin release

Questions 122 to 123

A 48-year-old woman with insulin-dependent diabetes mellitus reports to her physician with nausea, leg weakness, and finger numbness. She is being treated for hypertension and congestive heart failure with propranolol, a β-adrenergic antagonist. She has previously been diagnosed with stage 3 kidney failure.

122. When checking the patient's electrolyte status, which of the following condition is most likely expected?

A. Hypercalcemia
B. Hyperkalemia
C. Hypomagnesemia
D. Hypophosphatemia
E. Hypouremia

123. After careful analysis, the medical care for this patient includes the following list of interventions: insulin, glucose, sodium bicarbonate, a β_2 adrenergic agonist, plus one additional. Which of the following is the most likely one?

A. Aldosterone receptor antagonist
B. Carbonic anhydrase inhibitor
C. Mannitol injection
D. Saline solution IV
E. Thiazide diuretic

124. A patient with renal failure develops symptoms of fatigue, elevated heart rate, pale skin and mucous membranes, and dizziness. These symptoms are most likely caused by the loss of which substance that is normally produced in the kidneys?

A. Bicarbonate
B. Erythropoietin
C. Prostaglandins
D. Renin
E. Vitamin D

7.8 Answers and Explanations

98. Correct: 6, 6, 9 (E)

For divalent ions, one millimole equals two milliequivalents, so 3 mM (millimolar) Mg^{2+} translates into 6 mEq/L. For monovalent ions, one millimole equals one milliequivalent, so that 3 mM Cl^- translates into 3 mEq/L. Since $MgCl_2$ dissociates into two sets of 3 mM Cl^-, this number has to be multiplied by 2, or 6 mEq/L of Cl^-. The osmolarity of a 3 mM $MgCl_2$ solution is its concentration (3 mM) times the number of the three osmotically active particles: 3 × 3 = 9 mOsm/L.

99. Correct: 125 ml (B)

(**B**) Approximately one-fourth of an administered load of normal saline remains in the vascular compartment. Approximately three-fourths diffuses into the interstitial space. Because its osmolality is close to that of plasma, normal saline entirely remains in the extracellular space, so it is widely considered as a good plasma volume expander. (**A, C, D, E**) These estimates are not correct.

100. Correct: 15 (C)

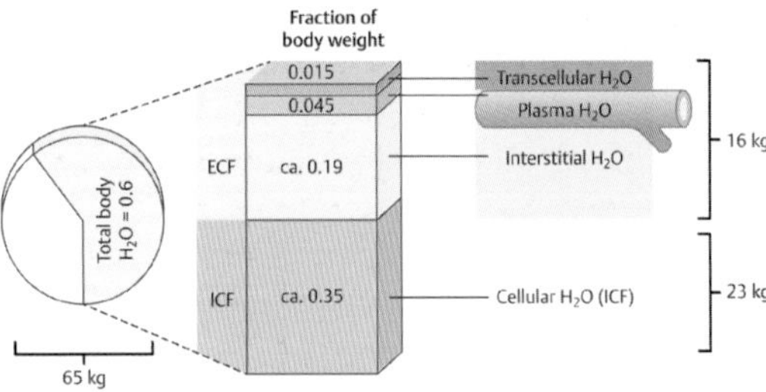

Since inulin does not cross cell membranes, it equilibrates in the extracellular fluid. Using the formula "Volume = amount/concentration" leads to 150 mg/(10 mg/L) = 15 L. This is a typical ECF volume for a lean young adult person as seen in the image (**A, B, D, E**) are incorrect choices.

101. Correct: The plasma volume is smaller (D)

Evans blue is a tracer for plasma volume, since it avidly binds to albumin. When the dye is dissolved in an isotonic solution such as 0.9% saline, there will be no compartmental fluid shift, and the color intensity is inversely related to plasma volume. When a blue solution is added to a large volume of plasma, the plasma color barely changes. When a blue solution is added to a small volume of plasma, plasma becomes blue. For direct comparisons, measurements need to be made at a given time after dye injection, since physiologically a small fraction of intravascular albumin passes to the interstitial space per unit time. (**A**) If the plasma volume of the second person were larger, the Evans blue solution would be more dilute compared to the first person. (**B, C, E, F**). Evans blue is a tracer substance for plasma, so there are no color changes in the interstitial or intracellular fluid compartments and no conclusions about their volumes can be drawn.

102. Correct: Hypotonic volume expansion (D)

Adding fluid without excretion leads to body fluid volume expansion. Mannitol is small enough to diffuse throughout the extracellular fluid (ECF), so ECF volume increases (see image). On the other hand, mannitol is large enough not to cross cell membranes and act as an osmotically active particle. The solution must have been hypotonic, since ECF osmolality decreased (see image, $[Na^+]\downarrow$). Intracellular fluid (ICF) volume increased and ICF osmolality decreased (see image, $[K^+]\downarrow$), as water shifted into cells along the osmotic gradient, until equilibrium between ICF and ECF had been reached. Plasma protein concentration decreased due to the increase in ECF volume. (**A, C, E**) Volume contraction is a decrease in the volume of body fluids, which is not the case after adding a mannitol solution. (**B**) In the case of a hypertonic mannitol solution, ECF and ICF osmolality would have been increased and ICF volume would have been decreased as water shifted from ICF to ECF. (**F**) In the case of an isotonic mannitol solution, there would have been no water and osmolality changes in the ICF.

103. Correct: 45.7, 14.4, 31.3 (D)

D_2O is used to measure total body water (TBW):

TBW = (Amount of D_2O injected – Amount of D_2O excreted)/[D_2O]
= [200 mCi – (20% of 200 mCi)]/(3.5 mCi/L)
= [200 mCi – 40 mCi]/(3.5 mCi/L)
= 160 mCi/(3.5 mCi/L) = 45.7 L

Mannitol is used to measure extracellular volume (ECF):

ECF = (Amount of mannitol injected – Amount of mannitol excreted)/[mannitol]
= [400 mg – (10% of 400 mg)]/(25 mg/L)
= [400 mg – 40 mg]/(25 mg/L)
= 360 mg/(25 mg/L) = 14.4 L
Intracellular fluid volume (ICF) = TBW – ECF = 45.7 L – 14.4 L = 31.3 L

104. Correct: C (C)

A 0.25% sodium chloride solution is hypotonic. It may be used as hydration fluid to dilute the intracellular concentration of hemoglobin and avoid red blood cell sickling. The patient will have a decrease in plasma osmolarity due to the infusion of the hypotonic solution, an increased extracellular fluid (ECF) due to the infusion of 1 L of fluid, and increase in intracellular fluid (ICF) due to osmosis of the hypotonic solution. (**A**) Box A represents an increase in ICF and ECF, with no change in plasma osmolarity. (**B**) Box B represents an increase in ECF, with no change in ICF or plasma osmolarity. (**D**) Box D represents an increase in ECF, a decrease in ICF, and an increase in plasma osmolarity. (**E**) Box E represents a decrease in ICF and ECF, with an increase in plasma osmolarity.

105. Correct: Sodium Chloride, 3% (E)

A 3% sodium chloride solution is hypertonic (513 mEq Na^+ and 513 mEq Cl^- → 1,026 mOsm/L). When added to the intravascular fluid compartment, it equilibrates with the interstitial fluid compartment. This extra solute in the extracellular fluid compartment (ECF) will cause water to move from the intracellular fluid compartment (ICF) to the ECF, so there will be a fluid expansion of more than 2 L. (**A, B, D**) A 5% dextrose solution (280 mM → 280 mOsm/L), lactated Ringer's (130 mEq Na^+, 4 mEq K^+, 3 mEq Ca^{2+}, 109 mEq Cl^-, 28 mEq lactate → 273 mOsm/L), and 0.9% sodium chloride (154 mEq Na^+ and 154 mEq Cl^- → 308 mOsm/L) are all isotonic (correction by the osmotic coefficient has been neglected), so that the 2 liters will remain in the ECF without any water shifts from the ICF. (**C**) Half-normal saline, or 0.45% NaCl, is hypotonic (clinically defined as a solution with an electrolyte content less than 250 mEq/L). When administered intravenously, some of the ECF will move to the ICF and less than 2 liters will remain.

106. Correct: D (D)

Box D represents an increase in extracellular fluid (ECF), a decrease in intracellular fluid (ICF), and an increase in plasma osmolarity. The patient will have an increase in plasma osmolarity due to the inability to excrete the normal solute load in the urine, and an increased ECF due to the inability to excrete water in the urine. The ICF will be reduced because water will move from the intracellular space to the extracellular space due to osmosis. (**A**) Box A represents an increase in ICF and ECF, with no change in plasma osmolarity. (**B**) Box B represents an increase in ECF, with no change in ICF or plasma osmolarity. (**C**) Box C represents an increase in ICF and ECF, with a decrease in plasma osmolarity. (**E**) Box E represents a decrease in ICF and ECF, with an increase in plasma osmolarity.

107. Correct: Uremia (E)

Plasma urea would be increased due to the reduced ability of the kidneys to filter the blood and excrete urine. (**A**) Kidney dysfunction causes imbalances in electrolytes, especially potassium, phosphorus, and calcium. High potassium (hyperkalemia), not hypokalemia, is a particular concern. (**B, D**) Blood volume and plasma sodium would be increased (not decreased) due to the reduced ability of the kidneys to filter the blood and excrete water and solutes in the urine. (**C**) Inability of failing kidneys to excrete phosphorus causes its levels in the blood to rise, not decrease.

108. Correct: Suffering from 21β-hydroxylase deficiency (D)

21β-hydroxylase deficiency, in its most common form, leads to salt wasting due to decreased aldosterone levels, which make the kidneys excrete more NaCl than water. Consequently, extracellular fluid (ECF) volume and ECF osmolality decrease, further augmented by a shift of water into the intracellular fluid (ICF). The hematocrit (Hct) increases. (**A**) The syndrome of inappropriate release of antidiuretic hormone (SIADH) leads to excessive renal water reabsorption, resulting in an increase of ECF volume, decrease of ECF osmolality, and dilution of red blood cells. On the other hand, fluid shifts from ECF into ICF, increasing the volume of red blood cells. The Hct is unchanged due the two offsetting effects. (**B**) Congestive heart failure leads to fluid retention and fluid expansion. ECF volume increases, and Hct decreases. (**C**) Excess intake of salt, here as pickled vegetables, leads to increased ECF osmolality, increased thirst, and, as a consequence, increased ECF volume, augmented by fluid shift from ICF to ECF. Hct is decreased. (**E**) Sweating leads to ECF volume loss and increased ECF osmolality, since sweat is hypotonic. This leads to fluid shifts from ICF to ECF. Thus, the concentration of red blood cells in blood increases and their cellular volume decreases, with the result that Hct remains unchanged.

109. Correct: Increased secretion of K^+ in the collecting duct (B)

In the collecting duct, high levels of potassium can be secreted if needed (up to 180%), as in the case of a high-potassium diet. This is where the primary regulation of potassium secretion occurs. Urine that is high in potassium can directly (or indirectly via sensory neuron excitation) lead to depolarization of the bladder wall detrusor muscle membrane. This results in random muscle contractions and urge incontinence. (**A, E**) Only ~ 20% of potassium is reabsorbed by the loop of Henle, but little or none is secreted there. (**C**) Potassium is secreted by principal cells that are present in the late (not early) distal tubule. (**D**) Approximately 67% of filtered potassium is reabsorbed in the proximal tubule, and the handling of potassium in the proximal tubule is not impacted by a high-potassium diet.

110. Correct: 0.33 (B)

The filtered load of Na^+ can be determined as 1 mEq/min, by multiplying plasma Na^+ concentration (0.2 mEq/mL) with GFR as determined by inulin clearance (5 mL/min). The proximal tubule is responsible for about 67% of Na^+ reabsorption, while the descending limb of the loop of Henle is relatively impermeable to solutes. Hence, the predicted Na^+ remaining in the tubular fluid at the end of the descending limb of the loop of Henle is 33%, or 0.33 mEq/min. (**A, C, D, E**) These results are incorrect.

111. Correct: Excessive vomiting (D)

There are several mechanisms that contribute to hypokalemia after excessive vomiting: First, the loss of gastric acid (HCl) leads to hypochloremic (loss of Cl^-) metabolic alkalosis (initially, loss of H^+ leaves HCO_3^- in blood unbalanced; maintained by volume contraction). To compensate for alkalosis, protons are shifted out of cells in exchange for K^+. Second, volume contraction increases aldosterone, which increases K^+ secretion by renal principal cells. Third, K^+ is enriched in gastric juice compared to plasma, so that there is a direct net loss during vomiting. (**A, E**) ACE inhibitors decrease aldosterone, and hypoaldosteronism can lead to hyperkalemia (not hypokalemia). (**B**) β receptor blockers shift K^+ out of cells by decreasing the activity of Na-K-ATPase. Hyperkalemia might ensue. (**C**) The classic and most common form of congenital adrenal hyperplasia due to *CYP21A* mutation leads to low aldosterone levels, which results in hyperkalemia (not hypokalemia). (**F**) Traumatic rhabdomyolysis is caused by injury to skeletal muscle and leakage of cellular content into blood. Leakage of intracellular K^+ causes hyperkalemia, which is augmented by backup of K^+ in serum due to injured kidneys. Kidneys become injured by released myoglobin, which directly and indirectly damages renal tubules.

112. Correct: Glomerular hydrostatic pressure (C)

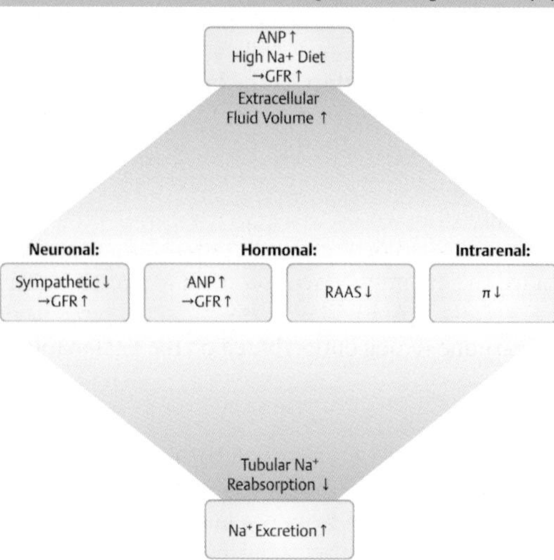

To maintain normal sodium balance after high sodium intake (no weight change), nervous, hormonal, and intrarenal mechanisms operate together to suppress sodium-retaining systems and to activate natriuretic systems (image). The only increase is in glomerular hydrostatic pressure (P_{GC}) and, consequently, glomerular filtration rate (GFR). Increased P_{GC} is a result of both decreased sympathetic activity (via dilation of afferent arterioles) and increased atrial natriuretic peptide (ANP, via constriction of efferent arterioles). These neuronal and hormonal responses are part of reactions that start with the activation of pressure receptors by the increased extracellular fluid (ECF) volume in response to the high sodium intake. (**A, B**) The renin-angiotensin-aldosterone system (RAAS) is decreased (not increased) in response to the woman's ECF volume expansion. Decreased RAAS contributes to sodium homeostasis, because it decreases Na^+ reabsorption in the proximal tubule and collecting ducts and hence increases Na^+ excretion. (**D**) Increases in ECF volume decrease (not increase) peritubular capillary oncotic pressure (π) via dilution. This pressure decrease contributes to sodium homeostasis in the woman by inhibiting proximal tubule Na^+ reabsorption. (**E**) Sympathetic nerve activity is decreased (not increased) in the brainstem in response to activation of low-pressure receptor reflexes.

113. Correct: Parathyroid hormone (D)

This patient has bilateral kidney stones. The most common types of kidney stones contain calcium oxalate, which can form when phosphate levels are low, due to a more acidic environment. Parathyroid hormone (PTH) inhibits the Na^+-dependent transporter for phosphate in the proximal tubule, so an increase in plasma PTH will increase phosphate excretion in the urine, causing hypophosphatemia. (**A, B, C, E**) Aldosterone, angiotensin II, antidiuretic hormone, and renin have little impact on typical kidney stone development.

114. Correct: A thiazide diuretic (C)

A thiazide diuretic is helpful since it decreases urinary Ca^{2+} excretion. The diuretic inhibits the Na-Cl cotransporter, which reduces Na^+ influx into the renal epithelial cells. The resulting intracellular negativity increases the driving force for Ca^{2+} reabsorption through calcium channel TRPV5. A thiazide diuretic may also increase the activity of the basolateral Ca-Na exchange, thus fostering Ca^{2+} reabsorption through a steeper transcellular Ca^{2+} gradient. (**A**) A high-oxalate diet is not helpful, since oxalate is excreted in urine, where it readily forms crystals with calcium and increases the likelihood of kidney stone formation. Diet normally contributes about half of human oxalate; the rest is from metabolism. (**B**) "Steroid medicine" refers to glucocorticosteroids, which can be part of cancer treatment. When taken at high dose, or for a long time, they lead to bone loss by increasing apoptosis of osteoblasts and inhibiting their proliferation/differentiation. This is counterproductive when bone metastases are most likely the cause of hypercalciuria. (**D**) In general, severe restriction of dietary calcium intake has not been proven beneficial for hypercalciuria. In particular, patients with advanced cancer commonly suffer from appetite and weight loss, so that palliative care aims at supporting any food intake. (**E**) Vitamin D increases gastrointestinal calcium absorption, augmenting (not alleviating) hypercalciuria. It is proposed that it also mobilizes calcium from bone, but this role at physiologic/pharmacologic concentrations is still unclear.

115. Correct: Increased serum osmolarity and hypotension (D)

Both increased serum osmolarity and decreased blood pressure are adequate stimuli for the release of antidiuretic hormone (ADH) from the posterior pituitary into blood. Both are indications of low blood volume. The high serum osmolarity is usually caused by a higher concentration of solutes in a smaller volume of blood, and low blood volume causes hypotension. (**A, B, C, E, F**) These choices include only one or no stimulus to increase ADH release. In the case that there are conflicting triggers such as increased osmolarity and volume expansion (i.e., blood pressure increase); the osmolarity signal is more powerful and ADH would increase.

116. Correct: Increased antidiuretic hormone synthesis (E)

Synthesis of antidiuretic hormone (ADH) is increased in response to hypothalamic osmoreceptors that sense the increased extracellular osmolality after infusion of a hypertonic solution. Hyperosmolality is a more powerful stimulus than the increase in blood volume, which inhibits ADH release, so that overall ADH increases. (**A**) Hydration and serum osmolality have no measureable effects on androgen production. (**B**) Atrial natriuretic peptide would be increased, not decreased, due to stretching of the atrial wall by increased blood volume. (**C, D**) Increased blood volume inhibits (not increases) renin, angiotensin, and aldosterone synthesis.

117. Correct: ↑, ↓, ↑, ↑, ↓ (C)

Excessive sweating causes volume contraction, which stimulates the renin-angiotensin-aldosterone system. Increased aldosterone will increase Na^+ reabsorption in the distal nephron, leading to a decrease in Na^+ excretion in urine (column 5). This is further supported by angiotensin II, which increases proximal Na^+ reabsorption, and there is an increased fractional Na^+ reabsorption due to the altered Starling forces (increased colloid pressure and decreased hydrostatic pressure) in peritubular capillaries. A decrease in blood volume will decrease atrial natriuretic peptide (ANP). Sweat is hypotonic to plasma. Hence, excessive sweating causes hyperosmotic dehydration. The increase in plasma osmolarity will induce ADH release, thus increasing water reabsorption in the distal nephron, which will produce a more concentrated urine (increased urine osmolarity). (**A, B, D, E**) Each of these choices has an incorrect set of answer choices.

118. Correct: ↓, ↓, ↓ (F)

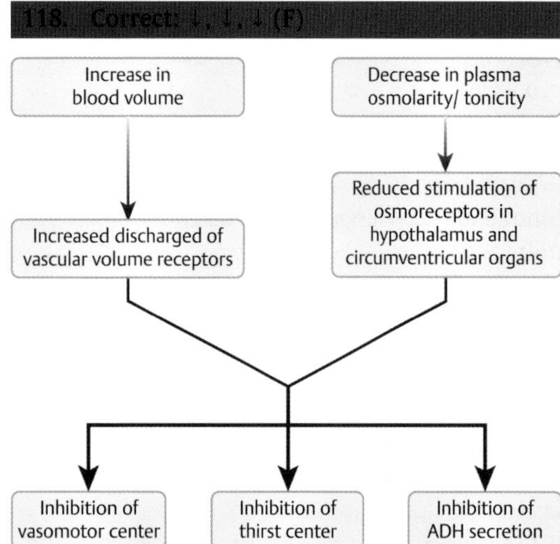

The water will appear in the bloodstream within minutes and be completely absorbed within an hour or so. More than one-fourth of the water will remain in the blood vessels and elevate blood volume (image). The activity of stretch-sensitive vascular baroreceptors will be increased and a neural cascade will be initiated, which leads to the activation of the cardioinhibitory (cardiac decelerator) center and the inhibition of the vasomotor (cardiac accelerator) center in the brainstem. The ultimate result is decreased heart rate, cardiac contractility, systemic vascular resistance, and venous elastance. The decreased plasma osmolarity/tonicity is recognized by osmoreceptors in the brain, which reduces the activity of the thirst center (groups of not well-defined osmo-sensitive hypothalamic neurons). The primary osmoreceptors that inhibit the release of antidiuretic hormone (ADH) lie outside of the blood-brain barrier in one of the circumventricular organs called the organum vasculosum of the lamina terminalis (OVLT). (**A–E**) All of these answer choices have at least one wrong option based on the explanation.

119. Correct: Collecting duct sodium channels (A)

This person is severely dehydrated (hypotensive, sympathetic activity) due to severe fluid loss from diarrhea. This activates several sodium-retaining mechanisms in the kidney. One is the activation of the renin-angiotensin-aldosterone system (RAAS), which leads to aldosterone release. Aldosterone stimulates the insertion of sodium channels on the apical membrane of the aldosterone-sensitive distal part of the nephron and the collecting duct, so sodium reabsorption is increased. (**B, D**) The extreme amount of fluid loss will override renal autoregulatory mechanisms, so that blood flow through the vasa recta and fluid flow through the renal tubule will be decreased (not increased). (**C**) Renal sodium excretion will be decreased, mediated by multiple sodium-retaining renal tubular mechanisms. (**D**) Antidiuretic hormone will increase the deposition of urea in the renal interstitium, so that renal urea excretion will decrease (not increase).

120. Correct: 100, 120/80, 120, 80/65, 130, 12, 900 (D)

The woman experiences hypovolemia and orthostatic hypotension. In the supine position her blood pressure is normal, but it drops when standing, since gravity pools blood in leg and trunk veins and the blood pressure regulatory systems are overwhelmed. Pulse is inversely related to blood pressure, so it is lower when supine, then increases on standing when blood pressure drops, as a compensatory mechanism to maintain blood pressure. With severe dehydration from persistent vomiting and diarrhea, fluid and electrolyte loss can lead to hyponatremia (plasma sodium < 135 mEq/L). While multiple sodium-retaining mechanisms will be activated, the plasma Na^+ concentration will not overshoot (i.e., > 145 mEq/L). Urine sodium concentration will be very low (normal 40–220 mEq/L/24 h) due to the Na^+ loss in vomit and stools and the activated renal Na^+-retaining mechanisms. After 12 hours of fluid intake restriction (or inability to keep fluids down in this patient's case), the urine osmolality will exceed 850 mOsm/kg of water due to the effects of the urine-concentrating function of antidiuretic hormone. (**A, B, C, E, F**) Each of these choices has an incorrect set of answer choices.

121. Correct: Insulin injection (B)

The internal K^+ balance consists of the short-term regulation of total body K^+ by altering the distribution between extracellular fluid (ECF) and intracellular fluid (ICF). This is distinguished from the external K^+ balance, which consists of the long-term regulation of body K^+ stores, primarily through renal K^+ excretion. Insulin binds to insulin receptors on cells and activates GLUT4 transporters, which transport glucose into the cell. This increases ATP production, which powers the Na-K pump, which moves K^+ into the cell, affecting the internal K^+ balance. (**A**) β-adrenergic receptors on cells utilize a cAMP-dependent signaling cascade to activate Na-K pumps, which increases intracellular K^+. Hence, antagonizing those receptors inhibits this action. (**C**) In metabolic acidosis, more than one-half of the excess hydrogen ions are buffered inside cells. Electroneutrality is maintained in part by the movement of K^+ from ICF to ECF, potentially resulting in hyperkalemia. (**D**) Plasma hyperosmolarity shifts K^+ out of cells as part of the water flow moving from ICF to ECF. (**E**) Renin release leads to aldosterone release, which, when in excess, can lead to hypokalemia by affecting the external (not internal) K^+ balance.

122. Correct: Hyperkalemia (B)

There are multiple physiological mechanisms that favor hyperkalemia in the woman. First, low insulin activity (insulin is not produced in type 1 and is used improperly by the body in type 2 diabetes mellitus) might lead to hyperkalemia, since insulin shifts K^+ into body cells. Second, hypertension leads to low renin and consequently low production of aldosterone, which minimizes K^+ secretion by renal principal cells. Third, nonselective β blockers such as propranolol block β_1 adrenoceptor-mediated renin release. Additionally, they decrease uptake of K^+ into all body cells via β_2 adrenoceptor-mediated effects. While neither mechanism alone necessarily leads to hyperkalemia, they make it more likely in patients with moderate renal failure who cannot excrete K^+ properly. (**A**) Hypo- (not hyper-) calcemia is likely to be present in moderate renal failure due to decreased renal production of 1,25-dihydroxycholecalciferol (calcitriol, or active vitamin D). Serum Ca^{2+} can be normal due to increased Ca^{2+} release from bone, but never high. (**C**) Renal handling of magnesium is highly adaptable, and plasma Mg^{2+} levels often remain normal until end-stage renal disease. Then, typically hyper- (not hypo-) magnesemia is seen. (**D**) Hyper- (not hypo-) phosphatemia is a common complication of the loss of renal function due to the reduction in glomerular filtration and renal excretion. (**E**) Elevated (not decreased) serum urea concentration is a hallmark of prerenal chronic kidney disease.

123. Correct: Thiazide diuretic (E)

It should be recognized that the three prescribed medical interventions target hyperkalemia by moving K^+ into the intracellular space: insulin (glucose is given to avoid hypoglycemia) and β_2 agonists shift K^+ into cells by increasing the activity of Na-K-ATPase. Sodium bicarbonate treats metabolic acidosis, which occurs when K^+ is exchanged with H^+ across cell membranes. Since intracellular K^+ storage is transient, some form of treatment to remove K^+ from the body is also required. This can be done by a thiazide diuretic since it leads to increased renal K^+ excretion. (**A**) Aldosterone receptor antagonists belong to the category of K^+-sparing diuretics, which are indicated for diuresis when loss of body K^+ is unwanted. (**B**) A carbonic anhydrase inhibitor increases bicarbonate excretion, which is counterproductive for a patient with susceptibility to metabolic acidosis due to hyperkalemia. (**C**) Mannitol injection as diuretic is incorrect, because hyperosmolarity favors hyperkalemia. It can be understood as K^+ exiting cells together with water along the osmotic gradient. (**D**) Isotonic volume expansion is not indicated in a hypertensive person with diminished renal excretory ability.

124. Correct: Erythropoietin (B)

The patient experiences classic symptoms of anemia, which are most likely caused by the loss of erythropoietin, the renal hormone that promotes the normal production of red blood cells. (**A**) Bicarbonate is not produced, but rather reabsorbed, in the kidney. Moreover, a loss in bicarbonate would present with acidosis. (**C**) Loss of renal prostaglandins would impair local vasodilation and potentially accelerate the progression of renal failure, but it cannot be directly linked to anemia. (**D**) Renin activates the renin-angiotensin-aldosterone systems, so a loss of renin leads to hyporeninemic hypoaldosteronism. This is not the best answer, since it would lead to hyperkalemia and acidosis (not anemia per se). (**E**) Loss of active vitamin D due to renal failure leads to secondary hyperparathyroidism and fragile bones.

7.9 Questions

125. A 71-year-old man experiencing chest pain and difficulty breathing waited 4 hours before finally calling 911 for help. The man was diagnosed with acute myocardial infarction and was hypotensive for several hours following the infarction. Over the next week, his urine output decreased and plasma creatinine increased. He underwent hemodialysis, and his urine output gradually returned to normal. Which of the following substances was most likely responsible for the initial elevation in plasma creatinine and decrease in urine output?

A. Antidiuretic hormone
B. Atrial natriuretic peptide
C. Endothelin
D. Erythropoietin
E. Renin

126. A 78-year-old man presented with a hematocrit of 55%, and at repeat testing one month later with a hematocrit of 61%. At that time, laboratory studies showed elevated plasma erythropoietin levels. Which of the following could have caused this elevation?

A. Experiencing polycythemia vera
B. Renal loss of plasma proteins
C. Suffering chronic kidney disease
D. Taking a hypoxia-inducible factor inhibitor
E. Taking an HIF prolyl hydroxylase inhibitor

7.10 Answers and Explanations

125. Correct: Endothelin (C)

This patient experienced acute kidney failure with tubular necrosis (ATN) from the period of hypotension following his myocardial infarction. The hypotension reduced renal perfusion, causing damage to the nephron endothelial cells, which reduced the amount of nitric oxide and prostaglandins (vasodilators) and increased the release of endothelin (a vasoconstrictor). Vasoconstriction of the renal vasculature reduces renal blood flow, glomerular filtration rate, and therefore urine output, which in turn reduces creatinine clearance and increases plasma creatinine. (A, E) Antidiuretic hormone and renin would decrease urine output, but would not affect plasma creatinine. (**B**) Atrial natriuretic peptide would increase urine output. (**D**) Erythropoietin would increase red blood cell production and not affect urine output or plasma creatinine.

126. Correct: Taking a HIF prolyl-hydroxylase inhibitor (E)

The adequate trigger for erythropoietin (EPO) production in kidney is systemic hypoxia. Central mediators of this process are the hypoxia inducible factors HIF-1 and HIF-2. When hydroxylated, they are targeted for degradation, so that inhibition of HIF prolyl hydroxylase stabilizes HIF. This leads to elevated EPO levels, increased erythropoiesis, and increased hematocrit. (**A**) In polycythemia vera, the presence of a neoplastic blood disorder increases the number of red blood cells, which results in compensatory suppression (not elevation) of EPO. (**B**) The presence of abnormal quantities of protein in urine indicates renal disease or excessive production of small proteins that cannot be handled by the kidney. In the first case, EPO would be decreased; in the second case, EPO would be normal (not increased). (**C**) In chronic kidney disease renal synthesis of EPO is decreased (not increased) due to loss of functional renal mass, resulting in anemia, not polycythemia. (**D**) HIF inhibitors (prospective anticancer drugs) decrease (not increase) erythropoietin expression.

7.11 Questions

127. Which of the following is a characteristic of intrarenal (or intrinsic) acute kidney injury?

A. Decreased fractional excretion of sodium
B. Decreased serum BUN to creatinine ratio
C. Difficulty urinating, flank pain, and blood in urine
D. Extracellular volume depletion
E. Urine production of 1 L per day

128. You attend to three patients with acute renal injury. Patient 1 has a history of lupus erythematosus and presents with peripheral edema, hypertension, proteinuria, and hematuria. Patient 2 has a history of enlarged prostate and presents with fever, lower back pain, and trouble urinating. Patient 3 has a history of congestive heart failure and presents with a blood pressure of 90/60 mm Hg, a pulse of 110 bpm, dizziness, and fatigue. The patient's renal plasma flow and glomerular filtration rate are substantially reduced.

Based on the signs and symptoms, what type of acute renal injury does each patient most likely have?

	Prerenal acute renal injury	Intrarenal acute renal injury	Postrenal acute renal injury
A.	Patient 1	Patient 3	Patient 2
B.	Patient 1	Patient 2	Patient 3
C.	Patient 2	Patient 3	Patient 1
D.	Patient 2	Patient 1	Patient 3
E.	Patient 3	Patient 2	Patient 1
F.	Patient 3	Patient 1	Patient 2

129. Which of the following best characterizes the presentation of a patient with prerenal acute kidney injury due to decreased kidney perfusion?

	Renal blood flow	Glomerular filtration rate	Angiotensin ii	Catecholamines	Fractional excretion of sodium	Serum BUN to creatinine ratio
A.	↑	↑	↑	↑	↓	↑
B.	↓	↓	↓	↓	↑	↓
C.	↓	↓	↑	↔	↓	↔
D.	↓	↓	↓	↔	↑	↔
E.	↓	↓	↑	↑	↓	↑

130. A 16-year-old boy living in the United States developed pain in his knee while playing soccer. The boy's physical examination showed high blood pressure, stress fractures, anemia, elevated BUN, and elevated serum creatinine. Renal ultrasonography revealed kidney scarring. Serum electrolytes were as follows:

Sodium:	160 mEq/L
Potassium:	4.0 mEq/L
Chloride	105 mEq/L
Calcium (total):	10 mg/dL
Phosphorus:	10 mg/dL

A diagnosis of genetic reflux nephropathy was made. The treatment included antibiotics and careful monitoring of kidney function. He was advised not to play heavy sports for some time and counseled for his diet. The dietary recommendation for the young man most likely included the use of which of the following?

A. Calcium salt
B. Iodized table salt
C. Pickling salt
D. Potassium salt
E. Sea salt

131. A third-year resident joins the hospital morning rounds late, after the presentation of the history of a 76-year-old man was already completed. The patient's physical exam showed tachycardia, lung rales, and pitting edema on extremities. His laboratory assessment included hypernatremia, hyperalbuminemia, elevated BUN, and elevated serum creatinine. The renal function tests were remarkable for decreased FENa and decreased FEUrea. From the following choices, which is the most likely history of the patient that resulted in his clinical presentation?

A. Benign prostatic hypertrophy
B. Congestive heart failure
C. Hepatitis B
D. High-dose chemotherapy
E. Renal colic

132. As part of perioperative fluid therapy, a patient receives an infusion of D5 $^{1}/_{2}$NS at a rate of 100 mL/hour. Extensive blood analysis before the operation was normal. The patient's urinary output is averaging only 35 mL/hour 1 day after the operation, so the fluid infusion rate is increased to 125 mL/hour. Nevertheless, urine output declines to 20 mL/hour 2 days after the operation and to 15 mL/hour 3 days after the operation. At day 3, the following laboratory values are obtained:

Urine:

Na^+ concentration:	85 mEq/L

Blood:

pH	7.25
Pco_2	30 mm Hg
HCO_3^-	15 mEq/L
K^+	5.8 mEq/L
Phosphate	10 mg/dL
BUN	90 mg/ dL
Creatinine	9 mg/dL

Which of the following is the most likely diagnosis?

A. Acute kidney injury
B. Excessive sodium intake
C. Fluid volume deficit
D. Gastrointestinal bleeding
E. Prerenal disease

133. A 68-year-old woman is diagnosed with stage 3 chronic kidney disease. Her daily excretion of acid is measured as 50 mEq/d. Based on her diet, she generates about 70 mEq of acid per day. Her serum bicarbonate level is 24 mEq/L and remains stable. From the following choices, which next test or treatment makes the most sense?

A. Collect a stool sample
B. Don't respond for now
C. Infuse potassium
D. Order a bone scan
E. Prescribe an aldosterone blocker

134. A 62-year-old woman with chronic kidney disease feels a vague abdominal pain. Laboratory investigation indicates that her glomerular filtration rate is 40 mL/min, serum bicarbonate is 15 mEq/L, and serum pH is 7.20. Which of the following best describes the cause of her acidosis?

A. Impaired ability to excrete metabolic acids
B. Increased production of uric acid
C. Increased renal synthesis and excretion of ammonia
D. Lack of respiratory compensation
E. Reduced production of new bicarbonate

135. A 63-year-old African American man presents with generalized fatigue and lethargy. He has powdery white deposits on his skin. For the past 10 years, he has suffered from hypertension. Laboratory studies show a normochromic, normocytic anemia. Estimated glomerular filtration rate is 20 mL/min/1.73 m^2. The white skin deposits are identified as urea-containing crystals. Which of the following sets of additional serum findings will most likely be present in this patient?

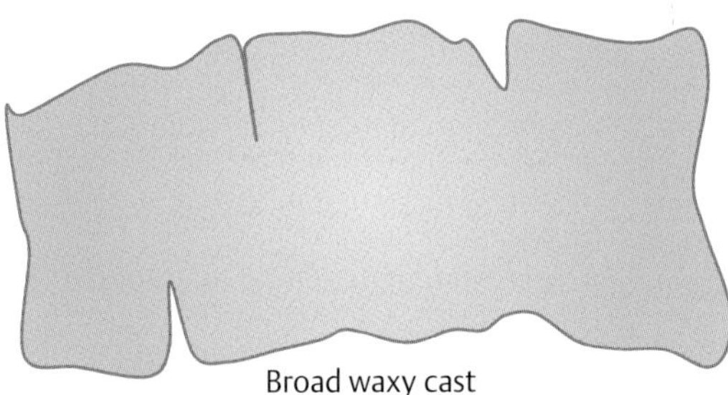
Broad waxy cast

	Serum phosphorus	1,25-Dihydroxycholecalciferol	Erythropoietin	Urinary casts (image)
A.	↑	↓	↑	↓
B.	↑	↑	↓	↓
C.	↓	↓	↓	↑
D.	↓	↓	↓	↑
E.	↑	↓	↓	↑

7.12 Answers and Explanations

127. Correct: Decreased serum BUN to creatinine ratio (B)

Intrarenal, or intrinsic, acute kidney injury (for instance, due to toxins, ischemia, or nephritis) leads to tubular damage, which prevents reabsorption of urea, so that the serum BUN to creatinine ratio is decreased, as compared to a normal ratio in a healthy kidney or in postrenal kidney disease. (**A**) Fractional excretion of Na^+ is increased (not decreased), since the tubular damage prevents Na^+ reabsorption and a higher fraction of filtered load is present in urine. (**C**) Difficulty urinating, flank pain, and blood in urine are characteristic signs of postrenal kidney injury due to an obstruction in the urinary tract below the kidney. They may be part of intrarenal injury but are not characteristic. (**D**) Intrarenal kidney injury is due to damage to the kidney itself, not due to damage as a result of extracellular volume depletion and insufficient kidney perfusion. (**E**) One liter (~ 34 oz) of urine per day is within the normal range (0.8 to 2 L) for an adult drinking 2 liters of fluid.

128. Correct: Patient 3, patient 1, patient 2 (F)

Prerenal acute renal injury results from conditions outside of the kidney that reduce blood flow to the kidney. Patient 3 has congestive heart failure, which fits this category. Intrarenal acute renal injury results from conditions inside the kidney that reduce kidney function. Patient 1 has lupus, which is an autoimmune disease that attacks tissues in the body, including in the kidneys, and affects renal function. Postrenal acute renal injury results from obstruction in the urinary tract system. Patient 2 has an enlarged prostate, which obstructs the urethra and causes urine backup into the kidney, and thus acute renal injury. (**A, B, C, D, E**) Each of these answer choices has at least one wrong answer.

129. Correct: ↓, ↓, ↑, ↑, ↓, ↑ (E)

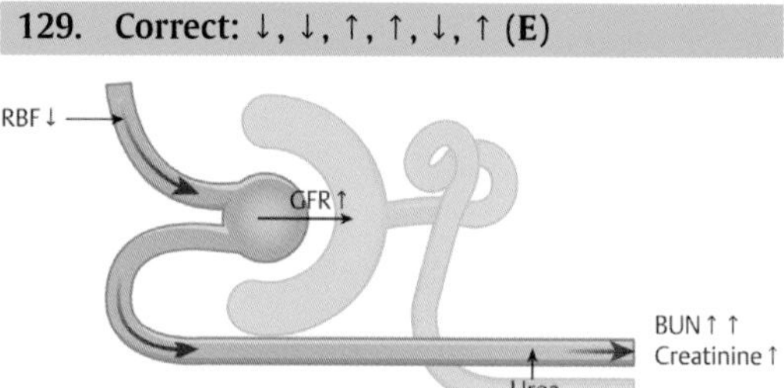

The most common cause of prerenal acute kidney injury is decreased perfusion such as caused by excessive diarrhea, vomiting, or congestive heart failure. Hence, renal blood flow (RBF) and glomerular filtration rate (GFR) are decreased. Angiotensin II (AngII) and catecholamine (Cat) releases are increased in response to the low effective arterial blood volume. Both lead to increased filtration fraction, which increases oncotic pressure of peritubular capillaries (π_C). This, together with the decrease in peritubular capillary hydrostatic pressure (P_C), increases proximal tubular Na^+ reabsorption as a body compensatory response. Fractional excretion of Na^+ (FENa) is decreased, since fractional Na^+ reabsorption is increased in response to the altered Starling forces (increased π_C and decreased P_C). Serum BUN: creatinine (BUN:Cr) ratio is increased since the increased fractional reabsorption of Na^+ concomitantly increases the passive reabsorption of urea. As a consequence, blood urea nitrogen increases proportionally more in blood than creatinine does (image). It is important to note that the table shows changes that led to kidney injury (RBF, GFR), as well as changes that reflect the body's response to prevent kidney injury as long as possible (AngII, Cat, FENa, BUN:Cr). (**A, B, C, D**) These answers have one or more incorrect changes.

130. Correct: Calcium salt (A)

The use of calcium salt is recommended, despite the fact that serum Ca^{2+} levels are normal. This is to replenish depleted body Ca^{2+} stores and, more importantly, to bind dietary phosphate and lower gastrointestinal phosphate reabsorption. The rationale is as follows: The heightened activity level of the adolescent boy in the presence of genetic reflux nephropathy (urine backflow into the ureter instead of outflow through the urethra) led to kidney injury (Na^+ retention and hypertension), as well as anemia due to low erythropoietin. Elevated BUN and serum creatinine indicate a substantial decrease in glomerular filtration. This leads to a backup of phosphorus, which inhibits renal 1-alpha hydroxylase. Low activity of the enzyme leads to low amounts of vitamin D (1,25-dihydroxycholecalciferol). Low vitamin D leads to insufficient gastrointestinal Ca^{2+} reabsorption and parathyroid hormone–induced Ca^{2+} release from bone. The consequences are stress fractures and pain. (**B**) Iodized table salt (NaCl), the most commonly used salt, is contraindicated when hypertension is present. (**C**) Pickling salt is also NaCl and thus contraindicated. In comparison to table salt, it has no additives, such as iodide or anticaking agents. (**D**) Potassium salt is not the best choice since serum potassium is normal. While a healthy kidney can deal with a wide range of dietary K^+, it makes no sense to challenge the boy's stressed kidney. (**E**) Sea salt is produced from evaporation of seawater. It includes a variety of electrolytes, of which about one-third are in the form of sodium salts. This makes it inappropriate for a patient with Na^+ retention.

131. Correct: Congestive heart failure (B)

In the presence of azotemia (elevated BUN and serum creatinine), renal diagnostic indices such as the fractional excretion (FE) of Na^+ and urea help to establish whether it is due to prerenal, intrarenal, or postrenal causes. Decreased FENa and FEUrea point toward a prerenal problem, which decreases blood flow to the kidneys. Congestive heart failure (supported by the evidence of tachycardia and pulmonary and systemic edema) best fits this description. The decrease in effective arterial blood volume (EABV) activates baroreceptor reflexes, which lead to sympathetic activation and multiple kidney mechanisms that attempt to restore EABV: Sympathetic nerve activity increases salt reabsorption directly (not well understood) and indirectly by stimulating renin release, which results in angiotensin II and aldosterone release and their support mechanisms for salt and water reabsorption. Sympathetic-induced vasoconstriction of afferent and, to a somewhat lesser degree, efferent arterioles decreases renal plasma flow and to a lesser extent glomerular filtration, which results in increased filtration fraction and increased sodium reabsorption via Starling forces. All these and other mechanisms, such as antidiuretic hormone (ADH) release, lead to increased reabsorption of salt, water, urea, and creatinine, so their excreted amount in relation to their filtered amount decreases. (**A, E**) Benign prostatic hypertrophy and renal colic can cause postrenal azotemia since the obstruction of flow by external pressure from the prostate tissue or by renal stones leads to increased hydrostatic pressure in the Bowman's capsule and opposes glomerular filtration. Most important diagnostics of this condition, such as anuria and pain, are missing, making postrenal kidney injury not the best choice. (**C**, **D**) The hepatitis B virus and high-dose chemotherapy and the hepatitis B virus are well known to cause damage to the kidney itself, which leads to high (not low) FENa and FEUrea. Glomerular and/or tubular damage leads to functional decline in the ability of the nephrons to filter and reabsorb substances, so Na^+ and urea are lost in urine.

132. Correct: Acute kidney injury.

The fall in urine output, the increase in blood creatinine and urea nitrogen, and the presence of hyperkalemia (> 5.5 mEq/L) and hyperphosphatemia (> 4.5 mEq/L) all point to acute kidney injury. Metabolic acidosis (low pH, HCO_3^-, and Pco_2) develops in response to the decreased ability for acid excretion, together with the increased acid production due to perioperative ischemia. (**B**) Half normal saline ($^1/_2$NS) contains 77 mEq/L of Na^+, which equals 231 mEq of Na^+ intake per day (77 multiplied by 3 L/d). This is higher than the recommended intake of 100 mEq/d, but it is not high enough to justify kidney injury, considering an average daily intake of 150 to 250 mEq/d on a Western diet. (**C**) If the high serum values of K^+, phosphate, BUN, and creatinine stemmed from fluid volume deficit, the kidneys would maximally preserve Na^+ and a very small amount (< 20 mEq/L) would be present in urine. (**D**) Gastrointestinal bleeding could explain the elevated BUN due to absorbed blood proteins but not account for other findings such as oliguria or increased creatinine. (**E**) Typical signs of prerenal disease secondary to volume depletion are low (not high) urine sodium concentration and increased (not normal) serum BUN: creatinine ratio. Moreover, adequate fluid therapy (5% dextrose in half-normal saline is a typical maintenance fluid in surgical units) would be expected to reverse the signs of volume depletion.

133. Correct: Order a bone scan (D)

The woman has a net acid gain, since 20 mEq per day are not excreted by her failing kidneys. The normal serum HCO_3^- levels indicate that the extra acid thus far has been buffered. Large amounts of skeletal bicarbonate buffers are present in bone. This could lead to bone demineralization in a woman who is, agewise, susceptible to osteoporosis. A bone scan is justified. (**A**) The gastrointestinal tract is not compensating for systemic acid-base imbalances by excreting acid in stools. (**B**) Chronic metabolic acidosis is a serious concern in the management of chronic kidney disease, which aims at slowing down the progression toward end-stage renal disease. (**C**) Metabolic acidosis can lead to hyperkalemia, since K^+ leaves cells in exchange for H^+ that is intracellularly buffered. Serum K^+ may be normal or even decreased due to renal loss by an injured kidney. Without laboratory values, K^+ infusion is not a good next treatment. (**E**) An aldosterone antagonist belongs to the class of K^+-sparing diuretics. First, there is no immediate need for a diuretic, and second, the choice would depend on the assessment of her total body K^+ stores.

134. Correct: Impaired ability to excrete metabolic acids (A)

Acidosis develops in chronic kidney disease (CKD) because the kidney cannot excrete the acids produced by metabolism of food. This is primarily due to reduced renal production and secretion of ammonia, the most important mechanism to replenish serum bicarbonate buffer. (**B**) Uric acid is the byproduct of purine nucleotide catabolism. CKD is not linked to excessive breakdown of DNA or RNA. (**C**) Ammonia production and secretion is reduced in CKD, not increased, primarily due to loss of functional renal mass. (**D**) The lungs are compensating for the metabolic acidosis by blowing off CO_2, but this is not sufficient to fix the acid-base imbalance. (**E**) Bicarbonate production is not reduced, but it is being used as a buffer for the excess acid from metabolism; thus levels are low.

135. Correct: ↑, ↓, ↓, ↑ (E)

The patient suffers from advanced kidney disease, as indicated by the severe decrease in glomerular filtration rate and uremic frost. The latter is caused by nitrogen waste products that are secreted by sweat glands and crystalize on the skin. Chronic hypertension points towards chronic kidney disease, which presents with the following common features: Hyperphosphatemia due to a decreased filtered load of phosphorus; bone disease due to decreased synthesis of 1,25-dihydroxycholecalciferol, leading to secondary hyperparathyroidism; and normochromic, normocytic anemia due to decreased renal synthesis of erythropoietin. These are consequences of the decreased number of functioning nephrons. In the remaining functioning nephrons, tubules become dilated, which favors cast formation in the distal convoluted tubules or the collecting ducts. When casts remain in the nephron for some time due to the low urine output, they become granular and ultimately waxy. The image, as part of the question, shows the form of a broad waxy cast, typical for end-stage chronic renal disease. (A, B, C, D) These choices have one or more unlikely findings.

Chapter 8

Gastrointestinal System

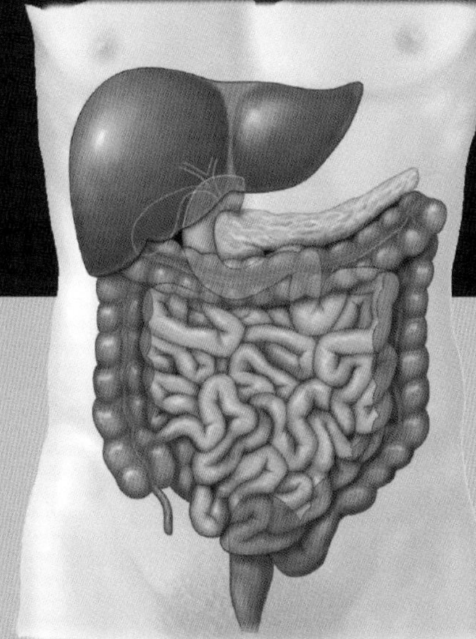

LEARNING OBJECTIVES

- Understand the structure of the gastrointestinal tract and how it is regulated by neurotransmitters, neuropeptides, and peptide hormones.
- Describe the roles of the mouth, esophagus, and stomach in regards to motility, secretions, and digestion and absorption. Use basic science principles related to these gastrointestinal sections to interpret common diseases and appropriate therapeutic approaches.
- Describe the roles of the small and large intestine in regards to motility, secretions, and digestion and absorption. Be able to apply general basic science processes to common gastrointestinal disorders and their treatments.
- Describe the major secretions of the exocrine pancreas and understand their functions and regulation. Explain the role of the liver for fat and bilirubin metabolism. Describe the composition of bile, the role of bile acids and salts, and the importance of the enterohepatic circulation.

8.1 Questions

Easy	Medium	Hard

1. A patient has a family history of multiple endocrine neoplasia type 1 (MEN1). Since he has suffered from abdominal pain for several months and experienced dark stool, an exploratory abdominal computed tomography (CT) scan was performed. A small pancreatic/duodenal mass was seen. His urine output was normal, and glucose was absent from urine. Serum potassium and glucose were normal. If the tumor were a functional islet cell tumor, what is the most likely initial diagnosis?

A. Gastrinoma
B. Glucagonoma
C. Insulinoma
D. Pancreatic polypeptidoma
E. Somatostatinoma

2. Gastrin gene knockout (GAS-KO) mice do not produce gastrin-17 ("little gastrin") in response to food. As a direct consequence, which of the following substances will most likely be diminished in these animals?

A. Amino acids
B. Bile acids
C. Fatty acids
D. Hydrochloric acid

3. A patient presents with intermittent symptoms of chronic diarrhea, steatorrhea, vomiting blood, abdominal pain, and weight loss for weeks. He does not respond to various antacid treatments. There is no history of significant nonsteroidal anti-inflammatory use. He tests negative of Helicobacter pylori and hypoglycemia. The suspicion of a gastrinoma arises. Tests confirm basal gastric acid hypersecretion and high levels of blood gastrin. What is the most likely cause of these findings?

A. A functional neoplasm in the antrum
B. A secreting beta-cell islet tumor
C. Atrophy of fundal gastric epithelium
D. High blood levels of secretin
E. Excess short chain fatty acids in stool

4. A horse with a primarily brown coat had a normal pregnancy but delivered an all-white foal. The veterinarian recognizes it as a genetic disease caused by the mutation of the endothelin receptor type B gene, which in humans causes Hirschsprung's disease. Assuming that the resultant gastrointestinal abnormalities in horses and humans are alike, without intervention, the foal will die from the lack of which of the following activities?

A. Colonic circular muscle contraction
B. Enteric inhibitory motor function
C. Gastroileal reflex
D. Receptive relaxation
E. Retrograde colonic movement

5. A 35-year-old obese female presents with a chief complaint of nonradiating epigastric abdominal pain and nausea. Her social history is significant for moderate alcohol use, excessive caffeine intake, and smoking one pack of cigarettes daily. Her medical history reveals that she has been taking nonsteroidal anti-inflammatory drugs (NSAIDs) for the past 3 months for a knee sprain. She also keeps a large supply of antacid tablets (histamine receptor blockers) at her bedside. She wears a hormone-releasing patch to avoid pregnancy. The abundance of independent disease risk factors from her history lead to an initial diagnosis of gastroesophageal reflux disease. The mechanism of which of the following risk factors is correctly described?

A. Antacid tablets, since hypochlorhydria may worsen acid reflux
B. Being obese, since a high body mass index lowers intragastric pressure
C. Contraceptive patch, since progestins weaken lower esophageal sphincter tone
D. Nicotine and caffeine, since they stiffen lower esophageal sphincter muscles
E. NSAIDs, since they cause dizziness so that patients frequently lie down

6. A patient with irritable bowel syndrome has written down information that he found when browsing public resources related to the disease. His physician supports which of the following statements regarding the enteric nervous system?

A. It contains as many neurons as present in the adult healthy brain.
B. It is present in the gastrointestinal tract from the esophagus to the anus.
C. Its ganglia are directly innervated by the central nervous system.
D. Its myenteric plexus primarily control secretion and absorption.
E. Its neurons are either postganglionic sympathetic or parasympathetic neurons.

7. A hiker consumes a mushroom containing the poisonous alkaloid muscarine. One hour later she begins to exhibit clinical signs of mushroom poisoning. Which of the following is the most likely sign of this poisoning?

A. Blood vomiting
B. Bradycardia
C. Dry mouth
D. Flatulence
E. Hypochlorhydria

8. A 32-year-old male patient presents with severe chronic abdominal pain and steatorrhea. His basal secretion rate of gastric acid is 12 mmol/hr (normal 1–5 mmol/hr). His serum gastrin level is 1,213 pg/mL (normal 50–150 pg/mL). After a test meal, the gastrin level does not increase significantly. He is scheduled for upper gastrointestinal endoscopy and a computed tomography (CT) scan. In the meantime, a pharmacologic antagonist of which of the following agents would make the most clinical sense to alleviate the symptoms?

A. Cyclooxygenase
B. Histamine
C. Prostaglandin
D. Secretin
E. Somatostatin

9. In search of novel acid-neutralizing compounds, a therapeutic peptide is injected intravenously in dogs; then pancreatic sodium bicarbonate secretion is measured in the presence and absence of additional vagal stimulation. The results are shown in the image and resemble the normal humoral response of a natural peptide. The drug peptide is most likely an analogue of which of the following natural peptides?

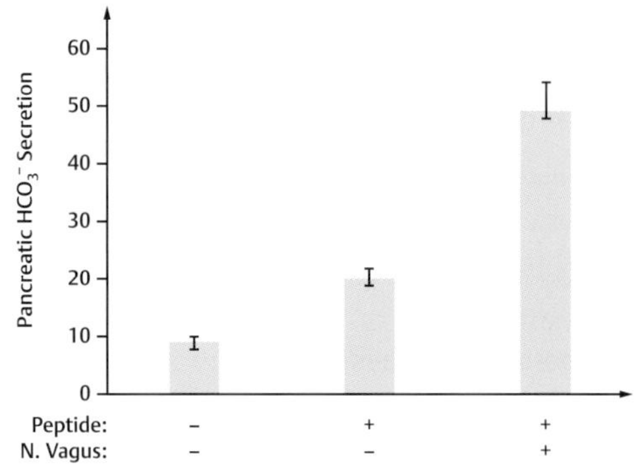

A. Gastrin
B. Gastrin-releasing peptide
C. Enkephalin
D. Secretin
E. Vasoactive intestinal peptide

10. Which of the following hormones is produced in the duodenum in response to digestion products and stimulates the pancreas in a true hormonal fashion to produce an enzyme-rich secretion?

A. Cholecystokinin
B. Gastrin
C. Glucose-dependent insulinotropic peptide
D. Secretin
E. Vasoactive intestinal peptide
F. Pancreatic polypeptide

11. The following diagram shows a bowel portion with rhythmic segmentation, which results from the collaborative action of an intestinal smooth muscle layer and the rhythmic activity of inhibitory neurons. If 1, 2, and 3 represent three inhibitory enteric neurons, which of the following neurons is currently inactive?

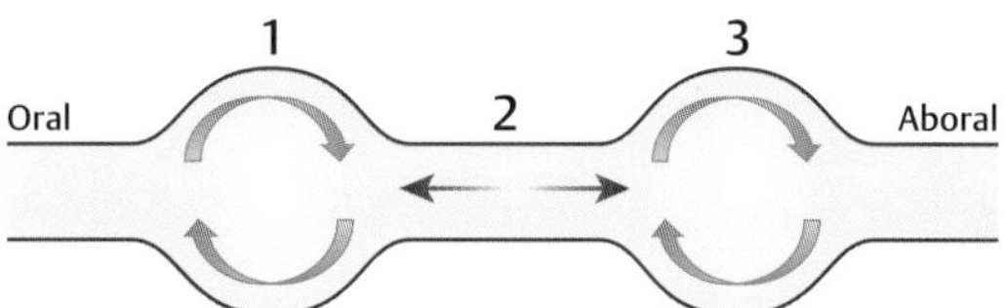

A. 1 and 2
B. 2 only
C. 2 and 3
D. 1 and 3
E. 1, 2, and 3

12. An investigator researches the acid production of the stomach in response to ingestion of distinct foods/drinks and certain behaviors. For which of the following situations does she record the lowest production of stomach acid?

A. Binging on low-alcohol beer
B. Craving a delicious apple pie
C. Dieting with high-protein shakes
D. Drinking a jar of cranberry juice
E. Eating ten hot dogs in five minutes
F. Having an espresso coffee

13. A 36-year-old man has a plasma level of vasoactive intestinal peptide (VIP) of 50 times the normal value. The patient most likely suffers from which of the following?

A. Hyperchloremic metabolic acidosis
B. Hyperkalemic metabolic acidosis
C. Hypochloremic metabolic acidosis
D. Hypochloremic metabolic alkalosis
E. Hypokalemic metabolic alkalosis

14. A newspaper is running an article on diabetes mellitus type 2. The reporter calls a physician to get input on GIP, formerly known as gastric inhibitory peptide. Which of the following is a true statement that can be printed about GIP?

A. It increases in serum in response to insulin.
B. It is released into the duodenum in the presence of food.
C. It is structurally related to gastrin and cholecystokinin.
D. Its degradation is inhibited by an oral anti-diabetic drug.
E. Its release is strongly stimulated by soy proteins.

15. Which of the following is expected to be directly diminished in gastrin gene knockout mice in response to food?

A. Acetylcholine
B. Cholecystokinin
C. Gastrin-releasing peptide
D. Histamine
E. Somatostatin

16. A 5-year-old child is diagnosed with pyloric stenosis due to the complete absence of electrical slow waves at the gastroduodenal junction. The pediatric gastroenterologist explains to the parents that in the bowel section where food transits from the stomach to the small intestine, a certain type of cell that initiates motility is missing. Which of the following is most likely the missing cell type?

A. Enteric mast cells
B. Enteroendocrine cells
C. Interstitial cells of Cajal
D. Parietal cells
E. Secretomotor neurons

17. In patients with clinical suspicion of Zollinger-Ellison syndrome (gastrin-secreting tumor), a positive secretin stimulation test supports the diagnosis. The test is positive when there is a quick and substantial increase in serum gastrin upon secretin injection. The behavior of the gastrin-producing tumor cells in regards to gastrin release compares to the physiological response of normal gastrin-producing cells in which of the following ways?

A. It is different since they are stimulated by secretin.
B. It is different since they respond to serum secretin.
C. It is similar except they respond significantly faster.
D. It is similar except they respond significantly stronger.
E. It is similar except that their response is less predictable.

18. An 18-year-old man severs his spinal cord at T5 in an automobile accident. When a mass movement propels bowel contents from the colon into the rectum, which of the following actions in the rectum and anus will occur in this patient?

	Contraction of the rectum	Relaxation of the internal anal sphincter	Contraction of the external anal sphincter
A.	No	Yes	No
B.	No	No	Yes
C.	Yes	No	Yes
D.	Yes	Yes	No
E.	Yes	Yes	Yes

19. In a patient with long-standing gastrointestinal problems, an electrode was implanted on the serosal surface of the upper jejunum at the time when the patient was undergoing surgery for removal of the gall bladder. After recovery from surgery, the electrode records slow waves at a frequency of 11 per minute. A manometric sensor was then used to measure the frequency of peristaltic contractile events per minute at the site of the implanted electrode. Which of the following is the number of contractions per minute that would be interpreted as normal physiologic activity?

A. 0 without food
B. 11 and lower
C. Exactly 11 at any time
D. 11 and higher at any time
E. 11 and higher with food

20. A newborn has a grossly distended abdomen, fails to pass meconium (earliest stool) within the first 48 hours of life, and vomits repeatedly. Analysis of a rectal biopsy provides a diagnosis of Hirschsprung's disease. The absence of which type of cell in the biopsy is diagnostic?

A. Capillary endothelial cells
B. Enteric ganglion cells
C. Lymphatic endothelial cells
D. Red blood cells
E. Smooth muscle cells

21. A 72-year-old retiree presents with constipation and hard stool. She describes it "like sausage but with cracks on the surface." Her past history includes chronic essential hypertension, tachycardia, hypothyroidism, and acid reflux, for which she takes various medications. Which of the following medication categories is the most likely to cause her constipation if it were due to a drug-induced inhibition of intestinal motility?

A. Antihypothyroid medications
B. Cholinergic agonists
C. L-type calcium channel blockers
D. Proton pump inhibitors
E. Thiazide diuretics

22. A 25-year-old medical student eats a fast food meal with a cheeseburger, french fries, and a chocolate shake. This meal stimulates the release of a hormone that is secreted by duodenal and jejunal K cells in response to carbohydrate and fat digestion products. Which of the following is the most likely hormone?

A. Cholecystokinin
B. Gastrin
C. GIP (Glucose-dependent insulinotropic peptide)
D. Motilin
E. Secretin

8.2 Answers and Explanations

Easy	Medium	Hard

1. Correct: Gastrinoma (A)

The pancreatic islet cell tumor cells are most likely producing gastrin, which leads to ulcers (blood in stool) and abdominal pain. About one-fourth of Zollinger-Ellison-type gastrinomas are linked to multiple endocrine neoplasia type 1. (**B**) Lack of glucosuria makes an alpha cell tumor, producing glucagon, unlikely. (**C**) Lack of hypoglycemia makes a beta cell tumor, producing insulin, unlikely. (**D**) While pancreatic endocrine tumors often release pancreatic polypeptide (PP), excess PP is not related to any clinical symptoms. Hence, without measuring serum PP, an initial diagnosis cannot be made. (**E**) A tumor producing somatostatin inhibits the secretion of many hormones, among them insulin. This leads in most patients to the development of diabetes mellitus, which is not supported by normal glucose values.

2. Correct: Hydrochloric acid (D)

The 17-amino-acid-long gastrin-17 (G17) is the classical gastrin that is released by antral G cells, in order to stimulate hydrochloric acid secretion from parietal cells directly and indirectly. It is also called little gastrin to distinguish it from the 34-amino-acid-form (G34, or big gastrin), which is more frequently released by duodenal rather than gastric cells. (**A**) While the lack of acidity and concomitant lower amount of pepsin would somewhat diminish protein digestion and amino acid production in the stomach, the intestinal phase of protein digestion is more relevant physiologically. Hence, an amino acid shortage as a direct consequence of achlorhydria is not expected in mice (and not seen in people). (**B, C**) Cholecystokinin (not gastrin) shortage could lead to diminished presence of bile acids and fatty acids.

3. Correct: High blood levels of secretin (D)

Hypersecretion of gastrin causes excess stomach acid secretion which acidifies the duodenum. This strongly stimulates secretin release, and as a result, excessive gastrointestinal secretions may lead to chronic diarrhea. The patient's pain and vomiting of blood are due to ulcers. His weight loss is due to maldigestion. (**A, B**) Excess gastrin production that fails to respond to a variety of antacid treatments strongly suggests an extrinsic (not antral) gastrinoma. These often occur by pancreatic islet cells that are not beta cells. The lack of hypoglycemia due to hyperinsulinemia further supports a non-beta cell tumor. (**C**) Gastrin causes hypertrophy (not atrophy) of parietal and other gastric epithelial cells. (**E**) Steatorrhea is due to the presence of undigested fat (not digested fat products such as fatty acids).

4. Correct: Enteric inhibitory motor function (B)

Hirschsprung's disease (HD) causes problems with passing stool due to the congenital lack of enteric ganglion cells in the large intestine. The most common (type 2) form of the disease affects only the last part of the colon and is caused by a mutation of the endothelin receptor type B gene. The normal function of colonic enteric neurons is to inhibit circular smooth muscle contraction, and the lack of this inhibition causes continuous constriction. Lethal white syndrome (LWS) is the analogous disease in horses. Without intervention, the foal will die from the inability to pass feces. (**A**) HD/LWS results in continuous (not lacking) colonic circular muscle contraction, since the whole GI tract functions as a self-excitable electrical syncytium due to the presence of pacemaker cells and gap junctions between cells. (**C**) The gastroileal reflex, which is initiated by food in the stomach and leads to peristalsis in the ileum, is still present in HD/LWS. (**D**) Receptive relaxation, the ability of a gastrointestinal section to expand with only slightly increasing intraluminal pressure, is a characteristic of the orad stomach, not the large intestine. (**E**) Some retrograde movement in the colon is normal, and the lack of it would increase colonic transit rate, opposite to HD/LWS.

5. Correct: Contraceptive patch, since progestins weaken lower esophageal sphincter tone (C)

Progestins are synthetic progestogens, substances that bind to and activate the progesterone receptor. They are known to worsen heartburn and gastroesophageal reflux disease (GERD), partly by weakening the lower esophageal sphincter tone. Estrogens are also linked to the disease, but the major underlying mechanism is not yet fully understood. (**A**) Antacid tablets cause hypochlorhydria, which alleviates acid reflux. They are a common type of medication taken by heartburn sufferers. (**B**) Obesity increases the risk of GERD, at least partly by increasing (not decreasing) intragastric pressure. (**D**) Nicotine and caffeine are known to relax smooth muscle and hence weaken (not stiffen) lower esophageal sphincter muscles. (**E**) While NSAIDs can cause dizziness as side effects, it is their ability to cause ulcers that makes them a risk factor for GERD.

6. Correct: It is present in the gastrointestinal tract from the esophagus to the anus. (B)

The enteric nervous system (ENS) is a network of neurons embedded in the wall of the whole gastrointestinal (GI) tract. Dysfunction of enteric neurons can lead to pathologies in any part of the GI tract, from esophageal atresia to slow-transit constipation. (**A**) The ENS contains more than 100 million neurons, which is as much as or more than present in the spinal cord, but about 1,000 times less than present in the adult human brain. (**C**) The two enteric ganglia, the myenteric and submucosal ganglia, receive no direct innervation from the central nervous system (CNS), which is different from the sympathetic and parasympathetic ganglia. (**D**) The neurons of the myenteric plexus primarily control GI motility and sphincter tonus, while the neurons of the submucosal plexus primarily control secretion and absorption. (**E**) The ENS is a separate division of the autonomic nervous system, the other divisions being the sympathetic and parasympathetic. While some enteric neurons are indeed postganglionic parasympathetic neurons, postganglionic sympathetic neurons synapse onto enteric neurons. In addition, there are many more neurons present, including sensory neurons, own standing motor neurons, and interneurons.

7. Correct: Bradycardia (B)

Muscarine is a nonselective agonist for muscarinic acetylcholine receptors and, hence, mimics excessive parasympathetic system (PS) activation. When acting on the heart, it can cause serious bradycardia. Although gastrointestinal (GI) irritations are likely consequences of most food poisoning, vomiting blood due to excessive PS stimulation is unlikely. (**C**) PS activation causes excessive salivation, not a dry mouth. (**D**) Flatulence, or the presence of undigested food in the colon leading to bacterial overgrowth and gas production, is not a likely symptom after PS activation, and if so, would be expected to occur later than 1 hour. (**E**) PS stimulation may lead to excessive GI secretions, not low stomach acid production (hypochlorhydria).

8. Correct: Histamine (B)

Significantly increased gastric acid production and hypergastrinemia that is not altered after a meal suggests Zollinger-Ellison syndrome (ZES). This is different from peptic ulcers that are not caused by a tumor, since they may present with normal acid and/or gastrin production, but gastrin production in response to a meal is typically increased. When a tumor produces too much gastrin (detectable by CT scan), parietal cell mass increases and the stomach produces too much acid. Painful peptic ulcers ensue (detectable by endoscopy). The excess acidity exceeds the duodenal neutralizing capacity, and at a low pH, digestive enzymes and bile malfunction and steatorrhea may ensue. Slowing down acid production (e.g., by a histamine receptor antagonist makes sense until the diagnosis is confirmed). (**A, C**) Blocking the enzyme cyclooxygenase, which forms prostaglandin, or a direct antagonist of prostaglandin would eliminate the inhibitory action on gastric acid secretion and hence not make much sense. (**D**) Blocking secretin would inhibit alkaline secretions that help neutralize the acidity. Moreover, ZES tumor cells respond oppositely to normal cells in regards to gastrin release in that they are stimulated (not inhibited) by secretin. (**E**) An antagonist of somatostatin, a natural inhibitor of acid production and secretion, would not make sense.

9. Correct: Secretin (D)

The novel peptide is most likely an analogue of secretin, whose normal action is to stimulate water and alkali secretions from pancreas and liver, in order to neutralize acid. The aqueous secretion is augmented in the presence of vagal stimulation through both cholinergic muscarinic and noncholinergic transmission. (**A**) Gastrin release is not required for normal pancreatic secretion. (**B, E**) Gastrin-releasing peptide and vasoactive intestinal peptide both stimulate pancreatic exocrine secretion, but they function as neurotransmitters rather than humoral substances. (**C**) Enkephalins typically inhibit gastrointestinal secretion.

10. Correct: Cholecystokinin (A)

Cholecystokinin (CCK) is produced by mucosal cells of the duodenum and jejunum in response to digestion products of fat and protein. When CCK binds to receptors on pancreatic exocrine cells, pancreatic juice that is rich in digestion enzymes is released. (**B**) The main stimulators for gastrin secretion are vagus nerve excitation, distention of the stomach, and protein digestion products. Gastrin promotes acid production and mucosal growth. (**C**) The release of glucose-dependent insulinotropic peptide (GIP) is stimulated by duodenal glucose and leads to insulin secretion. (**D**) The strongest stimulator for secretin release is acidic chyme, and it results in the release of bicarbonate-rich pancreatic juice. (**E**) Vasoactive intestinal peptide indeed stimulates pancreatic secretion; however, it acts as a neurotransmitter in the enteric nervous system and is mainly released by mechanical and neuronal stimulation (not nutrients). (**F**) Pancreatic polypeptide is indeed released by digestion products among other triggers, but it inhibits (not stimulates) pancreatic secretion.

11. Correct: 2 only (B)

One has to first recall that rhythmic segmentation involves the circular muscle layer only, in contrast to peristalsis, which requires both circular and longitudinal smooth muscle. When circular muscles contract, a propulsive segment is created (center of image) that squeezes the luminal content into receiving segments in both directions, oral and aboral (left and right side of image). For circular muscles to contract, inhibitory motor neurons must be turned off. Although the requirement of disinhibition for contraction to occur initially feels like an unusual arrangement, without inhibitory neurons, the whole gastrointestinal tract would continually be in action due to the electrically connected smooth muscle cells. In other words, switching off enteric inhibitory neurons is critical to creating distinct motility patterns. (**A, C, D, E**) Any answer that contains neurons 1 and/or 3 is incorrect, since these inhibitory neurons that innervate receiving segments are turned on in order to avoid contraction of circular muscle.

12. Correct: Drinking a jar of cranberry juice (D)

Cranberry juice is acidic (~pH 2.5). It will lower stomach pH, so somatostatin is released. Somatostatin inhibits acid production by indirectly inhibiting gastrin release and by directly inhibiting parietal cell action. (**A**) Alcoholic beverages with low ethanol content, such as beer, are strong stimulants of gastrin release and gastric acid secretion. (**B**) Craving for delicious food leads to gastric secretion even without food entering the stomach and is called the cephalic phase of gastric secretion. (**C, F**) Protein digestion products and caffeine stimulate G cells to secrete gastrin and stomach acid production. (**E**) Activating stretch receptors by a large amount of ingested food within a short time triggers a reflex that leads to acid release by parietal cells.

13. Correct: Hyperchloremic metabolic acidosis (A)

Very high plasma levels of vasoactive intestinal peptide (VIP) result in severe diarrhea, since VIP is a potent stimulator of gut cyclic adenosine monophosphate (cAMP) production, leading to watery secretions. Biliary, pancreatic, and duodenal secretions are all alkaline in order to neutralize the acidity of gastric secretion. Hence, diarrheal stools have a higher bicarbonate concentration than plasma, with the net result of metabolic acidosis. Gastrointestinal bicarbonate secretion is in exchange for chloride, which is added to blood and favors hyperchloremia. (**B**) Diarrheal volume depletion activates the renin-angiotensin-aldosterone system. In the epithelial cells of the colon, aldosterone initiates sodium uptake from the gut lumen in exchange for potassium secretion, which is taken from blood. Hence, diarrhea leads to hypokalemia (not hyperkalemia), augmented by aldosterone's increased actions at the kidney's principal cells. (C, D, E) Diarrhea leads to excess chloride and shortage of bicarbonate and potassium in blood, as explained.

14. Correct: Its degradation is inhibited by an oral anti-diabetic drug (D)

The main function of glucose-dependent insulinotropic peptide (GIP) is to stimulate insulin release. GIP is rapidly degraded by the enzyme dipeptidyl peptidase 4. DPP-4 inhibitors are a class of anti-diabetic drugs that can be taken orally by type 2 diabetics in order to lower blood glucose via the GIP-induced insulin release. (**A**) GIP triggers insulin release, but the reverse is not true. (**B**) GIP is a hormone and hence released into blood, not the lumen of the gastrointestinal tract. (**C**) It is structurally related to secretin, not to gastrin and cholecystokinin. (**E**) Although release of GIP might be triggered by certain amino acids, the strongest triggers are glucose and long-chain fatty acids, not soy proteins.

15. Correct: Histamine (D)

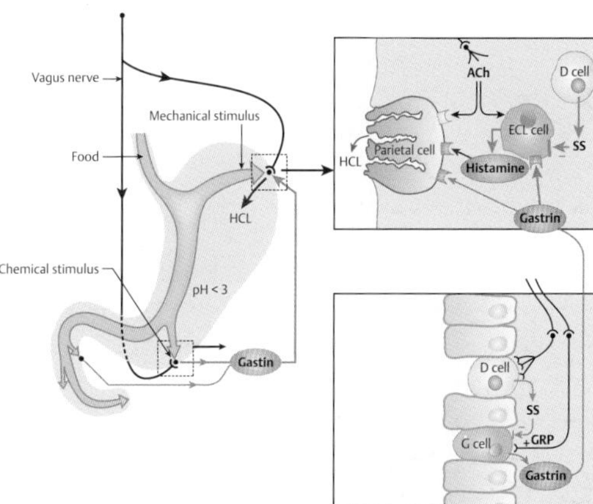

In gastrin gene knockout mice, gastrointestinal G cells cannot produce gastrin (image, lower right). This leads to low histamine release from fundic enterochromaffin-like (ECL) cells (image, upper right), which leads to lower acid production by parietal cells. This gastrin-histamine pathway seems to be the major mechanism for normal stomach acid secretion in response to food. (**A**) Acetylcholine (ACh), the vagal neurotransmitter, binds to parietal cells to induce acid release, independently of gastrin (image, upper right). (**B**) Although cholecystokinin (CCK) is involved in stomach acid regulation, the main stimuli for CCK are fat and protein digestion products, which are still produced in gastrin gene knockout mice. (**C**) Gastrin-releasing pepide (GRP) is an enteric neurotransmitter that stimulates G cells (image, lower right) and should not be affected, even though the G cells cannot produce gastrin. (**E**) Somatostatin (SS) is released by D cells to inhibit gastrin release (image, lower right) and acid secretion (image, upper right), but these mechanims are not directly affected by malfunctioning gastrin genes.

16. Correct: Interstitial cells of Cajal (C)

Slow waves are rhythmically rising and falling membrane potentials that originate in the interstitial cells of Cajal (ICC). From there, the potentials spread to the surrounding smooth muscle cells, where they induce contraction if the membrane potential exceeds a certain threshold and calcium channels are opened. Without the pacemaker activity of ICCs, slow waves will be absent. (**A, B**) Enteric mast cells and enteroendocrine cells communicate with enteric nerves in a paracrine or endocrine fashion through the release of histamine and gastrointestinal peptides. Their lack can affect the amplitude and duration of slow waves but not eliminate them. (**D**) Lack of parietal cells would lead to achlorhydria (lack of stomach acid), not lack of slow waves. (**E**) Secretomotor neurons regulate the movement of water and electrolytes across the gut mucosa. They are part of reflex circuits through which harmful substances are propelled with large amounts of fluid through the gut for fecal excretion. A lack of these cells might alter motility and stool consistency, but not abolish slow waves.

17. Correct: It is different since they are stimulated by secretin. (A)

Under normal physiological conditions, secretin inhibits gastrin release from antral G cells. In the abnormal gastrin-producing cells of patients with Zollinger-Ellison syndrome, secretin stimulates the release of gastrin by modulating adenylate cyclase activation. Hence, the secretin-stimulating test is used to diagnose gastrinomas and distinguish them from other causes of hypergastrinemia. (**B**) Despite the opposite end result in regard to gastrin release, both normal G cells and abnormal gastrinoma cells are responsive to secretin. (**C, D, E**) In regards to gastrin release, the behavior of gastrinoma cells is not similar to the physiological normal behavior of G cells.

18. Correct: Yes, yes, yes (E)

A patient with a spinal cord injury at T5 loses voluntary control of abdominal muscles, but spinal sacral reflexes are still intact, due to the rectrosphincteric reflex. The reflex is triggered by rectal wall distention when a mass movement moves bowel contents into the rectum. It leads to peristaltic contractions in the descending colon, sigmoid colon, and rectum, moving the bowel contents toward the anus. At the same time, the internal anal sphincter relaxes and the external anal sphincter contracts. However, the patient will not be able to sense the fullness of the rectum and hence would be unable to control the external anal sphincter voluntarily (i.e., further contract or relax it to delay or allow defecation). This will lead to both constipation and incontinence in these patients. (**A, B, D, E**) These choices are incorrect for an injury above T5.

19. Correct: 11 and lower (B)

The frequency of slow waves determines the maximal frequency of gastrointestinal contractions. However, only when the amplitude of the slow wave reaches a certain threshold potential there is a muscle contraction. In the presence of inhibitory neurotransmitters, hormones, or paracrine factors, the slow wave threshold might not be reached, in which case no contraction occurs. Hence, there can be fewer than 11 contractions per minute. In the presence of stimulatory neurotransmitters, hormones, or paracrine factors, the amplitude and duration of the slow wave are increased, which translates into more spike potentials on top of the slow wave. This increases the strength of the contractions but not the frequency of the contractions per minute. Hence, there cannot be more than 11 contractions. (**A, C, D, E**) These are incorrect choices based on the explanation.

20. Correct: Enteric ganglion cells (B)

In Hirschsprung's disease, enteric ganglion cells are absent in the myenteric and submucosal plexus. This lack eliminates intrinsic impulses that relax gastrointestinal (GI) smooth muscle, so that extrinsic, mainly GI-constricting stimuli, dominate. The result is obstruction in the affected area, most commonly in the late colon. (**A, C, D, E**) The absence of endothelial cells, red blood cells, or smooth muscle cells is not diagnostic for Hirschsprung's disease.

21. Correct: L-type calcium channel blockers (C)

Calcium channel blockers, typically used as blood pressure medications, inhibit smooth muscle contraction in that they prevent the rise of intracellular calcium. When gastrointestinal (GI) smooth muscle contraction is inhibited, constipation may ensue. (**A**) Since thyroid hormones regulate the metabolic activity of almost every cell, constipation due to smooth muscle hypoactivity is common in patients with hypothyroidism. Antihypothyroid medications would alleviate the symptoms. (**B**) Cholinergic agonists mimic parasympathetic action. They might be prescribed to treat tachycardia and could stimulate (not inhibit) GI smooth muscle activity. (**D**) Proton pump inhibitors inhibit the H^+/K^+-ATPase enzyme system, which inhibits gastric acid production, not intestinal motility. (**E**) Diuretics, independent of the class, may cause constipation due to dehydration, not inhibition of intestinal motility.

22. Correct: GIP (Glucose-dependent insulinotropic peptide) (C)

Glucose-dependent insulinotropic peptide (GIP) is the gastrointestinal hormone whose release by K cells is mediated by the presence of glucose or fatty acids in duodenum and jejunum. GIP leads to insulin release and most likely regulates fat metabolism. (**A**) Cholecystokinin release by I cells is triggered by fat and protein digestion products. (**B**) Gastrin release by G cells is stimulated by protein digestion products. (**D**) Control of motilin secretion by the presence of food is largely unknown. (**E**) Secretin release by S cells is stimulated by fatty acids and acidity.

8.3 Questions

23. Healthy adults were given a high-fat test meal, and the percent of food that remained in the stomach was measured every 20 minutes after meal ingestion. The image shows the average results of control test subjects (red line) and of subjects who were given an experimental drug (blue line) at doses that simulated a normal physiologic response. The drug is most likely a receptor agonist of which of the following gastrointestinal hormones?

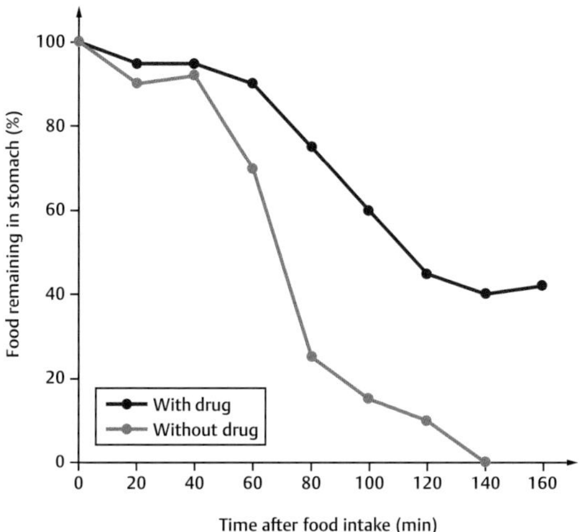

A. Cholecystokinin
B. Gastrin
C. GIP
D. Motilin
E. Secretin

24. The stomach contents of a murder victim are evaluated in a forensic laboratory in an attempt to estimate the time of death. It is found that the chyme has a low pH, a high osmolarity, and a high fat content. Which of these components have to be considered since they contribute to slowing down the emptying of the stomach?

	Acidity	Hyperosmotic solutions	Fatty acids
A.	Yes	Yes	No
B.	Yes	No	No
C.	Yes	Yes	Yes
D.	No	No	Yes
E.	No	Yes	Yes

25. A resident in training for abdominal radiography needs to recall which of the following gastrointestinal motility patterns applies best to the fundus, or orad region, of the stomach in the presence of food.

A. Heavy peristalsis
B. Mixing to homogenous chyme
C. Receptive relaxation
D. Retropulsive motility
E. Rhythmic segmentation

26. A diabetic patient attends an educational session and learns that which of the following delays the emptying of food from the stomach and increases belching?

A. Decreased duodenal motility
B. Decreased pyloric tone
C. Increased motility of the proximal stomach
D. Increased peristalsis of the distal stomach
E. Increased volume of meals

27. A patient is prescribed an anticholinergic drug, with a potential side effect on salivary production, to treat her chronic obstructive pulmonary disease. Which of the following is the most likely side effect experienced by the patient?

A. Bitter taste
B. Dry mouth
C. Gleeking
D. Spitting
E. Weight gain

28. Considering the rate of gastrointestinal (GI) alcohol absorption in a given person, which of the following is most effective in preventing intoxication when ingesting a total alcohol content of 30% (v/v) over 30 minutes?

A. Consuming it in a few shots
B. Drinking a glass of sugar water
C. Drinking high-fat beverages
D. Talking as much as possible
E. Rubbing the abdomen frequently

29. A woman with a body mass index of 45 enrolls in a study measuring postprandial serum levels of hormones involved in regulating hunger and satiety. Which of the following appetite-stimulating hormones or humoral factors is inadequately suppressed in this obese patient after eating?

A. Ghrelin
B. Glucagon-like peptide 1
C. Leptin
D. Neuropeptide Y
E. Peptide YY

30. To better understand episodes of uncontrolled hyperphagia in people with bulimia nervosa, the mechanisms for gastric accommodation are studied. Which of the following is normally the primary stimulus for this receptive relaxation pattern of the stomach?

A. Elevated serum motilin
B. Elevated serum secretin
C. Food in the intestine
D. Food in the stomach
E. Low pH in the stomach

31. A 60-year-old Caucasian man has an immunologic disease that has selectively destroyed the parietal cells of his stomach over several years. Which of the following would be expected for this patient?

A. High plasma secretin levels
B. Low plasma gastrin levels
C. Malnutrition due to inadequate protein digestion
D. Peptic ulcer disease
E. Pernicious anemia

32. A 43-year-old woman complains about an intermittent radiating pain in the left chest for 3 weeks. She also mentions a chronic cough. The pain is more prominent when lying down on her back compared to sitting. At night, she sleeps better with multiple pillows. Symptoms occur shortly after eating spicy food. Examination reveals a white coating on the tongue. Body temperature is 37.2°C; blood pressure 118/83 mm Hg; heart rate 80 beats per minute; and respiratory rate 16 breaths per minute. Heart and lung sounds are normal. The following tests were ordered and all came back normal: electrocardiogram (ECG), exercise stress test, white blood cell (WBC) count, and creatine kinase MB1 (CK-MB1) serum levels. Which of the following conditions is the most likely initial working diagnosis?

A. Congestive heart failure
B. Duodenal ulcer disease
C. Gallstones
D. Gastroesophageal reflux disease
E. Mild myocardial infarction

33. A 59-year-old Caucasian female complains of heartburn after meals and a sour taste in her mouth. The symptoms have become progressively worse over the past six months. Symptoms are worse when she lies down or bends over. The patient occasionally drinks a glass of wine, but does not smoke. She denies dysphagia, vomiting, abdominal pain, melena (blood in stool), and weight loss. Past medical history and family history are noncontributory. On physical exam, her height is 5 feet 6 inches (179 centimeters), and her weight is 220 pounds (100 kilograms), with a "pear-shaped" body type. Her blood pressure is 144/90 mm Hg. All other parameters are unremarkable. Which of the following is most appropriate to consider as treatment?

A. Antagonizing histamine-2 receptors
B. Forming mucosal polymer layers
C. Ingesting inert polymers
D. Inhibiting gastrointestinal motility
E. Suppressing the immune system

34. The digestive action of α-amylase in saliva is favored by which of the following pH ranges?

A. 1 to 10
B. 3 to 6
C. 6 to 7
D. 7 to 10
E. Not pH dependent

35. Excess gastric production of which of the following substances, either directly or indirectly, impairs the stomach's ability to protect itself from the destructive effects of hydrochloric acid?

A. Bicarbonate
B. Intrinsic factor
C. Lipase
D. Mucus
E. Pepsin

36. A 5-week-old baby boy presents to the emergency department with projectile vomiting after each meal for the past 3 days. The physical exam reveals a palpable "olive" in the epigastric region. Which of the following descriptions of the infant's vomit supports the diagnosis of congenital hypertrophic pyloric stenosis?

A. Bright red streaks
B. Coffee-ground
C. Dark red or brown
D. White and milk-like
E. Yellow green

37. A 53-year-old woman with severe duodenal ulcers tests negative for Helicobacter pylori. Her ulcers are recalcitrant to treatment with histamine-2 (H2) receptor blockers. She has no history of significant non-steroidal anti-inflammatory drug (NSAID) use. Tests confirm basal gastric acid hypersecretion and high levels of blood gastrin. Which of the following gastrointestinal sign or symptom is most likely additionally present?

A. Diarrhea due to nonabsorbed food binding water
B. Gastric epithelial atrophy due to high levels of gastrin
C. Pancreatic atrophy due to high levels of secretin
D. Steatorrhea due to excess fecal fat digestion products
E. Stomach pain due to intestinal vitamin B12 malabsorption

38. A group of pigs is used as a human model and are colonized with Helicobacter pylori. The pigs are fed a mixed meal with urea added, and their gastric content is sampled. The samples will likely reveal a change to which of the following measurements, compared to samples from the bacteria-free control pigs?

A. Higher levels of CO_2
B. Higher levels of gastrin
C. Higher levels of somatostatin
D. Lower levels of gastric acid
E. Lower levels of urease

39. The contraction of which of the following muscles aids in the ejection of gastric contents during vomiting?

A. Antral muscles
B. Distal esophageal muscles
C. External intercostal muscles
D. Pectoral muscles
E. Proximal jejunal muscles

40. A 56-year-old man complains of increasing difficulty swallowing over the past 3 years. A radiograph taken after swallowing barium shows a distended esophageal body. A manometric study supports the diagnosis of achalasia. Which of the following correctly describes the physiological changes associated with achalasia?

	Elevated pressure of upper esophageal sphincter	Diminished peristalsis in upper esophagus	Diminished peristalsis in mid to lower esophagus	Elevated pressure of lower esophageal sphincter before swallowing	Incomplete or absence of lower esophageal sphincter relaxation after swallowing
A.	Yes	Yes	No	Yes	Yes
B.	Yes	Yes	Yes	Yes	No
C.	No	No	No	No	No
D	No	No	Yes	Yes	Yes
E.	No	No	Yes	No	No

41. Dogs and cats instinctively lick their wounds, while such behavior in humans is atypical. If humans were to lick their wounds, which of the following constituents of human saliva would be most beneficial?

A. Angiotensin-converting enzyme
B. Lingual lipase
C. Lysozyme
D. Nucleic acids
E. Ptyalin

42. The image depicts a parietal cell. Which of the following correctly identifies the substances labeled X, Y and Z?

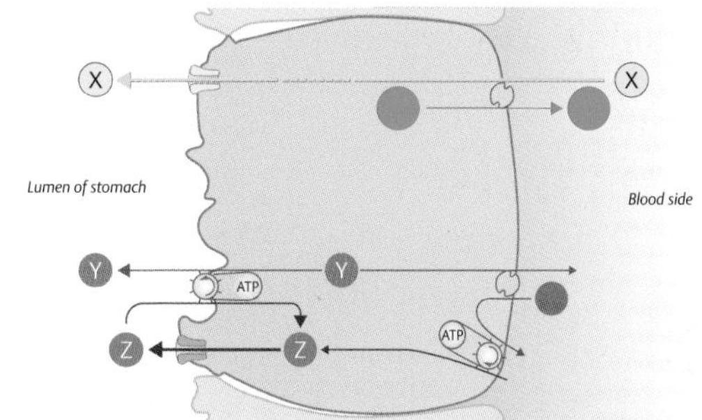

	X	Y	Z
A.	K^+	Na^+	H^+
B.	Cl^-	Na^+	K^+
C.	HCO_3^-	Cl^-	H^+
D.	H^+	Cl^-	Na^+
E.	Cl^-	H^+	K^+

43. Administration of which of the following therapeutic agents most likely leads to increased salivation?

A. Adrenergic receptor antagonist
B. Area postrema chemoreceptor agonist
C. Cholinergic receptor antagonist
D. Na^+-K^+-ATPase inhibitor
E. Secretin analogue

44. The treatment of choice for a 60-year-old man with duodenal ulcers is to inhibit the gastric phase of gastric secretion. From the following, which is the most effective drug category to achieve this?

A. Anticholinergic
B. Antigastrin antibodies
C. H_2 receptor blocker
D. Proton pump inhibitor
E. Prostaglandin E_2
F. Somatostatin

45. Patients with the following diseases all have potential problems with chewing and swallowing. For which of the diseases is a defect in smooth muscle control the cause of the motility problems?

A. Achalasia
B. Amyotrophic lateral sclerosis
C. Multiple sclerosis
D. Parkinson's disease
E. Poliomyelitis

46. A 63-year-old man suffers from chronic dry mouth. He was diagnosed six months ago with a third degree heart block and was prescribed atropine for the associated bradycardia. He is scheduled for a pacemaker. He has not changed his diet recently but admits to being an avid dairy eater. He says that he becomes very tired when walking. He uses a high-fat balm for his cracked lips. Salivary testing indicates that salivary flow does not increase with food intake. History and physical, including blood tests, are otherwise unremarkable. Which of the following is the most likely cause for his lack of saliva production?

A. Atropine
B. Dairy intake
C. Exercise
D. High-fat balm
E. Hypertonic saliva

47. A catheter with a pressure-sensor tip is inserted through the nose of a 79-year-old man and moved an unknown distance towards the stomach. Between swallows, the recorded pressure is subatmospheric and decreases and increases in response to inspiration and expiration, respectively. Which of the following is the most likely location of the pressure sensor?

A. Esophagus close to stomach
B. Lower esophageal sphincter
C. Main body of the esophagus
D. Orad stomach
E. Upper esophageal sphincter

48. Since hypochlorhydria becomes more prevalent with increasing age, the physician of a retirement community informs residents about the phasic regulation of gastric acid secretion. In this regard, which of the following is a correct statement?

A. During the cephalic phase, food in the stomach elicits acid secretion.
B. During the gastric phase, alcohol and caffeine inhibit acid secretion.
C. During the gastric phase, fat in the stomach elicits acid secretion.
D. During the gastric phase, gastric distention enhances acid secretion.
E. During the intestinal phase, gastrin acts as a paracrine factor to increase acid secretion.

8.4 Answers and Explanations

23. Correct: Cholecystokinin (A)

The drug substantially delayed gastric emptying by activating gastrointestinal hormone receptors at doses that are comparable to their normal physiologic activation. Under these circumstances, activation of cholecystokinin receptors leads to a strong inhibition of gastric emptying. (**B, D, E**) Gastrin, GIP (formerly known as gastric inhibitory peptide, now named glucose-dependent insulinotropic peptide), and secretin all require a very high dose to demonstrate their effect to delay gastric emptying. Hence, their physiologic significance is questionable. (**D**) Motilin increases gastrointestinal motility in the interdigestive phase in between meals.

24. Correct: Yes, yes, yes (C)

All three components need to be taken into account to estimate the rate at which gastric contents are emptied from the stomach. The more acidic the gastric content, the slower the rate of emptying. Hyper- and hypotonic solutions empty slower than isotonic saline. The rate of emptying also depends on the chemical composition of the chyme. Carbohydrates empty faster than protein and fat empties most slowly. (**A, B, D, E**) These choices are incorrect.

25. Correct: Receptive relaxation (C)

The orad (toward the mouth) stomach region is part of the gastric reservoir, where there is a motility pattern called receptive relaxation. When food enters, the stomach walls relax and the now larger reservoir is receptive to accommodate food. Despite the addition of food, the internal stomach pressure increases only slightly. (**A**) Heavy peristalsis is present in the body of the stomach and in the small intestine. (**B, D**) In the distal, antral part of the stomach, heavy mixing creates a homogenous chyme that can pass through the pylorus. Large particles cannot pass; instead they are ground and repulsed back into the lumen (retropulsive motility). (**E**) Rhythmic segmentation is a common motility pattern in the small and also large intestine caused by circular muscle contractions.

26. Correct: Increased volume of meals (E)

The major control mechanism for gastric emptying is sensing the amount and composition of food in the duodenum and providing hormonal and neuronal feedback to the stomach. Large volumes of food delay gastric emptying so as not to overwhelm the digestive and absorptive capacity of the small intestine. This is a normal response, but it might be aggravated in diabetic patients with autonomic neuropathy. (**A**) Decreased duodenal motility decreases duodenal pressure and hence the resistance of stomach contents to being propelled through the pyloric sphincter. The consequence is increased (not decreased) gastric emptying. (**B**) Decreased pyloric tone creates a wider opening of the gastroduodenal junction and hence increases (not decreases) the amount of passing food. (**C**) Increased motility of the proximal stomach counteracts the function of this gastrointestinal part for storing food and hence increases (not delays) gastric emptying. (**D**) The more intense the peristalsis of the distal stomach, the greater the force for pushing gastric content through the pyloric sphincter.

27. Correct: Dry mouth (B)

Since saliva production is stimulated by the parasympathetic nervous system, anticholinergic drugs decrease saliva production. This causes side effects such as dry mouth, difficulty swallowing, and increased infections. (**A**) Anticholinergic drugs decrease saliva production, which lowers taste in general but does not specifically cause a bitter sensation. (**C, D**) Gleeking (projection of saliva when compressing the salivary gland) and spitting are behaviors associated with large amounts of saliva, not small amounts such as caused by anticholinergic drugs. (**E**) Since saliva aids in normal chewing, tasting, and swallowing, people with dry mouth syndrome often lose (not gain) weight.

28. Correct: Drinking high-fat beverages (C)

Alcohol is reabsorbed by diffusion in the stomach and small intestine. At an alcohol concentration of about 20–25% (v/v) and above, the rate of absorption is faster in the small intestine, due to its large surface area and rich blood supply, than in the stomach. Since dietary fat keeps the GI contents longer in the stomach, it will be the most effective in preventing drunkenness. (**A**) Bolus drinking aggravates drunkenness because the higher the alcohol concentration, the higher the rate of absorption due to a larger concentration gradient between GI lumen and blood. (**B**) Adding dietary volume slows gastric emptying in general, but liquids empty significantly more rapidly than solids. Moreover, duodenal fat is a stronger stimulus than carbohydrates to delay gastric emptying. (**D**) In the best-case scenario, talking may increase a person's metabolic rate of alcohol elimination, so the resultant increased concentration gradient may increase (not decrease) the reabsorption rate. (**E**) Frequently rubbing the abdomen may in the best case increase GI motility, which may increase the rate of absorption.

29. Correct: Ghrelin (A)

Ghrelin is produced in the hypothalamus and the stomach and stimulates appetite. In a lean person, plasma ghrelin is decreased after eating. In an obese person, this normal response is blunted, and there is typically less postprandial ghrelin suppression. (**B**) Glucagon-like peptide 1 (GLP1) is released from intestinal cells in response to ingested food. It acts synergistically with other gastrointestinal signals to cause satiety (not appetite). (**C**) Leptin is secreted by adipocytes and acts at the hypothalamus to decrease (not increase) food intake. (**D**) Neuropeptide Y is indeed a very strong orexigenic (i.e., appetite-stimulating) signal. However, it is a neurotransmitter (not a hormone) that is released in response to ghrelin by first-order hypothalamic neurons to act on second-order hypothalamic neurons. (**E**) Peptide YY (also known as peptide tyrosine tyrosine) reduces hunger and instills satiety (not appetite) by delaying gastric emptying and inhibiting gastric acid secretion.

30. Correct: Food in the stomach (D)

When food distends the proximal stomach in a healthy person, it produces a vagovagal reflex by which noncholinergic, nonadrenergic fibers relax the stomach. About 2 liters of food can be accommodated in the stomach with maximal receptive relaxation. Eating disorders such as bulimia nervosa impair this normal response. It is suggested that when the food is more rapidly directed toward the stomach body, this leads to a diminished sense of fullness and episodes of uncontrolled hyperphagia. (**A, B, E**) Gastric accommodation is a vagovagal reflex that is initiated by the activation of gastric mucosal mechanoreceptors, not by hormones (such as motilin or secretin) and not by stomach acidity. (**C**) Gastric accommodation is part of the gastric (not intestinal) phase of digestion.

31. Correct: Pernicious anemia (E)

Parietal cells produce intrinsic factor, which plays a key role in intestinal vitamin B_{12} absorption, a vitamin that is involved in DNA synthesis. Thus, vitamin B_{12} deficiency impairs proliferating cells and leads to anemia, since there are about 2.5 million new red blood cells produced per second. The anemia is called pernicious (bad) since it had a fatal outcome in the past. Average onset in Caucasian adults is 60 years. (**A**) Without parietal cells, there will be little acid in stomach and duodenum, so secretin levels are expected to be low (not high). (**B**) Elevated stomach pH leads to decreased release of somatostatin, which results in increased (not low) gastrin plasma levels. (**C**) Although about 10% of protein digestion occurs in the stomach by acid-dependent pepsin, there is a great excess of pancreatic proteolytic enzymes, so malnutrition due to inadequate protein digestion is not expected. (**D**) Peptic ulcer disease develops due to disruption of the gastroduodenal mucosal defense mechanisms and/or excess acid secretion (which is not the case here).

32. Correct: Gastroesophageal reflux disease (D)

Gastroesophageal reflux disease is the most likely diagnosis. The dependence of the symptoms on body position and dietary intake, the chronic cough, and the coating of the tongue are all consistent with this working diagnosis. The nerves that supply the heart also supply the esophagus and can cause similar pain symptoms. (**A**) Patients with congestive heart failure would show hypertension, lung or ankle edema, difficulty breathing, or tiredness. (**B**) In duodenal ulcers, epigastric pain classically appears 2–3 hours after eating. It usually occurs on an empty stomach and is relieved by eating. A white coating on the tongue is not expected. It cannot be excluded, but it is not the most likely working diagnosis. (**C**) When symptomatic, gallstones cause episodic pain in the right upper part of the abdomen, often after eating a fatty or greasy meal. (**E**) Chest pain associated with myocardial infarction typically does not change when changing body position. Moreover, serum CK-MB1 and leukocytes would be expected to be elevated. Changes on the ECG and the exercise stress test are likely.

33. Correct: Antagonizing histamine-2 receptors (A)

History and physical point towards gastroesophageal reflux disease (GERD). The absence of abdominal pain, dysphagia, and bloody stool make inflammatory diseases, disorders due to abnormal motility, and cancer less likely. Central obesity (pear-shaped body and a body mass index of about 36) has been linked to GERD, most likely due to the belly fat causing pressure on the stomach. This link is strongest in white females. Histamine H_2 receptor antagonists decrease acid production and hence are useful in the treatment of GERD. (**B**) Polymers that form a protective mucosal layer are used when there are signs of ulceration, which is not supported in the patient due the lack of pain and blood. (**C**) Inert polymers such as polyethylene glycol are used as osmotic laxatives. Hence, they are an appropriate treatment for constipation, not GERD. (**D**) Enhancing (not inhibiting) normal gastrointestinal motility in the form of a prokinetic has been shown to be beneficial for GERD. (**E**) Immunosuppressive drugs are part of the treatment of inflammatory gastrointestinal disease, not GERD.

34. Correct: 6 to 7 (C)

The pH of saliva changes from slightly acidic at rest to slightly basic at maximal flow rate. Accordingly, the optimum pH for the enzymatic activity of salivary amylase is from 6 to 7. Above and below, the enzyme gets denatured and its reaction rate declines. (**A, B, D**). In acidic or alkaline conditions, the digestive action of saliva amylase is not favored. (**E**) The action of amylase is, like that of every other enzyme, pH dependent.

35. Correct: Pepsin (E)

Pepsin is a gastric protease for the digestion of dietary proteins in the stomach. When in excess, it can "self-digest" the stomach's mucosal defense barrier, which then allows back-diffusion of hydrogen ions into the gastrointestinal (GI) wall causing epithelial cell injury. (**A, D**) Bicarbonate and mucus production of GI epithelial cells are two mechanisms that help protect (not impair) the stomach wall against stomach acid. (**B, C**) Intrinsic factor and gastric lipase are produced by the stomach but do not contribute to the stomach's protection against acid but rather aid in the small intestinal reabsorption of vitamin B_{12} and the gastric emulsification of fat, respectively. Symptoms due to excess production are unknown.

36. Correct: White and milk-like (D)

The narrowing (stenosis) of the pyloric sphincter limits the passage of food from the stomach to the small intestine. Close to non-digested breast milk backs up and leads to projectile vomiting by the baby. Congenital hypertrophic pyloric stenosis is a condition that becomes symptomatic shortly after birth. The etiology is multifactorial and involves the lack of nitric oxide synthase in a large subset of cases. It is more common in males and the thickened pyloric sphincter can be palpated as an olive-shaped mass. (**A**) Bright red streaks would point to fresh blood in the vomit. (**B**) Coagulated blood in vomitus makes it appear like coffee ground. (**C**) Dark red or brown vomitus indicates that it comes from the lower GI tract and has undergone oxidation. (**E**) Yellow to greenish vomitus indicates the presence of bile. The absence of bile in vomitus is a diagnostic sign for pyloric stenosis.

37. Correct: Diarrhea due to nonabsorbed food binding water (A)

Multiple facts point towards a gastrinoma as the cause of the patient's duodenal ulcers. These include (1) increased baseline secretion of gastrin and gastric acid, (2) unresponsiveness to physiologic inhibition of proton secretion via H_2 blockers, (3) lack of *H. pylori*, and (4) no history of NSAID use. A patient with gastrinoma likely experiences osmotic diarrhea due to nonabsorbed food that binds water. Maldigestion by inactive digestive enzymes prevents food from being absorbed. The duodenal enzymes are inactive due to the low pH from excess stomach acid. (**B**) There is gastric epithelial growth (not atrophy) due to excess gastrin. (**C**) There is pancreatic growth (not atrophy) due to high levels of secretin, which is secreted in response to the high acidity. (**D**) Steatorrhea is present in stool due to undigested (not digested) fat as a result of inactive pancreatic lipases. (**E**) Stomach pain is due to the ulcers. Vitamin B_{12} malabsorption manifests as anemia, weakness, and numbness.

38. Correct: Higher levels of CO_2 (A)

Helicobacter pylori (Hp) colonize the stomach and metabolize urea into NH_3 and CO_2. Increased CO_2 is the basis of a human diagnostic *Hp* test, in which radioactively labeled urea is ingested and radioactive CO_2 is measured in exhaled air that has equilibrated with the increased stomach CO_2. (**B**) *Hp* colonization increases gastrin secretion into blood (not the stomach) due to an inhibition of gastric somatostatin secretion. (**C**) *Hp* inhibits (not increases) gastric mucosal somatostatin secretion. (**D**) Gastric acid secretion into the stomach lumen is increased (not decreased) due to a higher level of serum gastrin. (**E**) *Hp* contains urease to metabolize urea, so its content will be high (not low) in experimental compared to control pigs.

39. Correct: External intercostal muscles (C)

Ejection of stomach contents during vomiting involves the external intercostal muscles, which contract, together with abdominal skeletal muscles, to force the chyme into the mouth. (**A**) The projectile ejection of food is not produced by the contraction of stomach muscles itself. (**B**) Distal esophageal smooth muscles relax to create a passage for food to be ejected. (**D**) Pectoral muscles are not involved in the vomiting reflex. (**E**) Vomiting is preceded by a retrograde contraction wave that starts in the proximal jejunum, which forces small intestinal content into the relaxed stomach. Minutes later, retching and vomiting occurs.

40. Correct: No, no, yes, yes, yes (D)

Achalasia is a motility disorder that can affect various places in the gastrointestinal tract. Difficulty of swallowing points to the most common form of esophageal achalasia, which is caused by the degeneration of distal esophageal inhibitory enteric neurons and leads to a dominance of stimulatory influence on lower (not upper) esophageal smooth muscle. The consequences are diminished peristalsis in the mid to lower part of the esophagus and a hypertensive lower esophageal sphincter, which does not relax after a swallow. (**A, B, C, E**) These choices are incorrect.

41. Correct: Lysozyme (C)

Human saliva contains antibacterial agents such as lysozymes, thiocyanates, and immunoglobulin A, which supports the licking of wounds in order to avoid infection. On the other hand, there are bacteria present in the mouth which may infect a wound when licked. (**A**) Angiotensin-converting enzyme is not present in saliva. Furthermore, it would break down bradykinin and limit its vasodilatory role in wound healing. On the other hand, kallikreins that help convert kininogen into bradykinin are present in saliva. (**B**) Digestion of fat by the lingual lipase is not a mechanism known to improve wound healing. (**D**) While extracellular nucleic acids (DNA and RNA) are found in serum, a biological role in ultrafiltrates such as saliva has not been established, and their contribution to wound healing would be a stretch. (**E**) Digestion of carbohydrates by the salivary α-amylase ptyalin is not helpful for cleaning or healing wounds.

42. Correct: Cl^-, H^+, K^+ (E)

The function of the parietal cell is to secrete HCl into the stomach lumen. First, H^+ enters the stomach lumen via a proton pump. It uses the energy from ATP hydrolysis to drive H^+ into the lumen against its concentration gradient in exchange for K^+. Hence, Y and Z are H^+ and K^+, respectively. H^+ is created inside the cell, primarily through the dissociation of carbonic acid into H^+ and HCO_3^- and to a smaller extent through the dissociation of water. K^+ enters the cell in exchange for Na^+ (the orange unlabeled circle). Second, Cl^- diffuses into the stomach lumen through a conductance channel. Hence, X is Cl^-. It enters the cell on the basolateral membrane in exchange for bicarbonate (the blue unlabeled circle). (**A, B, C, D**) These are incorrect choices that can easily be eliminated once the characteristic H-K-ATPase has been identified.

43. Correct: Area postrema chemoreceptor agonist (B)

An agonist that activates the chemoreceptors in the area postrema in the medulla induces vomiting. This stimulates saliva production, a reflex to protect teeth from aspirated stomach acid. (**A, C**) Administration of adrenergic and cholinergic receptor antagonists can decrease salivary production, since both sympathetic and parasympathetic are known to stimulate salivation. (**D**) Many of the salivary epithelial cell transporters rely on the presence of a basolateral Na+-K+-ATPase, so that pump inhibition would decrease salivation production. (**E**) Salivary secretion is exclusively under neural control, so that administration of a secretin analogue would not increase salivation.

44. Correct: Proton pump inhibitor (D)

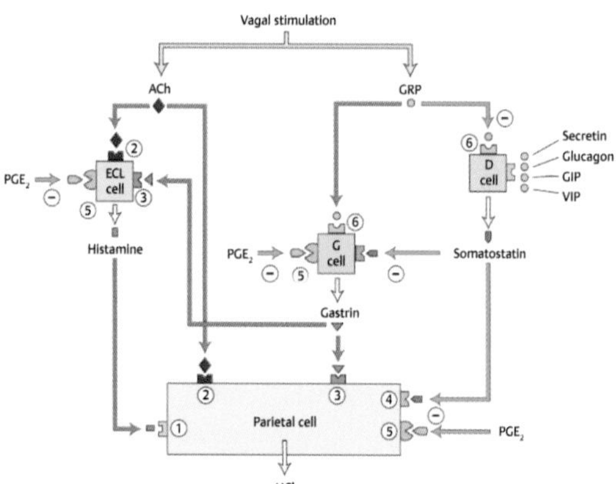

The final step for parietal cell acid secretion (image, arrow toward HCl) is to use energy from ATP hydrolysis to move protons from the cell cytoplasm to the stomach lumen in exchange for potassium ions moving from the stomach lumen into the cell cytoplasm. When this so-called proton pump is inhibited, acid production is maximally reduced. (**A, B, C**) There are multiple physiologic agents that directly and indirectly stimulate parietal cell signal transduction, which ultimately leads to proton pump activation. These include acetylcholine binding to M_3 receptors (image, circle 2), gastrin binding to CCK_B receptors (image, circle 3), and histamine binding to H_2 receptors (image, circle 1). Individually blocking these mechanisms at the receptor level (anticholinergic; antigastrin antibody; H_2 receptor blocker) will only partially inhibit gastric acid secretion. (**E, F**) Prostaglandin E_2 (PGE_2) and somatostatin have an inhibitory influence on the cAMP signaling pathway of parietal cells, and hence diminish gastric acid secretion. However, activating one inhibitory pathway has a smaller effect than inhibiting the end step of all pathways, the secretion of protons into the stomach lumen.

45. Correct: Achalasia (A)

Achalasia is a disorder of the enteric nervous system that impairs the contraction of lower esophageal smooth muscles and the relaxation of the lower esophageal sphincter. All other diseases are degenerative diseases of the brain or motor nerves that interfere with the control of skeletal muscle contraction. (**B, C, D, E**) Amyotrophic lateral sclerosis (motor neuron disease), multiple sclerosis (demyelination disease), Parkinson's disease (dopamine imbalance), and poliomyelitis (viral disease) all affect skeletal muscles and hence can impair gastrointestinal motility that involves skeletal muscle, such as swallowing and chewing.

46. Correct: Atropine (A)

Atropine inhibits parasympathetic activity in order to increase the patient's heart rate. A common side effect is dry mouth by inhibiting salivary production. (**B**) While dairy products might be involved in changing food perception, there is no scientific evidence that dairy products decrease saliva production or produce thick saliva, despite the widely held belief. (**C**) Walking exercise activates the sympathetic nervous system, which stimulates (not inhibits) saliva production. (**D**) A lip balm has no influence on salivary secretion. (**E**) There is no indication for normal hypotonic saliva to become hypertonic, such as for instance by hyperglycemia.

47. Correct: Main body of the esophagus (C)

Close to the whole length, but certainly the upper two-thirds, of the esophagus are above the diaphragm and hence within the thoracic cavity. This means that intraesophageal pressure is equal to intrathoracic pressure, which is subatmospheric. The respiratory changes in esophageal pressure are representative of changes in intrapleural pressure, the pressure surrounding the lung within the pleural space. It decreases during inspiration as the thoracic cavity expands and increases as the thoracic wall recoils during expiration. (**A**) Just before entering the stomach, the esophagus passes through the diaphragm. That makes its intraluminal pressure positive, similar to abdominal pressure, and it increases (not decreases) with inspiration. (**B, D**) The lower esophageal sphincter and the orad stomach lie in the abdominal cavity and are minimally sensitive to respiratory changes. (**E**) The upper esophageal sphincter is insensitive to respiratory motion.

48. Correct: During the gastric phase, gastric distention enhances acid secretion. (D)

During the gastric phase, acid secretion is enhanced by gastric distention, which is sensed by mechanoreceptors that consequently elicit enteric reflexes that stimulate gastrin release. This ability to produce acid and initial motility even in the absence of amino acids and peptides is important for the stomach's role in digestion. (**A**) The cephalic phase occurs before food enters the stomach, while food is being eaten, smelled, tasted, and thought about. (**B**) Alcohol and caffeine are known to stimulate (not inhibit) gastric acid secretion. (**C**) The gastric phase of gastric acid secretion is stimulated by the presence of amino acids and peptides, not fat. (**E**) During the early intestinal phase, gastric acid secretion is further stimulated by gastrin, which has been released by duodenal G cells. Independent of the origin, gastrin acts in a true hormonal fashion via blood (not by a paracrine pathway) on parietal cells.

8.5 Questions

49. At a routine office visit, the parents of a 6-month old baby girl describe that during breastfeeding, the baby pulls up her legs and starts crying. Typically, it is accompanied by a bowel movement, after which she stops crying. The baby is well nourished, her skin looks healthy, and the parents deny any abnormality in the baby's diaper content. An increase in which of the following is the most likely explanation?

A. Gastric lipase
B. Breast milk allergy
C. Gastrocolic reflex
D. Infantile colic
E. Serum cholecystokinin

50. A mother worries because her 3-year-old daughter swallows chewing gum. Which of the following is the best explanation for ingestion of chewing gum not being problematic?

A. It is eliminated by a power propulsion wave.
B. It is eliminated by interdigestive motility.
C. It is fully digested by bacteria.
D. It is fully digested by pancreatic enzymes.
E. It remains but does not cause any problem.

51. The toxin of Vibrio cholerae enters intestinal epithelial cells where it activates the Gα subunit of G proteins, which increases intracellular synthesis of cAMP. High intracellular concentration of cAMP leads to the opening of which ion channel, located at which part of the epithelial cell membrane?

	Ion channel type	Epithelial cell membrane
A.	Chloride	Apical
B.	Sodium	Apical
C.	Water	Basolateral
D.	Chloride	Basolateral
E.	Water	Apical

52. A 38-year-old female is scheduled for surgical removal of her terminal ileum. Which of the following is the most likely postoperative complication considering the functional lack of this gut portion?

A. Chvostek sign
B. Megaloblastic anemia
C. Pancreatitis
D. Peripheral edema
E. Scurvy

53. A 3-year-old child presents with chronic diarrhea. The father explains that she is an extremely picky eater and ingests a lot of dairy ice cream. A fecal osmolality test reveals the results shown in the image, which represents the contributions of solutes A–E to total fecal osmolality. The red area E represents which of the following?

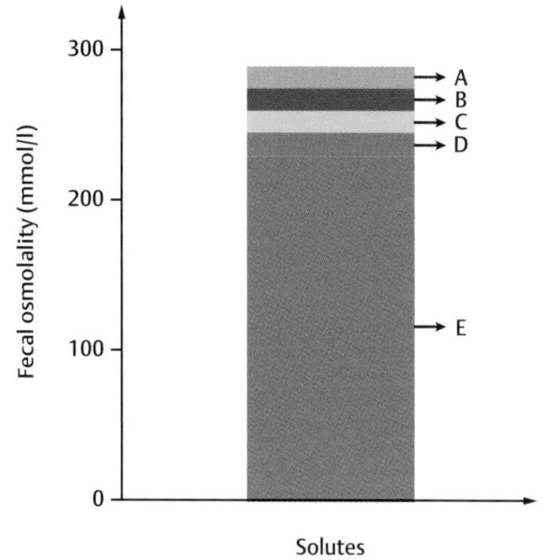

A. Bicarbonate
B. Chloride
C. Potassium
D. Sodium
E. Unmeasured osmoles

54. A 79-year-old female patient, living in a nursing home, was placed on long-term intravenous feeding for two months. Endoscopic examination of her gastrointestinal tract revealed atrophy of the gastrointestinal mucosa and the exocrine pancreas. A decrease in which of the following gastrointestinal peptides would further aggravate her situation?

A. Gastrin
B. Glucagon-like peptide 1
C. Glucose-dependent insulinotropic peptide
D. Pancreatic polypeptide
E. Somatostatin

55. A 9-year-old boy presents with weight loss and diarrhea. His tongue becomes sore and blistery after eating oatmeal or rye bread, which leads to the diagnosis of celiac disease. The physician discusses other possible effects of this disease with the parents and describes that muscle spasms and paresthesia are possible symptoms associated with malabsorption of which of the following nutritional substances?

A. Calcium
B. Carbohydrates
C. Fats
D. Iron
E. Water

56. As a competitive weight lifter, an 18-year-old woman desperately tries to gain weight by eating more carbs. Unfortunately, she notices that with this diet she has significantly lost weight over the past year. In addition, she experiences gastrointestinal distress, including flatulence, steatorrhea, and diarrhea after eating bread, cereal, or pasta. A stool sample and intestinal biopsy are obtained and sent for detailed analysis. The intestinal biopsy shows villous atrophy, crypt hyperplasia, and significant lymphocyte infiltration. Which of the following would most likely be decreased in the stool sample?

A. Antibodies
B. Brush border cells
C. Carbohydrates
D. Fat
E. Nitrogen

57. A 14-week-old baby is admitted to the emergency department with chronic watery diarrhea. The mother is breast-feeding and reports that the problem has existed since birth. History reveals the family traveled 60 miles to visit the baby's grandparents one month ago but otherwise have not traveled. The mother said that her pediatrician did blood tests two days ago, which all came back normal. Current tests show that the baby's stool has a low pH but is otherwise unremarkable. It is decided to switch to intravenous nutrition, and shortly thereafter the diarrhea stops. What is the most likely cause or mechanism for the diarrhea?

A. Exudative diarrhea
B. Infectious diarrhea
C. Osmotic diarrhea
D. Secretory diarrhea
E. Traveler's diarrhea

58. Which of the following is the gastrointestinal division with the least ability for storage?

A. Cecum
B. Duodenum
C. Gallbladder
D. Proximal stomach
E. Rectum

59. In an adult person on an average nonlimiting diet, which of the following minerals is most completely absorbed when ingested as part of food?

A. Calcium
B. Magnesium
C. Iron
D. Sodium
E. Sulfate

60. A 52-year-old patient is found to have elevated serum somatostatin levels derived from a duodenal tumor of D-cell origin. Which of the following conditions is also most likely to result from this tumor?

A. Fecal occult blood
B. Gallstones
C. Gastric pH below 1.0
D. Hypermotility
E. Hypoglycemia

61. Japanese rice is especially sticky when cooked. Which of the following enzymes are necessary for the digestion of this type of rice to monosaccharides?

A. Amylases, α-dextrinases, and maltases
B. Amylases and α-dextrinases only
C. Amylases and maltases only
D. Amylases of saliva and pancreas only
E. Cannot be digested to monosaccharides

62. On average, the gastrointestinal tract of a healthy adult person, eating a healthy Western diet, has to deal with 8–10 liters of fluid per day. Which of the following is correct in regards to this fluid load?

A. Most comes from drinking and eating.
B. Most comes from hepatic secretions.
C. Most is absorbed against its concentration gradient.
D. Most is absorbed in the large intestine.
E. Most is absorbed in the small intestine.

63. You notice that one of your friends has lost weight over the past year. As you are studying with her while eating pizza and breadsticks, she obviously experiences gastrointestinal discomfort. On questioning, she explains that she is not trying to lose weight, but avoids eating since it leads to embarrassing episodes of flatulence and diarrhea. Which of the following would most likely be decreased in this woman?

A. Intestinal bacteria
B. Intestinal crypts
C. Intestinal haustra
D. Intestinal villi
E. Peyer's patches

64. Doctors without Borders are setting up a camp in an area recently struck by an earthquake. A large number of people suffer from muscle cramps and profuse, watery stools, most likely due to cholera. For oral rehydration therapy, the powder from commercial packages is mixed with chemically purified water. When the patients drink these solutions, it will promote their intestinal sodium absorption by cotransport of which of the following?

A. Calcium
B. Citrate
C. Glucose
D. Magnesium
E. Potassium

65. Which of the following factors found in serum causes vasoconstriction of gastrointestinal blood vessels?

A. Angiotensin II
B. Bradykinin
C. Cholecystokinin
D. Glucagon
E. Vasoactive intestinal polypeptide

66. In regards to the cellular mechanisms of gastrointestinal electrolyte absorption, which of the following statements is correct?

A. Ca^{2+} absorption requires 25-hydroxycholecalciferol.
B. Cl^- absorption is accompanied by HCO_3^- absorption.
C. Fe^{2+} absorption is in the form of free iron or heme.
D. K^+ absorption in the colon is enhanced by aldosterone.
E. Na^+ absorption is by cotransport with proteins.

67. A 2-month-old infant presents with a failure to thrive. The parents note that her stool is foul and has a slippery texture. In addition, the girl experiences symptoms consistent with vitamin E deficiency, such as a distended abdomen, muscle weakness, and scoliosis in the spine. A genetic test reveals a mutation affecting the microsomal triglyceride transfer protein (MTP) gene. This gene mutation prevents the function of which of the following?

A. Apolipoprotein B
B. Bilirubin
C. Lingual lipase
D. Pancreatic lipase
E. Phospholipase A2

68. A 64-year-old male presents with complaints of urgent bowel movement. He recalls that he had similar problems several years ago but denies such complications for the past year. He typically voids 2 to 3 times per day. He has noticed several times small amounts of blood in his stool, which he recognized because it was bright red. He sometimes has diarrhea at night, but the stool can also be hard, in which case it is very painful to pass. He has tried over-the-counter hemorrhoid creams without relief. For many years, he has eaten a high-fiber diet. He has not noticed blood in his urine or in his mouth after brushing his teeth. There is no sign of right upper quadrant tenderness or ascites. The whites of his eyes are not tinted. His vital signs, complete blood count, serum electrolytes, clotting tests, and renal profile are unremarkable. From the following, which is the most likely diagnosis to be considered?

A. Acute liver disease
B. Constipation
C. Crohn's disease
D. Diverticulosis
E. Ulcerative colitis

69. A patient with irritable bowel syndrome is scheduled for a hydrogen and methane breath test. The day before the test, he is asked to eat a special diet and then completely fast for 12 hours before ingesting a standard sugar load. During the breath test, exhaled air is collected and sampled for the concentration of hydrogen and methane for 1 hour. An increase from normal indicates which of the following?

A. Abnormal cytokine profile
B. Bacterial overgrowth
C. Increased gut permeability
D. Innate immune defect
E. Presence of fungi

70. A thorough investigation of a patient with vague signs of dyspepsia reveals abnormally low levels of motilin. Endoscopy confirms an absence of the migrating myoelectric complex. Further testing will most likely reveal an increase in which of the following?

A. Duodenal motility
B. Gastric emptying
C. Intestinal bacteria
D. Mass movements
E. Swallowing

71. A 2-month-old baby boy presents with vomiting, diarrhea, and failure to thrive. On investigation, edema and ascites are found. Blood values show hypoproteinemia. Several attempts with different protein diets are unsuccessful, but the administration of pancreatic enzymes alleviates the symptoms. A genetic profile reveals a rare deficiency of an intestinal brush border enzyme. Which of the following enzymes is most likely defective?

A. Carboxypeptidase
B. Chymotrypsin
C. Enteropeptidase
D. Pepsin
E. Trypsin

72. Vitamin K plays a key role in blood clotting. Which of the following is true regarding active vitamin K?

A. Deficiency is often due to inadequate intake.
B. Excess can be due to anticoagulant drugs.
C. It is abundantly present in bread, rice, and meat.
D. It is a group of similar fat-soluble vitamins.
E. Overload is treated by frequent bleeding.

73. The terminal ileum was removed from a 50-year-old man during excision of a tumor. About 3 years later, the patient presents with extreme tiredness. He is also very pale. Hemoglobin is 9 g/dL (normal 12–16 g/dL), and MCV (mean corpuscular volume) is 110 µm3 (normal 80–100 µm3). For treatment, he is given a vitamin supplement with which of the following active ingredients?

A. Ascorbic acid
B. Cholecalciferol
C. Cobalamin
D. Folic acid
E. Retinol
F. Thiamine

74. A 34-year-old woman broke her hip bone when getting out of the car and falling onto the pavement. Her past history shows that a year ago, she suffered from primary biliary cholangitis, which led to destruction of her bile ducts and disruption of bile flow. Her history is otherwise unremarkable, and she denies being tired. The results from a bone density scan shows significantly reduced bone mineral density for her age. There are no other remarkable findings from her exam. She is most likely deficient in which factor?

A. Iron
B. Folate
C. Vitamin B_{12}
D. Vitamin C
E. Vitamin D

75. A 3-year-old girl presents with bouts of cramping, diarrhea, and abdominal pain. She has no fever, and lactase deficiency is suspected. After an overnight fast, she performs a lactose challenge test. She is asked to drink a quart of low-fat milk, and it will be determined whether her gastrointestinal symptoms appear within the next hour. What is the reason for not using high-fat milk for this test?

A. It would blunt the symptoms.
B. It would inhibit the activity of lactase.
C. It would take longer to reach the small intestine.
D. It would unnecessarily cause fatty, greasy stool.
E. It would unnecessarily support obesity.

76. Medical students prepare a poster about intestinal digestion and absorption for a community health fair. Which of the following statements can be added as correct?

A. After absorption, lipid-soluble vitamins are attached to monoglycerides within enterocytes.

B. Free fatty acids traverse brush border mucosal cell membranes by facilitated diffusion.

C. Glucose and sucrose bind to the same transporter at the brush border mucosal cell membranes.

D. The uptake of fructose into an intestinal epithelial cell is independent of a sodium gradient.

E. Trypsin is present within the membrane brush border mucosal cell membrane.

77. A patient presents with severe constipation. A barium enema study reveals an almost total absence of mass movements from the transverse to the sigmoid colon. From the following choices, which is the most likely cause for the patient's constipation?

A. Denervation of the external anal sphincter

B. Damage to the colonic submucosal plexus

C. Destruction of the colonic myenteric plexus

D. Excess vasoactive intestinal peptide (VIPoma)

E. Ingestion of inert, nondigestible particles

78. A pharmaceutical company is developing a drug that activates proteolytic digestive enzymes that are released as zymogens by the pancreas. Which of the following most important natural activators does the company want to mimic?

A. Bile pigment

B. Brush border peptidase

C. Enterokinase

D. Hydrochloric acid

E. Pepsin

79. In an adult with a healthy lifestyle, which of the following is a correct statement in regards to the person's gastrointestinal bacteria?

A. Their colonic concentration is typically > 10^9/ mL.

B. Their duodenal concentration is half compared to the colon.

C. Their pharmacological eradication is asymptomatic.

D. They are primarily of the aerobic type.

E. They contribute < 1% to total fecal dry weight.

8.6 Answers and Explanations

49. Correct: Gastrocolic reflex (C)

The gastrocolic reflex initiates colonic motility when there is food in the stomach in order to make room for more food. It is the reason why babies often have bowel movements during or immediately after feeding. Some babies experience stronger reflexes, which makes them cry. (**A**) Gastric lipase is an important enzyme in babies for the digestion of milk fat. When increased, it would lead to steatorrhea. (**B**) An allergy would lead to weight loss and signs of an immune response such as a skin rash. In addition, most babies are allergic to something the mother is eating, not the milk itself. (**D**) Infantile colic is when a healthy infant cries for more than 3 hours, which is not supported here. It typically has subsided by 4 months of age. (**E**) Cholecystokinin increases immediately after start of breastfeeding and peaks again 30–60 min later to induce satiety. Inappropriately increased levels are associated with nausea and taste aversion (not defecation).

50. Correct: It is eliminated by interdigestive motility. (B)

Every type of chewing gum has a gum base that is not digestible. Indigestible substances are swept out between meals as part of the interdigestive motility (migrating myoelectric complex). Swallowed gum might also be propelled forward with the help of digestive motility that has been evoked due to the chewing motion. (**A**) Substances that are recognized by the body as harmful initiate giant propulsive contractions independent of the slow wave rhythm. This is not the case for gum base. (**C, D**) While some ingredients such as fats, preservatives, and sweeteners are digested by bacteria and enzymes, gum always contains a nondigestible base. (**E**) Undigested food does not remain in the GI tract—certainly not for 7 years as a popular saying suggests.

51. Correct: Chloride, apical (A)

The apical membrane chloride channel of small intestinal cells is usually closed. It is physiologically opened by intracellular cAMP, which is produced when a bioactive substance (e.g., a hormone) binds to the basolateral membrane of the cell and initiates G-protein signaling. Cholera toxin mimics this normal response. Excess chloride secretion into the gut lumen leads to excess water and electrolyte secretion and consequently severe voluminous diarrhea. (**B, C, E**) cAMP opens chloride (not sodium or water) channels. (**D**) Apical (not basolateral) chloride channels are opened by cAMP to stimulate intestinal fluid secretion.

52. Correct: Megaloblastic anemia (B)

Vitamin B_{12} can be absorbed only in the terminal ileum. In its absence and after hepatic stores have been depleted, thymidine synthase function is impaired, which diminishes DNA synthesis. This leads to the development of giant cells (megaloblasts) in all rapidly dividing cells such as erythroid precursor cells. Anemia ensues. (**A**) Chvostek sign is the clinical sign that occurs in hypocalcemia and, potentially, hypomagnesemia. Both calcium and magnesium are primarily absorbed in the upper small intestinal parts. (**C**) The lack of the terminal ileum affects vitamin B_{12} and bile salt reabsorption. Neither is related to pancreatitis. (**D**) Peripheral edema can be due to low protein in blood as a result of poor protein digestion and/or peptide/amino acid absorption. However, this is largely completed before the luminal contents reach the terminal ileum. (**E**) Scurvy is the disease due to the deficiency of vitamin C. As a water-soluble vitamin, its absorption is not affected by the removal of the terminal ileum.

53. Correct: Unmeasured osmoles (E)

An osmotic stool analysis is useful to support a suspicion of osmotic diarrhea, without causing the child further discomfort. The child's history suggests lactose intolerance, which leaves undigested lactose in stool, where it attracts water and causes chronic diarrhea. In the fecal osmolality test, lactose is not measured; hence it increases the millimolar concentration of the unmeasured osmoles. Unmeasured osmoles are obtained by subtracting the osmolality of the measured solutes from 290 mOsm/kg, since fecal osmolality is equal to serum osmolality when stool leaves the colon. (**A, B, C, D**) Bicarbonate, chloride, potassium, and sodium are the major osmoles of a stool sample and normally account for at least two-thirds of the total fecal osmoles. Sodium and potassium are typically measured, and their concentration is doubled to account for the contributing anions bicarbonate and chloride. The amount-of-substance concentration decreases in osmotic diarrhea and increases in secretory diarrhea.

54. Correct: Gastrin (A)

In addition to stimulating hydrochloric acid secretion, the second physiologic action of gastrin is its trophic effect on the gastrointestinal mucosa and exocrine pancreas. In its absence, these tissues will atrophy unless exogenous gastrin is administered. (**B, C, D**) These peptides have no trophic actions at physiologic concentrations. Glucagon-like peptide 1 is released after a meal and induces satiety, inhibits secretion of glucagon, and supports the release of somatostatin. Glucose-dependent insulinotropic peptide stimulates insulin release. Pancreatic polypeptide mainly functions as negative feedback regulator for pancreatic secretions. (**E**) Somatostatin reduces DNA and RNA synthesis, as well as mucosal and pancreatic protein content. Hence, low somatostatin stimulates growth.

55. Correct: Calcium (A)

The greatly diminished absorptive surface in celiac disease leads to malabsorption of nutrients in general. Since calcium is difficult to reabsorb, celiac patients often experience symptoms of hypocalcemia, such as muscle spasm and tingling due to nerve hyperexcitability (paresthesia). (**B**) The inability to absorb carbohydrates manifests as weight loss as experienced by the boy. (**C**) Fat malabsorption is fairly common in patients with celiac disease and manifests as steatorrhea. (**D**) Iron, like calcium, is difficult to absorb, and lack of it may lead to anemia. (**E**) Decreased electrolyte absorption leads to decreased water absorption. The increased osmotic load in the gastrointestinal lumen manifest as diarrhea, as experienced by the boy.

56. Correct: Brush border cells (B)

The results of the intestinal biopsy confirm that the woman has celiac disease, an autoimmune disorder that damages the gastrointestinal (GI) lining when carbohydrates with gluten proteins are eaten: The villi are atrophied, while the crypts have become deeper. The latter are filled with lymphocytes that have infiltrated the intestinal lining. Normally, intestinal cells are permanently renewed, so the remnants of dead cells that are shed from the tips of the villi end up in stool. In the patient, there are significantly fewer villi, so that fewer cells will be present in the stool sample. (**A**) Celiac patients produce antibodies that are diagnostic when present in serum. These antibodies are also secreted into the GI lumen and can be present in stool. Many antibodies are digested along the bowel passage, so they might not appear in stool, but they are certainly not decreased. (**C, D, E**) The enormous decrease in absorptive area leads to malabsorption, so increased (not decreased) amounts of carbohydrates, fat, and nitrogen can be found in stool.

57. Correct: Osmotic diarrhea (C)

The fact that the diarrhea disappeared after intravenous nutrition points to malabsorption of an ingested nutrient. Human milk contains lactose, and lactose intolerance is fairly common. Unabsorbed lactose binds water, causing osmotic diarrhea. In children and adults, it is diagnosed with a lactose challenge test, but this is not done in babies to avoid further aggravation of diarrhea and dehydration. Large-intestinal bacteria feast on lactose and produce compounds that acidify the stool. (**A**) Exudative diarrhea derives from inflammation or ulceration of the gastrointestinal system. The stool is likely to contain mucus, pus, serum proteins, and/or blood. (**B, D, E**) These types of diarrhea would not resolve with intravenous nutrition. Moreover, in the case of an infection, normal blood work would have shown increased white blood cells. Secretory diarrhea is due to excessive secretion or inhibited absorption of electrolytes, infections, drugs, or a hormone-secreting tumor. None of these is supported by the vignette. Traveler's diarrhea could have been from microbial contamination of water when traveling, but symptoms would not have been occurring since birth.

58. Correct: Duodenum (B)

The function of the duodenum is to further digest and efficiently absorb the partially digested food from the stomach. Chyme is normally delivered at a rate that ensures rapid digestion and absorption. Thus, the duodenum is not an important storage site for food or partially digested food. Peristaltic waves reinforce the movement of chyme toward the jejunum, and this action is interrupted occasionally by segmentation, which helps mix the chyme with the digestive secretions, thereby increasing the rate of digestion. (**A**) The cecum contains bacteria, to which food is exposed when the ileocecal sphincter opens and chyme is temporarily stored inside the blind pouch, before being pushed upward into the ascending colon. It is of minor importance for human digestion. (**C**) The function of the gallbladder is to concentrate and store bile until needed for digestion. (**D**) The proximal stomach is distended by food and forms a balloonlike pouch to store food without a significant increase in intraluminal pressure. (**E**) As the last part of the digestive tract, the rectum is the place for temporary storage of feces until the person voluntarily proceeds with defecation.

59. Correct: Sodium (D)

Sodium absorption is tightly coupled to water absorption, which leads to isotonic gastrointestinal chyme. Often, even more sodium than water is absorbed. since the colon secretes potassium in exchange for sodium absorption. (**A, B**) Calcium and magnesium absorption are about 30–40% efficient. Many factors influence their availability for absorption. For instance, calcium forms insoluble complexes with phosphate ions, while phytates and oxalates can have a negative impact on absorbable magnesium. (**C**) Only 10–20% of dietary iron is absorbed, and iron deficiency is present in all societies. (**E**) Sulfate is poorly absorbed by the human gastrointestinal tract. Hence, it is used as an osmotic laxative. As part of medication, it serves as a "nonabsorbable" anion.

60. Correct: Gallstones (B)

Somatostatin (SS) inhibits secretion and activity of cholecystokinin (CCK). The lack of CCK inhibits gall bladder contraction, and the resultant static bile is more likely to crystallize and provide the nucleus for gallstones. (**A**) Blood in stool is unlikely since SS inhibits a wide range of GI functions, including motility, secretions, and hormones. Hence, SS analogues can be used in the treatment of aggressive conditions that might lead to GI bleeds. (**C**) SS inhibits gastrin secretion, which leads to hypochlorhydria, with a pH unlikely below 4.0. (**D**) SS reduces smooth muscle contractions and inhibits motilin, leading to digestive and interdigestive hypomotility (not hypermotility). (**E**) SS inhibits insulin release, leading to hyperglycemia and diabetes mellitus in almost all patients with excess SS.

61. Correct: Amylases, α-dextrinases, and maltases (A)

Japanese rice is a short-grain rice with a very high amylopectin-to-amylose ratio. This results in the rice being much stickier when cooked compared to longer-grain forms of rice. The digestion of amylopectin (branched starch) and amylose (linear starch) begins with the action of salivary α-amylase and continues with pancreatic amylase in the small intestine. Amylases hydrolyze amylose to maltose and maltotriose and hydrolyze amylopectin to maltose, maltotriose, and α-dextrin. Maltases further digest maltose and maltotriose to glucose, but α-dextrinases are necessary to fully digest amylopectin to monosaccharides. (**B, C, D**) Without maltases or α-dextrinases, poly- and disaccharides would remain. (**E**) Amylopectin can be completely digested into absorbable glucose units. It is the branched form of starch and is a main food group for human nutrition.

62. Correct: Most is absorbed in the small intestine. (E)

The small intestine absorbs about 85% of the fluid and hence is the primary site of fluid absorption in the gastrointestinal tract. (**A**) On average, a healthy adult person ingests about one-fifth of the daily fluid load, or 2 liters of fluid, per day. (**B**) The hepatic secretions that enter the gastrointestinal lumen are through bile, which accounts for about half a liter per day. (**C**) Water is transported across the intestinal membrane by osmosis, not active transport. (**D**) After the majority of fluid has been reabsorbed in the small intestine, most of the remaining 15% is reabsorbed by the large intestine. Only about 100 milliliters (1%) of water is excreted per day.

63. Correct: Intestinal villi (D)

The woman is most likely suffering from celiac disease. Gastrointestinal pain and signs of malabsorption such as diarrhea, weight loss, and flatulence when eating gluten-containing carbohydrates are hallmark signs. In the disease, an immune response to gluten damages small intestinal villi, and villous atrophy causes malabsorption. (**A**) The number of intestinal bacteria is increased since they thrive from nonabsorbed food. They are the major reason for her flatulence. (**B**) In celiac patients the intestinal crypts are not decreased but rather become deeper, and crypt cells secrete fluid in response to undigested food and irritation. (**C**) Haustra are the permanent folds of the colon. Their number is not decreased. Their contraction pattern might be altered but not decreased by the presence of nonabsorbed food. (**E**) Peyer's patches are gastrointestinal accumulations of immune cells. Their number and/or size is increased in celiac patients due to an increased immune response.

64. Correct: Glucose (C)

Sodium is absorbed by intestinal epithelial cells via the sodium-glucose cotransporter SGLT1. The transporter is driven by a sodium gradient from the gut lumen into the cell, which is created by Na-K-ATPases at the basolateral sides of the intestinal cells. (**A**) Sodium absorption is not mediated or regulated by calcium absorption. The latter is regulated by the body's calcium stores. (**B**) While sodium-dependent citrate transporters are known to exist, citrate absorption is probably regulated by the acid-base balance and not known as a route to increase intestinal sodium absorption. (**D**) Magnesium is poorly absorbed, and magnesium salts are even used as osmotic laxatives. (**E**) Potassium absorption across the intestinal mucosa is largely passive through lateral spaces and tight junctions and is not coupled with sodium reabsorption.

65. Correct: Angiotensin II (A)

Angiotensin II is a potent vasoconstrictor of mesenteric blood vessels. Under stressful situations the vasoconstrictor action of angiotensin II redirects blood flow from the gastrointestinal circulation to more essential circulations such as the coronary and cerebral circulations. (**B**) Bradykinin is a ubiquitous vasodilator in response to inflammation and acts via nitric oxide and prostacyclin. (**C**) Cholecystokinin, the hormone supporting digestion and absorption, additionally acts as vasodilator and hence increases mesenteric blood flow. (**D**) Glucagon improves blood flow to the intestine, especially after situations of vasoconstriction or mesenteric ischemia. (**E**) Vasoactive intestinal polypeptide is a potent vasodilator and increases gastrointestinal blood flow.

66. Correct: Fe^{2+} absorption is in the form of free iron or heme. (C)

Fe^{2+} is absorbed at the brush border as free Fe^{2+} by an iron transporter. It can also be endocytosed in the form of heme, in which case Fe^{2+} is liberated inside the cells and essentially follows the same pathway for export as absorbed inorganic iron. Some heme might also be transported intact into the circulation. (**A**) Ca^{2+} absorption requires active vitamin D, or 1,25-dihydroxycholecalciferol (not 25-hydroxycholecalciferol). (**B**) Cl^- transport is using a Cl^-/HCO_3^- antiporter, not cotransporter. (**D**) K^+ is actively secreted (not absorbed) in the colon under the influence of aldosterone. As in the renal principal cell, aldosterone increases luminal membrane Na^+ channels, which increases Na^+ absorption in exchange for K^+ secretion. (**E**) Na^+ is absorbed by several mechanisms. One major route is by cotransport with amino acids (not proteins).

67. Correct: Apolipoprotein B (A)

Mutation of the microsomal triglyceride transfer protein gene affects the assembly of apolipoproteins of class B. The function of these proteins is to stabilize chylomicrons and very-low-density lipoproteins. When these lipid transport vessels become unstable, they fall apart and cannot support the normal absorption and transport of dietary fats and lipid-soluble vitamins such as vitamin E. Hence, abetalipoproteinemia leads to the presence of nonabsorbed lipids in stool and symptoms from deficiency of lipid-soluble vitamins. (**B**) Bilirubin is a waste product derived from the dismantling of hemoglobin. It is excreted in bile and has no function in digestion, absorption, or transport of lipids. (**C, D, E**) While the boy's steatorrhea could stem from malfunctioning lipases or phospholipases, vitamin E does not need to be digested by these enzymes. Hence, there would be no symptoms of vitamin E deficiency.

68. Correct: Ulcerative colitis (E)

Ulcerative colitis is the most likely diagnosis to consider and to confirm with further tests. It is a chronic inflammatory disease of the large intestine that flares up episodically. It causes irritation and sores that lead to the described problems of changes in bowel movements. Bright red blood points towards a source of bleeding close to the stool exit. (**A**) Acute liver disease is not the most likely consideration, due to the lack of abdominal tenderness, ascites, jaundice, or clotting problems. (**B**) Constipation is the difficult, infrequent, or incomplete passage of stool, which is not supported in this patient. Moreover, a low-fiber (not high-fiber) diet is the most common cause of constipation. (**C**) Crohn's disease is, like ulcerative colitis, an inflammatory bowel disease, but it affects various parts of the GI tract, rather than being restricted to the colon. (**D**) Diverticulosis is the presence of small outpouchings in the large intestinal wall that is most frequent in people who eat a low-fiber diet. It is asymptomatic if not inflamed, in the latter case it is called diverticulitis.

69. Correct: Bacterial overgrowth (B)

In humans, hydrogen and methane are exclusively produced by intestinal bacteria, primarily anaerobic bacteria that are normally present in the colon. In the case of bacterial overgrowth, these bacteria also live in the small intestine, leading to excess production of gas, which diffuses into blood and out of pulmonary vessels into alveoli. A higher concentration is then measured in exhaled air. (**A, C, D, E**) Irritable bowel syndrome can be caused by and/or can lead to an abnormal cytokine profile, increased permeability of the gut, innate immune defects, and the presence of fungi. However, neither of these symptoms or causes can be derived from a positive hydrogen/ methane breath test.

70. Correct: Intestinal bacteria (C)

The migrating myoelectric complex (MMC) consists of characteristic peristaltic waves that occur about every 90 minutes between meals. They sweep out undigested food residue to avoid bacterial overgrowth. (**A**) The MMC typically starts in the stomach, and these peristaltic waves travel slowly the entire length of the small intestine to the ileum. Hence, an absence of the MMC does not increase duodenal motility. (**B, D, E**) Gastric emptying, mass movements, and swallowing belong to the digestive phase and will not be affected by the absence of the interdigestive MMC.

71. Correct: Enteropeptidase (C)

Enteropeptidase (also called enterokinase) is a protease that is present in and secreted by the intestinal brush border membrane. It converts pancreatic trypsinogen to trypsin, which then activates the rest of the pancreatic proteases. Pancreatic enzymes are necessary for normal digestion of proteins and polypeptides into absorbable amino acids and di- and tripeptides, so enteropeptidase deficiency causes hypoproteinemia and failure to thrive. Low oncotic pressure leads to edema and ascites. Undigested proteins cause vomiting and osmotic diarrhea. (**A, B, E**) Carboxypeptidase, chymotrypsin, and trypsin are pancreatic enzymes, not intestinal brush border enzymes. (**D**) Pepsin is a protease that is secreted by cells of the stomach, not the small intestine.

72. Correct: It is a group of similar fat-soluble vitamins. (D)

Like many other vitamins, "vitamin K" consists of a number of structurally similar compounds. Vitamin K is fat-soluble and stored in fat tissue. (**A**) Vitamin K deficiency is rarely due to diet. (**B**) Anticoagulants such as warfarin block the recycling of used vitamin K, so that active vitamin K levels are low (not high) when taking blood-thinning medication. (**C**) Vitamin K is abundant in green leaves, fruits, vegetables, and nuts (not bread, rice, and meat). (**E**) Iron (not vitamin K) overload is treated by frequent bleeding.

73. Correct: Cobalamin (C)

The removal of the terminal ileum limits the ability to absorb vitamin B_{12}. Vitamin B_{12} deficiency results in a low red blood cell count (low hemoglobin) with macrocytic red blood cells (increased MCV). The 3-year latency of the symptoms can be understood, since the storage of vitamin B_{12} in the liver is thought to be sufficient to maintain normal blood levels up to 3–6 years. The active ingredient of vitamin B_{12} supplements is cobalamin (in the form of either cyanocobalamin or methylcobalamin). (**A, B, D, E, F**) Ascorbic acid (vitamin C), cholecalciferol (vitamin D), folic acid (vitamin B_9), retinol (vitamin A), and thiamine (vitamin B_1) are all primarily absorbed in the duodenum (not the terminal ileum).

74. Correct: Vitamin D (E)

Without sufficient bile, absorption of the fat-soluble vitamin D is reduced. Vitamin D deficiency initially leads to hypocalcemia, which increases parathyroid hormone. This causes calcium to be released from bone, which normalizes serum calcium but leads to demineralized bones that easily break on impact. (**A, B, C**) Iron, folate (vitamin B_9), and vitamin B_{12} deficiency lead to anemia and fatigue, which is not supported by the clinical vignette. Bile is not necessary for their absorption. (**D**) Deficiency of the water-soluble vitamin C leads to scurvy with early symptoms of malaise and lethargy. Fatigue may also stem from anemia, since vitamin C deficiency limits iron absorption and folate activation.

75. Correct: It would take longer to reach the small intestine. (C)

When a lactase-deficient person drinks skim milk after an overnight fast, the onset of gastrointestinal symptoms occurs within minutes to one hour, when lactose has reached the small intestine and cannot be digested there by lactase. Since fat delays gastric emptying, high-fat milk would take longer than skim milk to reach the small intestine, which would unnecessarily extend the time for diagnosis. (**A**) If at all, fat might aggravate (not blunt) the symptoms by initiating more digestive motility. (**B**) Fat has no direct effect on the activity of lactase. (**D**) Lactose intolerance does not affect fat d igestion, and steatorrhea is not expected. (**E**) A clinical test is optimized for diagnosis, not treatment of a chronic disease such as obesity.

76. Correct: The uptake of fructose into an intestinal epithelial cell is independent of a sodium gradient. (D)

Fructose is primarily absorbed by GLUT5, a facilitated transporter that functions independent of a sodium gradient. (**A**) Lipid-soluble vitamins are not digested and therefore not reconstituted within enterocytes. (**B**) Free fatty acids pass through the brush border mucosal cell membranes by simple diffusion. No transporters are necessary. (**C**) Glucose is a monosaccharide that binds to the sodium-glucose-linked transporter SGLT1 for reabsorption, while sucrose needs to be digested to glucose and fructose before absorption. (**E**) Trypsin is an endopeptidase that is released as trypsinogen by the pancreas into the duodenal lumen and hence is not an integral protein of the brush border.

77. Correct: Destruction of the colonic myenteric plexus (C)

The myenteric plexus innervates the circular and longitudinal muscle layers of the gastrointestinal (GI) tract and, in the colon, controls mass movements. These are peristaltic waves that occur a few times per day and move large amounts of large intestinal content from one segment into the next. Without a mass movement of material into the sigmoid colon, defecation is not initiated and constipation ensues. (**A**) Denervation of the external anal sphincter would result in loss of voluntary control of the anal sphincter. Mass movements, on the other hand, are under autonomic control. (**B**) Damage to the submucosal plexus would result in loss of control of GI secretions and the muscularis mucosa but have only a minor effect on the circular and longitudinal muscle layers. (**D**) Excess vasoactive intestinal peptide due to a tumor (VIPoma) leads to watery diarrhea, since VIP increases GI secretions as well as small and large intestinal motility. (**E**) Inert, nondigestible particles osmotically bind water and support bowel evacuation (not constipation).

78. Correct: Enterokinase (C)

Enterokinase (also called enteropeptidase) activates trypsinogen that has been released by the pancreas into the gastrointestinal lumen to become trypsin. Trypsin then catalyzes the formation of additional trypsin and activates other proteolytic enzymes such as procarboxypeptidase, proelastase, and others. Hence, it makes sense to mimic the first step in this catalytic chain. (**A**) Bile salt (not bile pigment) is discussed to control the release of enterokinase. (**B**) Brush border peptidase is an already active enzyme that is integrated into the enterocyte cellular membrane near amino acid transporters, since it converts di- and tripeptides to amino acids. (**D, E**) In the presence of hydrochloric acid, pepsinogen that is released by chief cells (not pancreatic cells) is cleaved to become pepsin. Previously secreted pepsin then activates additional pepsinogen to become pepsin in the stomach.

79. Correct: Their colonic concentration is typically >10^9/ ml. (A)

The bacterial density in the colon in a healthy adult is typically higher than 10^9, and up to 10^{12} bacteria per milliliter. This dense colonization has recently raised considerable interest since there is increasing evidence that humans not only tolerate the gut bacteria but significantly benefit from them. (**B**) The duodenum contains only a very small amount of bacteria compared to the colon. The bacterial concentration increases in the distal parts of the small intestine, but is still less than 1–5% of the colonic concentration. (**C**) Eradication of the normal bacteria flora by drugs such as antibiotics causes negative health effects and favors the growth of harmful species. Humans with no gut flora can survive, but are not healthy. (**D**) Less than 1% of the gut bacteria are of the aerobic type. Since the majority require low or no oxygen to grow, they are difficult to study outside of the human body. (**E**) Bacteria make up about one-third of the total fecal dry mass. Epithelial cell and food rests make up most of the remainder.

8.7 Questions

80. As part of a large grant studying pancreatic adenocarcinoma, baseline data of pancreatic exocrine secretion are obtained from healthy people. Which of the following findings is expected?

A. Its enzyme concentration is increased with pancreatic polypeptide.
B. Its HCO_3^- concentration increases with increasing Cl^- concentration.
C. Its HCO_3^- concentration increases with secretin stimulation.
D. Its Na^+ and K^+ concentrations increase with increasing flow rate.
E. Its osmolality is less than 100 mOsm/kg at average flow rate.

81. A chronic alcoholic is urged to abstain from alcohol, because of which of the following consequences of liver failure?

A. Absorption of all nutrients will be impaired.
B. Plasma levels of ammonia will rise.
C. Plasma oncotic pressure will rise.
D. Severe hyperglycemia will develop.
E. The chance for venous thrombosis will rise.

82. As part of a study that aims to find better medical solutions for people with gallbladder stones, 6 hours after a meal, a fluid sample A is taken from the gallbladder of healthy subjects, and a fluid sample B is taken from their common hepatic duct. The concentration of which of the following is decreased in sample A compared to sample B?

A. Bicarbonate
B. Bile salt
C. Bilirubin
D. Cholesterol
E. Potassium

83. The plasma concentration of which of the following substances is the major aspect that controls the de novo synthesis of bile acids by the liver?

A. Bile acids
B. Cholecystokinin
C. Fat
D. Gastrin
E. Secretin

84. A patient complains of residue in her underwear. She also notes her stool floats and smells worse than normal. From her history, it is known she had a bowel resection of the terminal ileum one month ago. She evades answering the question whether she follows the dietary guidelines that were provided after the surgery. It is explained that her symptoms are not unexpected and most likely due to the decrease in which of the following?

A. Bile reabsorption in the small intestine
B. Bile release into the small intestine
C. Cholecystokinin release
D. De novo bile acid synthesis
E. Pancreatic lipase secretion

85. Based on the history and physical, a patient is suspected to have biliary obstruction. An increase in which of the following would support this suspicion?

A. Bile salt enterohepatic circulation
B. Dark reddish stool
C. Destruction of red blood cells
D. Lipid content in feces
E. Unconjugated bilirubin

86. Which of the following is generated by the liver to aid in fat metabolism?

A. Bile salts
B. Chylomicrons
C. Colipase
D. Lymph
E. Vitamin K

87. A patient presents with severe itching, jaundice, unexpected weight loss, and general fatigue. Which of the following urine or stool findings would support the physician's initial thought of a posthepatic (also called extrahepatic) cause of jaundice?

A. Black, tarry stool
B. Clay-colored urine
C. Dark-colored stool
D. Dark-colored urine
E. Urobilinogen in urine

88. The image shows the bile circulation cycle. It is present on the wall of a patient investigation room. The failure of the hormone cholecystokinin to be released into blood will directly affect which of the following parts of the cycle?

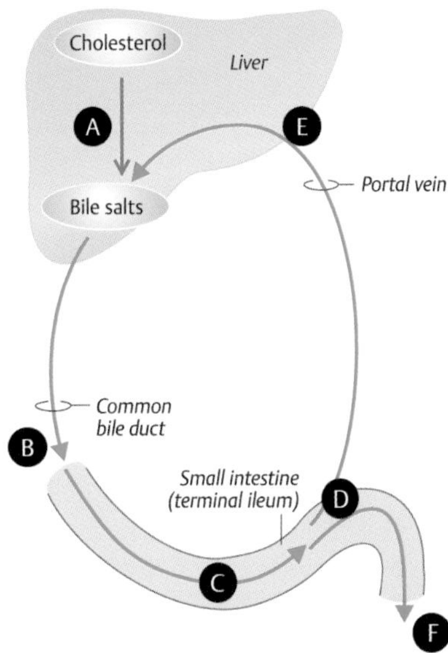

A. A
B. B
C. C
D. D
E. E
F. F

89. A 21-year-old woman presents at the primary care office with a yellow staining of her sclerae. She is not very concerned since she has had multiple similar experiences since she was 12 years old, typically when under stress or when ill. Currently, she is stressed because she just moved to the city. In between episodes she is asymptomatic. She has been diagnosed with a genetic liver disorder (the name escapes her). The patient's laboratory values are as follows, compared to the reference values in parentheses:

Hematocrit:	43%	(36.1–44.3%)
Reticulocytes	1.2%	(0.5–1.5%)
Serum total bilirubin	1.92 mg/dL	(< 1.17)
Serum direct bilirubin	0.29 mg/dL	(0–0.3)
Urine bilirubin	Undetectable	(< 0.01)

Which of the following is most likely responsible for her periodic jaundice?

A. Intermittent bile duct obstruction
B. Reduced activity of UDP glucuronyltransferase
C. Decreased secretion of conjugated bilirubin
D. Genetic susceptibility to gallstone formation
E. Genetic susceptibility to hemolytic anemia

90. A 65-year-old male presents with a 1-week history of abdominal pain, especially in the right upper quadrant. He also reports nausea, itching, and fatigue but denies blurred vision or light-headedness. Physical examination shows scleral icterus and diffuse jaundice. A complete blood count with differential shows no abnormalities. The following blood values are available:

Total bilirubin:	3.4 mg/dL	(< 1.12)
Direct bilirubin:	1.2 mg/dL	(0.0–0.3)
Alkaline phosphatase:	280 IU/L	(44–147)
C-reactive protein:	20 mg/dL	(0–10)

Which of the following is the most likely cause of his jaundice?

A. Crigler-Najjar syndrome
B. Gallstones
C. Gilbert's syndrome
D. Hemolysis
E. Ruptured spleen

91. A very thin 65-year-old white male comes to the office for a full body checkup. He says he lost weight 3 years ago when he and his wife switched to a strict vegan diet, and that his weight has remained low ever since. The comprehensive physical exam is unremarkable except for minor abdominal tenderness. On questioning, he denies having problems with stool evacuation. Instead, he states that his stool smells "strong." His stool sample is negative for occult blood, but it appears abnormally pale. Serum amylase, serum lipase, and C-reactive protein are all normal. Which of the following is most likely responsible for his pale stools?

A. Acute pancreatitis
B. An upper GI bleed
C. Constipation
D. Partial biliary obstruction
E. Ulcerative colitis

92. A 35-year-old female presents with fat digestion problems but denies colicky abdominal pain. Since abdominal ultrasonography is inconclusive, cholescintigraphy is ordered. For the latter, a radioactive chemical is intravenously injected into the patient. After the chemical has time to disperse, a radiographic body picture is taken. It shows radioactivity in the liver, bile ducts, and gallbladder, but minimally in the intestine. Injection of which of the following hormones aids in determining the lack of intestinal bile as a problem of the gallbladder or the bile ducts?

A. Cholecystokinin
B. Estrogen
C. Pancreatic polypeptide
D. Somatostatin
E. Vasoactive intestinal peptide

93. A 23-year-old African American college student with sickle-cell trait presents with pallor, fatigue, and shortness of breath. She is distressed since she wants to run the college's summer half-marathon in 1 week. Which of the following lab results were most likely obtained from this patient?

	Plasma bile acids/ salts	Plasma direct bilirubin	Plasma indirect bilirubin	Hematocrit
A.	↔	↓	↑ ↑ ↑	↑
B.	↓	↔	↑	↓
C.	↓	↔	↔	↔
D.	↓	↔	↑	↑
E.	↔	↑ ↔	↑ ↑ ↑	↓

94. Which of the following bile components quantitatively constitute the largest percentage of total bile solute in an adult person on a normal mixed Western diet?

A. Bile salts
B. Bilirubin
C. Cholesterol
D. Fatty acids
E. Phospholipids
F. Proteins

95. A 5-week-old baby has been undergoing daily phototherapy for jaundice since day 2 after a full-term birth. So far, there are no signs of neurological impairment (kernicterus), but there is also no normalization of the skin and eye color. Total bilirubin values are continually 10–15 times higher than normal. Direct bilirubin levels are unmeasurable. Which of the following best explains the condition?

A. Biliary tree abnormality
B. Defective basolateral membrane hepatocyte bilirubin transporter
C. Deficiency in UDP glucuronyltransferase
D. Lack of gallbladder contraction
E. Normal physiological jaundice of the newborn

96. Secondary bile acids are which of the following?

A. Formed by small intestinal enterokinases
B. Not subject to enterohepatic circulation
C. Primary bile acids conjugated to glycine or taurine
D. Produced by bacterial action in the colon
E. Secreted primarily in adulthood

8.8 Answers and Explanations

80. Correct: Its HCO_3^- concentration increases with secretin stimulation. (C)

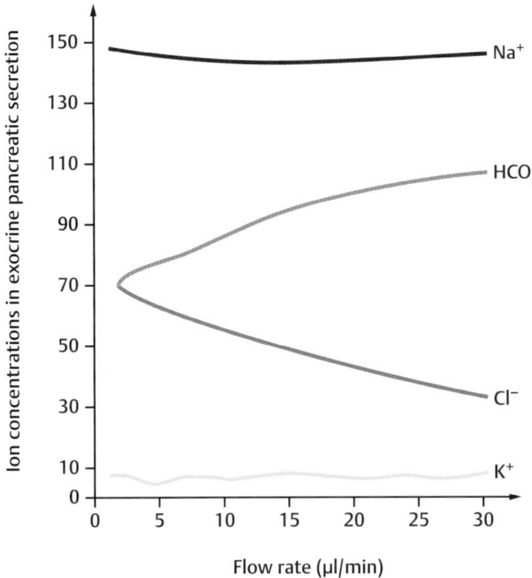

The epithelial cells of the pancreatic ducts secrete most of the aqueous component of the pancreatic secretion. Secretin increases the quantity and bicarbonate concentration, which increases threefold above basal levels during high secretory rates. (**A**) Pancreatic polypeptide is released by the pancreatic islet cells and inhibits pancreatic secretion. (**B**) Bicarbonate and chloride concentrations vary reciprocally, so that with increasing HCO_3^-, there is decreasing Cl^- (image). (**D**) Na^+ and K^+ concentrations of pancreatic secretion are largely independent of flow rate. (**E**) Pancreatic secretion is isotonic and hence approximately 300 mOsm/kg.

81. Correct: Plasma levels of ammonia will rise. (B)

Plasma ammonia levels will rise, because the liver's normal role to convert ammonia from disassembled amino acids into urea is diminished. (**A**) Absorption of fat will indeed be impaired, because the liver's bile production will slow or cease. However, absorption of carbohydrates and proteins will not be affected. (**C**) The plasma oncotic pressure will fall because the hepatic synthesis of plasma proteins will be impaired in liver failure. (**D**) Severe hypoglycemia (not hyperglycemia) will develop, because the liver plays a central role in maintaining plasma glucose. (**E**) The synthesis of clotting factors decreases, so the chance for venous thrombosis will not rise.

82. Correct: Bicarbonate (A)

During the interdigestive period, bile is diverted into the gallbladder. The gallbladder removes Na^+ and water, thereby concentrating other bile constituents. While bile on average is slightly alkaline, it becomes more acidic the longer it is stored in the gallbladder. The gallbladder acidifies bile by removing Na^+ in exchange for H^+ ions. The protons are buffered by bicarbonate, so that gallbladder bile contains about one-fourth as much HCO_3^- as liver bile. (**B, C, D**) Bile constituents such as bile salts, bilirubin, and cholesterol are all five- to tenfold concentrated when bile is stored in the gallbladder. (**E**) Potassium is severalfold more concentrated in the gallbladder, since water removal is primarily due to removing sodium and chloride. The same applies to the calcium concentration.

83. Correct: Bile acids (A)

Bile acids are produced *de novo* from cholesterol, primarily in hepatocytes that surround the central hepatic vein. The rate-limiting enzyme in the biosynthetic pathway is cholesterol 7-α-hydroxylase (CYP7A1), whose gene transcription is inhibited by bile acids. This means that the plasma concentration of bile acids regulates their own hepatic synthesis. With the emerging understanding that bile acids regulate not only their own homeostasis but also that of other molecules such as glucose, their potential role as hormones is receiving attention. There is an alternate bile acid synthesis pathway of lesser importance (~ 5%), whose regulation is not well understood. (**B, C, D, E**) The hormones cholecystokinin, gastrin, and secretin, as well as fat, are not involved in regulating the bile acid pool.

84. Correct: Bile reabsorption in the small intestine (A)

About 90% of bile acids/salts are reabsorbed in the terminal ileum by a sodium-bile cotransporter. With each regular meal, the total amount circulates twice between intestine and liver (with a greasy meal, up to six times). Hence, it is not unexpected that soon after ileal bowel resection the patient experiences symptoms of insufficient lipid absorption and excess lipid excretion, especially if she does not follow a low-fat diet. (**B**) The release of bile from the liver into the small intestine is not affected. (**C**) Cholecystokinin is released by cells in the duodenum and proximal jejunum in response to digestive products of dietary fat and proteins (not bile acids/salts) (**D**) After ileal bowel resection, the patient's pool of bile acids/salts in the portal vein decreases. This is sensed and increases (not decreases) hepatic *de novo* bile acid synthesis. (**E**) The secretion of pancreatic lipase is regulated by cholecystokinin, which is not altered as explained in answer C.

85. Correct: Lipid content in feces (D)

Biliary obstruction refers to the blockade of any duct that carries bile from the liver to the gallbladder or from the gallbladder to the small intestine. In either case, bile does not reach the gastrointestinal lumen to aid in the absorption of dietary lipids, so the lipid content in feces increases. (**A**) With bile duct obstruction less (not more) bile salts would undergo enterohepatic circulation. (**B**) Biliary obstruction causes pale-colored (not dark-colored) feces due to the lack of bile pigments. (**C**) The lifetime of red blood cell destruction is not affected by biliary 91 obstruction. (**E**) Regardless whether the cause of biliary obstruction is intrahepatic (e.g., viral hepatitis) or extrahepatic (e.g., gallstones), it predominantly causes conjugated (not unconjugated) hyperbilirubinemia.

86. Correct: Bile salts (A)

The liver generates *de novo* the portion of bile acids/salts that is daily lost in feces. This is quantitatively 15–30% of the total pool of about 2–4 grams of bile salts that circulate continuously in the enterohepatic circulation. (**B**) Chylomicrons are generated in endoplasmic reticulum of small-intestinal enterocytes. (**C**) Colipase is generated and secreted by the pancreas in an inactive form and activated by contact with trypsin in the intestinal lumen. (**D**) Lymph is generated when interstitial fluid is taken up by blind-ending lymph bulbs. (**E**) Vitamin K is generated by the liver but does not contribute to fat metabolism.

87. Correct: Dark-colored urine (D)

In a posthepatic obstruction of bile flow, water-soluble conjugated bilirubin backs up in hepatocytes and spills over into urine, to which it imparts a dark color. Accumulation of bilirubin in skin and eyes accounts for itching and jaundice. Malabsorption of lipid-soluble nutrients leads to the patient's unexpected weight loss and fatigue. (**A**) Black, tarry stool is typically due to digested blood, indicating a blood source upstream of the small intestine. (**B, C**) Stool (not urine) is pale or clay-colored due to the lack of bilirubin products such as stercobilin. (**E**) Urobilinogen is formed by bacteria in the small and large intestine from conjugated bilirubin. Normally, about 90% is excreted in feces and 10% in urine after being reabsorbed. Hence, in a posthepatic bile obstruction, when no bile enters the intestine, no urobilinogen is found in urine.

88. Correct: B (B)

Cholecystokinin (CCK) regulates the release of bile into the small intestine via the common bile duct. It does so by directly stimulating the contraction of the gallbladder and by relaxing the sphincter of Oddi, so that bile salts are ejected into the intestinal lumen. (**A**) CCK has no direct effect on the *de novo* synthesis of bile salts from cholesterol. (**C**) CCK has no direct action on the formation or action of micelles in the intestinal lumen. (**D**) CCK does not regulate the reabsorption of bile acids/salts via the sodium cotransporter. (**E**) CCK has no direct effect on the reuptake of bile acids/salts into hepatocytes. (**F**) CCK has no direct effect on the excretion of bile in stool.

89. Correct: Reduced activity of UDP glucuronyltransferase (B)

The patient most likely has Gilbert's syndrome (GS), which normally has no serious consequences but can cause mild jaundice at stressful times. It is caused by the reduced activity of the liver enzyme UDP glucuronyltransferase. The enzyme conjugates glucuronic acid to bilirubin, which makes the latter more water-soluble and ready to be excreted via bile. Hence, in GS there is less bilirubin elimination and a backup of total serum bilirubin. The hyperbilirubinemia is primarily due to unconjugated, indirect bilirubin, which is evident in the patient by her normal direct, conjugated bilirubin values. (**A**) Bile duct obstruction would lead to increased direct bilirubin. (**C**) Conjugated bilirubin is synonymous with direct bilirubin, which is normal in her case. (**D**) Stones in gallbladder or other parts of the biliary tract would lead to increased direct bilirubin. (**E**) Hemolytic anemia would increase her reticulocyte count.

90. Correct: Gallstones (B)

Biliary obstruction due to gallstones leads to jaundice with primarily elevated levels of direct (conjugated) bilirubin, since the cause for the backup is “after” the liver, which conjugates bilirubin to glucuronic acid. Such posthepatic jaundice also presents with significantly elevated alkaline phosphatase. Right upper quadrant tenderness is due to the liver and gallbladder being present in this abdominal area. C-reactive protein is elevated due to acute cholecystitis. (**A, C**) Crigler-Najjar syndrome and Gilbert's syndrome are the severe and the mild manifestation, respectively, of genetic disorders that involve the absence of, or a defect in, the liver enzyme UDP glucuronyltransferase. This leads to backup of primarily indirect (unconjugated) bilirubin. (**D**) Fatigue due to hemolytic anemia presents with primarily elevated unconjugated bilirubin, since the degradation of red blood cells exceeds the ability of the liver to clear bilirubin as hemoglobin waste product. (**E**) A week-long pain with normal blood count and no signs of shock (such as blurred vision or light-headedness) could point only to an injured rather than ruptured spleen. Even this is unlikely, since it would cause pain predominantly in the left upper abdominal quadrant. Liver and bilirubin values would not be affected.

91. Correct: Partial biliary obstruction (D)

The typically dark brown color of stool is due to stercobilin, a metabolite of bilirubin that has been transformed by intestinal bacteria. Hence, in biliary obstruction, when bilirubin does not reach the intestine, it results in pale, clay-colored stools. Without bile, one might also expect fat absorption problems and fatty stools, but considering the patient's low-fat vegan diet, it results only in a strong smell. (**A**) Acute pancreatitis almost always presents with elevated amylase and lipase, and typically with elevated C-reactive protein. (**B**) An upper gastrointestinal bleed would result in black tarry stool. (**C**) Constipation would be infrequent, irregular and/or difficult evacuation of feces. Stool is usually dry and hard. (**E**) Ulcerative colitis is an intense inflammatory reaction of the large intestine, so C-reactive protein would likely to be elevated. Additionally, patients often experience frequent stools that contain blood and mucus.

92. Correct: Cholecystokinin (A)

Cholecystokinin (CCK) is the hormone that causes gallbladder contraction. If the patient after intravenous CCK injection shows reduced ejection of radioactive bile from the gallbladder into the intestinal lumen, a disease with the gallbladder itself is likely. If, on the other hand, after CCK injection, the patient's gallbladder contracts causing colicky pain but there is no bile ejection, a bile duct obstruction by gallstones, tumors, parasites, or blood clots is likely. (**B**) Although estrogen receptors have been found in the gallbladder, no direct effect on gallbladder contractility is known. (**C, D, E**) Pancreatic polypeptide, somatostatin, and vasoactive intestinal peptides are known to inhibit gallbladder motility and would not be helpful to distinguish between an obstruction and a problem related to the gallbladder itself.

93. Correct: ↔, ↑↔, ↑↑↑, ↓ (E)

The red blood cells in people with sickle cell trait are susceptible to deform and sickle with exercise that can cause temporary hypoxic conditions, such as training outdoors in summer. Such sickled cells easily break apart when squeezing through capillaries (low hematocrit), leading to signs of hemolytic anemia such as pallor, fatigue, and shortness of breath. When the hemolysis exceeds the capacity of the liver to clear the metabolites derived from the heme molecules, it results in increased serum bilirubin, primarily indirect bilirubin. Plasma bile acids/ salts are unchanged, since their enterohepatic circulation is not affected and their *de novo* synthesis is regulated in the liver by the presence of bile acids/ salts in blood. (**A, C, D**) These choices are unlikely due to the patient's sign of anemia. (**B**) There is no obvious reason for the patient's bile acids/salts to be low.

94. Correct: Bile salts (A)

Bile composition is complex and varies based on the diet of the individual. However, the largest percentage is always bile salts (50–60%). (**B**) Bilirubin (about 3% of total solute) is the most common end product of body metabolism that is excreted in bile. (**C, D, E**) Cholesterol, fatty acids, and phospholipids (mainly phosphatidylcholine), constitute about 9%, 12%, and 3% of bile, respectively. When released by hepatocytes, they, together with bile salts, form the aggregates that are called mixed micelles. Cholesterol in excess is also excreted via bile. (**F**) Bile proteins are about 7% of total bile solute. Some plasma proteins passively enter bile. Most proteins are actively secreted from blood (e.g., immunoglobulins), liver (e.g., lysosomal enzymes), and biliary tract/ gallbladder cells (e.g., alkaline phosphatase, mucin).

95. Correct: Deficiency in UDP glucuronyltransferase (C)

The baby most likely suffers from Crigler-Najjar syndrome. The deficiency of UDP glucuronyltransferase in hepatocytes prevents the formation of conjugated bilirubin, the form that is primarily transported into bile. Hence, unconjugated bilirubin builds up in blood. Normally, it cannot be excreted in urine since it is bound to albumin. Phototherapy modifies it so that some can be excreted—enough to prevent it from being transported into the brain to cause brain damage (kernicterus), but not enough to resolve the jaundice and icterus. (**A, D**) Biliary tree abnormality and lack of gallbladder contraction would lead to elevated serum conjugated bilirubin after about 2 weeks, when the baby's liver has matured to perform the conjugation. (**B**) With a defective bilirubin transporter at the basolateral membrane of hepatocytes (Dubin-Johnson syndrome), unconjugated bilirubin can still enter the hepatocyte and be conjugated. It would then reflux back into blood. (**E**) Normal physiological jaundice resolves within 2 weeks for a baby born at full term and does not rise to 10 times above normal.

96. Correct: Produced by bacterial action in the colon (D)

Inside the colon, the primary bile salts cholate and chenodeoxycholate are acted upon by bacteria. Bacteria dehydroxylate and convert primary bile acids/ salts into the secondary bile acids deoxycholic acid and lithocholic acid, respectively. (**A**) Small-intestinal enterokinases activate digestive enzymes that have been released in inactive forms. (**B**) Secondary bile acids are reabsorbed and subject to enterohepatic circulation. (**C**) Primary bile acids that are conjugated to glycine or taurine are called bile salts (not secondary bile acids). (**E**) Children have the microbial flora in the colon that produces secondary bile acids.

Chapter 9

Endocrine System

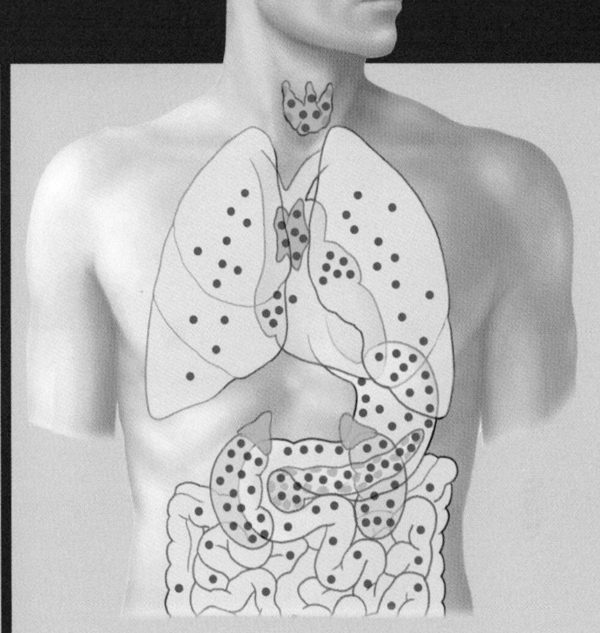

LEARNING OBJECTIVES

- Understand the general principles of endocrinology, including hormone synthesis, serum transport, and signaling, in order to use this knowledge for diagnosis and treatment.
- Understand the functions of hypothalamic and pituitary hormones and their roles in maintaining body homeostasis. Use this knowledge for diagnosis and treatment of various diseases.
- Understand the role of pancreatic hormones in energy metabolism and apply this knowledge to various diseases caused by endocrine dysfunction.
- Understand the synthesis, functions, and regulation of thyroid hormones and apply this knowledge to the diagnosis and treatment of hypothyroid and hyperthyroid conditions.
- Understand the synthesis, functions, and regulation of adrenal gland hormones and use this knowledge for diagnosis and treatment of adrenal gland–related disorders.
- Understand the hormonal regulation of calcium and phosphate homeostasis and apply this knowledge to bone diseases and conditions with dysregulation of calcium and phosphate homeostasis.

9.1 Questions

Easy	Medium	Hard

1. Clinical studies that examine the effectiveness of l-tyrosine as a dietary supplement to increase cognitive performance have thus far shown inconclusive results. Nevertheless, advertisements for l-tyrosine supplements are common. Physicians should discourage patients with which of the following conditions from taking tyrosine supplements without supervision?

A. Addison's disease
B. Congenital adrenal hyperplasia (21-beta form)
C. Graves' disease
D. Hashimoto's disease
E. Type 1 diabetes

2. Patient A is a 61-year-old woman with kidney stones, osteoporosis, constipation, frequent urination, and depression. Patient B is a 12-year-old obese boy with short stature, short fingers, developmental delay, and a hyperexcitable facial nerve. Blood tests for patient A reveal elevated parathyroid hormone, serum calcium, and alkaline phosphatase, and low levels of phosphorus. Blood tests for patient B show elevated parathyroid hormone and serum phosphate and low serum calcium. Which of the following are the expected urinary cAMP levels of patient A and patient B?

	Patient A	Patient B
A.	Increased	Increased
B.	Increased	Decreased
C.	Increased	No change
D.	Decreased	Increased
E.	Decreased	Decreased
F	Decreased	No change

3. A new long-acting insulin analogue is tested for potential carcinogenicity. As part of drug development, tests for abnormal cell growth must always be included since an insulin analogue carries the risk of enhancing signaling of which of the following hormones?

A. Glucagon
B. Insulin-like growth factor 1
C. Thyroid hormone
D. Thyroid-stimulating hormone
E. Thyrotropin-releasing hormone

4. In a research study with healthy people, the half-lives of four hormones in serum were measured and the following average results were recorded:

Hormone 1: 1–3 minutes
Hormone 2 4–6 minutes
Hormone 3 8–24 hours
Hormone 4: 7 days

Which of the following are the four measured hormones?

	Hormone 1	Hormone 2	Hormone 3	Hormone 4
A.	Angio-tensin II	Insulin	Total T_3	Total T_4
B.	Total T_4	Angio-tensin II	Insulin	Total T_3
C.	Total T_4	Total T_3	Angio-tensin II	Insulin
D.	Insulin	Total T_3	Total T_4	Angio-tensin II
E.	Angio-tensin II	Total T_3	Insulin	Total T_4

5. An in vitro insulin dose-response curve was created from a patient with multiple endocrine neoplasia. For that test, glucose in the form of [14C-U] 2-deoxyglucose was added to freshly isolated adipocytes, and glucose transport was quantified in the presence of increasing insulin concentrations. The image shows the patient's results (red dashed line) in comparison to controls (black solid line). Compared to controls, which of the following best describes the patient's insulin responsiveness and insulin sensitivity?

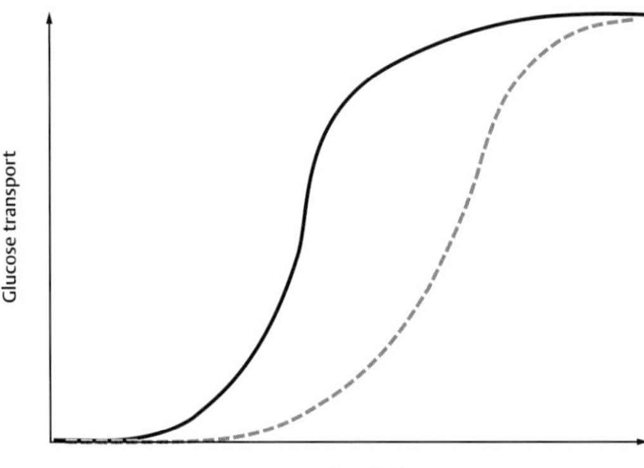

	Insulin responsiveness	Insulin sensitivity
A,	↓	↔
B.	↓	↑
C.	↓	↓
D.	↔	↓
E.	↔	↑

6. A 68-year old woman with type 2 diabetes mellitus and hypothyroidism, who occasionally uses a hydrocortisone topical cream, asks about the potential to administer thyroxine and insulin through the skin. The physician's answer includes information about the chemical versatility of hormones. To which chemical classes of hormones do cortisol, thyroxine (T4), and insulin belong, respectively?

	Cortisol	Thyroxine (T_4)	Insulin
A.	Steroid hormones	Amino acid derivatives	Peptide hormones
B.	Protein hormones	Amino acid derivatives	Steroid hormones
C.	Catecholamines	Amino acid derivatives	Peptide hormones
D.	Steroid hormones	Peptide hormones	Catecholamines
E.	Catecholamines	Peptide hormones	Steroid hormones
F.	Protein hormones	Peptide hormones	Catecholamines

9.2 Answers and Explanations

Easy | Medium | Hard

1. Correct: Graves' disease (C)

Tyrosine is the precursor for epinephrine, dopamine, and thyroxine. When a person with hyperthyroidism from Graves' disease takes tyrosine supplements, thyroxine concentrations can further increase to dangerous levels. (**A, B**) Addison's disease and congenital adrenal hyperplasia (21-beta form) typically present with low cortisol, and patients are known to be especially symptomatic in stressful situations. Some studies indicate that tyrosine improves performance under stressful condition, so these are not the best answers. (**D**) Patients with chronic Hashimoto's disease typically have hypothyroidism, so supplements with thyroid hormone precursor are not contraindicated. (**E**) There is no obvious overlap between tyrosine and insulin.

2. Correct: Increased, decreased (B)

Patient A has primary hyperparathyroidism leading to hypercalcemia. Typical signs and symptoms are summarized by the following mnemonic: stones (kidney stones), bones (osteoporosis), groans (gastrointestinal problems such as constipation), thrones (polyuria), and overtones (personality changes including depression). Serum calcium is high and serum phosphate is low, confirming a primary parathyroid hormone (PTH) disorder. Since PTH signals via cAMP, this molecule can be found at higher levels in urine. Increased concentrations of renal tubular cAMP lead to polyuria.

Patient B has hypocalcemia causing a positive Chvostek sign (hyperexcitable facial nerve), short stature, short fingers, and developmental delay. He also has elevated serum phosphate. Hypocalcemia and hyperphosphatemia would be expected with low PTH, but PTH concentrations are increased. Such pseudohypoparathyroidism (also called end-organ resistance to PTH) is due to an abnormal G_s protein (the patient resembles type 1a Albright hereditary osteodystrophy), resulting in low PTH-mediated cAMP, and low cAMP levels in urine. Note that urinary cAMP can help distinguish between primary and secondary PTH disorders. (**A, C, D, E, F**) These choices are incorrect.

3. Correct: Insulin-like growth factor 1 (B)

Insulin and insulin-like growth factor 1 (IGF-1) both bind to receptors that act via tyrosine kinase signaling mechanisms. Pharmacologic insulin signaling can unintentionally activate IGF-1-dependent mitogenic pathways and increase cell proliferation, hence the potential for carcinogenicity. (**A**) Insulin inhibits glucagon and hence glucagon signaling. (**C**) Thyroid hormone binds to intracellular receptors that act as transcription factors and directly regulate gene expression. (**D, E**) Thyroid-stimulating hormone (TSH) signaling is via cAMP, and thyrotropin-releasing hormone (TRH) signaling is an IP_3 mechanism. Neither of these signaling pathways directly interacts with tyrosine kinase signaling pathways activated by growth factors.

4. Correct: Angiotensin II, insulin, Total T3, Total T4 (A)

Angiotensin II and insulin are water-soluble peptide hormones. They have a short half-life, which is proportional to the size of the molecule. Angiotensin II consists of 8 amino acids in a single chain and hence has a shorter half-life than insulin, which is composed of 51 amino acids in the form of two chains. Triiodothyronine (T_3) and thyroxine (T_4) are lipid-soluble hormones. They are carried in blood bound to albumin and special carrier proteins. Hence, their half-life is long and proportional to the affinity for the protein carrier. T_4 is the main hormone released by the thyroid gland. It is tightly bound to thyroxine-binding globulin (TBG) and, in this form, is delivered to target tissue, where T_3 is produced. T_3 is the most potent thyroid hormone and is only loosely bound to TBG. Hence, based on the binding affinity, T_4 has the longest half-life (days) and T_3 has a shorter half-life (hours). (**B, C, D, E**) These choices are incorrect.

5. Correct: ↔, ↓ (D)

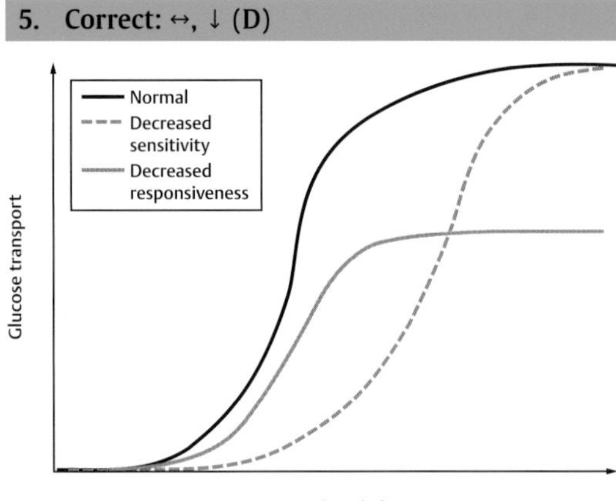

The patient's dose-response curve is shifted to the right, but maximum glucose uptake is still reached at very high insulin levels. This indicates decreased insulin sensitivity with normal insulin responsiveness. Insulin responsiveness is defined by the maximal effect of insulin, which is here not different from that of the control patients. If responsiveness were decreased, the dose-response curve would be flattened, as shown in the green line in the image. It is affected when there is a defect in insulin receptor signaling, when there is a change in the number of target cells or receptors per cell, or when an inhibitor is present. The patient exhibits decreased insulin sensitivity, since a higher insulin concentration is required for a half-maximal response. This can be seen since the number of insulin molecules that bind to the receptor at a given dose is reduced and the insulin response (in this case glucose transport) is reduced. Most often, it means that there is a decrease in receptor affinity for insulin. It would also be seen when there is excessive hormone degradation or when a competitive hormone is present. (**A, B, C, E**) These choices are incorrect.

6. Correct: Steroid hormones, amino acid derivatives, peptide hormones (A)

Cortisol, and the closely related metabolite cortisone, are steroid hormones. Steroid hormones are derived from cholesterol and are generally insoluble in water. Their names typically end with "-ol" or "-one," including cortisol, aldosterone, testosterone, progesterone, and estradiol. Thyroxine is an amino acid derivate. Amino acid–derived hormones are derived from tyrosine or tryptophan (thyroxine is derived from tyrosine), and usually have names ending in "-ine." They are typically water soluble and include epinephrine, norepinephrine, and thyroxine. Insulin belongs to the class of peptide hormones. Peptide hormones have a polypeptide chain and include growth hormone, oxytocin, insulin, and many others. Transcutaneous thyroxine and insulin delivery is challenging because it requires the association of the lipid-insoluble hormones with lipid-soluble vehicles. (**B, C, D, E, F**) These choices contain the wrong combination of answers.

9.3 Questions

7. A 75-year old woman complains of bilateral temporal hemianopsia, and imaging of the head reveals a suprasellar granular cell tumor. The tumor is excised, and immunohistochemical studies using biomarkers are performed in order to determine the tumor cell origin. A positive reaction for which of the following hormones would indicate that the tumor is of neuroectodermal origin?

A. Adrenocorticotropic hormone
B. β-endorphin
C. Luteinizing hormone
D. Oxytocin
E. Thyroid-stimulating hormone

8. A male soldier experienced severe head trauma that resulted in permanent interruption of his hypothalamohypophyseal portal vessels. Which of the following would be expected to develop?

A. Acromegaly
B. Excessive aggressiveness
C. Hyperpigmentation
D. Hyperprolactinemia
E. Hyperthyroidism

9. A 17-year-old boy previously sustained a severe fracture at the base of his skull while skateboarding. He presents with increased thirst and polyuria. His urine is pale in color with a low specific gravity. He has a blood pressure of 98/50 mm Hg, has tachycardia, and is very weak. An analogue of which of the following hormones is most likely prescribed for treatment?

A. Adrenocorticotropic hormone
B. Aldosterone
C. Androstenedione
D. Angiotensin II
E. Antidiuretic hormone

10. A patient with excessive thirst undergoes a 6-hour water deprivation test. The patient is deprived of water beginning at time 0 (baseline). Synthetic antidiuretic hormone (ADH) is given to the patient after 3 hours. Urine osmolality is measured every hour with the following results:

Time	Urine osmolality (mOsm/kg)
0 (baseline)	200
1 h	200
2 h	200
3 hr (ADH given)	200
4 h	400
5 h	600
6 h	800

What is the patient's diagnosis?

A. Central diabetes insipidus
B. Nephrogenic diabetes insipidus
C. Osmotic diuresis
D. Primary polydipsia
E. SIADH

11. A 30-year-old woman is diagnosed with galactorrhea from both breasts. She is not pregnant and has never been pregnant. The nipple discharge started two weeks ago, after she was in a car accident. She had a concussion and is still having headaches. The galactorrhea is most likely a result of which substance not reaching the pituitary gland?

A. Dopamine
B. Gonadotropin-releasing hormone
C. Growth hormone–releasing hormone
D. Oxytocin
E. Thyrotropin-releasing hormone

12. As part of an anti-doping educational session for athletes, the normal functions of various hormones are introduced. Which of the following hormones is best described as follows: "Increases lipolysis, stimulates protein synthesis, decreases glucose uptake, and supports calcium retention?"

A. Cortisol
B. Glucagon
C. Growth hormone
D. Insulin
E. Parathyroid hormone

13. A 50-year-old man is concerned about changes in his appearance. He has not seen a doctor for the past 8 years. His feet and hands have grown larger, his jaw is protruding, and his face is looking strangely "out of shape." He has slight difficulty breathing, frequent headaches, fatigue, impotence, and excessive sweating. Magnetic resonance imaging (MRI) reveals a 1.5-cm mass on the anterior pituitary. An oral glucose tolerance test is given. Which of the following is a positive test result that supports the patient's signs and symptoms?

A. Increased serum ghrelin
B. Failed growth hormone suppression
C. Failed insulin-like growth factor 1 increase
D. Increased serum glucose
E. Increased somatostatin

14. As part of a Big Data study, deidentified patient records were selected into four categories (labeled 1–4 in the image) based on plasma osmolality and plasma antidiuretic hormone (ADH) levels. In a first step, it was assumed that each patient had one of the following four diagnoses: central diabetes insipidus, nephrogenic diabetes insipidus, syndrome of inappropriate ADH secretion, or primary polydipsia. In a second step, additionally available patient values were used to support the assumption. A patient in which of the following categories should have hyperosmotic urine?

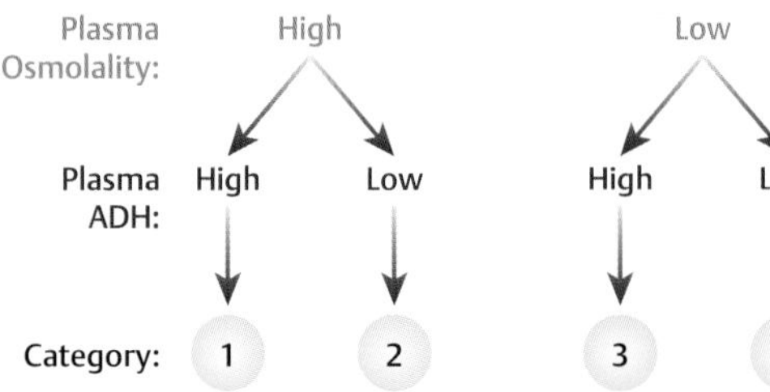

A. 1
B. 2
C. 3
D. 4

9.4 Answers and Explanations

7. Correct: Oxytocin (D)

Oxytocin is the hormone that is released by the posterior pituitary, which is derived from neuroectoderm. The posterior pituitary is called the neurohypophysis because it is formed from neuroectoderm and is, functionally, an extension of the hypothalamus. (**A, B**) Adrenocorticotropic hormone (ACTH) and β-endorphin are both products of the precursor proopiomelanocortin (POMC) and secreted by the anterior pituitary, which is of oral ectodermal origin. (**C, E**) Luteinizing hormone (LH) and thyroid-stimulating hormone (TSH) are from the anterior pituitary, which is not derived from nervous tissue.

8. Correct: Hyperprolactinemia (D)

Prolactin release is tonically inhibited by dopamine (also called prolactin-inhibiting factor), which is produced in the hypothalamus. Without dopamine reaching the pituitary via hypothalamohypophyseal portal vessels, hyperprolactinemia can develop. (**A**) In this patient, hypothalamic growth hormone–releasing hormone (GHRH) cannot reach the pituitary, so excessive growth hormone release and acromegaly are not expected. (**B**) Since hypothalamic gonadotropin-releasing hormone (GnRH) cannot activate luteinizing hormone (LH) and follicle-stimulating hormone (FSH) release, excess testosterone and potential aggressiveness are not expected. Moreover, hyperprolactinemia inhibits GnRH release. (**C**) One would not expect hyperpigmentation, since it results from increased production of POMC, which is produced through the influence of hypothalamic corticotropin-releasing hormone (CRH). (**E**) With hypothalamic thyrotropin-releasing hormone (TRH) not reaching the pituitary, one does not expect hyperthyroidism. The lack of TRH might slightly blunt hyperprolactinemia, since TRH normally stimulates prolactin release, but the effect is small compared to the lack of dopamine.

9. Correct: Antidiuretic hormone (E)

The patient presents with the typical symptoms of central diabetes insipidus. He is very thirsty (polydipsia), but cannot drink enough to make up for the renal fluid loss (polyuria, low-osmolality urine). Hypovolemia leads to a decrease in blood pressure and baroreceptor-induced tachycardia. Hence, desmopressin, a modified form of vasopressin (also called antidiuretic hormone) will be prescribed. (**A**) Adrenocorticotropic hormone (ACTH) leads to the synthesis of glucocorticoids and androgen, with no direct impact for water balance and unnecessary side effects. (**B**) Aldosterone would unnecessarily affect his acid-base and potassium status. (**C**) Androstenedione is irrelevant for water balance and would unnecessarily impact testosterone homeostasis. (**D**) Angiotensin II does not address the root problem and could cause hypertension and other unnecessary side effects.

10. Correct: Central diabetes insipidus (A)

In the fluid deprivation test, the patient is not able to concentrate urine after water restriction (urine remains at 200 mOsm/kg from time 0 to 3 hours), but is responsive to treatment with exogenous ADH, which causes water reabsorption. Thus, urine concentrates from 200 mOsm to 800 mOsm from 3 to 6 hours. This suggests that the kidneys are functioning properly, but that the patient's pituitary gland is defective in secreting ADH. The disease is called central diabetes insipidus. (**B**) In a patient with nephrogenic diabetes insipidus, urine would never be concentrated in the fluid deprivation test, since the kidney is unresponsive to ADH. (**C**) If the polydipsia was due to osmotic diuresis, the baseline urine osmolality would be higher, due to a normally functioning kidney plus the presence of an osmotically active compound (e.g., hyperglycemia). (**D**) During a water deprivation test of a patient with primary polydipsia (excessive fluid intake), urine osmolality would continually increase starting at time zero, since both kidney and pituitary are functioning normally. (**E**) In a patient with the syndrome of inappropriate antidiuretic hormone secretion (SIADH), urine would be inappropriately concentrated (hyperosmolar in relation to plasma), so a fluid deprivation test would not be appropriate. A water load test could be performed instead to confirm the failure to dilute urine.

11. Correct: Dopamine (A)

In nonpregnant women, dopamine normally suppresses the release of prolactin by lactotrophs of the anterior pituitary. Dopamine, which is synthesized in hypothalamic neurons, reaches the anterior pituitary cells either by transport through long portal veins or by axonal transport within periventricular dopaminergic neurons along the pituitary stalk and through short portal vessels. Any disruption of these pathways, such as may be caused by traumatic brain injury, can lead to low pituitary dopamine and the consequent disinhibition of prolactin release. The resultant hyperprolactinemia leads to galactorrhea. (**B, C, D, E**) Hypothalamic gonadotropin-releasing hormone (GnRH), hypothalamic growth hormone–releasing hormone (GHRH), posterior pituitary oxytocin, and hypothalamic thyrotropin-releasing hormone (TRH) are all known to support prolactin release. Hence, if these substances do not reach the pituitary lactotrophs, galactorrhea is not expected.

12. Correct: Growth hormone (C)

Growth hormone increases lipolysis and protein synthesis as part of its anabolic function. In times of stress, it decreases glucose uptake and contributes to the maintenance of blood glucose concentration. Growth hormone supports calcium retention as part of its growth-promoting and bone-forming function. (**A**) Cortisol increases lipolysis and decreases glucose uptake by muscle and fat, but it decreases protein synthesis. This leads to the release of amino acids from liver and muscle, which are substrates for gluconeogenesis. (**B**) Glucagon promotes degradation of fat as described, but also decreases protein synthesis. (**D**) Insulin decreases lipolysis and increases glucose uptake. (**E**) Parathyroid hormone increases calcium serum concentrations but has none of the described metabolic functions.

13. Correct: Failed growth hormone suppression (B)

The patient presents with typical symptoms of acromegaly due to excess growth hormone (GH) from a pituitary adenoma. GH is a stress hormone and, as such, part of the defense system against hypoglycemia. Negative feedback from hyperglycemia, such as that provided by the oral glucose tolerance test, normally inhibits GH secretion. Hence, the failure of hyperglycemia to suppress GH secretion is diagnostic of autonomous GH secretion due to an adenoma. (**A**) After oral glucose ingestion, serum ghrelin normally decreases, leading to a decrease in GH release. If ghrelin were to increase, acromegaly would be due to this abnormal response of ghrelin to glucose, rather than due to a pituitary adenoma. (**C**) GH stimulates insulin-like growth factor 1 (IGF-1). Hence, failed IGF-1 suppression (not increase) would support a GH-producing pituitary adenoma, as explained in B. (**D**) Serum glucose normally increases after eating glucose and cannot be used for the diagnosis of acromegaly. (**E**) Somatostatin is the natural GH-inhibiting factor. It would not increase after a glucose dose.

14. Correct: 3 (C)

Among the given four diagnoses, the only patients with a hyperosmotic urine are the ones with syndrome of inappropriate antidiuretic hormone secretion (SIADH). These patients present with high plasma ADH, which increases water reabsorption. This leads to low plasma and high urine osmolality. (**A, B, D**) If the patients indeed were diagnosed with nephrogenic diabetes insipidus (high plasma osmolality and high ADH), central diabetes insipidus (high plasma osmolality, low ADH), or primary polydipsia (low plasma osmolality, low ADH), they all should have hyposmotic urine. Any deviation would justify a subcategory, such as high plasma osmolality, high serum ADH, and hyperosmotic urine for patients with water deprivation.

9.5 Questions

15. A 45-year old man has routine bloodwork at his annual checkup. His hemoglobin A1c (HbA1c) is 6.9%. His fasting plasma glucose level is 135 mg/dL. His urine is negative for glucose and ketones. A C-peptide test is scheduled in one week. A drug with which of the following actions is most likely to increase the C-peptide levels in the patient's blood?

A. Increases insulin sensitivity of target tissues
B. Inhibits dipeptidyl peptidase-4 (DPP-4)
C. Inhibits glucagon-like peptide-1 (GLP-1)
D. Inhibits small intestinal sodium/glucose symporter
E. Opens pancreatic β cell KATP channels

16. A 45-year old man with diabetes mellitus type 2 is prescribed an incretin drug that mimics endogenous glucagon-like peptide-1 (GLP-1) activity. Which of the following is a function of the drug?

	Insulin secretion	Glucagon release	Gastric motility	Gastric emptying
A.	Increase	Increase	Increase	Increase
B.	Increase	Decrease	Increase	Increase
C.	Increase	Decrease	Decrease	Decrease
D.	Decrease	Decrease	Decrease	Decrease
E.	Decrease	Increase	Increase	Increase
F.	Decrease	Increase	Decrease	Decrease

17. A patient with poorly controlled diabetes mellitus has an elevated level of hemoglobin A1c (HbA1c). How many months will this patient have to control his blood glucose levels in order to return his HbA1c levels back to normal?

A. 1
B. 2
C. 3
D. 4
E. 5

18. Which of the following stimulates the secretion of both insulin and glucagon from the pancreas?

A. A protein shake recommended for a bodybuilder
B. Epinephrine injection to treat a severe allergic reaction
C. Deep-fried food available at the county fair
D. Hyperglycemia due to corticosteroid medication
E. Hypoglycemia due to prolonged starvation

19. An 18-year-old patient is hospitalized with symptoms of uncontrolled diabetes mellitus type 1, including polyuria, polydipsia, and polyphagia. A serum sample shows the following values:

[K^+]	4.5 mEq/	(normal 3.5–5.0 mEq/L)
[Na^+]	135 mEq/	(normal 134–143 mEq/L)
[Glucose]	500 mg/d	(normal 70–110 mg/dL)
Arterial blood pH	7.0	(normal 7.35–7.45)

Which of the following will most likely be present in the patient?

A. Decreased serum aldosterone
B. Decreased total body K^+
C. Increased serum HCO_3^-
D. Increased total body Na^+
E. Increased total body water

20. A 55-year-old female sees her family doctor with a red blistering rash around the mouth. She reports weight loss but says it is because "eating isn't fun anymore." Her vital signs are normal. Her serum laboratory results are as follows. Normal reference values are in parentheses:

Total calcium	9.2	(8.5–10.5) mg/dL
Potassium	4.2	(3.5–5.0) mEq/L
Sodium	138	(135–145) mEq/L
Glucose (fasting)	162	(65–110) mg/dL
Albumin	3.8	(3.5–5.5) g/dL
RBC	3.18	(3.9–5.6) × 10^{12}/L
Hct	35	(36–48) %
Hgb	11.2	(11.5–15.5) g/dL
MCV	85	(80–95) fL
MCH	29	(27–34) pg

A hormone-producing tumor is suspected. Which of the following cell types is most likely hypertrophied?

A. Pancreatic islet α cells
B. Pancreatic islet β cells
C. Thyroidal parafollicular cells
D. Adrenal zona fasciculata cells
E. Adrenal chromaffine cells

21. A 52-year-old man is diagnosed with multiple endocrine neoplasia syndrome. Ultrasound analysis and functional studies reveal hypersecretory tumors of the parathyroid and pancreatic islet β cells. Computed tomography reveals a pituitary adenoma. He has hyperprolactinemia. With the information given, which of the following laboratory serum values can be expected for this patient?

	Sodium (Na^+)	Potassium (K^+)	Calcium (Ca^{2+})	Bicarbonate (HCO_3^-)	Blood urea nitrogen (BUN)	Creatinine	Glucose (Fasting)
A.	Low	High	Normal	Low	High	High	High
B.	Low	High	Normal	Low	High	High	Normal
C.	Normal	Normal	High	Normal	Normal	Normal	Low
D.	Normal	Low	High	Normal	Normal	Normal	Low
E.	High	Low	High	High	Low	Low	Low
F.	High	Low	Low	High	Low	Low	Low

22. A 16-year-old female college student presents with weight loss, extreme tiredness, nausea, and vomiting. She states, "I'm not a party girl," and denies drug or excessive alcohol use. Her aunt was diagnosed with diabetes mellitus in childhood. The patient's urine is positive for glucose and ketones. Blood serum values are not yet available. Based on the most likely diagnosis, which of the following finding is expected in this patient?

A. Blood pressure is high.
B. Breathing pattern is normal.
C. Heart rate is decreased.
D. Mucous membranes are moist.
E. Serum bicarbonate is low.

23. A 15-year-old girl with a 4-year history of diabetes mellitus type 1 is admitted to the hospital because of diarrhea for the past 18 hours. Her respiratory rate is 32/min and blood pressure is 90/50 mm Hg. Her serum glucose concentration is 300 mg/dL and her arterial pH is 7.20. Which of the following is the most likely additional finding in this patient?

A. Decreased adrenal aldosterone production
B. Decreased renal ammonia production
C. Decreased serum osmolality
D. Increased arterial PCO^2
E. Increased renal net acid secretion

24. In a healthy young woman, which of the following metabolic changes (hepatic glucose uptake, muscle glucose uptake, and hormone-sensitive lipase activity) are expected during exercise as compared to resting, and postprandial as compared to the postabsorptive state?

	Hepatic glucose uptake		Muscle glucose uptake		Hormone-sensitive lipase	
	Exercise	Postprandial	Exercise	Postprandial	Exercise	Postprandial
A.	↑	↑	↑	↑	↑	↑
B.	↑	↑	↓	↓	↑	↑
C.	↓	↓	↑	↑	↓	↓
D.	↓	↑	↑	↑	↑	↓
E.	↑	↓	↑	↑	↓	↑

9.6 Answers and Explanations

15. Correct: Inhibits dipeptidyl peptidase-4 (DPP-4) (B)

This patient has type 2 diabetes mellitus, based on an HbA1c level above 6.5% and a fasting blood glucose level above 126 mg/dL. The lack of glucosuria and ketonuria indicates that he still has functioning pancreatic β cells, and treatment aims to stimulate them to release insulin and C-peptide. Glucagon-like peptide-1 (GLP-1) and glucose-dependent insulinotropic peptide (GIP) are hormonal agents that stimulate β cells. They are normally degraded by the enzyme dipeptidyl peptidase-4 (DPP-4), which means that DDP-4 inhibitors increase the hormonal lifetime and action. Measuring C-peptide (instead of or in addition to insulin) can be helpful since its plasma levels are five times higher than those of insulin, because its half-life is five times longer. Moreover, a baseline level is helpful for later comparison when the patient might be on insulin therapy. (**A**) Increasing target tissue insulin sensitivity has little effect on insulin/C-peptide secretion. (**C**) Inhibiting GLP-1 would decrease the stimulation of β cells. (**D**) Inhibiting the intestinal sodium/glucose symporter, and hence gastrointestinal glucose absorption, would not affect or lower insulin/C-peptide release. (**E**) Closing (not opening) of K_{ATP} channels depolarizes pancreatic β cells, leading to the secretion of insulin and C-peptide.

16. Correct: Increase, decrease, decrease, decerase (C)

Glucagon-like peptide-1 (GLP-1) receptor agonists belong to the pharmacological class of incretin mimetics and act like endogenous GLP-1. GLP-1 (also GLP-2 and glicentin) is normally produced in ileal L cells from the pre-pro-hormone for glucagon. GLP-1 has a short lifetime, but it is a potent anti-hyperglycemic hormone that stimulates insulin secretion and suppresses glucagon release. It also decreases gastric motility and delays gastric emptying, which causes increased satiety. (**A, B, D, E, F**) These are incorrect choices for the functions of GLP-1.

17. Correct: 4 (D)

HbA1c is a glycosylated form of hemoglobin that is produced when blood glucose levels are high. Once hemoglobin is glycosylated, it cannot be reversed. The average life span of red blood cells (RBCs) in the human body is about 120 days (4 months). With good glycemic control, it will take that long to renew the RBCs and reduce HbA1c back to normal. This is why HbA1c is used as a measure of average blood glucose levels and longer-term blood glucose control. (**A, B, C, E**) These choices do not accurately reflect the typical lifespan of an RBC.

18. Correct: A protein shake recommended for a bodybuilder (A)

A protein-rich meal leads to the release of insulin and glucagon. Since excess amino acids are not stored and would be excreted in urine, glucagon stimulates their conversion to glucose in the liver via gluconeogenesis. Insulin stimulates the uptake of this glucose in muscle and liver to store it as glycogen. (**B**) Epinephrine inhibits insulin secretion and stimulates glucagon secretion. (**C**) Fatty acids stimulate insulin release and inhibit glucagon secretion. (**D**) Hyperglycemia stimulates insulin release and insulin inhibits glucagon release. (**E**) Hypoglycemia stimulates glucagon release and does not alter (or may slightly inhibit) insulin release.

19. Correct: Decreased total body K^+ (B)

The majority of patients with diabetic ketoacidosis (low pH) are markedly K^+-depleted due to a number of factors: (**1**) renal loss due to osmotic diuresis, favored by negatively charged urinary ketone bodies, (**2**) gastrointestinal loss due to vomiting, (**3**) elevated aldosterone caused by volume depletion, (**4**) K^+ shifts out of cells favored by hyperosmolality, insulin deficiency, glycogenolysis, and proteolysis. (**A, E**) Polyuria due to osmotic diuresis leads to volume depletion, which activates the renin-angiotensin-aldosterone system. Hence, one expects increased serum aldosterone and decreased total body water. (**C**) Serum HCO_3^- will be decreased (not increased) in a patient with acidemia. (**D**) Total body Na^+ will most likely be decreased (not increased) due to excess renal Na^+ loss. On the other hand, serum Na^+ can be low (shift of intracellular water to the outside due to hyperosmolality), high (renal loss of water in excess of Na^+), or normal (as a combination of both processes).

20. Correct: Pancreatic islet α cells (A)

Pancreatic islet α cells produce glucagon. Hyperglucagonemia causes hyperglycemia and diabetes mellitus type 2. Weight loss is likely due to glucagon stimulating lipolysis and proteinolysis. Anemia (normocytic normochromic) is likely due to glucagon's catabolic action on the bone marrow. The rash, called necrolytic migratory erythema, is a common sign of a glucagonoma, but this knowledge is not necessary to answer the question. (**B**) Pancreatic β cells produce insulin. Hyperinsulinemia causes hypoglycemia (not hyperglycemia). (**C**) Thyroidal parafollicular cells produce calcitonin. Excess calcitonin causes hypocalcemia (not normal serum calcium). (**D**) Adrenal zona fasciculata cells produce cortisol. Hypercortisolism produces signs of Cushing's syndrome, among them hypernatremia and hypokalemia (patient's values are normal). (**E**) Adrenal chromaffine cells produce catecholamines. Sympathetic overactivity leads to increased heart rate and blood pressure (patient has normal vital signs).

21. Correct: Normal, low, high, normal, normal, normal, low (D)

For multiple endocrine neoplasia syndrome, the specific tumors will dictate the clinical presentation. For type 1 disease, hypersecretory tumors are almost always present at the parathyroid gland, frequently at the pancreas, and sometimes at the pituitary. In this patient, all three tumors are present, so that there is primary hyperparathyroidism (resulting in hypercalcemia), hyperinsulinemia (causing low fasting glucose and K^+ levels), and hyperprolactinemia. Hyperprolactinemia does not lead to electrolyte abnormalities or kidney impairment. Hence, plasma sodium, HCO_3^-, BUN, and creatinine should not be affected. Low serum bicarbonate would also be possible, because HCO_3^- buffers H^+ that shifted out of cells in exchange for K^+. (**A, B, F**) These choices do not contain high serum calcium and low fasting serum glucose levels. (**C**) Hyperinsulinemia is commonly associated with hypokalemia. (**E**) Low BUN and serum creatinine cannot be expected.

22. Correct: Serum bicarbonate is low. (E)

The most likely diagnosis of the patient is diabetes mellitus type 1 (high blood glucose, ketone bodies, family history). There are signs of metabolic acidosis (nausea, vomiting). Hence, serum bicarbonate would be low due to neutralizing H^+. (**A**) Blood pressure could be low (not high) due to dehydration. (**B**) Respiration would be deep, and the respiratory rate could be increased as a compensatory response to metabolic acidosis. (**C**) Heart rate could be high (not decreased) due to sympathetic activation in response to starving cells. (**D**) Mucous membranes would be dry (not moist) due to dehydration.

23. Correct: Increased renal net acid secretion (E)

The patient is severely dehydrated (evident as low blood pressure) and acidemic (pH 7.20) due to the combination of losing alkaline fluid (diarrhea) and development of ketoacidosis (increased respiration in the presence of high serum glucose). The kidneys respond with increased renal net acid secretion. (**A**) Dehydration stimulates renin, which increases (not decreases) aldosterone production. Additionally, acidemia increases serum potassium levels, which further stimulates aldosterone release. (**B**) An important mechanism of renal net acid secretion is to increase (not decrease) renal ammonia production. (**C**) Serum osmolality is increased (not decreased) due to excess serum glucose and ketones. (**D**) Acidemia stimulates hyperventilation, so arterial P_{CO_2} is decreased (not increased).

24. Correct: ↓, ↑. ↑. ↑. ↑ ↓ (D)

Exercise increases glucagon and epinephrine release, which both decrease hepatic glucose uptake. After a meal (postprandial), insulin is released, which increases hepatic glucose uptake. In exercise, epinephrine increases muscle glucose uptake. Moreover, working muscle cells increase glucose uptake by upregulating plasma membrane GLUT4 molecules, independent of hormonal activity. Postprandially, insulin is responsible for the increased muscle glucose uptake. Last, during exercise, epinephrine increases the activity of hormone-sensitive lipase, while insulin decreases the enzyme activity. Overall, for exercise, hormones mobilize nutrients to provide energy to skeletal and cardiac muscle, while after a meal, hormones facilitate body nutrient storage.

9.7 Questions

Questions 25 to 27

A 53-year-old male has a 10-year history of fatigue, depression, weight gain, and cold intolerance. His symptoms are not improved with antidepressants. For the past 3 years, he has been living by himself. His diet consists mainly of fast food and ice cream. On exam, he has a small goiter. His lab values are as follows:

Total triiodothyronine (TT_3)	< 0.1 nmol/	(0.9–28 nmol/L)
Total thyroxine (TT_4)	< 10 nmol/	(50–150 nmol/L)
Thyroid-stimulating hormone (TSH)	110 mIU/	(20 mIU/L)
Albumi	636 µmol/	(640 µmol/L)

25. The patient's serum levels of thyroid-stimulating hormone (TSH) are elevated because of the lack of which of the following?

A. An appropriate antidepressant
B. Dietary iodine
C. Physical exercise
D. Pituitary feedback inhibition
E. Social and family support

26. Which of the following is most likely increased in this patient?

A. Basal metabolic rate
B. Blood pressure
C. Body temperature
D. Heart rate
E. Growth hormone
F. Oxygen consumption

27. What test is used to correct the patient's total serum thyroxine levels (TT4), to estimate free thyroxine levels?

A. Serum reverse T3 test
B. Serum thyroglobulin test
C. T3 resin uptake test
D. Thyroglobulin antibody titer
E. TSH receptor antibody titer

Questions 28 to 29

As part of a thyrotropin-releasing hormone (TRH) stimulating test, TRH is injected into a healthy adult at time zero and peripheral blood samples are taken at 0 minutes, 20 minutes, and 60 minutes to measure thyroid-stimulating hormone (TSH).

28. In a healthy adult with a TSH baseline level of 2 mU/L at time zero, which of the following is expected for the TSH levels 20 minutes and 60 minutes after TRH administration?

	20-minute serum TSH (mU/L)	60-minute serum TSH (mU/L)
A.	2	15
B.	2	45
C.	15	45
D.	15	10
E.	15	2

29. In the TRH stimulation test described in question 28, in which of the following conditions would TSH be expected to rise promptly 20 minutes after TRH administration?

A. Primary hyperthyroidism
B. Primary hypothyroidism
C. Secondary hypothyroidism
D. Secondary hyperthyroidism
E. Tertiary hyperthyroidism

30. A 21-year-old woman presents with weight loss, nervousness, sweating, and fatigue. Her neck examination shows a soft, diffuse, nonnodular midline mass that is mobile on swallowing. Mild exophthalmia is also noted. Her resting pulse is 100/min and blood pressure 135/90 mm Hg. The patient's thyroid function tests are as follows:

Serum TSH	0.2 mU/	(0.5–5.0 mU/L)
Total thyroxine (TT_4)	14 µg/d	(5–12 µg/dL)

Which of the following diseases best fits this patient's clinical presentation?

A. Addison's disease
B. Conn's disease
C. Cushing's disease
D. Graves' disease
E. Hashimoto's disease
F. Secondary hypothyroidism
G. Thyroid carcinoma

31. A 45-year old woman presents with a 6-month history of excessive tiredness, unexpected weight gain, constipation, galactorrhea, and amenorrhea. Laboratory values show elevated concentrations of thyroid-stimulating hormone (TSH) and follicle-stimulating hormone (FSH). A pregnancy test is negative. She denies any head injuries, and brain magnetic resonance imaging (MRI) is normal. Which of the following serum levels of thyrotropin-releasing hormone (TRH) and gonadotropin-releasing hormone (GnRH) are expected?

	TRH	GnRH
A.	Normal	Increased
B.	Normal	Decreased
C.	Decreased	Normal
D.	Decreased	Increased
E.	Increased	Decreased
F.	Increased	Normal

32. Clinical trials determined that a new drug had the undesirable effect of stimulating thyrotropin-releasing hormone (TRH) receptors. Which of the following is the most likely side effect experienced by male patients who took the medication?

A. Constipation
B. Decreased libido
C. Hair loss
D. Premature ejaculation
E. Pretibial myxedema

33. A patient with hypothyroidism is prescribed a synthetic thyroxine analogue, 50 µg orally each day. He reads about the multiple functions of this drug and wants to understand the mechanism of action. To which of the following does the drug bind, in order to activate its cellular mechanism of action?

A. Nuclear thyroid hormone receptors in order to regulate DNA transcription
B. Iodine in order to be transported across cell membranes
C. Plasma membrane receptors in order to activate secondary messengers
D. Retinoid X nuclear receptors in order to bind iodine
E. RNA polymerase in order to bind to nuclear receptors

9.8 Answers and Explanations

25. Correct: Pituitary feedback inhibition (D)

The patient suffers from symptoms of hypothyroidism such as fatigue, weight gain, depression, and cold intolerance. In areas without iodine deficiency, the most common cause is chronic autoimmune hypothyroidism (Hashimoto's thyroiditis), a persistent inflammation of the thyroid with nonspecific symptoms that often overlap with signs of depression. The thyroid gland is gradually destroyed by antibody-mediated immune reactions, leading to low thyroid hormone T_3/T_4. The lack of negative feedback inhibition leads to progressively elevated thyroid-stimulating hormone (TSH). (**A, C, E**) Lack of an appropriate antidepressant, lack of physical exercise, and lack of social or family support all may aggravate the symptoms of hypothyroidism but are not the cause for elevated TSH. (**A**) Comfort food is typically high in iodized salt. Dairy products are high in iodine as well. Hence, lack of iodide to synthesize thyroid hormones is not likely the cause of elevated TSH.

26. Correct: Blood pressure (B)

Many people with hypothyroidism have high blood pressure. The absence of vasodilatory thyroid hormones leads to increased vascular tone and increased peripheral vascular resistance, which results in increased diastolic blood pressure. People with hypothyroid disorders are typically overweight, and the concomitant increase in arterial stiffness may also lead to increased systolic blood pressure. It is further supported by high serum cholesterol due to the lack of T_3, but it may be offset by decreased cardiac output. (**A, C, F**) In a patient deficient in thyroid hormones the rate of intermediary metabolism decreases, thereby decreasing (not increasing) basal metabolic rate, body temperature, and oxygen consumption. (**D**) Hypothyroidism leads to decreased (not increased) heart rate, by directly affecting the cells of the sinoatrial node and by indirectly decreasing the actions of catecholamines. (**E**) Thyroid deficiency would decrease (not increase) growth hormone.

27. Correct: T3 resin uptake test (C)

The T_3 resin uptake test is the traditional test used to calculate free thyroxine concentrations. Free (unbound) T_4 typically represents less than 0.05% of the total thyroxine in serum. There are no tests that measure free thyroxine directly. The T_3 resin uptake test measures the binding capacity of thyroid hormones in serum and hence is an indirect measure of thyroid-binding proteins including thyroid-binding globulin (TBG). The test is used to calculate the estimated concentration of free T_4. In the presence of low TT_4 such as for the given patient, a low T_3 resin uptake confirms hypothyroidism, while a high T_3 resin uptake would indicate TBG deficiency and a potential liver problem. (**A**) Reverse T_3 is the metabolically inactive form of T_4. Inactivation occurs in the liver (and kidney), so a positive serum reverse T_3 test is used when an illness outside of the thyroid is suspected. This is not supported in this patient (normal serum albumin). (**B**) Thyroglobulin (Tg) is produced by thyroid follicular cells to store thyroid hormone within the gland's follicular lumen. The Tg test is used to monitor follicular cell activity (not free thyroxine levels). (**D, E**) The presence of antibody against Tg or the TSH receptor points to Hashimoto's disease as the cause of primary hypothyroidism but does not provide information on free serum hormone levels.

28. Correct: 15,10 (D)

In a healthy person, thyrotropin-releasing hormone (TRH) stimulates thyroid-stimulating hormone (TSH) release, and TSH increases from baseline of 2 to about 15 mU/L. This response is expected to happen within 20 min, since TSH is preformed and ready to be released upon stimulation. Sixty minutes after TRH stimulation, a decrease in serum TSH is expected. The half-lives of hypothalamic releasing hormones are very short (in the minute range), so there is no stimulatory TRH remaining after 1 hour. Conversely, the half-lives of pituitary stimulating hormones are longer (in the hour range), so some TSH remains active after 1 hour. The thyroid hormones bring the TSH levels toward normal via negative feedback regulation, but have not reached baseline levels after 1 hour. (**A, B**) Twenty minutes into the test, TSH is increased (not unchanged) upon TRH stimulation. (**C**) After 20 minutes, TSH is indeed increased from baseline, however, after 60 minutes, TRH's effect has subsided and TSH will not further increase. (**E**) Sixty minutes into the test, about half of TSH is still present and negative feedback regulation has not yet normalized TSH levels back to baseline.

29. Correct: Primary hypothyroidism (B)

In primary hypothyroidism, the thyroid gland fails to produce thyroid hormones, but the pituitary responds normally. Hence, administration of TRH produces a prompt increase in TSH. (**A**) In primary hyperthyroidism, the gland produces excess thyroid hormone (T_3/T_4) that strongly suppresses TSH release. Administration of TRH causes little or no changes in TSH serum concentrations. (**C, D**) In secondary hypo- or hyperthyroidism, the pituitary does not produce TSH or produces too much TSH. Stimulation by external TRH does not alter the pituitary activity. (**E**) Tertiary hyperthyroidism means that the hypothalamus already produces excess TRH, and a TRH stimulation test is inappropriate. However, in tertiary hypothyroidism (not a choice), TSH would increase, although probably with a delayed response time.

30. Correct: Graves' disease (D)

The patient's symptoms (weight loss and fatigue) suggest hyperthyroidism and are confirmed by elevated total T_4 (TT_4) and low thyroid-stimulating hormone (TSH). The presence of a midline mass indicates a small goiter. The presence of exophthalmia suggests Graves' disease, in which autoantibodies stimulate the TSH receptor and hence act like endogenous TSH. (**A**) Addison's disease presents with symptoms of low cortisol and aldosterone and no changes in T_4. (**B**) Conn's disease is an aldosterone-producing adenoma, with no changes in T_4. (**C**) Cushing's disease presents with high cortisol levels and symptoms of hypercortisolism, which are not present here. (**E**) Hashimoto's disease presents with low T_4 and high TSH. (**F**) Secondary hypothyroidism presents with low TSH and low T_4. (**G**) Thyroid carcinoma presents with firm, nontender nodules in the thyroid. Exophthalmia is not present. The thyroid hormone levels can vary (eu-, hyper-, and hypothyroidism may occur) and hence are not diagnostic.

31. Correct: Increased, decreased (E)

The patient has signs and symptoms of secondary or tertiary hypothyroidism (tiredness, weight gain and constipation, but a low TSH). Secondary hypothyroidism is the inability of the pituitary to produce TSH. Tertiary hypothyroidism is the inability of the hypothalamus to produce TRH. She also has amenorrhea. Since her FSH is low, she is not in menopause. The most likely diagnosis is secondary hypothyroidism resulting in elevated TRH because increased TRH will cause hyperprolactinemia (and galactorrhea). Elevated prolactin will suppress GnRH, resulting in amenorrhea. If the problem were at the hypothalamus, TRH would be decreased, and low TRH would not cause hyperprolactinemia. Other reasons for excess prolactin, such as a tumor or head injury, are not likely due to the woman's history. (**A, B, C, D, F**) These combinations do not explain the patient's history and physical results.

32. Correct: Decreased libido (B)

In addition to pituitary thyrotrophs, lactotrophs also have receptors for thyrotropin-releasing hormone (TRH). Hence, drug-induced TRH stimulation leads to hyperprolactinemia, which consequently inhibits the hypothalamic-pituitary-gonadal sex hormone axis, leading to diminished sexual function and decreased libido. (**A**) Constipation is a common symptom of hypothyroidism (not hyperthyroidism). (**C**) Since thyroid hormones regulate protein metabolism, hair structure may be affected. Thin, brittle hair (and potentially hair loss) are seen in hypothyroidism (not hyperthyroidism). (**D**) Premature ejaculation can be a symptom of hypoprolactinemia (not hyperprolactinemia). (**E**) Pretibial myxedema is a rare but diagnostic complication of Graves' disease, an autoimmune disorder not likely to develop in the trial participants.

33. Correct: Nuclear thyroid hormone receptors in order to regulate DNA transcription (A)

Thyroid hormones act by regulating DNA transcription. The hormone binds to nuclear thyroid hormone receptors. The hormone-receptor complex then binds to thyroid hormone response elements on the DNA of target cells. (**B**) Like endogenous thyroxine, the synthetic drug analogue has iodine bound to it before it is transported across target cell membranes. For natural thyroxine, iodine binding occurs within the thyroid follicular lumina. (**C**) Thyroid hormones bind to intracellular/intranuclear receptors, not plasma membrane receptors. (**D**) Thyroid hormone can bind to retinoid X nuclear receptors before binding to thyroid hormone receptors. The whole complex then binds to DNA hormone response elements (not to iodine). (**E**) The complex of hormone, hormone receptor, and hormone response element recruits RNA polymerase and other biomolecules, in order to start DNA transcription (not nuclear receptor binding).

9.9 Questions

34. A patient with a pheochromocytoma is scheduled for surgical removal of the tumor. The day before the surgery, the patient is given large volumes of fluids and a high-salt diet to avoid which of the following perioperative situations?

A. Hyperglycemia
B. Hypotension
C. Palpitations
D. Perspiration
E. Vasoconstriction

35. An ultramarathon runner is brought to the emergency tent with extreme exhaustion and muscle pain. The urine is dark in color, but no blood is detected. Serum creatine kinase is critically elevated. The runner is transported to the hospital, where serum potassium and aldosterone are measured. Which of the following are the most likely values?

	Serum potassium	Serum aldosterone
A.	↑	↑
B.	↑	↓
C.	↑	↔
D.	↓	↑
E.	↓	↓
F.	↓	↔
G.	↔	↑
H.	↔	↓
I.	↔	↔

36. A person experiencing which of the following situations would be expected to present with parallel changes in serum aldosterone and cortisol (i.e., both increased, both decreased, or both unaffected)?

A. Addison's disease

B. Cushing's syndrome

C. High-potassium diet

D. Low-sodium diet

E. Suffering chronic abuse

37. A patient is diagnosed with hypertension caused by renal artery stenosis. Compared to a normotensive patient, what hormone-dependent changes would most likely be seen in the concentrations of serum potassium and bicarbonate?

	Serum potassium	Serum bicarbonate
A.	Decreased	Decreased
B.	Increased	Increased
C.	Decreased	Increased
D.	Increased	Decreased
E.	Decreased	Unchanged

38. A 15-year-old girl presents with a 3-week history of nausea and 2 months of unexpected weight loss. Menarche has not yet occurred. Her physical examination reveals immature secondary sexual development. Her temperature is 97.8°F, her pulse is 72 beats per minute, her respiratory rate is 14 breaths per minute, and her blood pressure is 138/89 mm Hg. Her gums are hyperpigmented. Laboratory tests reveal hypernatremia, hypokalemia, and low fasting blood glucose. Results from blood tests show an increased titer of autoantibodies that block the normal action of the target antigen. Which of the following autoantibodies is most likely found?

A. Antithyroglobulin

B. Antithyroperoxidase

C. Anti-TSH-receptor

D. Anti-17-α hydroxylase

E. Anti-21-β hydroxylase

39. Patients with the syndrome of inappropriate antidiuretic hormone (SIADH) often present with vague symptoms including confusion, nausea, and irritability. Which of the following laboratory results will support a provisional diagnosis?

A. Decreased blood sodium

B. Increased aldosterone

C. Increased blood osmolality

D. Increased blood urea nitrogen

E. Maximally diluted urine

40. A 2-week-old male infant is brought to the hospital in the evening after vomiting for most of the day. He appears underweight and dehydrated. Physical examination shows penile enlargement and subtle hyperpigmentation. He is hypotensive. Serum electrolyte levels were obtained:

Na^+:	120 mEq/L	(136–145 mEq/L)
K^+:	5.6 mEq/L	(3.5–5 mEq/L)
Cl^-:	90 mEq/L	(95–105 mEq/L)
Glucose:	55 mg/dL	(70–110 mg/dL)

Abdominal imaging shows bilateral adrenal hyperplasia. Further examination will most likely show which of the following serum levels compared to normal?

	Aldosterone	Cortisol	Corticosterone	Adrenocorticotropic hormone (ACTH)	Insulin	Growth hormone
A.	↓	↓	↓	↓	↓	↓
B.	↓	↓	↓	↑	↓	↑
C.	↑	↓	↓	↓	↑	↓
D.	↑	↓	↓	↑	↓	↑
E.	↑	↑	↓	↑	↑	↑
F.	↑	↑	↑	↑	↑	↓

41. A 50-year-old man presents with headache and weakness for several weeks. On investigation, he is hypertensive and hypokalemic. Serum aldosterone is elevated, so imaging is performed. The result shows an adenoma in the adrenal zona glomerulosa, so primary hyperaldosteronism is suspected. Additional tests are ordered. Which of the following changes to serum renin and serum angiotensin II would support the initial diagnosis?

	Serum renin	Serum angiotensin II
A.	↑	↑
B.	↓	↓
C.	↑	↓
D.	↓	↑
E.	↔	↔

42. The husband of a 63-year-old woman reports that his wife's personality has significantly changed over the past 2 years. Upon investigation, the woman also admits to having memory problems. Physical examination reveals centralized obesity, a round face, and thin limbs. Laboratory results show fasting hyperglycemia. The image shows the patient's adrenocorticotropic hormone (ACTH) concentrations (red line), compared to a control patient. Serum ACTH is measured every 10 minutes for one hour, and corticotropin-releasing hormone (CRH) is infused at the time of the arrows. Which of the following is the most likely diagnosis?

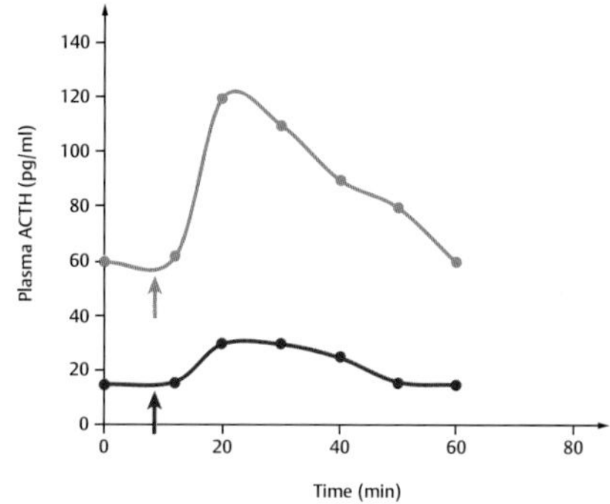

A. Addison's disease

B. Conn's disease

C. Cushing's disease

D. Glucocorticoid therapy

E. Hypopituitarism

43. A young patient with a liver disease asks the physician to comment on potential health concerns if he performs strenuous aerobic exercise. The physician's answer includes which of the following effects of epinephrine, cortisol, and glucagon on liver glycogen in response to acute stress?

	Epinephrine	Cortisol	Glucagon
A.	↓	↓	↓
B.	↓	↓	↑
C.	↓	↑	↓
D.	↑	↓	↑
E.	↑	↑	↓

44. A patient with a dislocated shoulder had it corrected under conscious sedation. The anesthesia drug that was used is known to impair the function of the pituitary-adrenal axis. Hence, one week later, the patient's adrenocorticotropic hormone (ACTH) and cortisol were measured in blood samples taken at the indicated times.

	Normal values	Patient, 7 a.m.	Patient, 7:30 a.m.	Patient, 7 p.m.	Patient, 7.30 p.m.
ACTH (pg/mL)	50–250	110	90	120	210
Cortisol (µg/dL)	6–23	15	15	20	23

Which of the following is the correct conclusion from the patient data?

A. Excessive pulsatility of ACTH
B. Inverted circadian rhythm
C. No abnormalities
D. Primary adrenal insufficiency
E. Secondary adrenal insufficiency

45. An increase in serum levels of which of the following electrolytes will directly increase aldosterone secretion?

A. Calcium
B. Chloride
C. Magnesium
D. Potassium
E. Sodium

9.10 Answers and Explanations

34. Correct: Hypotension (B)

Pheochromocytomas release excess catecholamines. The resulting sympathetic stimulation leads to hypertension and concomitantly to severe inhibition of the renin-angiotensin-aldosterone system. The consequence is excessive urinary fluid loss and volume depletion. Excision of the tumor causes a rapid removal of sympathetic stimulation. Fluid and salt loading before the operation avoids perioperative hypovolemia and hypotensive crisis. (**A, C, D, E**) Hyperglycemia, palpitations (tachycardia), sweating, and vasoconstriction are all adrenergic symptoms that are typical for a patient with a pheochromocytoma and are reduced by removing the tumor. These symptoms would not be improved by perioperative fluid and salt loading.

35. Correct: ↑, ↑ (A)

The elevation of serum creatine kinase during extreme exercise indicates rhabdomyolysis (skeletal muscle cell necrosis), which is supported by dark urine due to the presence of myoglobin. Damaged muscle cells release potassium into serum. Hyperkalemia stimulates aldosterone release, in order to promote renal potassium excretion. (**B–I**) These choices are incorrect.

36. Correct: Addison's disease (A)

(**A**) Addison's disease is a primary adrenal insufficiency in which the adrenal glands produce both less glucocorticoids (including cortisol) and mineralocorticoids (including aldosterone). (**B**) Cushing's syndrome causes elevated serum cortisol. This leads to hypertension, inhibition of renin, and, consequently, low serum aldosterone levels. (**C**) Serum potassium stimulates aldosterone release but does not affect serum cortisol. (**D**) Low serum sodium leads to hypotension, renin release, and elevation of aldosterone. Cortisol is not affected. (**E**) Psychological stress, such as suffering chronic abuse, activates the hypothalamo-pituitary-adrenal stress axis, with release of corticotropin-releasing hormone (CRH), adrenocorticotropic hormone (ACTH), and cortisol. While ACTH is necessary for optimal release of aldosterone, it is not a primary stimulant.

37. Correct: Decreased, increased (C)

For renal artery stenosis, the juxtaglomerular apparatus of the kidney senses low perfusion pressure. It activates the renin-angiotensin-aldosterone system, which causes hypertension due to vasoconstriction and salt retention. Aldosterone activates the basolateral Na-K-ATPase of renal tubular cells, leading to sodium reabsorption in exchange for potassium secretion. Serum potassium decreases. It is counterbalanced by potassium shifting out of cells, in exchange for hydrogen ions shifting into cells. Unmatched serum bicarbonate causes metabolic alkalosis. Secondly, aldosterone increases renal H^+ secretion via H-ATPase and HCO_3^- reabsorption via basolateral chloride-bicarbonate exchanger activity in renal type A intercalated cells, which aggravates metabolic alkalosis. (**A, B, D, E**). These choices are unlikely in the case of hyperaldosteronism.

38. Correct: Anti-17-α hydroxylase (D)

An antibody that blocks 17-α hydroxylase leads to decreased cortisol (low blood glucose, nausea, weight loss), increased adrenocorticotropic hormone (hyperpigmentation), and increased mineralocorticoid action (hypernatremia, hypokalemia). The increased mineralocorticoid is mainly 11-deoxycorticosterone (DOC), which might also lead to hypertension. Decreased 17-α hydroxylase activity also leads to decreased adrenal androgen production, which contributes to her primary amenorrhea and lack of sexual development. (**A, B, C**) Blocking thyroglobulin or thyroperoxidase would cause hypothyroidism and weight gain (not weight loss). Elevated antibody titers are most commonly found in Hashimoto's disease. Antithyroglobulin and anti-TSH receptor antibody of the blocking type may also be present in Graves' disease, which would not explain the patient's hypernatremia, hypokalemia, and hyperpigmentation. It is important to note that the typical antibody causing Graves' disease is anti-TSH receptor antibody of the stimulating type. (**E**) Blocking 21-β hydroxylase leads to low mineralocorticoids, which would cause hyponatremia and hyperkalemia and signs of virilization (not sexual underdevelopment).

39. Correct: Decreased blood sodium (A)

Patients with inappropriate oversecretion of antidiuretic hormone (SIADH) retain water, which leads to hyponatremia, a key feature of the disease. (**B**) The body responds to the water retention by decreasing (not increasing) serum aldosterone, which worsens hyponatremia. (C, D) The dilution of plasma decreases (not increases) blood urea nitrogen and blood osmolality. (**B**) Hyponatremia should lead to a maximally diluted urine due to inhibition of ADH. However, patients with SIADH have an inappropriately elevated urine osmolality—that is, less than maximally diluted urine.

40. Correct: ↓, ↓, ↓, ↑, ↓, ↑ (B)

The boy has the most common form of the congenital adrenal hyperplasias: 21-hydroxylase deficiency. Mutations of the *CYP21* gene result in low 21-hydroxylase enzyme activity. This results in decreased production of adrenal mineralocorticoids (aldosterone) and glucocorticoids (cortisol and corticosterone). Decreased aldosterone causes hyponatremia (Na^+ is low, boy is dehydrated) and hyperkalemia (K^+ is high; malaise and developing metabolic acidosis led to vomiting and weight loss). Underproduction of glucocorticoids causes low blood glucose and increased production of adrenocorticotropic hormone (ACTH). The ACTH precursor, proopiomelanocortin, is responsible for the observed hyperpigmentation. Vomiting further aggravates hypoglycemia, so insulin levels are low. Hypoglycemia and hypotension are physiological stressors that stimulate release of growth hormone. Penile enlargement is due to the overproduction of adrenal androgen in this disease. (**A, C, D, E, F**) These choices show one or more incorrect serum levels.

41. Correct: ↓, ↓ (B)

Excess aldosterone released by an adrenal adenoma (Conn's disease) increases renal tubular sodium reabsorption and results in plasma volume expansion. This leads to elevated blood pressure and headache. The high blood pressure is sensed in the kidney, and renin release is suppressed, which then leads to lower than normal angiotensin II levels. High aldosterone in the setting of decreased concentrations of renin and angiotensin is diagnostic for primary hyperaldosteronism. Elevated aldosterone also causes increased renal tubular potassium secretion, which may result in hypokalemia and muscle weakness. (**A**) Renin and angiotensin II are suppressed (not elevated) due to renal artery hypertension. (C, D) Renin is a proteolytic enzyme that forms angiotensin I, which is enzymatically transformed into angiotensin II, so the plasma changes of renin and angiotensin II are almost always in the same direction. (**E**) The renin-angiotensin system is altered (not unaffected) by blood pressure changes such as present in hyperaldosteronism.

42. Correct: Cushing's disease (C)

The patient has typical symptoms of hypercortisolism, which relate to cortisol's functions of degrading proteins and stimulating gluconeogenesis (central obesity, a round face, thin limbs, and hyperglycemia). Neuronal protein degradation leads to emotional lability and difficulty with memory. The adrenocorticotropic hormone (ACTH)-monitoring test shows that ACTH is elevated at baseline compared to normal, before the administration of corticotropin-releasing hormone (CRH). The most likely diagnosis is Cushing's disease, caused by a CRH-responsive pituitary adenoma that produces excessive amounts of ACTH. (**A**) Addison's disease would present with symptoms of cortisol deficiency. (**B**) Conn's disease leads to symptoms related to hyperaldosteronism. (**D**) A person on glucocorticoid medication would have these symptoms of excess cortisol but would have low ACTH. (**E**) Hypopituitarism could cause ACTH deficiency, which would lead to signs of adrenal insufficiency (not hypercortisolism).

43. Correct: ↓, ↑, ↓ (C)

In response to acute stress such as exercise, the levels of all three hormones are increased. Epinephrine (along with norepinephrine) causes a body response that includes a surge of energy as a result of glycogen breakdown. Cortisol is increased within minutes of strenuous exercise and counters insulin. Cortisol stimulates gluconeogenesis, using substrates produced by protein and lipid breakdown. Conversely to these catabolic actions resulting in glucose production, cortisol also stimulates glycogen synthesis in the liver, which decreases net blood sugar levels. Hence, under stress, cortisol becomes a relevant regulator of blood glucose. Glucagon is an antihypoglycemic hormone, decreasing glycogen in response to starvation and a wide variety of physiological and pathophysiological stress situations, including exercise. The physician's answer to potential health concerns of exercise for a patient with liver disease will depend on the type of liver disease. Also note that all stress hormones act interdependently. For instance, cortisol increases hepatic responsiveness to glucagon, while glucagon stimulates epinephrine and ACTH-induced cortisol release. This interaction, further complicated by additional hormones such as vasopressin as well as neuronal and immune regulation of somatic cells, leads to a variety, not always identical symptoms when acute (physiologically beneficial) stress becomes chronic stress. (**A, B, D, E**) These choices have one or more incorrect answers.

44. Correct: Inverted circadian rhythm (B)

The patient's serum adrenocorticotropic hormone (ACTH) and cortisol values are higher in the evening than in the morning, which is the opposite of the normal circadian rhythm. Such an inverted pattern could be observed for night workers and is not likely to be a side effect of the anesthetic. (**A**) ACTH and cortisol have pulsatile rhythms in the range of half-hour to one hour. These rhythms are superimposed on the circadian rhythm. Since all values are within the reference range, there is no excessive pulsatility. (**C**) The patient's blood values show normal pulsatility but abnormal circadian rhythm. (D, E) Primary (disorder of the gland) and secondary (low ACTH secretion) adrenal insufficiency both present with low levels of cortisol, which is not the case here.

45. Correct: Potassium (D)

Circulating potassium increases aldosterone secretion directly by depolarizing cells of the zona glomerulosa, which open voltage-gated calcium channels. This triggers the fusion of cellular vesicles with the plasma membrane and the release of its hormonal content. (**A, B, C, E**) In the absence of additional triggers, there are no known direct, clinically relevant effects of these electrolytes on zona glomerulosa cells.

9.11 Questions

46. A 60-year-old woman presents with daily pain and stiffness of the right knee with minimal exertion. Pain is worse with activity, but acetaminophen provides partial relief. She is 5 feet, 3 inches (160 centimeter) tall and weighs 125 pounds (57 kilograms). Physical exam is normal, except for knee pain upon standing. Blood chemistry and lipid profiles are unremarkable. Serum alkaline phosphatase levels are normal. Radiography of the right knee reveals joint space narrowing and osteophytes. Bone density scans are unremarkable. The patient's clinical presentation is most consistent with which of the following conditions?

A. Achondroplasia
B. Osteoarthritis
C. Osteopenia
D. Osteoporosis
E. Paget's disease

47. During a normal checkup of a 68-year-old patient with diabetes mellitus type 2, total serum calcium levels are slightly below the reference range. All other tests are normal. The patient denies numbness/tingling in hands, feet, mouth, and lips. Tendon reflexes are normal. Both Trousseau and Chvostek signs are absent. A serum sample is sent for retesting. In the meantime, which of the following conditions should be considered for further investigation?

A. Chronic kidney disease
B. Hyperalbuminemia
C. Hypophosphatemia
D. Parathyroid hormone–related peptide
E. RANKL and OPG expression*

*RANKL: receptor activator of NF-kB ligand, OPG: osteoprotegerin

48. A 52-year-old man with alcoholism, liver cirrhosis, and chronic fatigue presents with acute back pain and is diagnosed with a vertebral fracture. He also reports tingling and numbness of his skin. Ascites and a mild Trousseau sign are present. Insulin, glucagon, epinephrine, cortisol, growth hormone, thyroid hormone, and thyroid-stimulating hormone are all normal. Insulin-like growth factor 1 and reverse triiodothyronine (rT3) are reduced. Which of the following is most likely increased in this patient?

A. Albumin
B. Bone resorption
C. Serum calcium
D. Serum glucose
E. 1-25-dihydroxycholecalciferol

49. A 6-year-old boy is brought to the emergency department because of severe malaise. The family recently emigrated from Nigeria to Washington State. The boy's laboratory blood values are remarkable for a BUN of 75 mg/dL (normal 7–20 mg/dL) and creatinine of 5.8 mg/dL (normal 0.5–1 mg/dL). Serum calcium and parathyroid hormone levels are measured. Compared to normal, which of the following choices most likely depicts the boy's concentrations of serum calcium and parathyroid hormone?

	Parathyroid hormone	Serum calcium
A.	Increased	Decreased
B.	Increased	Increased
C.	Decreased	Decreased
D.	Decreased	Increased
E.	Decreased	Normal

50. The graph in the image demonstrates the normal relationship of the serum levels of two hormones in response to serum calcium. Which of the following are the correct names for hormone A and hormone B?

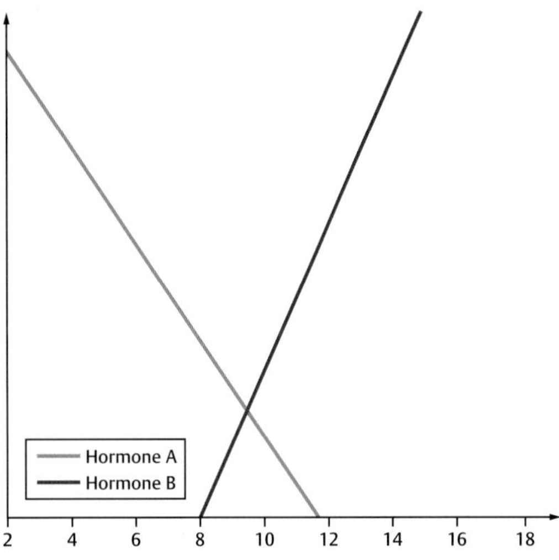

	Hormone A	Hormone B
A.	Calcitonin	Parathyroid hormone
B.	Calcitonin	Active vitamin D
C.	Parathyroid hormone	Calcitonin
D.	Parathyroid hormone	Active vitamin D
E.	Active vitamin D	Parathyroid hormone
F.	Inactive vitamin D	Parathyroid hormone

51. Calcitonin and parathyroid hormone both inhibit which of the following?

A. Osteoblast activity in bones
B. Osteoclast activity in bones
C. Renal tubular calcium reabsorption
D. Renal tubular phosphate reabsorption

52. Which of the following are typical symptoms in a patient with moderate to severe hypercalcemia?

A. Hypertension
B. Muscle fasciculations
C. Skeletal muscle cramps
D. Tingling, numbness
E. Vocal cord spasms

53. A 79-year old man presents with "aching bones." His pain is most pronounced in his back, pelvis, and lower extremities. The pain is dull and increases after weight-bearing activities. One year ago he was diagnosed with the skin disease actinic keratosis. Since then, he avoids sunlight. To improve his symptoms, it is recommended that he spend 1 hour a day outdoors in order to support which of the following chemical conversions?

A. 7-dehydrocholesterol to vitamin D3 (cholecalciferol)
B. Vitamin D3 (cholecalciferol) to vitamin D2 (ergocalciferol)
C. Vitamin D2 (ergocalciferol) to 25-hydroxycholecalciferol
D. 25-hydroxycholecalciferol to 1,25-dihydroxycholecalciferol
E. 25-hydroxycholecalciferol to 24,25-dihydroxycholecalciferol

54. A 77-year old white woman fell while getting out of her car. She does not report any symptoms, including pain. Dual-energy X-ray absorptiometry (DXA) of her hip shows a fracture of the femoral neck and decreased bone density. The patient's laboratory results are as follows:

Calcium	9.3 mg/d	(8.5–10.1 mg/dL)
Phosphorus	2.6 mg/d	(2.6–4.6 mg/dL)
Alkaline phosphatase	45 U/L	(19–71 U/L)
Urinary hydroxyproline	42 mg/d	(25–74 mg/dL)

Which of the following conditions is most likely present in the patient?

A. Osteoarthritis
B. Osteomalacia
C. Osteoporosis
D. Primary hyperparathyroidism
E. Pseudo-hypoparathyroidism

55. A patient presents with signs and symptoms of mild hypercalcemia for several months. Tests confirm that corrected/adjusted plasma Ca^{2+} and PO_4^{3-}, is elevated but parathyroid hormone (PTH) is low. There are no indications of kidney disease or alcoholism. Cancer screening one month ago was negative. Measuring which of the following substances would be most useful to understand this patient's condition better?

A. Serum albumin
B. Serum Mg^{2+}
C. Serum PTH-rp*
D. Serum vitamin D
E. Urinary cAMP
*PTH-rp: parathyroid hormone–related protein

56. A 72-year-old man presents with back pain for 1 week after shoveling snow. He also has mild right leg pain near the knee. On examination, he has a lumbar lordosis and slight bowing of both femur bones. Lab results show elevated alkaline phosphatase levels in the serum, and a bone scan and X-ray confirm a diagnosis of Paget's disease of bone. Based on this diagnosis, which of the following best describes the osteoclast and osteoblast activity in this patient?

	Osteoclast activity	Osteoblast activity
A.	↑	↑
B.	↑	↓
C.	↑	↔
D.	↓	↑
E.	↓	↓
F.	↓	↔

9.12 Answers and Explanations

46. Correct: Osteoarthritis (B)

Osteoarthritis is a degenerative joint disorder, and the prevalence increases with age. It most commonly affects joints of the knee, hip, hands, and lumbar and cervical spine. Patients have joint pain and stiffness that is typically worse with activity. Radiographs show loss of joint space, subchondral sclerosis, and osteophytes. (**A**) Achondroplasia is the most common type of short-limb disproportionate dwarfism, characterized by intrinsic abnormalities in the growth and remodeling of cartilage and bone. This can be ruled out because this patient has normal stature. (**C, D**) Osteopenia and osteoporosis are caused by age-related decreases in bone mass that occur secondary to an imbalance between bone resorption and bone formation. Osteoporosis is more advanced than osteopenia. These are unlikely because the patient's bone density scans are unremarkable. (**E**) Paget's disease is a bone remodeling disease that typically presents in men over the age of 50 years. New bone formation is disorganized, causing affected bones to be weak, resulting in pain, misshaped bones, and fractures. This is inconsistent with the patient's presentation. Additionally, the patient's serum alkaline phosphatase levels are normal.

47. Correct: Chronic kidney disease (A)

The patient does not show any signs of hypocalcemia such as paresthesias, tetany, and nerve hyperexcitability (absent Trousseau and Chvostek signs). Nevertheless, diabetes mellitus type 2 is a major risk factor for chronic kidney disease, which could lead to lower levels of active vitamin D and mild hypocalcemia. Any suspicion justifies further investigation. (**B**) Total serum calcium levels are correlated with the amount of serum proteins, primarily albumin, so low albumin (not high) could lead to low total calcium values. (**C**) Very high (not low) serum phosphate levels, such as seen in critically ill patients, can cause acute hypocalcemia, since phosphate avidly binds calcium. (**D**) Parathyroid hormone–related protein is produced in some tissues but does not play a major role in normal calcium/phosphate homeostasis in the adult. It can be part of cancer screening tests, for which there are no indications in this patient. (**E**) RANKL (receptor activator of NF-kB ligand) and OPG (osteoprotegerin) are critical signaling molecules to determine the relative activities of osteoblasts and osteoclasts in certain bone diseases, which is not necessary for this patient.

48. Correct: Bone resorption (B)

The patient has severe liver cirrhosis. His liver cells produce less insulin-like growth factor 1 in response to growth hormone and are not able to inactivate thyroid hormone to reverse triiodothyronine (rT_3). It is likely that other liver cell functions are affected as well. The patient's hypocalcemia (Trousseau sign, paresthesia) is likely due to liver cells that fail to produce 25-hydroxycholecalciferol (storage vitamin D). This leads to less active vitamin D and, consequently, low serum calcium. Hypocalcemia triggers the release of parathyroid hormone, which leads to bone resorption. While the calcium release from bone ameliorates hypocalcemia (evident as mild form of Trousseau sign), bones are more easily broken. (**A**) A patient with liver failure would present with low (not high) albumin, leading to edema and ascites. (**C**) A positive Trousseau sign points to hypocalcemia (not increased serum calcium). (**D**) Increased serum glucose is not likely, since insulin, glucagon, epinephrine, cortisol, and growth hormone are all normal. (**E**) A patient with reduced liver function presents with low (not increased) 1,25-dihydroxycholecalciferol.

49. Correct: Increased, decreased (A)

The boy has severely impaired kidney function (increased BUN and creatinine) and decreased sun exposure, resulting in decreased production of active vitamin D. This will cause low serum calcium and concomitant release of parathyroid hormone (PTH). (**B, D**) This patient has secondary hyperparathyroidism, which can cause serum calcium to be normal, but never high. (**C, E**) PTH is increased (not decreased) as a consequence of low concentrations of active vitamin D and hypocalcemia.

50. Correct: Parathyroid hormone, calcitonin (C)

Hormone A is parathyroid hormone (PTH), since parathyroid cells directly sense circulating calcium with the calcium-sensing receptor, and increasing calcium concentrations leads to decreased PTH. Hormone B is calcitonin, which increases when serum calcium increases. (**A, B**) Hormone A cannot be calcitonin since it increases with increasing serum calcium. (**D**) Active vitamin D, or 1,25$(OH)_2$, cannot be Hormone B, since active vitamin D increases with low (not high) serum calcium. Low calcium stimulates renal 1-α-hydroxylase, which catalyzes the conversion from inactive to active vitamin D. (**E, F**) Hormone B cannot be PTH, since PTH decreases with increasing serum calcium.

51. Correct: Renal tubular phosphate reabsorption (D)

Parathyroid hormone (PTH) and calcitonin have mostly reciprocal functions, with the aim of PTH to increase and calcitonin to decrease blood Ca^{2+} concentrations; however, both hormones inhibit renal tubular phosphate reabsorption. Calcitonin decreases serum calcium and serum phosphate concentrations. PTH increases serum calcium without phosphate, avoiding the formation of calcium phosphate crystals. In healthy people, calcitonin does not have a major role in the physiologic regulation of calcium homeostasis. (**A**) Both calcitonin and PTH activate (not inhibit) osteoblast activity. In the case of PTH, it is an indirect action that ultimately leads to bone resorption via formation of new osteoclasts. (**B**) Calcitonin inhibits osteoclast activity in bone, while PTH stimulates osteoclast activity. (**C**) Calcitonin inhibits and PTH stimulates renal tubular calcium reabsorption.

52. Correct: Hypertension (A)

Hypercalcemia increases smooth muscle contraction. This leads to vasoconstriction and increased total peripheral resistance. Renal vasoconstriction and renal calcium deposition decreases the kidney's ability to maintain blood pressure homeostasis and manifests as worsening hypertension. (**B, C, D, E**) Hypocalcemia (not hypercalcemia) causes increased excitability of excitable cells, including sensory nerves (tingling, numbness), motor nerves, and skeletal muscle. The latter leads to involuntary twitches (muscle fasciculations) and uncontrolled contractions (skeletal muscle cramps, vocal cord spasms). This is because low extracellular calcium destabilizes the closed formation of the voltage-gated sodium channel. The mechanism is not fully elucidated and may involve changes to the channel's voltage sensor, less calcium in the channel lumen, and moving the resting membrane closer to threshold potential.

53. Correct: 7-dehydrocholesterol to vitamin D3 (cholecalciferol) (A)

The patient's aching bones and history of lack of exposure to sunlight point toward bone demineralization due to low vitamin D and secondary hyperparathyroidism. The vitamin D precursor stored in the skin is 7-dehydrocholesterol. Under the influence of sunlight, it is converted to vitamin D_3. (**B**) Ergocalciferol is a vitamin D precursor mainly obtained through food or supplements (not by conversion from cholecalciferol). (**C**) The conversion of ergocalciferol to 25-hydroxycholecalciferol occurs in the liver and is not light-dependent. (**D, E**) The conversions of 25-hydroxycholecalciferol to 1,25-dihydroxycholecalciferol (active vitamin D) or 24,25-dihydroxycholecalciferol (inactive vitamin D) occur in the kidney and are not light-dependent.

54. Correct: Osteoporosis (C)

The woman most likely suffers from osteoporosis, since her bone scan shows reduced bone density. Her normal serum calcium, phosphorus, and alkaline phosphatase levels are in agreement with the diagnosis. Osteoporosis is typically asymptomatic until a fracture occurs. (**A**) In osteoarthritis, bone density is high or unaffected. (**B**) In osteomalacia, bone pain is common. Serum alkaline phosphatase is usually elevated, or calcium and phosphate are decreased. (**D**) Primary hyperparathyroidism would present with elevated serum calcium and, in most cases, reduced serum phosphate levels. (**E**) Pseudohypoparathyroidism would present with low serum calcium levels.

55. Correct: Serum vitamin D (D)

Low plasma parathyroid hormone (PTH) with elevated Ca^{2+} and PO_4^{3-} point toward a secondary problem, not originating in the parathyroid glands. With renal function being normal, measuring vitamin D would be most useful, since vitamin D intoxication due to supplements or medication could explain the presentation. (**A**) Corrected/adjusted plasma Ca^{2+} already takes the serum albumin levels into account. (**B**) Severe hypomagnesemia (alcoholism as most likely cause) can indeed inhibit PTH; however, this leads to a primary problem that would present with low Ca^{2+} and high PO_4^{3-}. (**C**) The production of parathyroid hormone–related protein (PTH-rp) and its release into the circulation is unlikely in the absence of malignancy. PTH-rp induces rapidly rising hypercalcemia (not mild symptoms for months), and high calcium suppresses endogenous PTH production. Patients typically have low (not high) PO_4^{3-}. (**E**) Urinary cAMP is most helpful for better understanding the presence of high (not low) plasma PTH, since it can help to distinguish between a primary hyperparathyroidism and receptor insensitivity.

56. Correct: ↑, ↑ (A)

Paget's disease is a bone remodeling disease that typically presents in men over the age of 50 years. Increased osteoclast activity causes excessive bone resorption. Osteoblast activity increases to provide new bone formation, but the bone remodeling is disorganized, causing affected bones to be weak, resulting in pain, misshaped bones, fractures, and arthritis in the joints near the affected bones. (**B, C, D, E, F**) These choices are incorrect.

Chapter 10

Reproductive System

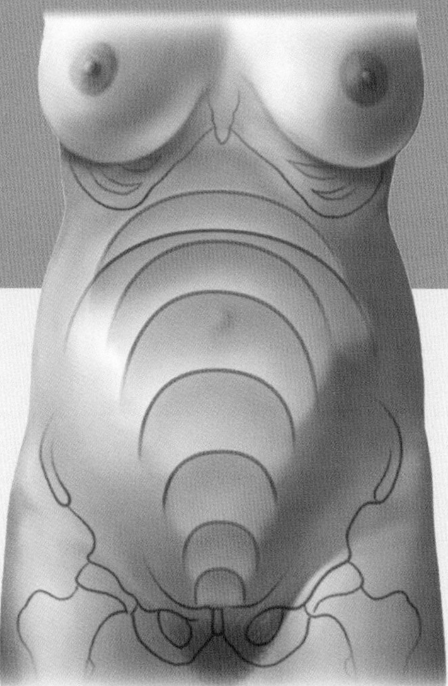

LEARNING OBJECTIVES

- Describe the determinants of genetic, gonadal, and phenotypic sex differentiation as well as the physiological changes during puberty.
- Discuss the physiological functions of the male reproductive system and be able to apply the knowledge to relevant daily and clinical situations.
- Discuss the physiological functions of the female reproductive system and be able to apply the knowledge to relevant daily and clinical situations.
- Describe the physiological changes in a pregnant woman and the mechanisms leading to childbirth. Have a basic understanding of the major phases in fetal development.

10.1 Questions

Easy	Medium	Hard

1. A mother educated herself since she is concerned about the sexual development of her son. She asks the physician, an increase in which of the following is the *primary* event in initiating his pubertal development?

A. Adrenal steroids
B. FSH/LH ratio
C. GnRH pulses
D. Morning erections
E. Size of testes

(FSH: Follicle-stimulating hormone; GnRH: gonadotropin-releasing hormone, LH: luteinizing hormone)

2. A congenital deficiency of the adrenal 21-β-hydroxylase enzyme (*CYP21A2* defect) causes which of the following symptoms?

A. Ambiguous genitalia in girls
B. Delayed puberty in boys
C. Hypopigmentation in boys
D. Impeded skeletal maturation
E. Lack of body hair in girls

3. A research study compares the amount of pubic hair in 10-year-old girls. When considering averages from large cohorts, girls with which of the following are expected to have the lowest physiologic amount of pubic hair?

A. A home at sea level
B. Addison's disease
C. High stress
D. Turner's syndrome (45, XO)
E. Overnutrition

4. Genetic testing of a fetus revealed a karyotype of 46, XY and a mutation in the androgen receptor. If the child were born with complete androgen receptor insensitivity syndrome, which of the following is expected?

	Testes	Ovaries	Vas deferens	Prostate	Cervix	Vagina
A	Present	Present	Absent	Absent	Present	Present
B	Present	Absent	Present	Female form	Absent	Present
C	Absent	Female form	Female form	Absent	Present	Absent
D	Absent	Present	Absent	Female form	Absent	Absent
E	Female form	Absent	Present	Absent	Present	Present
F	Female form	Female form	Female form	Female form	Absent	Present

5. A 15-year-old female patient is concerned since she has not started her menstrual periods. She is phenotypically female, and she dresses, behaves, and has the psychosocial outlook of a normal, well-adjusted teenage girl. On physical examination, she has normal female external genitalia, a blind-ending vagina, and no cervix. Imaging study reveals no uterus but intrapelvic gonads, which on biopsy turn out to be testicular tissue. Karyotyping shows that the patient is 46, XY. Which of the following is the most likely diagnosis?

A. Androgen insensitivity syndrome
B. Female Kallman's syndrome
C. Female pseudohermaphroditism
D. Müllerian agenesis
E. True hermaphroditism
F. Turner's syndrome

6. A newborn was born with ambiguous external genitalia, indicating either an enlarged clitoris or a very small penis. The pediatrician ordered various newborn screening tests, using blood from a heel stick and karyotype analysis. The blood results came back 2 days later and showed some abnormality. The genetic test results arrived 14 days later and revealed two X chromosomes. Which of the following is the most likely result from the blood analysis?

A. 5-α-reductase deficiency
B. 17-α-hydroxylase deficiency
C. Down's syndrome
D. Excess maternal androgen
E. Phenylketonuria

7. A 19-year old male is brought to the emergency room with an abdominal injury requiring surgery. During surgery, a small uterus is discovered. It is also observed that his testes have not descended. Later, he explains that he is bothered by the cryptorchidism, but that he had a normal childhood, is sexually active, and has no gender ambiguity in his life. He is muscular and does not look feminine. The most likely explanation for the presence of a uterus in this otherwise normal 46, XY male is that during the first 10 weeks of fetal development there was a decrease of which of the following?

A. 5-α-dihydrotestosterone
B. 5-α-reductase
C. Antimüllerian hormone
D. Estrogen
E. Luteinizing hormone

8. Which of the following is the most likely cause of amenorrhea due to hypergonadotropic hypogonadism?

A. Eating disorder
B. Hyperprolactinemia
C. Kallmann's syndrome
D. Pregnancy
E. Strenuous exercise
F. Turner's syndrome

9. A young man discusses with his physician that he seems incapable of conceiving a child with his wife. Upon physical examination, small and firm testes; moderate gynecomastia; poor beard growth; sparse body hair; long, thin arms and legs; narrow shoulders; and wide hips are found. Laboratory tests show decreased levels of testosterone and increased levels of luteinizing hormone (LH) and follicle-stimulating hormone (FSH). There are no spermatozoa in the ejaculate. Karyotyping and additional analysis would most likely indicate which of the following?

A. 45, X
B. 46, XY, complete androgen insensitivity syndrome
C. 46, XY, 11-β-hydroxylase deficiency
D. 47, XXY
E. 47, XYY

10. A couple wishes to conceive a child. The male receives testosterone supplementation because he had been diagnosed with androgen insensitivity syndrome (AIS) of the male phenotype. Considering that AIS inheritance follows an X-linked recessive pattern, which of the following is correct for a future child of the couple?

A. A boy would be a carrier for AIS.
B. A boy would have AIS.
C. A girl would be unaffected.
D. A girl would be a carrier of AIS.
E. A girl would have AIS.

11. Which of the following cells produce antimüllerian hormone in order to induce regression of paramesonephric (müllerian) ducts in a male fetus?

A. Fetal Leydig cells
B. Fetal Sertoli cells
C. Fetal spermatogonia
D. Maternal granulosa cells
E. Maternal theca cells
F. Syncytiotrophoblast

10.2 Answers and Explanations

Easy	Medium	Hard

1. Correct: GnRH pulses (C)

While the exact triggers of puberty are still mainly unknown, there is a predictable sequence of events. The one event that precedes all others is an increase in the pulsatile release of gonadotropin-releasing hormone (GnRH). (**A**) The increased release of adrenal androgen, called adrenarche, occurs between 6 and 10 years of age. It cannot be used as a sign of puberty, since it is independent of gonadal sex steroid production during gonadarche. (**B**) In adulthood, luteinizing hormone (LH) exceeds follicle-stimulating hormone (FSH), so that the FSH/LH ratio decreases (not increases) after puberty. (**D**) Morning erections are increased due to an increase in LH pulse frequency and amplitude, but for this increase to happen, GnRH pulsatility has to increase first. (**E**) Increased size of the testes is in response to the upregulated sex hormonal axis of GnRH, LH, and FSH and hence is not the initial event.

2. Correct: Ambiguous genitalia in girls (A)

Congenital deficiency of adrenal 21-β-hydroxylase presents with ambiguous genitalia in girls due to the increased production of adrenal androgens. The enzyme deficiency blocks cortisol synthesis and removes the negative feedback inhibition for adrenocorticotropic hormone (ACTH). Elevated ACTH causes adrenal hyperplasia and increased production of adrenal hormones that are unaffected by the enzyme block, such as androgens. (**B**) Increased androgen in boys leads to precocious (not delayed) puberty. (**C**) The disease leads to hyper- (not hypo-) pigmentation in boys and girls. This is due to increased production of α-melanocyte-stimulating hormone (α-MSH) that is part of proopiomelanocortin (POMC), the precursor for ACTH. (**D**) Excess androgen accelerates (not impedes) skeletal maturation and linear growth before closure of the epiphyseal growth plate. (**E**) Excess adrenal androgen in girls leads to hirsutism (not lack of body hair).

3. Correct: Addison's disease (B)

Pubic hair development (from Tanner stage 1 to 2/3) initially occurs due to adrenarche, which typically occurs in girls before age 10. While pubic hair still increases during puberty to Tanner stage 4, age 10 is the average age when puberty begins. Adrenarche is absent or decreased in Addison's disease, which is characterized by low production of all adrenal hormones, including androgens. (**A**) Living at high altitude is related to delayed puberty, but girls with a home at sea level will have no different adrenarche or gonadarche compared to average. (**C, E**) Girls living with high stress, such as in a household with an abusive parent, are known to have early puberty. Increased nutrition and body weight is the strongest external link to early puberty. Hence, in both cases the girls' pubic hair at age 10 has matured due to adrenarche and potentially early puberty. (**D**) A 10-year-old girl with Turner's syndrome will have typical adrenarche and hence typical (not decreased) development of pubic hair.

4. Correct: Present, absent, present, female form, absent, present (B)

Dependent on the type, androgen receptor mutation in the fetus can lead to mild, partial, or complete androgen insensitivity syndrome (CAIS). In a 46, XY child with CAIS, internal sex structures are male, though vastly regressed due to the missing influence of testosterone receptor signaling, while external sex structures are female, since testosterone is converted into estrogen by aromatase. In particular: testes are present due to the *SRY* gene on the Y chromosome. Ovaries are absent since *SRY* induces the expression of antimüllerian hormone (AMH), and fetal gonads develop into ovaries only in the absence of AMH. The vas deferens, which is a derivate of the wolffian duct, is present. The prostate, a derivate of the fetal urogenital sinus, is in female form (Skene's gland). The cervix is absent, since it is a derivative of the müllerian ducts. The lower portion of the vagina is present, since lack of testosterone leads to external female genitalia. (**A, C, D, E, F**) These are incorrect choices for a male with CAIS.

5. Correct: Androgen insensitivity syndrome (A)

Unambiguously female external genitalia with a male karyotype is characteristic for complete androgen insensitivity syndrome. There are regressed testes, but the lack of functioning androgen and the conversion of androgen to estrogen leads to a female phenotype. (**B**) Kallman's syndrome is characterized by low gonadotropin-releasing hormone (GnRH) release, leading to symptoms of hypogonadism such as immature sexual characteristics. (**C**) Female pseudohermaphroditism is a condition in which the person has ovaries but the external genitalia are male or ambiguous. (**D**) Patients with müllerian agenesis have a similar phenotype as the presented patient but have a 46, XX karyotype. (**E**) True hermaphroditism is the rare case in which both testicular and ovarian tissues are present. (**F**) Turner's syndrome is characterized by a karyotype of 45, XO, or rarer 45, X mosaicism (e.g., 45X/46XX).

6. Correct: Excess maternal androgen (D)

The presence of excess amount of androgen delivered via maternal blood can cause prenatal virilization of a genetically female fetus (46, XX). It leads to enlargement of the clitoris or even a small penis, since both derive from the genital tubercle. (**A**) 5-α-reductase deficiency results in low amounts of dihydrotestosterone, which in girls has no significant effect for female development. (**B**) 17-α-hydroxylase deficiency presents with low adrenal androgen and in girls is typically undetected until puberty, when the development of secondary sexual characteristics is delayed. (**C**) Virilization of genitalia, such as present in this case, is not part of Down's syndrome (trisomy 21). (**E**) Phenylketonuria is typically part of the newborn screening tests, but it would not manifest as virilization of female newborns.

7. Correct: Antimüllerian hormone (C)

Antimüllerian hormone (AMH) prevents the development of female internal structures. Hence, inadequate AMH can lead to a rudimentary uterus, which remains small because it is not supported by female hormones. Due to the XY genotype, testes have developed and there is production of testosterone and dihydrotestosterone (DHT), leading to external male genitalia and male sexual identity. (**A, B**) A decrease in 5-α-DHT per se, or a decrease in the enzyme 5-α-reductase, which converts testosterone into DHT, would lead to nontypical external male genitalia. (**D**) A decrease of estrogen during early male development is not known to be clinically relevant. (**E**) During the first 10 weeks of fetal development, the fetal brain does not yet produce luteinizing hormone (LH), and human chorionic gonadotropin (hCG) takes the role of LH to stimulate fetal cells to produce testosterone.

8. Correct: Turner's syndrome (F)

Chromosomal abnormalities such as Turner's syndrome are the most common cause of amenorrhea due to ovarian dysgenesis. Nonfunctional ovaries produce low estrogen and progesterone (hypogonadism), which increases follicle-stimulating hormone (FSH) and luteinizing hormone (LH) production by gonadotropes (hypergonadotropy). (**A, E**) Eating disorders such as extreme dieting or anorexia nervosa, and high levels of prolonged mental or physical stress, can lead to the decrease in the frequency and amplitude of gonadotropin-releasing hormone (GnRH) pulses, with the consequence of hypogonadotropic hypogonadism and amenorrhea. (**B**) Hyperprolactinemia decreases GnRH and leads to hypogonadotropic hypogonadism. (**C**) Kallmann's syndrome is the failure to produce GnRH, which leads to low LH and FSH, hence hypogonadotropic hypogonadism. (**D**) During pregnancy, there are low levels of FSH and LH due to increased estrogen and progesterone. Since amenorrhea during pregnancy is a normal occurrence, it is typically not described by this terminology, which describes abnormalities.

9. Correct: 47, XXY (D)

A 47, XXY karyotype leads to Klinefelter's syndrome. The male exhibits testicular atrophy (small, firm testes), in which abnormal Leydig cell function leads to decreased production of testosterone (poor beard growth) and increased luteinizing hormone (LH) levels, while loss of Sertoli cells leads to low inhibin production and elevated follicle-stimulating hormone (FSH) levels. The elevated gonadotropins stimulate estrogen production and feminization (gynecomastia, wide hips). Elevated estrogen, together with low dihydrotestosterone, leads to sparse body hair. (**A**) Patients with Turner's syndrome (45, monosomy X) are phenotypic females. (**B**) Patients with complete androgen insensitivity syndrome have female external genitalia and body appearance. Testes are located within the abdomen. (**C**) 11-β-hydroxylase deficiency presents with increased adrenal androgen (not signs of feminization). (**E**) 47, XYY is not characterized by distinct physical features. Fertility is normal. The extra Y may lead to increased growth.

10. Correct: A girl would be a carrier of AIS. (D)

Androgen insensitivity syndrome (AIS) includes diseases with mutations of the androgen receptor gene, which is located on the X chromosome. While it is rare for a 46, XY male with AIS to be fertile, it is not impossible with testosterone treatment. From such a father, a baby girl would receive one X chromosome and would be a carrier for the syndrome. (**A, B**) A boy would receive the X chromosome from the mother and hence neither have AIS nor carry the gene for AIS. (**C, E**) A girl would be a carrier for AIS (and not be unaffected). A girl would not have AIS. Being a carrier leads to minor, clinically often insignificant impact on sexual development.

11. Correct: Fetal Sertoli cells (B)

Sertoli cells of the fetal testes produce antimüllerian hormone (AMH) early in sexual differentiation to prevent the formation of the oviduct and uterus in genetic males. (**A**) Fetal Leydig cells produce testosterone and no AMH. (**C**) Fetal spermatogonia are germ cells that develop into sperm through spermatogenesis, which happens after sexual differentiation. (**D**) Maternal granulosa cells produce small amounts of AMH after puberty, but this is independent of pregnancy and not responsible for the sexual differentiation of the woman's child. (**E**) Maternal theca cells are not known to produce AMH. (**F**) A syncytiotrophoblast is a multinucleated tissue of embryonal and maternal cells, formed as barrier for maternal immune cells to reach the fetus independent of its sex.

10.3 Questions

12. The semen of a healthy normospermic adult male has which of the following characteristic, when obtained after 48 to 72 hours of sexual abstinence?

A. A sperm concentration of > 20 million/mL
B. An alkaline pH around 9.0
C. Small fatty acids as main energy source
D. Testosterone levels similar to serum
E. The highest fluid amount from the bulbourethral gland

13. Which of the following is a characteristic of Sertoli cells in the seminiferous tubules of the testes?

A. Luteinizing hormone receptors
B. Meiotic division
C. Production of estriol
D. Secretion of inhibin
E. Synthesis of testosterone

14. A 31-year-old male patient is known to have taken androstenedione as an over-the-counter anabolic supplement. Which of the following is expected to be increased in his urinary sample?

A. Estradiol
B. Follicle-stimulating hormone
C. 17-ketosteroids
D. Luteinizing hormone
E. Testosterone

15. The wife of a 38-year-old man urges him towards sterilization as a means of contraception. As part of the procedure, a portion of which semen-conveying duct is excised and bilaterally sealed?

A. Epididymis
B. Seminal gland duct
C. Urethra
D. Vas deferens
E. Wolffian duct

16. A pig farmer accidentally injected himself with a high dose of follicle-stimulating hormone (FSH). He is very concerned, since he read that FSH stimulates estrogen production in the testes. The physician explains that only a tiny amount of estrogen is produced that way and that it will not cause any feminization, but rather, the estrogen is necessary for which of the following?

A. *De novo* synthesis of androgens
B. Negative feedback to the brain
C. Production of dihydrotestosterone
D. Support of spermatogenesis
E. Testosterone release into seminiferous tubules

17. An 80-year-old man presents with urinary frequency. He describes that he wakes up at least five times a night with the compelling need to urinate, but then produces only a weak urinary stream and feels that he did not fully empty the bladder. Rectal and urinary tests suggest benign prostatic hypertrophy. Direct inhibition of the formation of which of the following androgens is an appropriate pharmacologic treatment for this condition?

A. 11-deoxycorticosterone
B. Dehydroepiandrosterone
C. Dihydrotestosterone
D. Epitestosterone
E. Androstenedione

18. A young couple has been trying to have children for the past two years. History and physical examination for the woman are normal. The man is difficult to talk to and responds aggressively, but denies any problems with libido and/or penile erection. He is very muscular and confirms that he does weightlifting frequently. His testes are small and soft. There is gynecomastia. His sperm count is low. Laboratory results indicate:

Testosterone:	1,936 ng/dL	(350–1,050)
Luteinizing hormone:	undetectable	(1–15 µU/mL)
Follicle-stimulating hormone:	1 µU/ml	(1–15 µU/mL)

Which of the following serum hormone levels is expected for this man, compared to normal?

	Testosterone/ epitestosterone ratio	Estrogen	Prolactin	Dopamine
A.	↔	↑	↔	↔
B.	↔	↓	↑	↑
C.	↑	↔	↓	↓
D.	↑	↑	↔	↔
E.	↓	↓	↑	↑
F.	↓	↔	↓	↓

19. An athlete is banned from competition since he has been convicted of long-term injections with testosterone. Such abuse would be expected to increase which of the following in the man compared to the time before the hormone injections?

A. Inhibin secretion by Sertoli cells
B. Serum creatinine levels
C. The rate of spermatogenesis
D. The size and mass of the testes
E. Testosterone secretion by Leydig cells

20. The research laboratory of a fertility clinic investigates various biomolecules for their ability to induce sperm capacitation. The molecules have most likely been isolated from the fluid of which of the following structures?

A. Epididymis
B. Ovaries
C. Seminal vesicles
D. Seminiferous tubules
E. Uterus

21. A physician considers the use of a drug that inhibits 5-α-reductase for a patient. Which of the following is the most likely warranted effect for this patient?

A. Decreasing male libido by inhibiting testosterone
B. Delaying male pattern baldness by inhibiting dihydrotestosterone
C. Depressing premature puberty by inhibiting luteinizing hormone
D. Increasing "maleness" by inhibiting male estrogen
E. Preventing prostate growth by inhibiting aldosterone

22. In females, a drug inhibits progesterone production by the corpus luteum by preventing luteinizing hormone (LH) from binding to its receptor in luteal cells. In males, which of the following is expected to be decreased in Sertoli cells when functional testicular tissue is exposed to the drug?

A. Cholesterol uptake from serum
B. *De novo* synthesis of inhibin
C. Production of androgen-binding protein
D. Stimulation of aromatase activity
E. Testosterone transport by apical membrane

23. Which of the following conditions is a likely cause for male infertility due to testicular azoospermia?

A. Cystic fibrosis
B. Kallman's syndrome
C. Klinefelter's syndrome
D. Testosterone doping
E. TRH*-producing tumor

*TRH: thyrotropin-releasing hormone

10.4 Answers and Explanations

12. Correct: A sperm concentration of > 20 million/mL (A)

A semen sample obtained after 48 to 72 hours of abstinence is considered normal when it has a volume of more than 2 mL with a sperm concentration higher than 20 million per mL. (**B**) Slight (rather than extensive) alkalinity of semen helps neutralize vaginal acidity. A normal pH of semen is 7.2 to 7.8. (**C**) Fructose (not fatty acids) is the main energy source for sperm cells. (**D**) While there seems to be a positive association between semen testosterone and sperm motility, the testosterone concentration in semen is drastically lower than in serum. (**E**) The largest amount of fluid (up to 75%) in semen arises from seminal vesicles. The bulbourethral gland produces a clear secretion known as pre-ejaculate.

13. Correct: Secretion of inhibin (D)

Sertoli cells secrete inhibin under the influence of follicle-stimulating hormone (FSH) receptor signaling. Serum inhibin then suppresses pituitary FSH release and hence creates a negative feedback loop. (**A**) Sertoli cells have FSH (not luteinizing hormone) receptors. (**B**) Sertoli cells are diploid cells that nurture and support sperm development, but do not undergo themselves meiotic division. (**C**) Sertoli cells produce small amounts of estradiol to support spermatogenesis. Estriol is the dominant hormone in pregnant females. (**E**) Sertoli cells are incapable of producing testosterone *de novo*.

14. Correct: 17-ketosteroids (C)

Androstenedione (Andro) in males is primarily produced in the adrenal cortex. In the past, it has been promoted in bodybuilding circles, but it is now on the list of controlled substances with significant health risks. Andro and other adrenal androgens are excreted in urine as 17-ketosteroids (17-KS). Hence, they would be increased with exogenous use of Andro. Clinically, the 17-KS test is used for the diagnosis of certain adrenal disorders but is not available as a doping test. (**A**) Andro is converted by aromatase into estrone (not estradiol), and a metabolite of it would be in urine. (**B, D**) Adrenal androgens have little if any feedback regulatory effect on follicle-stimulating hormone and luteinizing hormone. If so, they would be decreased, not increased. (**E**) Andro has no significant effect on increasing serum testosterone, so no increase in urine is expected.

15. Correct: Vas deferens (D)

The procedure for permanent sterilization of a male involves the bilateral excision of a part of the vas deferens and the sealing of the ducts. The vasa deferentia are relatively easy to access via simple surgery due to their length of about 1 foot (0.3 meters). (**A**) The epididymis is a duct that connects the testis and the vas deferens. Its excision would risk damaging the testis. (**B**) The seminal gland duct is the part where the coiled tubes of each seminal vesicle come together and empty into the vas deferens just before the prostate. Excision would risk damaging the prostate. (**C**) The male urethra conducts semen and urine, and excision would impair urination. (**E**) The wolffian duct is a urogenital structure of the male embryo and is not present in the male adult.

16. Correct: Support of spermatogenesis (D)

A small amount of testosterone is converted into estradiol in Sertoli cells under the influence of follicle-stimulating hormone (FSH), which is necessary for normal development of sperm. It is only a tiny amount. The main amount of male estrogens is produced by peripheral tissue such as fat cells. (**A**) *De novo* synthesis of testicular androgens happens in Leydig cells under the influence of luteinizing hormone (LH, not FSH). (**B**) Serum testosterone and inhibin are responsible for negative feedback inhibition of FSH and LH, and estrogens do not play any significant role. (**C**) The enzyme 5-α-reductase (not FSH-induced estrogen production) is necessary for production of dihydrotestosterone in androgen target tissue. (**E**) Testosterone is released into the lumen of seminiferous tubules when bound to androgen-binding protein, not under the influence of estrogen.

17. Correct: Dihydrotestosterone (C)

The symptoms of the man are consistent with benign prostatic hypertrophy, which is present in about three of four men by age 80. One type of medication blocks 5-α-reductase, the enzyme that converts testosterone to dihydrotestosterone (DHT) in the prostate. DHT is critical for prostate growth. (**A, B, D, E**) The hormones androstenedione (testes and adrenal gland), dehydroepiandrosterone (DHEA, adrenal gland), 11-deoxycorticosterone (mineralocorticoid of adrenal gland), and epitestosterone (inactive hormone, testes) have no or minor effects on prostate growth. Some of them are substrates for 5-α-reductase and hence slightly increase when this enzyme is inhibited.

18. Correct: ↑, ↑, ↔, ↔ (D)

The man's presentation (high serum testosterone with low luteinizing hormone [LH] and low follicle-stimulating hormone [FSH]) suggests the use of exogenous testosterone. It is fairly easy to obtain without prescription due to the ever-growing illicit offers of androgens as performance-enhancing drugs. Testosterone supports muscle growth (the man is very muscular) and affects male behavior (responds aggressively) but decreases endogenous production of testosterone (T) and epitestosterone (Epi), which affects the male reproductive system (small and soft testes, low sperm count). Hence, the T/Epi ratio is increased with exogenous testosterone, from a normal ratio of ~ 1:1 to usually > 6:1. Estrogen is elevated, since some extra testosterone is converted to estradiol, which leads to gynecomastia. Prolactin is unaffected, since testosterone has no feedback regulatory function to prolactin. Moreover, hypo- and hyperprolactinemia could lead to erectile dysfunction and affect libido, signs that are not present. Dopamine is unaffected, since there is no known feedback regulatory mechanism from testosterone to dopamine. (**A, B, C, E, F**) These contain one or more incorrect answers.

19. Correct: Serum creatinine levels (B)

The reason why athletes inject testosterone is that elevated plasma testosterone levels increase the mass and strength of muscles, especially when exercised by an athlete. In the absence of kidney dysfunction, the amount of creatinine that is spontaneously converted from creatine depends on the muscle mass. A higher skeletal muscle mass leads to higher serum creatinine levels. (**A, C, D, E**). The man's increased serum testosterone levels due to hormone injections inhibit via negative feedback the release of gonadotropin-releasing hormone, luteinizing hormone, and follicle-stimulating hormone, leading to declines in inhibin secretion by Sertoli cells, spermatogenesis, testicular size, and testosterone secretion by Leydig cells.

20. Correct: Uterus (E)

Capacitation is a biochemical event that improves the ability of sperm to fertilize a human egg by altering the membrane of the sperm head and maturing it for the consequent acrosome reaction. It normally happens to sperm within the female tract, supported by fluid secreted by the uterus. (**A, C, D**) Fluid from the epididymis, the seminal vesicles, or the seminiferous tubules does not induce capacitation. Rather, the sperm needs to be in contact with substances provided by the female tract. When provided to mature sperm, the chance for *in vitro* fertilization significantly increases. (**B**) Capacitation of sperm occurs during the passage of sperm in the female tract to the fallopian tubes, where fertilization occurs. Fluid released by the ovaries would be too far away to support this process.

21. Correct: Delaying male pattern baldness by inhibiting dihydrotestosterone (B)

The enzyme 5-α-reductase is present in skin, where it converts testosterone into dihydrotestosterone (DHT). Since DHT contributes to male pattern baldness, inhibiting the enzyme can be considered to treat male alopecia. (**A**) Testosterone is slightly accumulated (not inhibited) when the enzyme is inhibited that converts it to DHT. (**C**) 5-α-reductase inhibitors (5-ARIs) do not inhibit luteinizing hormone (LH) and depress premature puberty. Instead, their use leads to DHT deficiency, which would increase mean plasma LH due to lack of negative feedback. (**D**) 5-ARI may decrease (not increase) "maleness," due to some excess testosterone that has been converted into estrogen. (**E**) 5-ARI indeed can be considered to prevent prostate growth, but by inhibiting DHT production (not aldosterone). Aldosterone might slightly increase since it is known to be a substrate of 5-α-reductase.

22. Correct: Testosterone transport by apical membrane (E)

In females, granulosa and theca cells of the corpus luteum produce progesterone after luteinizing hormone (LH) binds to the cell membrane and starts intracellular signaling. In functional testicular tissue of males, LH binds to Leydig cells and induces production of testosterone. Some of the testosterone is transferred to Sertoli cells, which transport it, bound to androgen-binding protein, across the apical cell membrane into the lumen of the seminiferous tubules. Hence, if the drug inhibits LH binding to its receptor, there is less T accumulation in seminiferous tubular lumen. (**A**) Cholesterol uptake from serum for steroidogenesis occurs in Leydig cells (not Sertoli cells). (**B, C, D**) *De novo* synthesis of inhibin, production of androgen-binding protein, and stimulation of aromatase activity in Sertoli cells are under the influence of follicle-stimulating hormone. Sertoli cells do not have LH receptors.

23. Correct: Klinefelter's syndrome (C)

Testicular azoospermia is the complete lack of sperm due to a cause from within the testes. In Klinefelter's syndrome, the extra X chromosome(s) lead to low-functioning testes and infertility. (**A**) Cystic fibrosis causes male infertility most frequently due to the congenital absence of the vas deferens. Hence, it is a potential cause of posttesticular azoospermia. (**B**) Kallmann's syndrome is a form of hypogonadotropic hypogonadism, hence it can cause male infertility due to pretesticular azoospermia. (**D**) Doping with testosterone inhibits follicle-stimulating hormone and luteinizing hormone, so the cause for a lack of sperm in semen is pretesticular and not from within the testes. (**E**) Excess thyrotropin-releasing hormone (TRH) can lead to hyperprolactinemia. High prolactin leads to low gonadotropin-releasing hormone and potential pretesticular azoospermia.

10.5 Questions

24. An 18-year-old woman is very concerned about her fertility since she has had no menstrual bleeding for the past 6 months. Menarche occurred at age 14. Physical examination reveals that the woman is severely obese and has acne. She admits to being very hairy and to shaving her face. A pelvic ultrasound shows numerous small peripheral follicles in her ovaries. A blood sample is sent for hormonal analysis. Which of the following hormones is most likely to be within the normal reference range in this patient?

A. Androstenedione
B. Estrone
C. Follicle-stimulating hormone
D. Luteinizing hormone
E. Testosterone

Questions 25 to 27

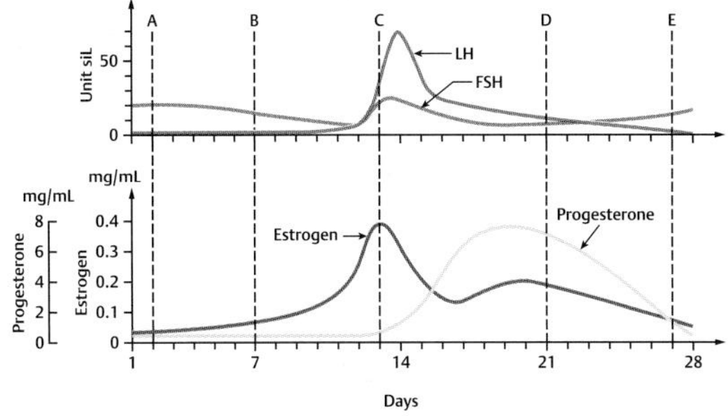

Use the image to answer questions 25, 26, and 27. The graph shows the plasma hormone levels of luteinizing hormone (LH, yellow line), follicle-stimulating hormone (FSH, red line), estrogens (purple line), and progesterone (blue line) during a 28-day cycle of a healthy woman.

25. At which time point is the highest concentration of progesterone receptors present in the endometrium?

A. A
B. B
C. C
D. D
E. E

26. If the egg of a woman is fertilized and develops into a zygote, what is the most likely time that it will implant in the endometrium?

A. A
B. B
C. C
D. D
E. E

27. The woman checks the amount and consistency of her cervical mucus daily. At which time does she produce the highest amount of watery and elastic mucus, a characteristic used for the spinnbarkeit and ferning tests?

A. A
B. B
C. C
D. D
E. E

28. The following are the measured serum concentrations of a particular hormone in a healthy adult woman measured at age 30 and age 52. The data are averages of 20 measurements on days 8, 13, and 22 of her regular 31-day menstrual cycles, and averages of 10 measurements after cessation of menstruation at age 52:

Age 30:
Day 8: 70 pg/mL
Day 13: 320 pg/mL
Day 22: 130 pg/mL
Age 52: 5 pg/mL

Which of the following hormones has been measured?

A. Estradiol
B. Follicle-stimulating hormone
C. Gonadotropin-releasing hormone
D. Luteinizing hormone
E. Progesterone

29. A study found that primates that ate fruit rich in phytoestrogens showed progesteronemia, which led to alterations in the primates' menstrual cycle length and endometrial histology. To investigate whether the progesterones also alter systemic parameters, as they do in humans, the researchers planned to monitor easily obtainable parameters. Which of the following makes the least sense?

A. Clotting tendency
B. Respiratory rate
C. Serum glucose
D. Urine sodium

30. In an adult woman with a normal menstrual cycle, estrogen levels in blood continually increase for 6–8 days after menstruation. What is the source of the estrogen?

A. Corpus luteum
B. Developing follicles
C. Endometrium
D. Ovarian stromal cells
E. Pituitary gonadotropes

31. A 24-year-old woman recorded her basal body temperature every morning before getting out of bed for one month starting with the first day of her menstrual period. The results are shown in the image. Which of the following can be concluded about her cycle that month?

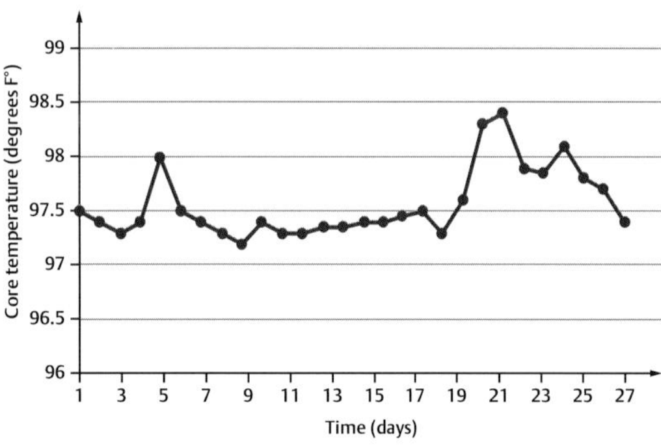

A. A normal female cycle
B. A premature ovulation
C. A short luteal phase
D. No ovulation
E. Two ovulations

32. The blood level of luteinizing hormone (LH) is measured daily in a 23-year-old healthy woman over a 28-day menstrual cycle (day 1 is the first day of menstrual bleeding) and plotted in the image. At times A and B, the blood levels of various hormones were measured. Which of the following hormones is expected to have the highest B/A blood concentration ratio?

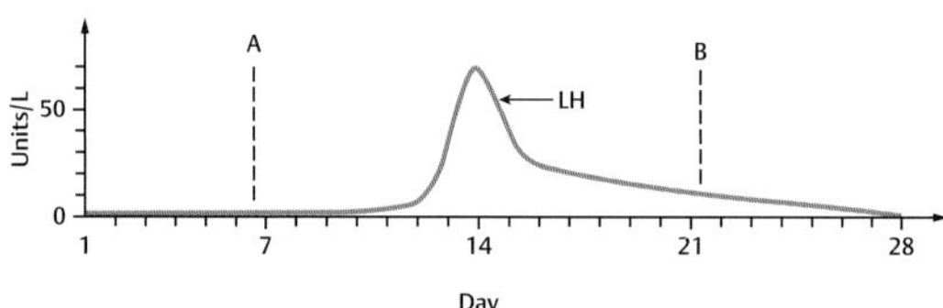

A. Dihydrotestosterone
B. Estradiol
C. Follicle-stimulating hormone
D. Progesterone
E. Testosterone

33. A 27-year-old female patient has problems with conception. An abdominal ultrasound scan shows no abnormalities, so a functional sex hormone test is ordered. For that, the biological cycle of the woman is hormonally shut down for a week. When synthetic analogues of follicle-stimulating hormone/luteinizing hormone (FSH/LH) are administered, changes in estradiol and progesterone are measured. When gonadotropin-releasing hormone (GnRH) is administered, changes in FSH and LH are monitored. Which of the following results would support the working diagnosis of a functional problem at the hypothalamus as the cause of the infertility?

	Change in serum estradiol and/or progesterone after FSH/LH	Change in serum FSH and/or LH after GnRH
A.	No change	No change
B.	Decrease	Increase
C.	Increase	Decrease
D.	Decrease	No change
E.	Increase	Increase

34. A 29-year old woman has difficulty conceiving. Her family history includes diabetes mellitus type 2. The physical exam reveals acne, hirsutism, hypertension, and multiple small cysts in the ovaries. Laboratory tests show an elevated plasma ratio of luteinizing hormone to follicle-stimulating hormone (LH/FSH), increased free testosterone, and increased fasting plasma glucose. Which of the following interventions would be most appropriate to improve her acne and hirsutism without further negatively affecting her fertility?

A. Blocking estrogen receptors
B. Blocking LH receptors
C. Decreasing 5-α reductase
D. Decreasing androgen-binding protein
E. Increasing sex hormone–binding globulin
F. Removing about half of her ovarian tissue

35. Home-use ovulation predictor kits measure two urinary hormones and display a "smiley face" when ovulation is predicted to occur. In addition to luteinizing hormone, which of the following hormones is most likely measured as part of the kit?

A. Estrone
B. Estrone-3-glucuronide
C. Follicle-stimulating hormone
D. Human chorionic gonadotropin
E. Progesterone

36. A 51-year old woman has had hot flashes and no menstrual bleeding for the past 4 months. When compared to average levels in menstruating women, her serum follicle-stimulating hormone, luteinizing hormone, and estrone levels are increased, and her serum estradiol and progesterone concentrations are decreased. Which of the following substances is the most likely source of the elevated estrone?

A. Nonovarian androstenedione
B. Nonovarian estradiol
C. Nonovarian testosterone
D. Ovarian estradiol
E. Ovarian estriol

10.6 Answers and Explanations

24. Correct: Follicle-stimulating hormone (C)

The woman most likely has polycystic ovary syndrome (PCOS), the most common cause of secondary amenorrhea (absence of menses for 6 months and previously menstruating). Her physical examination fits the general profile (obese, acne, hirsutism), and polycystic-appearing ovaries support the diagnosis. Obesity causes and/or contributes to the hormonal profile since it leads to insulin resistance. Excess insulin increases gonadotropin-releasing hormone (GnRH) pulse frequency, which increases luteinizing hormone (LH) over follicle-stimulating hormone (FSH). The resultant excess estrogen production inhibits FSH, so FSH is typically in the normal range. (A, E) Elevated LH stimulates the ovaries to make more androstenedione, which is converted to testosterone. (**B**) Aromatase in adipocytes converts excess androstenedione into estrone, which is normally very low. (**D**) Normally, in mid-cycle, an increase in estrogen leads to an abrupt LH surge. In PCOS, the excess amount of estrogen made in adipocytes leads to a steady increase in the concentration of LH.

25. Correct: C (C)

The concentration of endometrial progesterone (P) receptors is highest in the late proliferative phase (days 10–14). It allows endometrial cells to respond to P that is produced by the corpus luteum after ovulation. (**A**) During menstruation, serum P is low and a high endometrial P receptor concentration is unnecessary. (**B**) During the early proliferative phase (days 6–9), P receptor concentration still increases to reach a maximum before ovulation. (**D, E**) The P receptor concentration continually decreases during the early secretory phase (days 15–21) to reach its lowest concentration by the late secretory phase (days 22–28). Since implantation failed to occur, as evident in the graph by the declining serum P levels at the end of the cycle, the endometrium begins to detach.

26. Correct: D (D)

Implantation of a fertilized egg should occur on days 21 or 22 in a woman with a 28-day menstrual cycle. By then, the zygote has developed into a blastocyst (mass of cells with a fluid-filled cavity), from which the blastula can "hatch" and implant. The endometrium has fully grown under the influence of estrogen, and the uterine glands have become secretory under the influence of progesterone. Furthermore, progesterone suppresses uterine contractions that might endanger implantation. (**A, B, C**) Ovulation is around day 14, so implanation cannot happen prior to it. (**E**) At this time, the endometrium begins to detach, primarily due to the woman's decline in progesterone.

27. Correct: C (C)

High estrogen (and low progesterone) is responsible for the production of cervical mucus that promotes the transport of sperm. This includes large amounts of mucus in order to propel the sperm, supported by uterine contractions, through the female tract. Furthermore, the mucus has an elastic, sperm-permissive consistency. When touched with a piece of paper and lifted up vertically, the mucus can form a thread (spinnbarkeit test), and when placed on a slide and allowed to dry, it forms a pattern that looks like a fern (ferning test). (**A, B, D, E**) At these times, there is no maximal estrogen production, which is responsible for the production of large quantities of watery, elastic cervical mucus.

28. Correct: Estradiol (A)

In a 31-day menstrual cycle, the luteinizing hormone (LH) surge is about 14 days prior to menstruation (on day 17). Hence, days 8 and 13 are in the middle and the end of her follicular, preovulatory phase. Day 22 is in the middle of her luteal, postovulatory phase. The measurements are consistent with serum estradiol, which increases during the follicular phase, peaks shortly before ovulation, and decreases during the luteal phase. After menopause, when follicles are depleted, estradiol levels are markedly decreased. (**B, D**) Follicle-stimulating hormone (FSH) and LH are both increased after menopause compared to their premenopausal concentrations, due to the lack of negative feedback inhibition. (**C**) Gonadotropin-releasing hormone (GnRH) might not be changed much in early menopause. With age, GnRH pulse frequency decreases, but pulse amplitude increases due to lack of negative feedback inhibition. (**E**) Progesterone serum concentrations would be low on days 8 and 13 during the follicular phase and higher on day 22, during the luteal phase of the menstrual cycle.

29. Correct: Clotting tendency (A)

Estrogen (not progestogen) increase the tendency of blot clots, so that clotting tendency is not a good systemic indicator of progesteronemia. (**B, C, D**) The monitoring of these systemic parameters could be considered. They are easily obtainable and, in humans, are known to be altered by progesterone action. Progesterone receptor activation leads to an increased basal metabolism, which can be monitored as increased respiratory rate. Progesterone favors insulin release, which might lead to insulin resistance and development of diabetes mellitus, so that monitoring of serum glucose makes sense. Last, progesterone receptor signaling causes increased natriuresis, so that monitoring of urine sodium makes sense.

30. Correct: Developing follicles (B)

As menstruation ends around day 4 of the female menstrual cycle, selected ovarian follicles develop and mature under the influence of follicle-stimulating hormone (FSH). Maturation includes the proliferation of granulosa cells, which convert androgens to estrogen and release it into blood. (**A**) The corpus luteum is responsible for the estrogen production during the luteal phase of the menstrual cycle after ovulation. (**C**) The endometrium is affected by estrogen but does not produce it. (**D**) Ovarian stromal cells produce the tissue surrounding the follicles. They are not a source of estrogen in premenopausal women. (**D**) Gonadotropes of the anterior pituitary produce FSH and luteinizing hormone (LH), not estrogen.

31. Correct: A short luteal phase (C)

Ovulation has occurred when the basal body temperature has increased by at least 0.4°F to a temperature that is higher than the temperatures of the previous 6 days and when the temperature remains elevated for at least 48 hours. This is due to the increase in serum progesterone from the corpus luteum. It usually takes about 2 days after ovulation for the temperature to increase. Thus, ovulation has occurred on day 19. This is later than the typical time of ovulation on day 14. Normally, the temperature remains elevated throughout the typically 14-day luteal phase. For this woman, the temperature remains elevated until day 25, which indicates a short luteal phase. (**A**) A 6-day luteal phase will not allow implantation of an embryo and hence cannot be considered normal. (**B**) Elevated temperature for one day only, as seen on day 5, is not due to ovulation but more likely a measurement error or a day of illness. (**D**) The woman ovulates on day 19, as explained. (**E**) While uncommon, it is possible for a woman to ovulate more than once per cycle. However, this is not the case here, based on the temperature chart.

32. Correct: Progesterone (D)

In a normal menstrual cycle, serum progesterone is high at time B and low at time A, resulting in a high B/A ratio. (**A, E**) Serum testosterone and dihydrotestosterone do not follow the rhythmic changes of the female hormones throughout the female cycle and, hence, are not very predictable. They might be slightly elevated at time A, causing an increased libido before ovulation. (**B**) Estradiol is elevated at times B and A, so the B/A ratio would be lower than that for progesterone. (**C**) Follicle-stimulating hormone is low at time B and elevated at time A, leading to a low B/A ratio compared to progesterone.

33. Correct: Increase, increase (E)

For successful female reproductive function, it is critical that the hypothalamus release gonadotropin-releasing hormone (GnRH) in a pulsatile manner, with a correct timing of the pulse frequency and amplitudes during the menstrual cycle. To monitor GnRH pulsatility clinically is challenging, if not impossible. Hence, in a first step, the responsiveness of the pituitary and gonads is tested. When follicle-stimulating hormone/luteinizing hormone (FSH/LH) is administered, an increase in estradiol and/or progesterone is the appropriate response. When synthetic GnRH is administered, an increase in LH and/or FSH is appropriate. Positive results indicate that the pituitary is responsive and that the axis from the anterior pituitary to the gonads is intact, so that the fault most likely lies at the hypothalamic level. Without any obvious structural abnormalities, a functional problem in the hypothalamic pulse generation becomes likely. (**A, B, C, D**) These are incorrect choices.

34. Correct: Decreasing 5-α reductase (C)

The description is that of a woman with polycystic ovary syndrome (PCOS), and such patients often also experience peripheral insulin resistance (plasma glucose is elevated). Hormonal disturbances prevent the cyclic maturation of one dominant follicle and regression of the others, so the nonregressed ovarian follicles look like “cysts” on ultrasound. Elevated luteinizing hormone (LH), in relation to follicle-stimulating hormone (FSH), stimulates theca cells to produce androgen (her free testosterone is elevated), which is not fully aromatized by FSH-activated granulosa cells. Increased testosterone leads to increased dihydrotestosterone (DHT), which manifests as acne and hirsutism. Hence, inhibition of 5-α-reductase to lower DHT would improve the skin-related conditions. (**A, B**) Blocking estrogen receptors or LH receptors would not improve acne and hirsutism, while unpredictably affecting the delicate cyclic hormonal balances that are necessary for normal fertility. (**D**) Androgen-binding protein (ABP) is produced by male Sertoli cells. It is structurally similar to sex hormone–binding globulin (SHBG), which is present in males and females. Hence, pharmacologically decreasing ABP might also decrease SHBG, which would further increase free testosterone. (**E**) Increasing SHBG could potentially decrease free testosterone, but it would most likely also decrease free estrogen, which would negatively affect the woman's fertility. (**F**) One possible intervention is indeed the selective destruction of stromal/thecal cells to decrease androgen production, however, it involves 4–10 small punctures (ovarian drilling) and never removal of half of the ovarian tissue.

35. Correct: Estrone-3-glucuronide (B)

Luteinizing hormone (LH) is the most important hormone to monitor a woman's cyclic fertile interval, since it surges about 24 hours before ovulation. This surge defines the two most fertile days: the day before and the day after ovulation, since the released egg will survive about 24 hours. However, there are about 4 additional fertile days prior to the LH surge, because sperm can survive up to 5 days in cervical mucus. To best determine these days, estradiol levels are monitored, since they are responsible for triggering the LH surge and for stimulating the production of sperm-permissive cervical mucus. In urine, lipid-soluble estradiol is present in a metabolized, water-soluble form such as estrone-3-glucuronide. (**A**) Estrone is the least abundant estrogen in fertile females and is not monitored for fertility. (**C**) While follicle-stimulating hormone (FSH) also increases somewhat in midcycle, measuring this increase is not a reliable predictor of ovulation. (**D, E**) Human chorionic gonadotropin (hCG) and progesterone are used to predict and monitor pregnancy, after fertilization has occurred.

36. Correct: Nonovarian androstenedione (A)

Based on her age, amenorrhea, and vasomotor symptoms, this woman is likely in the perimenopausal transition. With increasing age, ovarian follicles become less sensitive to gonadotropin stimulation and produce increasingly less estradiol and progesterone. The resultant increase in follicle-stimulating hormone (FSH) and luteinizing hormone (LH) leads to some theca cell proliferation, where androstenedione is converted to estrone by aromatase. However, most androstenedione to estrone conversion in the postmenopausal woman is nonovarian and happens in adipose, muscle, and other cells. This is evident since estrone levels are relatively stable, even when the ovaries have been removed. (**B, D, E**) Estradiol and estriol are not converted into estrone, independent of their source. (**C**) Aromatization of testosterone leads to estradiol (not estrone).

10.7 Questions

37. Which of the curves in the image best approximates the plasma level of progesterone during a normal pregnancy?

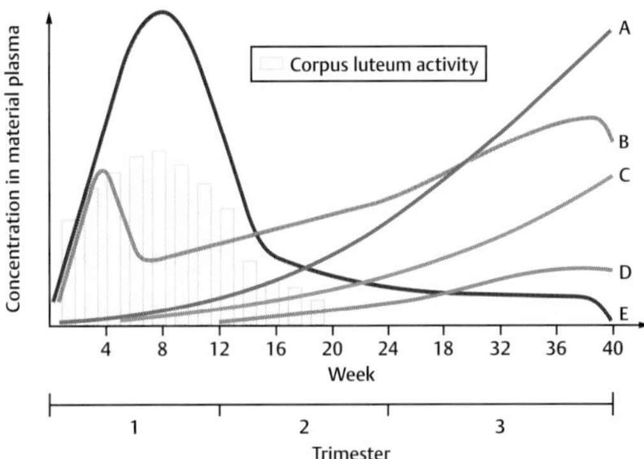

A. A
B. B
C. C
D. D
E. E

38. A 41-week pregnant woman presents to the hospital because of uterine contractions. She is frustrated because she has experienced uterine contractions for several days. Her cervix is only 3 centimeters dilated, and the amniotic sac is intact. During the evaluation, she experiences mild contractions every 6–10 minutes, each lasting 15–20 seconds. A synthetic analogue of which of the following could be given to increase the strength and frequency of her contractions?

A. Cortisol
B. Estrogen
C. Oxytocin
D. Prolactin
E. Prostacyclin

39. A woman does not lactate during normal pregnancy because lactation is inhibited by which of the following hormones?

A. Androgens
B. Estrogen
C. Growth hormone
D. Oxytocin
E. Prolactin

40. A breast pump kit includes a device to record the baby's cry, which is then played back when the mother pumps breast milk for storage and later use. The production and release of which of the following maternal hormone is triggered by the baby's sound and induces the milk let-down reflex?

A. Adrenocorticotropic hormone
B. Follicle-stimulating hormone
C. Growth hormone
D. Human chorionic gonadotropin
E. Human placental lactogen
F. Luteinizing hormone
G. Oxytocin
H. Prolactin
I. Thyroid-stimulating hormone

41. A 17-year-old woman calls her physician's office and asks for advice since she just had a positive result on a home pregnancy test. She states that she normally has regular menstrual bleeding every 29 days and that her menses was due 4–5 days ago. How many days have likely elapsed since fertilization of the embryo?

A. 4–5
B. 9–10
C. 18–19
D. 25–26
E. 33–34

42. A 44-year old woman presents to her physician complaining of no menstrual bleeding for 2 times. She says that she has not experienced this problem before, and that she usually experiences regular 28-day cycles. A urine pregnancy test is positive. She recalls that she had sexual intercourse several times about 8 weeks ago, although condoms were used. Blood tests are ordered for further analysis. Which of the following hormonal combinations would be expected if there is a normal pregnancy?

A. Increased estradiol and no change in progesterone
B. Increased prolactin and no change in progesterone
C. Increased human placental lactogen and increased progesterone
D. Increased human chorionic gonadotropin and no change in progesterone
E. Increased human chorionic gonadotropin and increased progesterone

43. A primigravid woman at 20 weeks of pregnancy is placed in a program that closely monitors her hormone status as pregnancy progresses. Which of the following hormones, measured in maternal blood or urine, is an indicator of normal communication between fetal and maternal tissue?

A. Dehydroepiandrosterone
B. Estradiol
C. Estriol
D. Estrone
E. Progesterone

44. Pregnant women typically experience which of the following as they progress through the first and second trimesters of pregnancy?

A. Decreased cardiac output due to the competition with the fetus
B. Gastrointestinal hypermotility to improve nutrient absorption
C. Increased vascular resistance to redirect blood to the core
D. Increased oxygen consumption to support the enlarging fetus
E. Metabolic acidosis due to the waste production by the fetus

45. For *in vitro* fertilization, the female menstrual cycle is exogenously controlled and stimulated utilizing several hormone treatments and assessments. A cycle begins by administering a receptor antagonist of Hormone 1, which stops the hypothalamic-pituitary-gonadal axis for one week. During that week, there will be daily injections of Hormone 2, which stimulates the development of large antral ovarian follicles. During the next week, ultrasound is used to monitor follicular growth, and Hormone 3 is expected to increase. When several 18-mm follicles are seen, Hormone 4 is injected to induce oocyte maturation. Mature eggs are retrieved just before ovulation and mixed with, or injected with, sperm *in vitro*. The fertilized eggs are incubated for 3 days. During this time, the woman is injected daily with Hormone 5. After the embryos are transferred back to the uterus, Hormone 6 is monitored to confirm potential pregnancy. Which of the following are Hormones 1–6?

	Hormone 1	Hormone 2	Hormone 3	Hormone 4	Hormone 5	Hormone 6
A.	GnRH	FSH	E	hCG	E	hCG
B.	FSH	LH	P	E	P	P
C.	LH	GnRH	hCG	P	hCG	E
D.	GnRH	FSH	E	hCG	P	hCG
E.	FSH	LH	P	E	E	P

E: Estradiol; FSH: Follicle-stimulating hormone; GnRH: Gonadotropin-releasing hormone; hCG: Human chorionic gonadotropin; LH: Luteinizing hormone; P: Progesterone

46. During the examination of a 2-hour-old infant born at term, the murmur of a patent ductus arteriosus is heard. During which timeframe after the baby's first breath is the ductus arteriosus expected to be functionally closed?

A. 1–5 minutes
B. 1–5 hours
C. 1–5 days
D. 1–5 weeks
E. 2–5 months

47. Which of the following is a sign or symptom of possible preeclampsia when occurring in late pregnancy?

A. Blood pressure > 140/90 mm Hg
B. Changes in appetite
C. Dehydration
D. Glucose in urine
E. Left QRS axis deviation

48. A physician-in-training looks over a 19-year-old patient's records the day before her appointment. Her chief concern is that she has had no menstrual bleeding for 3 months. Laboratory tests show that serum prolactin, estriol, estrogen, and progesterone are elevated. Luteinizing hormone (LH) and follicle-stimulating hormone (FSH) are decreased. With the given information, which of the following is the most likely diagnosis for the woman?

A. Aromatase inhibitor treatment
B. Functional hypothalamic amenorrhea
C. Hyperprolactinoma
D. Pregnancy
E. Polycystic ovary syndrome

49. A pregnant woman is required to take a medication. She is very concerned about the teratogenicity of the drug. Which of the following weeks after fertilization is the most vulnerable period for the development of the fetal heart?

A. Weeks 1–2

B. Weeks 3–6

C. Weeks 9–12

D. Weeks 13–20

E. Weeks 20–24

50. Which of the following is the most effective method to cause a medical abortion in the first 9 weeks of pregnancy?

A. Estradiol analogues

B. Progesterone receptor blockers

C. Progestins

D. Selective estrogen receptor modulators

E. Synthetic oxytocin

51. A 28-year old mother delivers a baby at 37 weeks of gestation with severe malformations in the head, brain, and the spinal cord. Overexposure to which of the following vitamins or vitamin analogues during the first trimester of her pregnancy could have caused these birth defects?

A. Vitamin A

B. Vitamin B

C. Vitamin C

D. Vitamin D

E. Vitamin E

10.8 Answers and Explanations

37. Correct: B (B)

Serum progesterone levels increase rapidly during the first 4–5 weeks of pregnancy, decrease slightly, then increase steadily until the last few weeks of pregnancy. The initial source of progesterone is the corpus luteum. The placenta is the predominant source after about 8–9 weeks. Progesterone concentrations decrease toward the late stages of pregnancy (different from estrogen). This is important since progesterone suppresses uterine contractility, so a decrease in this hormone is necessary for labor to occur. (**A**) This line represents estrogens, which are continually rising throughout pregnancy and do not decrease in the last week. (**C, D**) These lines represent placental corticotropin-releasing hormone (CRH) and human placental lactogen (hPL), both hormones that increase toward the end of pregnancy. (**E**) This line represents human chorionic gonadotropin (hCG), which is the predominant hormone during the first trimester. During this time, it acts in place of luteinizing hormone (LH), which is suppressed by the increasing levels of progestogen and estrogen.

38. Correct: Oxytocin (C)

This woman has been experiencing mild, slightly irregular contractions for several days. At 41 weeks of pregnancy, she is at “term” and would be postterm if pregnancy extended beyond 42 weeks. Synthetic oxytocin could be given (typically intravenously), since it will increase the frequency and intensity of uterine contractions. (**A**) While fetal cortisol is an important contributor to the onset of labor, its pharmacologic use would not strengthen her contractions. (**B**) While an increase in the estrogen/progesterone ratio is critical for normal labor and birth, estrogen levels remain elevated until delivery and supplementation would not be useful. (**D**) Prolactin does not play a critical role in uterine contractions. (**E**) Prostaglandins (not prostacyclin) physiologically facilitate parturition and can be used to induce labor.

39. Correct: Estrogen (B)

High levels of hormones that are produced by the placenta, such as progestogen and estrogen, inhibit lactation during pregnancy. Their abrupt decrease due to the removal of the placenta is critical for inducing lactation. Estrogen is considered the major inhibitor, since progestins can be given postpartum and have no effect on lactation. (**A**) While androgens can be used postpartum to increase the success rate of lactation suppression, they are not the natural regulators to inhibit lactation during pregnancy. (**C**) Growth hormone, produced by the anterior pituitary, is structurally similar to prolactin and supports breast development during pregnancy. It is not the main inhibitor of lactation. (**D**) Oxytocin is produced by the hypothalamus and supports the mother's well-being during pregnancy, the uterine contractions of delivery, and milk ejection after delivery. (**E**) Prolactin is produced by the anterior pituitary and supports breast development during pregnancy and milk production after delivery.

40. Correct: Oxytocin (G)

Oxytocin is critical for the milk let-down reflex. For the reflex to occur, paraventricular nuclei produce and release oxytocin in response to neuronal signals. These signals occur due to mechanical nipple sucking and due to the sound of the baby, the latter being used to support breast pumping. Milk let-down occurs since serum oxytocin stimulates the contraction of myoepithelial cells encircling mammary alveoli so that milk flows into the lactiferous ducts. (**A, B, C, D, E, F, I**) All of these hormones, adrenocorticotropic hormone (ACTH), follicle-stimulating hormone (FSH), growth hormone (GH), human chorionic gonadotropin (hCG), human placental lactogen (hPL), luteinizing hormone (LH), and thyroid-stimulating hormone

(TSH) are known to play a direct or indirect role in human lactation but are not clearly associated with the milk let-down reflex. (**H**) The sound of a crying baby also stimulates the release of prolactin, which is critical for milk production rather than milk ejection.

41. Correct: 18–19 (C)

Fertilization of the embryo occurs at the time of ovulation, which is 14 days prior to the expected time of menses. Hence, 18–19 days (14 plus 4–5 days) is the baby's approximate developmental age. (**A**) Conception is in midcycle, not at the expected time of menses, 4–5 days ago. (**B**) These days best align with the time that has elapsed since implantation of the fetus in the uterine wall. This happens about 7 to 10 days after ovulation. (**D**) The menstrual cycle time minus 4–5 days is inconsistent with fertilization and a physiologically irrelevant time. (**E**) These days represent the gestational age of her pregnancy. It is the time that has elapsed since the first day of the woman's last menstrual period.

42. Correct: Increased human chorionic gonadotropin and increased progesterone (E)

The woman's gestational age is roughly 10 weeks, since the fertilization happened about 8 weeks ago, 2 weeks after menstruation. At 10 weeks of gestation, both human chorionic gonadotropin (hCG) and progesterone are necessary to maintain pregnancy. During the first 8 weeks, concentrations of hCG double approximately every 2–3 days and maintain the corpus luteum until the placenta becomes the major site of hormone production around 10 weeks of gestation. Progesterone increases and helps to establish the placenta, among other functions. Although there might be a slight decline around weeks 4–6, the serum levels are always higher than in a nonpregnant woman. (**A, B, D**) Progesterone needs to be increased to maintain pregnancy. Decreasing progesterone concentrations are often a sign of a failing early pregnancy. (**C**) Human placental lactogen (hPL) typically just starts to increase at 10 weeks of gestation. It is not essential for pregnancy but helps to adjust the energy metabolism of the mother to the new physiological conditions.

43. Correct: Estriol (C)

Estriol concentration can be used to monitor fetal-placental health, since production of estriol requires transport of steroids from the placenta to the fetus and back. Thus, normal values in maternal blood or urine indicate a fetus with a normal metabolism and normal exchange with maternal tissue. (**A**) Dehydroepiandrosterone in sulfate form (DHEA-S) is secreted by the fetal adrenal cortex and cannot be used as marker for fetal maternal exchange before it is converted to estriol by the placenta. (**B, E**) Both estradiol and progesterone are vital for normal development of the fetus. However, their placental production does not require fetal tissue. (**D**) Estrone is primarily produced in menopausal woman and does not play a large role in pregnant women.

44. Correct: Increased oxygen consumption to support the enlarging fetus (D)

The hormonal changes in a pregnant woman prepare her body for carrying the enlarging fetus. These include an increase in oxygen consumption, which is achieved by increased tidal volume and decreased residual volume. (**A**) Pregnancy changes the maternal body so that it nurtures, rather than competes with, the fetus. Thus, cardiac output is increased due to elevated heart rate, stroke volume, and blood volume. (**B**) Pregnant women often experience gastrointestinal hypomotility and constipation. It is believed that a slower intestinal transit is an adaptation to optimize time for the absorption of nutrients and development of a healthy bacterial flora. (**C**) Progesterone decreases total peripheral resistance, leading frequently to postural hypotension and easy fainting. (**E**) Pregnant woman have a decreased P_{CO_2}, which facilitates gas transfer between mother and child. However, it also leads to low serum HCO_3^- and a state of metabolically compensated respiratory alkalosis (not acidosis).

45. Correct: GnRH, FSH, E, hCG, P, hCG (D)

Inhibiting the actions of gonadotropin-releasing hormone (GnRH) by a receptor antagonist stops the production of gonadotropins so that the woman's cycle can be controlled and manipulated with exogenous hormones. To stimulate follicular growth, follicle-stimulating hormone (FSH) is used. The growing follicles release estrogen, which at high concentrations induces the luteinizing hormone (LH) surge. Human chorionic gonadotropin (hCG) is similar to LH and is given exogenously. The increase in LH (or hCG) is critical for egg maturation. After mature eggs have been collected and fertilized, they are cultured and grown *in vitro* to the blastocyst stage. During that time, the endometrium is prepared by progesterone (**P**) injections. After one or more embryos are transferred into the uterus, if successful implantation occurs, the developing syncytiotrophoblast releases hCG, which can be detected in maternal blood 8 days after implantation. (**A, B, C, E**) These choices have the incorrect hormonal sequence.

46. Correct: 1–5 days (C)

The ductus arteriosus is kept patent in the fetus by low arterial oxygen content and circulating prostaglandin E_2 (PGE_2), which is produced by the placenta. After birth, the increase in arterial oxygen and the decrease in PGE_2 induces the functional closure of the duct, which may occur as early as 15 hours and is usually completed within 1–2 days after birth. Structural closure is much longer and usually not completed until 2–3 months after birth. If the ductus still causes left-to-right shunting of blood after a few months, it is considered to be patent. (**A, B, D, E**) These are incorrect times.

47. Correct: Blood pressure > 140/90 mm Hg (A)

The acute onset of hypertension in a patient with previously normal blood pressure is the most alerting sign for possible preeclampsia. The cause of this pregnancy complication is still not fully known, but is likely related to abnormal placental vasculature leading to placental hypoperfusion. The placenta then releases antiangiogenic factors that alter maternal endothelial cell function, resulting in hypertension and maternal organ dysfunction. (**B, C**) Changes in appetite and dehydration are possible in late pregnancy but are not characteristic for preeclampsia. (**D**) Some glucosuria can be normal in late pregnancy due to an increased renal plasma flow and glomerular filtration rate, or it can be a sign of gestational diabetes. (**D**) The elevation of the diaphragm in late pregnancy can change the position of the heart and cause left axis deviation in a woman without preeclampsia.

48. Correct: Pregnancy (D)

The most common cause of secondary amenorrhea is pregnancy. Her hormonal profile (high prolactin, estrogen, estriol, and progesterone; low LH and low FSH) and amenorrhea are consistent with a pregnancy in the late first trimester or early second trimester. Increased concentrations of estriol indicate placental production and nearly always indicate a pregnancy. (**A**) Aromatase inhibitor treatment can lead to menopausal symptoms including amenorrhea due to low (not high) estrogen. (**B, C**) Functional hypothalamic amenorrhea (for instance, caused by stress, weight loss, and/or excessive exercise) and an adenoma producing prolactin both inhibit or distort the pulsatile gonadotropin-releasing hormone (GnRH) release and hence can lead to low FSH and LH, but also low (not elevated) female sex hormones. (**E**) Women with polycystic ovary syndrome present with elevated estrogen and androgen, but typically also with an elevated (not suppressed) LH/FSH ratio.

49. Correct: Weeks 3–6 (B)

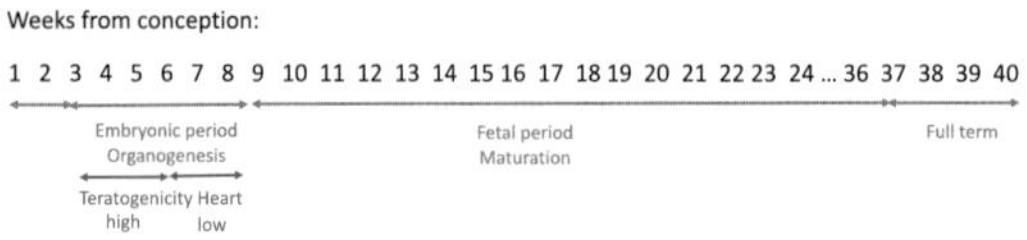

Teratogenicity is the capability of producing fetal malformation. The developing heart is most vulnerable during the early formation of the chambers between weeks 3 and 8 after fertilization (i.e., 5–10 weeks after the first day of last menses). Weeks 3–6 are especially vulnerable (see image). Heart development starts shortly before week 3, when passive diffusion becomes limiting for delivering nutrients and gases to all embryonic cells. Right after 3 weeks, the single endocardial tube of the heart is formed and the heart soon starts to beat, with blood circulating by week 4. Formation of the atrium and ventricle takes place during weeks 4–6. The interventricular septum develops during weeks 5–8. (**A**) During weeks 1 and 2, the embryo is usually not susceptible to teratogens. It is the time for the zygote to divide and implant and for the bilaminar embryo to be formed. (**C**) During weeks 9–12, the heart has done much of its development. The ears, eyes, teeth, palate, and external genitalia of the fetus are highly sensitive to teratogens during this time. (**D, E**) The most susceptible organ systems that remain sensitive to teratogens after week 13 are the central nervous system, eyes, and external genitalia (not the heart). The heart has completed its development by week 20, and by week 24, most organ systems are fully developed.

50. Correct: Progesterone receptor blockers (B)

Progesterone is critical to maintain pregnancy. Blocking progesterone receptors prompts detaching of the developing embryo from the uterine wall and increases uterine contractions, both leading to abortion. (**A**) Estradiol is involved in the development of the endometrial lining and hence cannot be used to induce abortion. (**C**) Progestins are synthetic analogues of progesterone. Since they act like progesterone, they cannot be used for abortion. (**D**) Selective estrogen receptor modulators (SERMs) selectively inhibit estrogen receptors in the hypothalamus. They can be used to inhibit the negative feedback of estrogen on follicle-stimulating hormone, or in the treatment of breast cancer, but not to trigger abortion. (**E**) The body does not respond to external oxytocin with uterine contractions until late pregnancy, when the density of oxytocin receptors is upregulated.

51. Correct: Vitamin A (A)

Vitamin A is critical for cell differentiation and hence is an essential nutrient in fetal development. However, exposures in excess of 10,000 international units per day (4 times the recommended dose) appears to be teratogenic and causes birth defects, especially during the first weeks after conception, when the mother might not know about the pregnancy. The critical periods to cause major morphological abnormalities for the nervous system are weeks 3 to 5, and organogenesis in general takes place between weeks 3 and 8. Functional defects to the brain can occur much later. (**B**) B vitamin (especially B_9 and B_{12}) deficiency (not overexposure) is known to contribute to neural tube defects. (**C, D, E**) These vitamins are necessary for normal fetal development, but there is no known correlation between excess intake and the development of structural birth defects.

Chapter 11

Multisystem Processes

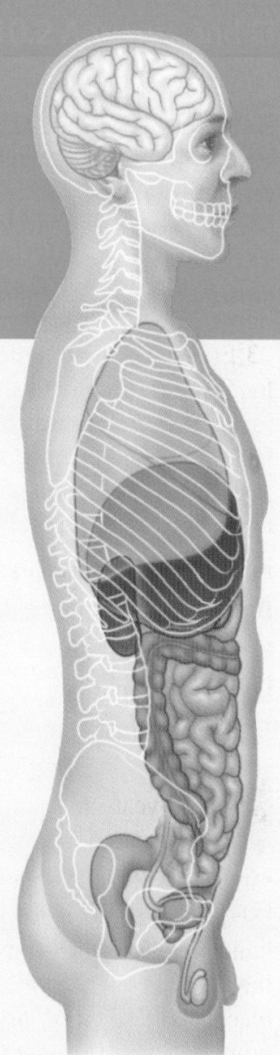

LEARNING OBJECTIVES

- Describe the role of the hypothalamus in temperature regulation and discuss the mechanisms responsible for heat production and heat loss during exercise, different weather conditions (hot, cold, humid, dry), and after acclimatization to hot/cold weather.
- Describe the relationship between nutrition and energy; discuss the requirement, sources, and expenditure of energy; and explain energy balance in the human body.
- Discuss the mechanisms of acid-base homeostasis and describe how to determine whether a disorder is an acidosis or alkalosis and whether it is of metabolic, respiratory, or mixed origin. Also, determine whether an acid-base disorder is compensated, whether an anion gap is present, and whether a respiratory condition is acute or chronic.

11.1 Questions

Easy	Medium	Hard

1. A 69-year-old man is watching television at home on a summer day. The indoor temperature is 73°F (22.8°C). He steps outside to talk to his neighbor for 20 minutes where the air temperature is 102°F (38.9°C). After several minutes he is sweating and feels overheated. An increase in which of the following is expected in response to standing in this outdoor air temperature for 20 minutes?

A. Hypothalamic PGE_2 production
B. Oxygen consumption
C. Resistance of cutaneous blood vessels
D. Secretion of norepinephrine
E. Skeletal muscle tone

2. A 21-year-old, healthy college student wakes up each day around 6 a.m. and goes to bed each night around 11 p.m. He has a normal circadian rhythm, typically does not drink alcohol, and eats a balanced diet. He does not exercise but meditates. Which of the following changes to his normal routine would produce the greatest increase in peak body temperature?

A. Drinking an alcoholic beverage
B. Drinking hot tea
C. Eating a high-carbohydrate meal
D. Fasting for 12 hours
E. Jogging for 30 minutes

3. A 10-year-old boy is sitting on a blanket in the shade with his mother after a leisurely walk. It is a 70°F (21°C) day with no breeze. The boy is wearing only shorts. While sitting in the shade, the majority of his body heat will be lost via which of the following mechanism?

A. Conduction
B. Convection
C. Radiation
D. Respiration
E. Evaporation

4. An American healthcare worker lived for several years in the Sahara Desert as caregiver for nomads who mostly live outdoors. Which of the following adaptations to this extremely hot environment is expected in the worker when compared to his previous life in the United States?

A. Decrease in the mass of brown adipose tissue
B. Decreases in plasma aldosterone levels
C. Increases in catecholamine levels
D. Increases in plasma thyroxine levels
E. Large increase in maximal rate of sweating

5. A 56-year-old woman is recovering in the intensive care unit from a kidney transplant when she develops a fever. Her rectal temperature is measured hourly, has risen from 97°F (36.1°C) to 102°F (38.9°C) over the last 3 hours, and is still rising. If her hypothalamic set point is 104°F (40°C), which of the following is expected to be observed in this patient when her body temperature is 102°F?

	Shivering	Sweating	Vasodilation
A.	Yes	Yes	Yes
B.	Yes	Yes	No
C.	Yes	No	Yes
D.	Yes	No	No
E.	No	Yes	Yes
F.	No	Yes	No
G.	No	No	Yes
H.	No	No	No

6. A man is sailing alone in the Caribbean and falls off his sailboat. The boat continues to sail forward and he cannot get back onboard. The water temperature is 80°F (26.7°C), and there is no land in sight, so he floats and scans the seas for another boat to rescue him. After 6 hours in the water, he begins to show signs of hypothermia. What is this man's primary mode of heat loss?

A. Conduction
B. Convection
C. Radiation
D. Respiration
E. Evaporation

7. A 7-month-old girl has tossed her blanket off while sleeping. The house temperature is 68°F (20°C). When checked on by the babysitter, the baby's skin is cool to the touch. Which of the following receptors are currently activated in this baby to increase heat production?

A. α-adrenergic
B. β-adrenergic
C. Metabotropic glutamate
D. Muscarinic acetylcholine
E. Nicotinic acetylcholine

8. A mother measured the rectal temperature of her 3-year-old daughter about 5 times a day for the past week, since she is suspicious of an undiagnosed illness. When she shows the values to the pediatrician, which of the following variations in body core temperature does the pediatrician explain as a normal average variation during a 24-hour period of time without any significant increase in physical activity?

A. 0.5°F (0.28°C)
B. 2.0°F (1.1°C)
C. 4.5°F (2.5°C)
D. 5.5°F (3°C)
E. 6.0°F (3.3°C)

9. After drinking a few cold beers, you measure your ear temperature and realize that it has decreased by 2°F (~1°C). In which brain region is this temperature change sensed and delivered to the thermoregulatory integration and control center?

A. Hypothalamus
B. Medulla oblongata
C. Midbrain
D. Pons
E. Thalamus

10. A 16-year old high-school student earns summer money by mowing lawns. After finishing his sixth yard for the day on a very hot day, he complains of fatigue, light-headedness, and nausea. When he loses consciousness, the homeowner calls for emergency help. The homeowner tells the responders the boy was acting agitated and disoriented before he passed out. The paramedics note a rapid heart rate and rising skin temperature and suspect heat stroke. Which of the following symptoms would confirm the suspicion?

A. Cool extremities
B. Dry skin
C. Pale skin
D. Profuse sweating
E. Reduced respiration rate

11. If the temperatures of the following women were representative of the average values of their respective cohorts, which of them will most likely have the lowest resting body temperature during a 24-hour period of time?

A. A 20-year-old pregnant woman
B. A 30-year-old healthy woman who is ovulating
C. A 40-year-old woman who has hyperthyroidism
D. A 50-year-old healthy woman
E. A 60-year-old woman who is generally healthy

12. A 27-year-old man is thrown from a raft while whitewater rafting in Colorado in May. He is in the water for 2 minutes while swimming to shore, where he waits for 15 minutes in wet clothes for the guide to reach him. The water temperature is 35°F. Which of the following mechanisms helps to maintain his core temperature while he waits for help?

A. Cutaneous vasodilation
B. Diving reflex
C. Increased thermoregulatory set point
D. Inhibition of catecholamine release
E. Shivering

13. A 10-year-old girl comes home from school feeling tired and irritable. Her oral temperature is 98.7°F (37.1°C). After two hours, she complains of achy muscles, at which time her temperature is measured again and is 101.1°F (38.4°C). Which of the following changes occurs at the beginning of the rising phase of the fever?

A. Behavioral thermoregulatory responses are inhibited.
B. Mean skin temperature is below normal.
C. Muscle blood flow is decreased.
D. Sweat secretion is stimulated.
E. Warm-sensitive neurons in the integration center are excited.

14. A mother brings her 12-year-old son for an examination. He complains of typical symptoms of the common cold for the past two days. Based on the expected changes to the boy's thermoregulatory set point, which of the following symptoms is he most likely experiencing?

	Feelings of	Heart rate	Muscle tone	Shivering
A.	Coldness	↑	↑	↑
B.	Coldness	↓	↔	↓
C.	Coldness	↔	↓	↑
D.	Warmth	↓	↑	↓
E.	Warmth	↑	↓	↑
F.	Warmth	↔	↔	↓

15. During the clinical morning session in the critical care unit, the anesthesiologist discusses the value of considering insensible water loss as part of a patient's best care. She refers to the loss of body water by which of the following processes?

A. Defecation
B. Perspiration
C. Respiration
D. Urination
E. Vomiting

16. An Olympian cyclist is training in cool climates in Northern Michigan for a cycling event that will take place in Las Vegas in September, when the average temperature is 95°F and the humidity around 20 percent. He plans to train for two weeks in Las Vegas before the race. Given the same level of activity, which of the following will be higher after 8 days of acclimatization to the weather, compared to the response on the first day of training in Las Vegas?

A. Antidiuretic hormone
B. Extracellular fluid volume
C. Heart rate
D. Sweat salt concentration
E. Thermoregulatory set point

17. A mountain climber who has been climbing for 2 hours sits on a large rock to rest. He just completed the most strenuous part of the climb and is perspiring. It is a cool (60°F, 15.6°C) and breezy day. Which of the following modes of heat loss is/are occurring in this climber while he rests?

	Conduction	Convection	Radiation	Evaporation
A.	Yes	Yes	Yes	No
B.	Yes	Yes	No	Yes
C.	Yes	Yes	Yes	Yes
D.	Yes	No	No	No
E.	Yes	No	Yes	No
F.	No	Yes	No	Yes
G.	No	Yes	Yes	Yes
H.	No	No	No	No
I.	No	No	Yes	Yes

18. A 30-year-old patient with an obsessive-compulsive disorder and no other health problems wakes up each day at 7 a.m. and goes to bed each night at 11 p.m. He has a normal circadian rhythm, sleeps soundly, and does not exercise. Assuming his normal routine, at which of the following times of day is his body temperature most likely highest?

A. 5 a.m.
B. 9 a.m.
C. Noon
D. 5 p.m.
E. 11 p.m.

19. A 4-year-old child is having a wellness visit before starting kindergarten. The nurse starts the appointment by measuring her temperature. Which of the following locations would provide the most accurate measurement of body core temperature?

A. In the anus
B. In the ear
C. In the mouth
D. In the nose
E. Under the arm

20. Which of the following human thermoregulatory responses is controlled by cholinergic sympathetic nerves?

A. Brown adipose tissue thermogenesis
B. Shivering thermogenesis
C. Sweat secretion
D. Thermoregulatory behavior
E. Vasomotion

21. Five clinicians at the same age and with similar body conditions are in a phone conference from five different geographical locations, while all sitting outside in the shade without any breeze. The clinicians are citizens of northern Canada and just recently moved. At which of the following locations will the individual suffer the least from the heat?

A. 90°F (32.3°C) with 50% humidity
B. 89°F (31.7°C) with 60% humidity
C. 88°F (31.1°C) with 70% humidity
D. 91°F (32.8°C) with 80% humidity
E. 90°F (32.2°C) with 90% humidity

11.2 Answers and Explanations

Easy	Medium	Hard

1. Correct: Oxygen consumption (B)

Oxygen consumption is the amount of oxygen extracted by the peripheral tissues during the period of one minute. The elevation in body temperature increases metabolic rate, which requires a greater oxygen consumption. (**A**) Hypothalamic prostaglandin E_2 (PGE_2) is a pyrogen that changes the thermoregulatory set point, which induces fever. This man may have hyperthermia (elevated body temperature), but it is not due to fever. (**C, D, E**) Increased cutaneous vessel resistance (vasoconstriction), increased skeletal muscle tone, and increased secretion of norepinephrine all serve to conserve and/or raise body temperature and therefore are not occurring in this man. The neurotransmitter for sympathetic-activated sweat glands is acetylcholine, not norepinephrine.

2. Correct: Jogging for 30 minutes (E)

Exercise increases the metabolic rate up to 15 times the basal rate, which directly increases body temperature more than any other answer choice option. (**A**) Alcohol can make one feel warmer because the blood vessels dilate and move warm blood closer to the surface of the skin, but over time, this actually lowers the core body temperature as heat is dissipated. (**B**) Drinking a hot beverage can increase body temperature minimally for a short period of time, but it will not exceed the heat produced by exercise. (**C**) The process of digesting, absorbing, and processing nutrients generates heat by increasing the metabolic rate by 10 to 20%. This food-induced thermogenesis is greatest after eating a high-protein meal and is less after eating carbohydrates and lipids. (**D**) Fasting reduces metabolism, which reduces heat production and lowers body temperature.

3. Correct: Radiation (C)

Every object emits energy in the form of electromagnetic radiation. The rate increases and the wavelength shortens with temperature. Warm or hot objects that are not hot enough to emit visible light emit infrared radiation, which can sometimes be felt as heat on the skin, as from a hot stove. Radiation is the principal way a resting human body loses heat in still air that is cooler than the skin temperature. The mean skin temperature of a healthy person (calculated as a weighted average of different skin areas) is around 33°C (91.4°F), so the boy loses heat to the environment. Radiation is the primary way of heat loss at rest. (**A**) The transfer of energy between two objects in direct contact is called conduction, such as heat loss from sitting on a cold chair (here the boy sits on a blanket). There is some conduction from the boy's skin to the air, but more heat is lost by convection. (**B**) Convection is the process of a fluid (air or water) carrying away the heat it has absorbed from a body. There is always some convection in air because warmer air rises above cooler air, but if there is no wind, as in this case, less heat is lost by convection than by radiation. (**D**) The body can lose a small amount of heat through respiration, which is actually an example of convection. (**E**) Evaporation occurs during sweating, as water evaporates from the skin. This becomes a major way of heat loss during exercise, but not at rest in temperature ambient conditions.

4. Correct: Large increase in maximal rate of sweating (E)

The efficiency of evaporation as a mechanism of heat loss depends on a number of factors, including whether or not the person is acclimated to the high temperatures. Nonacclimated individuals can produce only 1 L of sweat per hour, whereas acclimated individuals can produce 2 to 3 L of sweat per hour, which enables them to dissipate three times as much heat per hour through evaporation. Acclimatization to hot environments usually occurs over 7–10 days and enables individuals to reduce the threshold at which sweating begins, increase sweat production, and increase the capacity of the sweat glands to reabsorb sweat sodium, thereby increasing the efficiency of heat dissipation. (**A**) Brown adipose tissue is especially abundant in newborns and decreases in quantity as humans age. It is not affected by temperature acclimatization. (**B**) During acclimatization, plasma aldosterone is typically increased so that more sodium is reabsorbed from sweat ducts, but it normalizes again after some time. (**C, D**) Increased catecholamines and thyroxine levels occur in adaptation to cold (not heat) exposure. This adaptation typically takes longer and is mechanistically not as well understood.

5. Correct: Yes, no, no (D)

Since her hypothalamic set point is higher than her body temperature, she will experience symptoms associated with coldness and will exhibit compensatory responses to raise body temperature (to the set point). Therefore, she will exhibit shivering and vasoconstriction. She will not exhibit sweating or vasodilation, as these are compensations for lowering body temperature. (**A, B, C, E, F, G, H**) These answers do not contain the correct combination of choices.

6. Correct: Convection (B)

Convection is the process of a fluid, such as water or air, flowing by the skin and carrying away body heat. When the body is immersed in water, nearly all heat exchange occurs by convection. If it is not possible to keep body parts out of the water, treading water (not swimming) is the best strategy to increase survival time. Early signs of hypothermia include shivering, poor coordination, and mental sluggishness. (**A, C**) Heat is transferred by conduction between objects at different temperatures in direct contact, as when sitting on a cold floor. Warmer objects also radiate heat at a greater rate than cooler surrounding objects, leading to a net heat loss. Both of these processes transfer heat from the man's body to surrounding water, but this warms up the water too, limiting the heat loss unless the warmed water flows away and cold water flows in to replace it, which is convection. (**D**) The amount of heat lost through respiration (which involves convection of air) is minimal compared to the man's heat loss through convection of the water. (**E**) Evaporative heat loss occurs during sweating, which is not the case here.

7. Correct: β-adrenergic (B)

Newborn babies and infants experience a greater net heat loss than adults because they cannot shiver to maintain body heat. They rely on nonshivering thermogenesis, which is facilitated by greater amounts of brown adipose tissue. When cold-stressed, norepinephrine binds to β-adrenergic receptors on brown fat and reacts with lipases to break fat down into triglycerides, which are degraded to produce heat. (**A, C, D, E**) These receptors are not involved in brown fat tissue thermogenesis in babies.

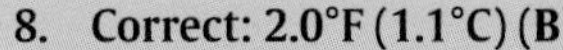

8. Correct: 2.0°F (1.1°C) (B)

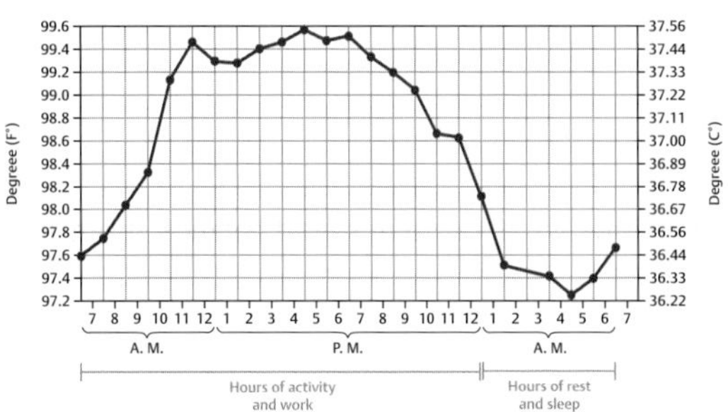

As shown in the image, the body temperature of a healthy person varies during the day between about 97.4°F and 99.5°F (~ 2.2°F), with lower temperatures in the morning and higher temperatures in the late afternoon and evening, as the body's needs and activities change. The variations are most prominent in children. (**A, C, D, E**) These values are not typical and at the lower or upper end of normal.

9. Correct: Hypothalamus (A)

The preoptic area of the hypothalamus contains cold- and warm-sensitive neurons. Cooling of the preoptic area elicits heating responses and behaviors (e.g., putting on clothing and shivering), while warming of this area elicits cooling responses and behaviors (e.g., vasodilation and seeking shade). Hence, it is believed that the sensors are at the same place as the thermoregulatory integration and control center. (**B**) The medulla oblongata is a continuation of the spinal cord within the skull, forming the lowest part of the brainstem and containing control centers for the heart and lungs. (**C**) The midbrain is the small uppermost part of the brainstem associated with vision, hearing, motor control, sleep/wake, and arousal. (**D**) The pons is the part of the brainstem that links the medulla oblongata and the thalamus. It contains nuclei that relay signals from the forebrain to the cerebellum, along with nuclei that deal primarily with sleep, respiration, swallowing, bladder control, hearing, equilibrium, taste, eye movement, facial expressions, facial sensation, and posture. (**E**) The thalamus is made up of two masses of gray matter lying between the cerebral hemispheres on either side of the third ventricle, relaying sensory information and acting as a center for pain perception.

10. Correct: Dry skin (B)

When heat gain exceeds heat loss, the body temperature rises. The hallmark symptom of heat stroke is a core body temperature above 104°F (40°C) together with neurologic dysfunction. The absence of sweating indicates that the heat stress moved from a state of heat exhaustion due to acute plasma volume loss (the boy was working for hours in the sun and is likely dehydrated) to a state where the hypothalamic regulatory mechanisms are not functioning any more, potentially due to direct heat damage to the brain. The lack of sweating with a rising skin temperature is not always present during heat stroke, but when present, it is a medical emergency, since it indicates the most severe form of heat-related illness. (**A**) Since the body's temperature control system is failing, the extremities and core will be warm/hot to the touch. (**C**) The skin will be dry, hot, and red, not pale. (**D**) Generally, sweating is absent in heat stroke; however, this is not always the case, particularly in exercise-induced heat stroke. (**E**) Respiration rate will be increased as a sign of severe sympathetic activity and as a mechanism for heat loss.

11. Correct: A 60-year-old woman who is generally healthy (E)

The resting metabolic rate decreases with age, which is why older individuals tend to have lower body temperatures and a smaller fluctuation in body temperature throughout the day. (**A**) Pregnancy raises body temperature due to increased progesterone. (**B**) Ovulation raises body temperature due to increased progesterone. (**C**) Hyperthyroidism increases metabolism due to increased circulating thyroxine, and thus raises body temperature. (**D**) A healthy woman at age 50 will have a normal circadian rhythm and body temperature range. If menopausal, her 24-hour average values might be higher due to nightly hot flashes.

The series of events that occur during the course of a fever, after pyrogens have raised the set-point temperature above normal, begin with vasoconstriction, piloerection, epinephrine secretion, and shivering. The vasoconstriction causes the mean skin temperature to fall below normal, in an effort to conserve heat. Eventually, the continuing rising body core temperature will inhibit the sympathetic centers that control cutaneous blood flow, and vasodilation occurs. (**A**) Behavioral thermoregulatory responses are not inhibited during fever induction, and the girl will seek the warmth of the bed. (**C, D, E**) At the beginning of the rising phase of a fever, when the body temperature is below the new set-point temperature, the body is trying to conserve heat to raise its temperature to the new set point. Hence, muscle blood flow is increased (not decreased) due to shivering, sweating does not occur, and the cold-sensitive (not warm-sensitive) neurons in the integration center are excited.

12. Correct: Shivering (E)

The temperature of the body is regulated by neural feedback mechanisms that provide information on core and skin temperature to the control center, where the sensed information is compared with the hypothalamic and the skin set points. If the sensed temperature is lower than the integrated set points, a variety of responses are initiated to conserve body heat and increase heat production. These include cutaneous vasoconstriction to decrease the flow of heat to the skin; the secretion of norepinephrine,

epinephrine, and thyroxine to increase heat production; and shivering to increase heat production in the muscles. (**A**) Cutaneous constriction, not vasodilation, would help to maintain core temperature. (**B**) The diving reflex is the body's physiological response to prolonged submersion in cold water, and includes selectively shutting down parts of the body in order to conserve energy for survival. This man was not submerged long enough for this reflex to occur. (**C**) The thermoregulatory set point is not altered when the body temperature changes in response to environmental factors. It is changed by pyrogens, which induce fever. (**D**) When body temperature drops, the secretion of catecholamines such as norepinephrine and epinephrine is stimulated to increase heat production.

13. Correct: Mean skin temperature is below normal. (B)

The series of events that occur during the course of a fever, after pyrogens have raised the set-point temperature above normal, begin with vasoconstriction, piloerection, epinephrine secretion, and shivering. The vasoconstriction causes the mean skin temperature to fall below normal, in an effort to conserve heat. Eventually, the continuing rising body core temperature will inhibit the sympathetic centers that control cutaneous blood flow, and vasodilation occurs. (**A**) Behavioral thermoregulatory responses are not inhibited during fever induction, and the girl will seek the warmth of the bed. (**C, D, E**) At the beginning of the rising phase of a fever, when the body temperature is below the new set-point temperature, the body is trying to conserve heat to raise its temperature to the new set point. Hence, muscle blood flow is increased (not decreased) due to shivering, sweating does not occur, and the cold-sensitive (not warm-sensitive) neurons in the integration center are excited.

14. Correct: Coldness, ↑, ↑, ↑ (A)

When sick with a bacterial or viral infection, the body's thermoregulatory set point is raised in response to pyrogens such as bacterial wall components and/or cytokines of the responding immune system. With a raised set point, the body perceives itself as suffering from hypothermia (colder than it should be). This initiates mechanisms to increase heat production and causes fever. They include the secretion of norepinephrine, epinephrine, and thyroxine to increase metabolism, which increases heart rate, as well as increased muscle tone and shivering to increase heat production in skeletal muscles. When the infection clears and the set point becomes normal again, the opposite occurs and the person behaves as if in a hot environment. (**B, C, D, E, F**) These choices do not contain correct combinations of answers.

15. Correct: Respiration (C)

Insensible water loss is solute-free water loss across the skin that cannot be avoided and hence is not sensed or perceived. An example is respiration, during which water evaporates into inspired air and is then breathed out. In clinical situations that requires an estimation of a patient's fluid balance, insensible water losses are often ignored or considered as constants. It is worth discussing whether care would improve if individual values were used for critically ill patients. (**A, B, D, E**) These are all considered sensible routes of water loss because they are measurable and sensed.

16. Correct: Extracellular fluid volume (B)

An acclimated individual begins sweating sooner and to a greater extent, but sweat contains less salt and more salt is retained. Thus, with adequate fluid intake (as expected by an Olympian athlete), the extracellular fluid volume is maintained at a higher level (up to 30%) than prior to acclimation. While complete heat adaptation requires up to 14 days, the plasma volume expansion is early during adaptation and starts declining again after about 8 days. (**A**) Antidiuretic hormone (ADH) is not a large player of heat adaptation. If at all, in the early phase, ADH would be suppressed by a larger plasma volume. (**C**) Heart rate is reduced (up to 25%) with acclimatization due to the reduced perceived exertion with exercise, which reduces central commands. It is the classic sign to demonstrate successful heat acclimatization. (**D**) Sweat salt concentration is reduced as sweat glands become more efficient at conserving salt. (**E**) The thermoregulatory set point does not change with heat acclimatization over weeks.

17. Correct: Yes, yes, yes, yes (C)

The mountain climber is losing heat via all four modes. As he sits on the rock, there is conductive heat loss from his body to the rock as well as to the air, both of which are cooler than his skin. Since it is a breezy day, there is convective heat loss. Since his body is warm, especially after exercise, it emits infrared radiation; since the air and other surroundings are cooler than his skin temperature, they emit less infrared radiation back toward him, so there is radiant heat loss. Since he just completed a strenuous part of the climb and is sweating, there is evaporative heat loss. (**A, B, D, E, F, G, H, I**) These choices contain incorrect combinations of answers.

18. Correct: 5 p.m. (D)

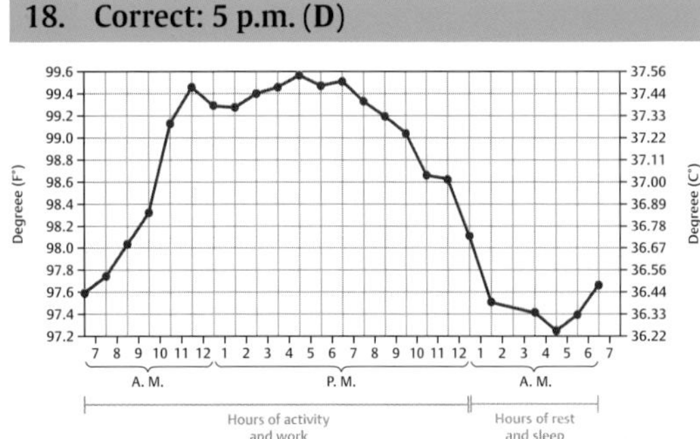

Body temperature normally fluctuates over the day, as controlled by a person's circadian rhythm and activity (see image), with the lowest levels around 4 a.m. and the highest level between 4 p.m. and 6 p.m. (for a person who sleeps at night and stays awake during the day like this patient). (**A**) Body temperature is close to its lowest point at 5 a.m. (**B**) Body temperature is increasing and close to its median point at 9 a.m. (**C**) Body temperature is close to its maximum point at noon, but still a bit lower than in the late afternoon. (**E**) Body temperature is decreasing and close to its median point at 11 p.m.

19. Correct: In the anus (A)

Rectal temperature (in the anus) is the most accurate, but is not used as often as the others due to the inconvenience. (**B**) Tympanic temperature (in the ear) runs higher than rectal measurements. (**C**) Oral temperature (in the mouth) is on average 0.5°C lower than rectal temperature. (**D**) Cranial temperature (in the nose) is more dynamic than the rectal. (**E**) Axillary temperature (under the arm) is typically lower than oral and can be variable.

20. Correct: Sweat secretion (C)

Sweat secretion is a sympathetic action; however, it is mediated by the release of acetylcholine from postganglionic neurons that act as muscarinic receptors at the sweat glands. This is one of the few cholinergic sympathetic actions in the body. (**A**) Nonshivering thermogenesis occurs in brown adipose tissue via the uncoupling of protons moving down their mitochondrial gradient from the synthesis of ATP, thus allowing the energy to be dissipated as heat. This is regulated by thyroid hormones and sympathetic adrenergic control. (**B**) Shivering thermogenesis is a somatic motor response to a drop in body temperature. The primary motor center for shivering in the hypothalamus is excited by cold signals from the spinal cord and skin when the body temperature falls even a fraction of a degree below a critical temperature level. (**D**) While changes in both skin and core temperatures have been implicated in mediating thermoregulatory behavior in humans (e.g., moving to a different spot, changing clothes), skin temperature (not sympathetic activity) is suggested to be the thermal input most likely inducing it. (**E**) Blood vessel dilation and constriction are mediated by epinephrine and norepinephrine, which are adrenergic substances mediating a sympathetic response.

21. Correct: 90°F (32.3°C) with 50% humidity (A)

The most efficient heat removal from the human body is by evaporation of sweat from the skin. However, high relative humidity reduces the gradient of water vapor pressure, which reduces the evaporation rate and hence the rate of heat removal from the body. Therefore, if the air temperature is approximately the same at the different locations, and there is no breeze, then the highest rate of heat loss from evaporation will occur at the lowest relative humidity. In everyday life, the heat index takes air temperature and relative humidity into account to estimate a person's comfort or, clinically, the likelihood of heat disorders with prolonged exposure to the outdoors. (**B, C, D, E**) Since these options have similar air temperatures but higher relative humidity, they will produce less heat loss from evaporation.

11.3 Questions

22. A patient with celiac disease is referred to a dietitian. At the consultation, which of the following food products is recommended for the patient to consume?

A. Barley
B. Bulgur
C. Rice
D. Rye
E. Spelt

23. A 2-year-old child from an immigrant family presents with a greenstick fracture of the radius bone. On exam, the child is noted to be short for her age, and a prominent bowing of the lower extremities is observed. A deficiency in which of the following vitamins is most likely responsible for this presentation?

A. Vitamin A
B. Vitamin B_6
C. Vitamin C
D. Vitamin D
E. Vitamin E

24. As part of a rehabilitation program of a cardiovascular clinic, patients recovering from a myocardial infarct are asked to step on and off a 5-inch (12.7-cm) high board for 30 minutes to the rhythm of slow music. Which of the following is the primary source of ATP production in the patients' recti femores?

A. Creatine phosphate
B. Glycogenolysis
C. Glycolysis
D. Ketone bodies
E. Oxidative phosphorylation

25. A 67-year-old woman with diverticulitis is asked to change to a low-meat diet with no indigestible fibers. Which of the following plant polymers can she use?

A. Amylopectin
B. Cellulose
C. Hemicellulose
D. Inulin
E. Pectin

26. A child developed chronic diarrhea when the mother switched from breast milk to formula. After testing out different formulas, it seems that the symptoms are present only when formula is given that contains high-fructose corn syrup. Which of the following ingredient should be avoided when feeding the baby?

A. Lactose
B. Maltose
C. Streptomycin
D. Sucrose
E. Trehalose

27. A 51-year old woman has been diagnosed with peripheral artery disease. She is shocked by this diagnosis and radically changes her lifestyle. She chooses a diet in which she ingests ten times more insoluble dietary fiber than recommended. The gastrointestinal binding of which of the following is an undesirable effect of such a diet?

A. Ammonia
B. Bile acids
C. Cholesterol
D. Heavy metals
E. Minerals

28. A nationally recognized male athlete, sprinting the 200-meter dash, will use which means of ATP production for the first third of the race?

A. Creatine phosphate dephosphorylation
B. Glycolysis
C. Myoglobin degradation
D. Oxidative phosphorylation
E. Pentose ribosylation

29. What is the nitrogen balance of a person who consumes a 3,500-kilocalorie diet containing 10% protein and who excretes a total of 12 grams of nitrogen?

A. –2
B. 0
C. +1
D. +2
E. +4

30. Which of the following describes the state of nitrogen balance for a normal, healthy 35-year-old person who consumes a diet that provides 75 g of protein and has a total nitrogen loss of 12 grams?

A. Negative nitrogen balance
B. Positive nitrogen balance
C. Zero nitrogen balance
D. Cannot be determined

31. The table shows five equicaloric meals containing different amounts of fat, carbohydrate, and protein (all in grams). Which meal has the highest thermic effect?

	Fat	Carbohydrates	Protein
Meal 1	10	81	8
Meal 2	31	52	30
Meal 3	18	63	21
Meal 4	22	12	12
Meal 5	20	46	57

A. 1
B. 2
C. 3
D. 4
E. 5

32. Which of the following elements requires the smallest intake in milligrams per day for an adult to stay healthy, assuming that it is ingested in an absorbable form?

A. Calcium
B. Chloride
C. Iron
D. Phosphorus
E. Potassium

33. Four individuals volunteer for a basal metabolism study. Before the study begins, the volunteers are evaluated for sex, age, height, and weight. The findings are shown:

	Sex	Weight (kg)	Height (cm)	Age (years)
Volunteer 1	Female	50	60	30
Volunteer 2	Female	90	70	60
Volunteer 3	Male	70	70	40
Volunteer 4	Male	90	60	60

Which volunteer has the highest basal metabolic rate (total calories per day)?

A. 1

B. 2

C. 3

D. 4

34. A product lists the following nutrition information:

Serving size	9 oz
Servings per package	1
Calories	242
Total carbohydrate	19 g
Total fat	10 g
Protein	19 g

What is the approximate percentage of calories from fat in this product?

A. 30%

B. 34%

C. 37%

D. 42%

E. 50%

35. A 29-year old women has noticed a significant decrease in her energy over the past few months. Before that time, she was a very active person, but now she is too tired to do much at the end of the day. Her iron panel shows low serum iron, ferritin, and transferrin saturation. Transferrin and total iron-binding capacity are high. A complete blood count reveals the following values:

Hb	8.0 g/dL
MCV	62 fL
MCH	19.0 pg/cell
MCHC	29 g/dL
WBC	5.3×10^9/L
Platelets	450×10^9/L

She is given oral iron replacement and is referred to a dietitian. At the consultation, she states that she is an avid salad eater. Considering her condition, which of the following salad dressing makes the most sense?

A. Balsamic vinaigrette

B. Caesar

C. Honey mustard

D. Ranch

E. Thousand island

36. As part of a clinical diet, 100 grams of fat needs to be substituted with proteins at the same caloric value. Which of the following is closest to be the correct amount of proteins in grams?

A. 45

B. 100

C. 130

D. 220

E. 460

37. A patient currently presents with severe fatigue. About 8 months ago, she started to experience shortness of breath, paroxysmal nocturnal dyspnea, and ankle edema. She dealt with it by herself; despite that, the symptoms became gradually worse. Two months ago, she experienced mesenteric ischemia, which required a small bowel resection. There are now 150 cm (59 inches) of her small intestine left, and the jejunal end is currently attached to the skin of her belly (end-jejunostomy). She is on total parenteral nutrition (TPN) but can also eat and drink. She has a stool output of 3 liters per day. A deficiency of which of the following vitamin or mineral is most likely to have created the current symptom of this patient with short bowel syndrome?

A. Chromium

B. Fluoride

C. Manganese

D. Vitamin E

E. Zinc

38. Which of the following substance has the largest discrepancy between its physiological energy that is derived through cellular respiration and its physical energy that is derived from the heat after combustion in a bomb calorimeter?

A. Ethanol
B. Glucose
C. Glycine
D. Palmitic acid
E. Sucrose

39. A 28-year-old lean man fell while mountain climbing and was rescued 5 days later. He had water but no food during the 5 days. He was taken to the hospital for treatment. His 24-hour urine urea nitrogen (UUN) was 5.0 grams. What was his approximate loss of mean muscle mass (in grams) during the past 5 days? (Assume the nonurea sources of nitrogen loss amount to 4 g).

A. 56 g
B. 156 g
C. 211 g
D. 281 g
E. 303 g

40. The action plan for a patient recovering from surgery includes physical activity of 8 metabolic equivalents (MET) for 15 minutes per week. Which of the following best describes the rate of energy expenditure by one MET?

A. 1 joule per pound of body weight per hour
B. 1 kcal per kg of body weight per hour
C. 1 milliliter O_2 uptake per kg per min
D. Maximum rate O_2 uptake
E. Total O_2 uptake per kg per day

41. A 20-year-old male athlete is training for an iron man competition. He weighs 180 pounds and ingests approximately 88 grams of protein per day. His physician orders a 24-hour urine urea nitrogen (UUN) test to check his nitrogen balance. The result of his UUN is 16 grams of nitrogen. What is this man's total nitrogen intake per day, total nitrogen loss per day, and nitrogen balance? (Assume the nonurea sources of nitrogen loss is 4 g).

	Total nitrogen intake (grams/day)	Total nitrogen loss (grans/day)	Nitrogen balance
A.	12	16	−6
B.	12	16	+6
D.	12	20	-6
E.	12	20	+6
F.	14	16	−6
G.	14	16	+6
H.	14	20	−6
I.	14	20	+6

11.4 Answers and Explanations

22. Correct: Rice (C)

Rice in all forms, including wild and brown rice, is a gluten-free food and is therefore a recommended food for patients with celiac disease. (**A, B, D, E**) Each of these items contains gluten and is not recommended for a patient with celiac disease. Gluten is part of the storage protein fraction of the endosperm of grains. It is composed of two classes of heterogenic proteins: glutenins and gliadins. The latter are the main components of food that are toxic and/or immunogenic for celiac patients. Barley is a grain often found in cereals and used for beer in the form of malt, the germinated and dried form of barley. Bulgur is a precooked wheat grain and a common ingredient of the vegan diet. Rye is a grain used in pumpernickel bread or alcoholic drinks. Spelt is an old grain used in many health foods.

23. Correct: Vitamin D (D)

This child most likely has rickets. It causes defective calcification of bones before epiphyseal plate closure due to the deficiency or the impaired metabolism of vitamin D, since vitamin D is required to adequately absorb calcium and phosphorus from diet. Rickets classically presents with bowed legs and short stature in toddlers. A greenstick fracture is a bent or cracked but not severed bone, like a bent green branch or stick. (**A**) Vitamin A deficiencies typically result in abnormal visual adaptation to darkness, dry skin, dry hair, and brittle fingernails. (**B**) Vitamin B_6 deficiencies can result in a variety of conditions, including peripheral neuropathy, seborrheic dermatitis, glossitis, and cheilosis. (**C**) Vitamin C deficiency typically results in scurvy, easy bruising, and joint/muscle pain. (**E**) Vitamin E deficiency typically results in muscle weakness and hyporeflexia and, in severe cases can cause blindness, arrhythmia, and dementia.

24. Correct: Oxidative phosphorylation (E)

For aerobic activities such as moving to music or long-distance running, the primary source of ATP production is aerobic metabolism of acetyl groups from glucose (via pyruvic acid) or fatty acid through the citric acid cycle and oxidative phosphorylation. Aerobic metabolism provides the least energy per unit time (~ 1 mole of ATP/minute), but it can generate ATP for periods of intense exercise lasting up to several hours. Generally speaking, most of the glucose used in aerobic metabolism is derived from the liver and can come from its glycogen storage. There is typically enough glucose stored as liver glycogen to supply skeletal muscle for hours (e.g., through 16 to 20 miles of a marathon or standing for an hour performing a surgical operation). (**A**) Creatine phosphate can quickly transfer the energy released by dephosphorylation to regenerate ATP from ADP, lasting for seconds. (**B, C**) Glycogenolysis (breakdown of glycogen stores) and glycolysis (breakdown of glucose) can make ATP for moderate bursts of activity, lasting for minutes. (**D**) Ketone bodies can also be used by muscle cells for aerobic metabolism, but they are particularly used when hepatic glucose reserves run low. This is not the goal for rehabilitation exercise.

25. Correct: Amylopectin (A)

Amylopectin is the major starch component in most plants. For instance, it makes up about 75 percent of wheat flour. It is a branched glucose polymer and can be completely digested to glucose, which is absorbed and used for nutrition. (**B, C, D, E**) These are all plant polymers that are indigestible by humans. They are used in human diet as indigestible fibers that increase the food transit time through the gut. A small percentage can be metabolized by bacteria of the lower intestinal tract, but as of now, this has not been shown to have any nutritive value. Cellulose and hemicellulose are found in wheat, rye, rice, and vegetables. Inulin is part of bananas and asparagus. It has clinical value in nephrology as an inert molecule for the body. Pectins are found in, for instance, citrus fruits, oat products, and beans. A low-fiber diet for diverticulitis makes sense to avoid further irritation due to increased motility.

26. Correct: Sucrose (D)

The child has most likely a hereditary fructose intolerance, for instance due to the deficiency of aldolase B, which hydrolyzes fructose-1-phosphate. Sucrose is a disaccharide composed of fructose and glucose. (**A**) Lactose is a disaccharide composed of galactose and glucose. (**B**) Maltose is made of two glucose molecules. (**C**) Streptomycin is an aminoglycoside that is highly polar and not absorbable. Hence, if used as an antibiotic drug, it cannot be given orally. (**E**) Trehalose is a disaccharide made of glucose. It is present in mushrooms, for instance, and has equal nutritional value to glucose since humans have trehalase as a brush border enzyme.

27. Correct: Minerals (E)

Dietary fibers bind minerals and trace elements, which limits the ability to absorb them. This is a side effect of concern only for a diet with very high fiber intake as in the person described. (**A**) Binding of ammonia to indigestible fibers is considered desirable, since fecal nitrogen excretion unburdens the liver and kidneys. (**B, C**) In peripheral artery disease the blood flow is obstructed by atherosclerotic plaques that contain fat and cholesterol. In people with such fat metabolism disorders a high-fiber diet is helpful, since it leads to increased excretion of bile acids and cholesterol. (**D**) Dietary fibers decrease the transit time of food, thereby limiting the absorption of heavy metals as a desirable effect.

28. Correct: Creatine phosphate dephosphorylation (A)

In exercise, as the intensity and duration of muscle activity increases, three sources of ATP are mobilized. The first source of ATP mobilized during increased activity comes from the transfer of phosphate from creatine phosphate (PCr) to ADP with the subsequent formation of ATP and creatine (Cr). Each creatine phosphate molecule yields one ATP molecule. This chemical reaction is very rapid and can quickly supply ATP for contraction at the rate of about 4 moles of ATP per minute. But the supply of creatine phosphate is limited and typically supports contractions for only 8–10 seconds; the standing world record for the 200-meter sprint is 19.19 seconds. In addition, to convert Cr back to PCr consumes an ATP molecule and so will occur only during times of adequate ATP supply. It is ideal for a short, intense burst of muscle activity, as in a short sprint or shooting a layup on the basketball court. (**B**) Glycolysis is the second form of energy mobilized in skeletal muscle, after creatine phosphate, and has a longer duration (minutes). (**C, E**) Myoglobin degradation and pentose ribosylation are not sources of energy in skeletal muscle tissue. (**D**) Oxidative phosphorylation is the third form of energy mobilized in skeletal muscle and has the longest duration (hours).

29. Correct: +2 (D)

"Ten percent protein" means that 10% of the 3,500 calories are from protein, so 350 calories are from protein. Protein provides 4 calories per gram, so 350/4 = 87.5 grams of protein intake. To convert the protein intake to nitrogen intake, divide the grams of protein intake by 6.25 g protein/g nitrogen, so 87.5/6.25 = 14 grams nitrogen intake. Fourteen g intake – 12 g loss = +2 nitrogen balance. (**A, B, C, E**) These choices do not contain the correct calculation.

30. Correct: Zero nitrogen balance (C)

The protein input can be converted to the nitrogen input by using the conversion factor of 6.25 g amino acids/g nitrogen. Hence, 75 grams of consumed protein/6.25 (g protein/g nitrogen) = 12 grams of nitrogen intake. Twelve grams of nitrogen intake minus 12 g of nitrogen loss equals a zero nitrogen balance. Note that the non-urea sources of nitrogen loss (typically a constant of 4 g) is included in the "total" nitrogen loss. (**A**) Nitrogen loss would have to be greater than the nitrogen intake to have a negative nitrogen balance. (**B**) Nitrogen loss would have to be less than the nitrogen intake to have a positive nitrogen balance. (**D**) The nitrogen balance can be calculated. It is the traditional method of determining dietary protein requirements of certain populations or individuals.

31. Correct: 5 (E)

The thermic effect of food, also called diet-induced thermogenesis, is related to the amount of energy expenditure above the basal metabolic rate required to process food for use and storage. In other words, the body must expend some energy to digest, absorb, and store the nutrients in the food. The thermic effect varies substantially for different food components; fats and carbohydrates are relatively easy to process and have very little thermic effect (about 5% of total energy). On the other hand, proteins are hard to process and have the largest thermic effect (about 25% of total energy). For instance, in a meal with 1,000 calories, 240 calories increase the basal metabolic rate through thermogenesis. Since meal 5 has the highest protein content, it will have the highest thermic effect. (**A, B, C, D**) are not the best choice because they have lower amounts of protein.

32. Correct: Iron (C)

Although iron is not easy to absorb and even adults on a balanced diet can become deficient in it, it is nevertheless a trace element. The daily recommended intake for adults on a 2,000-calorie diet is about 18 mg, which is significantly lower compared to the other elements. (**A, B, D, E**) These elements are major building blocks of the human body, and the daily recommended intake is between 1,000 mg (calcium and phosphorus) and 3,500 mg (chloride and potassium).

33. Correct: 4 (D)

The Mifflin–St. Jeor equation estimates basal metabolic rate by weighing the contribution of weight (factor of 10) and height (about factor of 6). It adjusts for age by subtracting it, weighted by a factor of 5. Last, there is a gender correction, which is a subtraction of the number 161 for women and the addition of the number 5 for men. The correct equation is as follows.

For women: BMR = 10 × weight (kg) + 6.25 × height (cm) – 5 × age (years) – 161

For men: BMR = 10 × weight (kg) + 6.25 × height (cm) – 5 × age (years) + 5

Since weight counts the most, and height and age are within 10–20 percent from each other, the male volunteer 4 will have the highest BMR. In detail,

(**A**) Volunteer 1 = (10 × 50 kg) + (6.25 × 60 cm) – (5 × 30 years) – 161 = 564
(**B**) Volunteer 2 = (10 × 90 kg) + (6.25 × 70 cm) – (5 × 60 years) – 161 = 876.5
(**C**) Volunteer 3 = (10 × 70 kg) + (6.25 × 70 cm) – (5 × 40 years) + 5 = 942.5
(**D**) Volunteer 4 = (10 × 90 kg) + (6.25 × 60 cm) – (5 × 60 years) + 5 = 980

34. Correct: 37% (C)

Fats contain 9 calories per gram, so 10 grams of fat × 9 calories per gram of fat = 90 calories in this product from fat. The question asks for the percentage of calories from fat, so this number must be divided by the total calories, which is 242. So, 90 calories/242 calories = 37.2% fat. (**A, B, D, E**) These calculations are incorrect.

35. Correct: Balsamic vinaigrette (A)

(**A**) The woman has a microcytic hypochromic anemia. Her iron panel confirms iron deficiency anemia. Anemia of chronic disease is excluded, since it would present with high ferritin levels. The treatment with iron tablets is consistent with this diagnosis. Hence, the dietitian will consider food that supports the intake of iron in the most absorbable form. Dietary iron is absorbed by enterocytes as ferrous iron (Fe^{2+}). Since acidity will reduce ferric iron (Fe^{3+}) to the absorbable form, a vinaigrette with acidity is most likely recommended. Adding fruit or a lemon zest will further help. (**B, C, D, E**) These contain less vinegar and hence are less acidic compared to a vinaigrette.

36. Correct: 220 (D)

The energy content of 1 gram of protein is 17 kJ (4 kcal), in comparison to 1 gram of fat, which is 37 kJ (9 kcal). This is about a factor of 2.2, so that 220 g of proteins are closest to be equicaloric to 100 g of fat. (**A**) This would be the correct answer if the conversion factor of 2.2 would be reversed, with the food energy of protein being higher than fat. (**B**) Fat is a more concentrated source of energy than protein. (**C**) This would be the approximate amount of alcohol that could replace the energy derived from fat. (**E**) This is the approximate amount of dietary fibers that would provide the same energy as 100 g of fat.

37. Correct: Vitamin E (D)

The patient's symptoms before the bowel resection are typical of progressive congestive heart failure (shortness of breath, worsening when lying down at night, ankle edema). Redirection of blood flow from the mesenteric vessels to perfuse body core organs caused mesenteric ischemia necessitating surgical bowel resection. In a person with short bowel syndrome, symptoms occur due to the loss of absorptive surface area and/or loss of specific transporters, cells, or hormones. This patient lost the colon, the ileum, and part of the jejunum. This primarily affects bile salt absorption and, consequently, absorption of lipids and lipid-soluble substances such as vitamin E. Vitamin E is an antioxidant. When deficient, oxidative damage to red blood cells can cause anemia (severe fatigue). (**A, B, C, E**) Most nutrients, including the listed trace elements, are absorbed in the proximal 100–150 cm of intestine. Hence, they are less likely to cause her symptom of fatigue. Moreover, their deficiency is typically related to anemia. Chromium deficiency has been associated with impaired glucose tolerance. The only association with low fluoride intake is dental caries. Manganese deficiency is extremely rare and causes skin and lipid problems. Zinc deficiency may result in impotence, immune dysfunction, and various skin lesions.

38. Correct: Glycine (C)

The nitrogen in amino acids is primarily catabolized into NH_3, which is a highly reduced molecule. Additionally, NH_3 is converted to, and excreted as, urea. Conversion of the NH_3 to urea is an endothermal reaction requiring the direct expenditure of 3 moles of ATP per mole of urea formed. In the bomb calorimeter, the glycine is combusted in an exothermal reaction that produces water and oxides of nitrogen. The released energy includes the energy stored in the reduced state of the nitrogen atom and the ATP energy used to create the molecular bonds of the urea molecule. In other words, the physiologically excreted urea still contains energy that is released in the calorimeter, which makes the physiological energy of glycine about three-fourths of its physical energy. (**A, B, D, E**) Alcohol (ethanol), carbohydrates (glucose, sucrose), and fats (palmitic acid) will be digested and catabolized in the body to CO_2 and H_2O, the same end products that are obtained in a calorimeter.

39. Correct: 281 g (D)

First, the man lost 9 g of nitrogen per day. He lost 5 g in the form of urinary urea, which is the largest fraction (~ 2%) of urinary solutes. This is lower than the normal of 12 to 20 g because the man had not eaten for 5 days. Additionally, he lost 4 g from non-urea sources (e.g., urinary ammonia and nitrogen in sweat, feces, hair, and skin). This is a constant number applicable to most situations. There are a few rare instances (e.g., total parenteral nutrition) when 3 g is more appropriate. Second, to convert the nitrogen loss to protein loss, multiply the total nitrogen loss by 6.25 g protein/g nitrogen, and account for the number of days: 9 g nitrogen/day × 6.25 g protein/g nitrogen = 56.25 g protein/day × 5 days = 281 g of protein loss. (**A, B, C, E**) These choices do not contain the correct calculation.

40. Correct: 1 kcal per kg of body weight per hour (B)

A metabolic equivalent (MET) is the rate of energy expenditure while sitting at rest. It is close to the expenditure of 1 kcal per kg of body weight per hour. Since MET is not readily understandable by many patients, in the clinics it is typically related to a particular activity. For instance, for a patient recovering from surgery who can use the toilet by him/herself, one MET is assigned. It takes about 4 METs to walk up a flight of stairs. Heavy exercise is typically more than 10 METs. When expressed in MET minutes, the time of the activity is taken into account. For instance, to reach 120 MET minutes, one can do a 4-MET activity for 30 minutes or an 8-MET activity for 15 minutes. (**A**) A MET is roughly 4.2 kilojoules per 2.2 pounds per hour. (**C, D**) A MET is taken by convention to be 3.5 milliliters oxygen uptake per kilogram of body weight per minute. This is an important conversion to relate oxygen expenditure to physical fitness, which can be determined by a person's maximum rate of oxygen uptake ($\dot{V}O_2max$). (**E**), The total O_2 uptake per kg per day could estimate a person's daily activity.

41. Correct: 14, 20, –6 (H)

To convert protein intake to nitrogen intake, divide by 6.25 g protein/g nitrogen. Hence, 88 g protein/day 6.25 g protein/g nitrogen = 14 g nitrogen intake/day. To obtain total nitrogen loss, add UUN and nitrogen from nonurea sources. Hence, 16 g nitrogen from UUN + 4 g other nitrogen loss = 20 g total nitrogen loss. The nitrogen balance is the difference between intake and loss. Hence, 14 g nitrogen intake/day – 20 g nitrogen loss/day = –6 g nitrogen balance. (**A, B, C, D, E, F, G, I**) These choices do not include the correct combination of answers.

11.5 Questions

42. Medical students discuss how best to demonstrate to high-school students the relevance of body buffers. They first create a list of facts about them. Which of the following is on their list?

A. Chemical buffers rid the body of H^+.
B. Excellent buffers are strong acids or bases.
C. Hemoglobin is an important buffer.
D. Urine is normally unbuffered.
E. Volatile body acid is not buffered.

43. As part of a clinical study, the study participants are sorted into groups A through D based on their arterial blood concentrations of CO_2 and HCO_3^-. A HCO_3^- concentration of 22–28 mEq/L and an arterial Pco_2 of 33–44 mm Hg is considered normal. Each study group is plotted on a graph (image) based on their HCO_3^- and Pco_2 concentrations. Which of the following indicates the correct metabolic disturbance for each group?

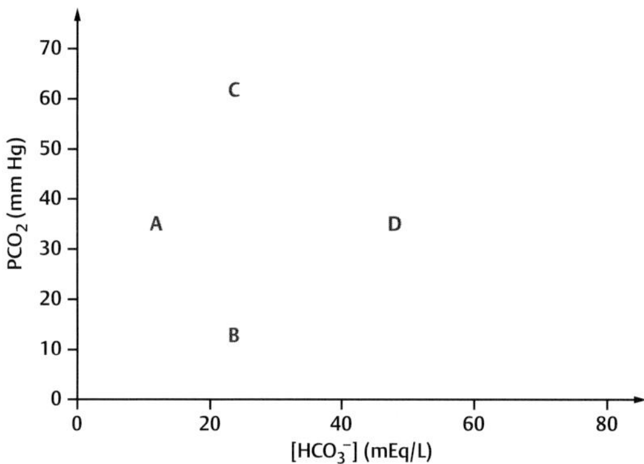

	Metabolic acidosis	Metabolic alkalosis	Respiratory acidosis	Respiratory alkalosis
A.	A	C	B	D
B.	A	D	C	B
C.	B	C	A	D
D.	C	A	D	B
E.	D	A	B	C

44. A website for high-altitude hikers explains that after a rapid ascent, one begins to hyperventilate, but that the kidney compensates for it. What is the renal response to this condition?

A. Decreased amount of urinary phosphate buffer
B. Decreased rate of renal tubular H^+ secretion
C. Diuresis to eliminate excess fluid
D. Increased ammoniagenesis
E. Increased rate of renal tubular H^+ secretion

45. A chemistry major and current medical student explains that the acid dissociation constants (pK_a) of some amino acid residues in plasma proteins are close to 7.4, whereas the pK_a of the CO_2/HCO_3^- system is only 6.1, but that nevertheless, the CO_2/HCO_3^- system is the body's most important buffer system due to which of the following?

A. It controls both CO_2 and HCO_3^-.
B. It has a set point in the hypothalamus.
C. It is faster compared to protein buffers.
D. It operates as a closed system.
E. It remains independent from other buffers.

46. Which of the following arterial blood values is expected in a mountain climber who has been residing at a high-altitude base camp below the summit of Mount Everest for one week?

	pH	Po_2 (mm Hg)	Pco_2 (mm Hg)	$[HCO_3^-]$ (mEq/L)
A.	7.18	95	25	9
B.	7.35	50	60	32
C.	7.53	40	20	16
D.	7.53	95	50	40
E.	7.62	40	20	20

47. A patient with chronic obstructive pulmonary disease (COPD) presents with severe diarrhea and the following lab values: pH 7.2, $Paco_2$ 60 mm Hg, and HCO_3^- 22 mEq/L. Which of the following acid-base disturbances is present?

A. Acute respiratory acidosis
B. Acute respiratory alkalosis
C. Chronic respiratory acidosis
D. Chronic respiratory alkalosis
E. Metabolic acidosis
F. Metabolic alkalosis
G. Respiratory acidosis and metabolic acidosis
H. Respiratory acidosis and metabolic alkalosis
I. Respiratory alkalosis and metabolic acidosis
J. Respiratory alkalosis and metabolic alkalosis

48. A patient was diagnosed 5 years ago with chronic renal failure. She comes to the clinic due to persistent nausea and vomiting. She says that these symptoms started 2 weeks ago and that she used baking soda as a remedy between meals and at bedtime. The symptoms did not change, but her ankles are now heavily swollen. Her physical examination reveals a blood pressure of 190/110 mm Hg, a heart rate of 100 bpm, bilateral crackles, and 2+ pitting edema on both feet and ankles. Laboratory values show:

Sodium	138 mEq/L
Potassium	4.0 mEq/L
Chloride	97 mEq/L (low)
Bicarbonate	24 mEq/L
Creatinine	14 mg/dL
Glucose	122 mg/dL
Ketones	Negative
pH	7.42
Pco_2	37 mm Hg
Po_2	78 mm Hg
Urine sample	pH 6.0; 3+ protein; granular casts

Which of the following is present?

A. Metabolic acidosis and metabolic alkalosis
B. Metabolic acidosis and respiratory alkalosis
C. Metabolic alkalosis and respiratory acidosis
D. No acid-base stress

49. A 17-year-old is brought to the emergency room at 10 a.m. He had been found 30 minutes earlier with a suicide note and an empty bottle of aspirin tablets. It is believed that he had no access to other medication. He was last seen at 5 p.m. the day before. A call to his phone at 8 p.m. was unanswered. The pH of an arterial blood sample is within normal range. Which of the following values for Pco_2 and HCO_3^- are most likely in case of an aspirin overdose?

	Arterial Pco_2	Arterial $[HCO_3^-]$
A.	High	High
B.	High	Low
C.	High	Normal
D.	Low	Low
E.	Low	High
F	Low	Normal

50. A patient's chart reads "muscle twitching and confusion," and as a side note "metabolic alkalosis." There is no information on the history or physical examination, nor are there any laboratory data. Which of the following is the most likely cause for the patient's symptoms?

A. Bartter's syndrome
B. Carbonic anhydrase inhibitor treatment
C. Cholera
D. Chronic kidney disease
E. Ethylene glycol poisoning
F. Primary hypoaldosteronism
G. Salicylate overdose

Questions 51 to 52

A 64-year old man presents with daily vomiting for the past 3 weeks and dizziness. He has been diagnosed with type 2 diabetes mellitus 4 years ago, and his records show that he has been in the hospital three times with diabetic complications during the past year due to noncompliance. His mouth is dry and his tongue is swollen. He says that he drinks as much as possible, but is nevertheless thirsty. His legs and feet are swollen. The complete metabolic panel shows an elevated BUN-to-creatinine ratio. The arterial blood gas analysis shows a pH of 7.51; Pco_2 of 46 mm Hg; and HCO_3^- of 34 mEq/L.

51. Which of the following acid-base disturbances is present in this patient?

A. Alkalemia but no alkalosis
B. Metabolic alkalosis and respiratory alkalosis
C. Metabolic alkalosis with respiratory compensation
D. Uncompensated metabolic alkalosis

52. Which of the following electrolyte imbalances is most likely expected for the patient?

A. Elevated anion gap
B. Hypercalcemia
C. Hyperchloremia
D. Hypokalemia
E. Hyponatremia

53. A 1-year-old child with pyloric stenosis presents with nonbiliary projectile vomiting. Which of the following changes in serum electrolyte and carbon dioxide are mostly likely seen?

	Serum chloride	Serum bicarbonate	Serum potassium	Serum Pco_2
A.	↑	↑	↑	↑
B.	↑	↑	↓	↑
C.	↓	↑	↓	↑
D.	↓	↓	↑	↓
E.	↓	↓	↓	↓

54. A 60-year-old man has a cardiac arrest, and cardiopulmonary resuscitation is performed. Epinephrine is administered. Measurements of blood gases and plasma electrolytes were obtained immediately after resuscitation and revealed the following values:

Arterial pH	= 7.30
Arterial P_{CO_2}	= 28 mm Hg
Plasma [Na^+]	= 140 mEq/L
Plasma [K^+]	= 6.0 mEq/L
Plasma [Cl^-]	= 100 mEq/L
Plasma [HCO_3^-]	= 14 mEq/L

Which of the following acid-base disturbances is present?

A. Metabolic acidosis with increased anion gap
B. Metabolic acidosis with normal anion gap
C. Mixed acid-base disturbance
D. Respiratory acidosis with increased anion gap
E. Respiratory acidosis with normal anion gap

55. A 15-year old boy had a streptococcal infection at age 6. At that time, his mother took him out of school and has tutored him at home ever since. The sister describes their mother as overprotective. The boy appears fearful and anxious. His physical exam is normal except for a blood pressure of 134/84 mm Hg, a pulse of 110 bpm, and a respiratory rate of 25 bpm. Laboratory studies are as follows:

Sodium	138 mEq/L
Potassium	3.3 mEq/L
Chloride	108 mEq/L
Bicarbonate	17 mEq/L
Creatinine	1.2 mg/dl
Glucose	80 mg/dL
Ketones	Negative
pH	7.52
P_{CO_2}	22 mm Hg
Urine sample	pH 7.5; protein, glucose negative

Which of the following is most likely present?

A. Acute metabolic alkalosis
B. Acute respiratory alkalosis
C. Chronic metabolic alkalosis
D. Chronic respiratory alkalosis
E. No acid-base disturbance

56. The following arterial blood values were measured in the hospital laboratory:

pH = 7.29 (normal 7.35–7.45)
P_{CO_2} = 26 mm Hg (normal 35–45 mm Hg)
Plasma [HCO_3^-] = 12 mEq/L (normal 23–26 mEq/L)

The blood sample was most likely from a patient fitting which of the following descriptions?

A. Diabetes mellitus; forgot to take insulin shots
B. Duodenal ulcers; self-treating with baking soda
C. Emphysema; 20-year history of smoking
D. Hysterical; was hyperventilating at admission
E. Infection; vomiting for past 2 days

57. During a trip to Mexico, an otherwise healthy woman develops severe diarrhea for 2 days and is admitted to the hospital overnight due to hypotension and syncope. If her acid-base status is depicted by point 4 of the Davenport diagram (image), what is her diagnosis?

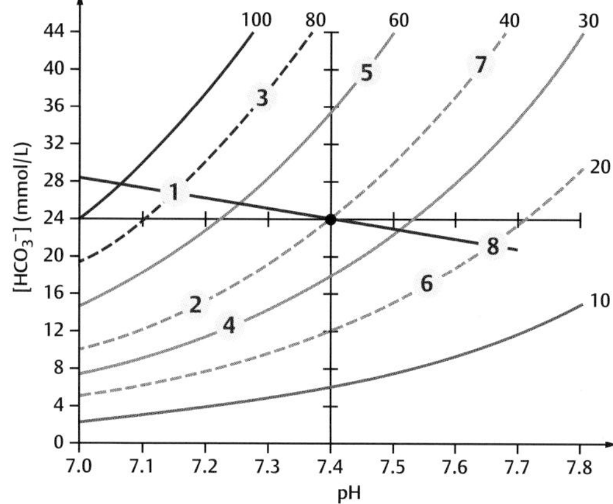

A. Partially compensated metabolic acidosis
B. Partially compensated metabolic alkalosis
C. Partially compensated respiratory acidosis
D. Partially compensated respiratory alkalosis
E. Uncompensated metabolic acidosis
F. Uncompensated metabolic alkalosis
G. Uncompensated respiratory acidosis
H. Uncompensated respiratory alkalosis

58. A 43-year-old woman with a history of severe diarrhea was admitted to the emergency department after fainting at the supermarket. Physical exam revealed decreased skin turgor. Arterial blood gas analysis revealed pH 7.21; P_{CO_2} 26 mm Hg; [HCO_3^-] 10 mEq/L; K^+ 2.2 mEq/L. A metabolic acidosis characterized by which of the following conditions is the correct diagnosis of her condition?

A. Secondary to hypokalemia
B. With increased anion gap
C. With respiratory acidosis
D. With respiratory compensation
E. Without compensation

59. There are currently several patients on the hospital floor recovering from severe acid-base disturbance. A new nurse-in-training wonders how long the patients will stay hospitalized. Which of the following processes will take the longest time to restore acid-base balance completely?

A. Extracellular buffering processes
B. Intracellular buffering processes
C. Renal excretion of acid
D. Renal excretion of base
E. Respiratory compensation

60. A 21-year-old college student, who lives at sea level and is unacclimated to high altitude, begins a climbing expedition on Mount Kilimanjaro. He reaches the first base camp at 9,000 feet (2,743 meters) above sea level on the first day, where he plans to stay for 5 days. Which point on the Davenport diagram (image) represents the climber's acid-base status 1 hour after reaching the first base camp?

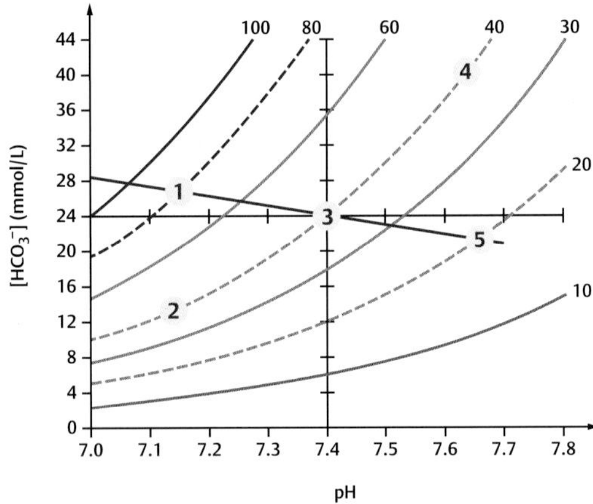

A. 1
B. 2
C. 3
D. 4
E. 5

61. A 41-year-old woman presents to the emergency department after vomiting gastric juices for a 24-hour period. Which of the following sets of arterial blood data is expected in this patient?

Patient	pH	P_{CO_2} (mm Hg)	$[HCO_3^-]$ (mEq/L)
A.	7.39	41	24
B.	7.55	25	21
C.	7.29	30	14
D.	7.51	49	38
E.	7.34	60	31

62. A woman with a history of severe diarrhea has the following arterial blood values:

pH = 7.24
P_{CO_2} = 25 mm Hg
$[HCO_3^-]$ = 10 mEq/L

Which of the following acid-base statuses best fits her laboratory findings?

A. Metabolic acidosis
B. Metabolic alkalosis
C. Respiratory acidosis
D. Respiratory alkalosis
E. Normal acid-base status

11.6 Answers and Explanations

42. Correct: Hemoglobin is an important buffer. (C)

Hemoglobin is an important buffer of plasma pH. When plasma P_{CO_2} is rising, CO_2 diffuses into red blood cells. It combines with H_2O to form carbonic acid. Carbonic acid dissociates into HCO_3^-, which diffuses into plasma, and H^+, which is buffered by hemoglobin. When H^+ binds to hemoglobin, oxygen is released (Bohr effect). An example where this makes sense is when exercising muscles produce excess CO_2 (and hence acidity) and require additional oxygen. This could be demonstrated in a high-school experiment. (**A**) Chemical buffers are the first line of defense of pH. They minimize pH changes but are not designed to rid the body of H^+. (**B**) Buffers are weak acids or weak bases. The term "weak" means that they are not fully dissociated, so the acid form (that can donate a hydrogen ion) and the base form (that can accept a hydrogen ion) are both present in an equilibrium in solution. (**D**) There are buffers in the urine, such as sodium phosphate and NH_3. Urine pH cannot fall below pH 4.5, and the way to get rid of more H^+ in urine is to create more buffers. (**E**) CO_2 is the only volatile acid of the body. It is buffered by HCO_3^- via carbonic acid and water.

43. Correct: A, D, C, B (B)

The primary disturbance in metabolic disorders is the abnormal HCO_3^- concentration; low in metabolic acidosis and high in metabolic alkalosis. The primary disturbance in respiratory disorders is the abnormal P_{CO_2}; increased in respiratory acidosis and decreased in respiratory alkalosis. (**A, C, D, E**) These choices have one or more false associations between acid-base disturbance and blood gas values.

44. Correct: Decreased rate of renal tubular H^+ secretion (B)

Hyperventilation experienced at high altitudes decreases arterial P_{CO_2}, which decreases H^+ and generates a respiratory alkalosis. Reducing both CO_2 and H^+ decreases renal proximal tubular cell H^+ secretion and thus HCO_3^- reabsorption. The filtered HCO_3^- load will exceed the rate of H^+ secretion (and hence HCO_3^- absorption), and the loss of excess bicarbonate is the renal response to correct the pH back to normal. (**A**) Urinary phosphate buffer (HPO_4^{2-}) binds H^+ for its elimination in urine. The amount of filtered phosphate is not regulated by the kidney but rather depends on diet and parathyroid hormone levels. (**C**) Diuresis would cause abnormalities of other electrolytes beyond HCO_3^-. (**D**) Ammoniagenesis is stimulated by decreased (not increased) pH in order to increase renal H^+ elimination. (**D**) An increased rate of renal tubular H^+ secretion would increase HCO_3^- reabsorption and worsen the alkalosis.

45. Correct: It controls both CO_2 and HCO_3^-. (A)

The pK_a is a measure of the ratio of the acid component to the base component of a buffer. A buffer works best when there is equal amount of conjugate acid and base, so that a physiological buffer ideally has a pK_a closest to pH 7.4. The CO_2/ HCO_3^- buffer has two advantages despite its unfavorable pK_a. First, both components are present in abundance (24 mmol of HCO_3^- and 1.2 mmol of CO_2). Second, CO_2 and HCO_3^- can be added to or removed from the body, which is under the control of the lung and kidney, respectively. (**B**) CO_2 is sensed in the medulla, HCO_3^- is potentially sensed in renal tubular cells. There is no integrating center in the hypothalamus known that compares the CO_2/HCO_3^- ratio to a set point. (**C**) The speed of the chemical reactions is not a criterion for the value of a buffer. The CO_2/HCO_3^- system might even be slightly slower compared to others due to the involvement of diffusion. (**D**) The CO_2/ HCO_3^- system operates as an open system as previously explained. (**E**) The CO_2/HCO_3^- system shifts H^+ back and forth with other buffer systems, hence buffering one another (isohydric principle).

46. Correct: 7.53, 40, 20, 16 (C)

The climber will experience respiratory alkalosis. The lower P_{O_2} at high altitude will stimulate breathing to offset the hypoxia. Carbon dioxide is driven from the blood faster than it is produced in the tissues, so P_{CO_2} falls and pH rises. As renal compensation occurs, the kidneys reabsorb filtered HCO_3^- less completely, thereby lowering plasma HCO_3^- concentration. (**A, B, D, E**) In these choices, one or more of the values are incorrect for respiratory alkalosis secondary to hypoxia.

47. Correct: Respiratory acidosis and metabolic acidosis (G)

Always first look at the pH. There is acidemia, since the blood pH is abnormally low. The clinical vignette indicates metabolic and respiratory problems; hence, look at the concentrations of either one, HCO_3^- or CO_2. The P_{CO_2} is high, which indicates respiratory acidosis, consistent with a person whose lungs are obstructed from blowing off CO_2. For 1 mm Hg increase in P_{CO_2}, one expects about 0.4 mEq/L increase in HCO_3^-. Hence, one would expect $20 \times 0.4 = 8$ mEq/L HCO_3^- above normal. This is not the case, so that there is an additional metabolic acidosis present, consistent with diarrhea. If you were to look first at HCO_3^-, you would arrive at the conclusion of metabolic acidosis (low pH and low HCO_3^-). For every 1 mEq/L decrease in HCO_3^-, one expects about 1.3 mm Hg decrease in P_{ACO_2}. Hence, one would expect the CO_2 level to be $2 \times 1.3 = 2.6$ mm Hg above normal. It is much higher, so that there is an additional respiratory acidosis present. (**A, B, C, D, E, F, H, I, J**) These are incorrect, as explained.

48. Correct: Metabolic acidosis and metabolic alkalosis (A)

The patient has two counterbalancing acid-base disorders: metabolic acidosis due to renal failure and metabolic alkalosis due to vomiting, which leaves the pH in normal range. The signs for renal failure are water retention and pitting edema; high blood pressure; elevated serum creatinine; and urinary protein and casts. The kidney's inability to excrete the daily acid load results in metabolic acidosis. Additionally, the acidosis can be inferred from the electrolyte pattern, which reveals an increased anion gap of 17 mEq/L. Since her pH is normal, there is a process that adds alkalinity. First, she ingests baking soda ($NaHCO_3$). Second, vomiting leads to metabolic alkalosis due to the loss of fixed H^+ from stomach acid. Long-term vomiting causes temporary volume depletion, which activates the renin-angiotensin-aldosterone system, in which angiotensin II stimulates HCO_3^- reabsorption. (**B, C**) There is no indication of a respiratory problem. The crackles are due to fluid backup in the lungs, a typical occurrence of a renocompromised person. (**D**) The patient is in acid-base stress despite normal pH, as explained.

49. Correct: Low, Low (D)

Salicylate metabolites stimulate the brain respiratory center. The resultant hyperventilation causes respiratory alkalosis, which leads to low P_{CO_2} and low HCO_3^- as compensatory response. In the time frame of 12–24 hours after ingestion, a metabolic acidosis develops due to complex interferences with cellular metabolic processes and accumulation of anaerobic products such as lactic acid and keto acids. This further decreases HCO_3^- and as compensation P_{CO_2}. Due to the combination of alkalosis and acidosis, the pH may be within the normal range. (**A, B, C, E, F**) These values are unlikely, as explained in the correct answer.

50. Correct: Bartter's syndrome (A)

Bartter's syndrome is a set of genetic mutations that directly or indirectly inhibit the renal tubular Na-K-Cl cotransporter. The resultant excessive distal Na^+ delivery increases distal tubular Na^+ reabsorption in exchange for the electrically equivalent ions K^+ and H^+. This, in turn, promotes hypokalemic metabolic alkalosis. (**B**) Carbonic anhydrase inhibitor treatment leads to decreased HCO_3^- absorption in the proximal tubule and hence may cause acidosis. (**C**) Cholera causes excessive diarrhea and metabolic acidosis. (**D**) One of the kidney's roles is to excrete the daily acid load, so that chronic kidney disease leads to acid retention and metabolic acidosis. (**E**) Ingestion of ethylene glycol (e.g., antifreeze) leads to metabolic acidosis, since it is metabolized to glycolic acid and other acid compounds. (**F**) Primary hyper- (not hypo)-aldosteronism may cause metabolic alkalosis. (**G**) Salicylate (e.g., as aspirin) overdose causes respiratory alkalosis due to hyperventilation and, secondly, metabolic acidosis due to interference with cellular metabolism.

51. Correct: Metabolic alkalosis with respiratory compensation (C)

Use the stepwise approach. Step 1: Alkalemia exists, since the blood pH is abnormally high. Step 2: The clinical vignette points toward metabolic disturbance, so next look at the HCO_3^- concentration. It is higher than normal. When pH and HCO_3^- are in the same direction (i.e., higher), there is metabolic alkalosis. Step 3: The P_{CO_2} is higher than normal, indicating that there is respiratory compensation. Step 4: HCO_3^- is about 10 mm Hg above normal. For adequate compensation, one expects an approximate increase of 7 ± 2 mm Hg (10 × 0.7 = 7) in P_{CO_2}. This is indeed the case, indicating a single acid-base balance. (**A**) The process that leads to alkalemia is called alkalosis, so both must exist. (**B**) If there were a respiratory alkalosis, the patient's P_{CO_2} would be lower than predicted by the calculation explained in A. (**C, D**) The patient has a single acid-base disturbance with adequate compensation, as explained.

52. Correct: Hypokalemia (D)

There are two mechanisms that favor hypokalemia. First, there is a net loss of protons, which favors the release of intracellular H^+ in exchange for K^+. Second, there are signs of dehydration due to vomiting (dry mouth, swollen tongue). Moreover, the elevated BUN:creatinine ratio indicates a prerenal cause such as hypovolemia for the acute failure of the kidneys, which have been weakened by the uncontrolled blood sugar. Dehydration leading to hypovolemia activates the renin-angiotensin-aldosterone system, which increases H^+ and K^+ secretion. (**A**) An elevated anion gap is associated with metabolic acidosis (not alkalosis). (**B**) In alkalemia, more free Ca^{2+} will bind to albumin in blood due to the free binding sites that normally would have been occupied by H^+. This may lead to hypocalcemia (rather than hypercalcemia). (**C**) Vomiting causes hypochloremic metabolic alkalosis due to the loss of stomach acid. (**E**) The patient's thirst indicates hypernatremia (not hyponatremia). Vomiting can lead to excess water loss relative to sodium.

53. Correct: ↓, ↑, ↓, ↑ (C)

Pyloric stenosis results from hypertrophy of the circular muscle of the pylorus, which prevents the flow of gastric content into the intestine and results in projectile vomiting that is free of bile. The loss of hydrochloric acid from the stomach causes hypochloremic (decreased serum chloride) metabolic alkalosis (increased bicarbonate). Renal compensation for this loss of H^+ involves preserving protons at the expense of K^+, and thus hypokalemia ensues (low serum potassium). Respiratory compensation for the metabolic alkalosis is hypoventilation, which increases serum P_{CO_2}. (**A, B, D, E**) These are incorrect choices.

54. Correct: Metabolic acidosis with increased anion gap (A)

The pH is low, and the acidosis is metabolic, since HCO_3^- is low and P_{CO_2} is low as a compensatory response. It is caused by accumulation of lactic acid due to hypoperfusion. It is worsened by epinephrine administration, since a β_2 agonist shifts K^+ into cells in exchange for H^+. The anion gap, (140 + 6) – (100 + 14) = 32, is higher than the normal gap. (**B**) Anaerobic metabolism produces the lactate anion, which increases the anion gap. (**C**) For every decrease in HCO_3^- (10 mEq/L), there is a 1.3 decrease in P_{ACO_2} (10 × 1.3 = 13; 40 – 13 = 27). The compensation is as expected, and data do not support additional disturbances. (**D, E**) Respiratory acidosis may happen due to inadequate ventilation of a nonintubated person. However, one would then expect a lower P_{CO_2}, as explained in C. The only acid in respiratory acid-base disorders is carbonic acid (and its acid form CO_2), so anion gaps do not apply.

55. Correct: Chronic respiratory alkalosis (D)

There is alkalemia since the blood pH is abnormally high. The history and vital signs of the clinical vignette point toward a chronic anxiety disorder with hyperventilation. This is supported by a low P_{CO_2}. In the chronic form of respiratory alkalosis, one expects for every mm Hg decrease in P_{CO_2} a 0.4-fold mEq/L decrease in HCO_3^-. Since P_{CO_2} is 18 below 40, one expects HCO_3^- to be around 17 (18 × 0.4 = 7.2 and 24 – 7 = 17), which is the case here. (**A, C**) The distinction between acute and chronic is not used for metabolic disorders, since the alterations in the breathing rates happen rapidly and most patients will present with some respiratory compensation. (**B**) In the acute form of respiratory alkalosis, renal compensation would not yet have occurred, so the HCO_3^- would be higher. (**E**) The abnormal pH indicates the presence of an acid-base disturbance.

56. Correct: Diabetes mellitus; forgot to take insulin shots (A)

The values indicate metabolic acidosis with respiratory compensation (low pH, HCO_3^- and CO_2). Uncontrolled insulin-dependent diabetes mellitus leads to cellular starvation, resulting in excessive production of ketone bodies (acetoacetic and β-hydroxybutyric acids) and development of diabetic ketoacidosis. (**B**) Baking soda is $NaHCO_3$ and likely causes alkaline blood. (**C**) Chronic obstructive pulmonary disease (COPD) produces respiratory acidosis due to inadequate ventilation and CO_2 accumulation. (**D**) Hyperventilation produces respiratory alkalosis due to excess elimination of blood CO_2 via the lungs. (**E**) Vomiting acidic gastric juice leaves unmatched base in blood and produces metabolic alkalosis.

57. Correct: Partially compensated metabolic acidosis (A)

Since the patient's pH is low, it is an acidosis, and since her HCO_3^- is low, it is due to a metabolic cause (diarrhea), so she has a metabolic acidosis. The metabolic acidosis is partially compensated because it shifted off of the normal P_{CO_2} isobar (40 mm Hg). (**B**) Partially compensated metabolic alkalosis is represented by point 5. (**C**) Partially compensated respiratory acidosis is represented by point 3. (**D**) Partially compensated respiratory alkalosis is represented by point 6. (**E**) Uncompensated metabolic acidosis is represented by point 4. (**F**) Uncompensated metabolic alkalosis is represented by point 7. (**G**) Uncompensated respiratory acidosis is represented by point 1. (**H**) Uncompensated respiratory alkalosis is represented by point 8.

58. Correct: With respiratory compensation (D)

The diarrheal intestinal bicarbonate loss resulted in a metabolic acidosis, with a blood HCO_3^- value of 10 mEq/L, which is about 14 mEq/L lower than normal. As a result, one would expect a 1.3-fold larger decrease in P_{CO_2}: 10 × 1.3 = 13. The actual decrease from normal is 14 mm Hg (40 – 14 = 26), which is close enough to conclude that adequate respiratory compensation has occurred. (**A**) When hypokalemia is the prime problem, one would expect as sequela metabolic alkalosis, since K^+ is shifted out of cells in exchange for H^+. In this case, the low K^+ is a consequence of fecal loss and potentially dehydration or hypovolemia. (**B**) The anion gap is normal in this case because in order to maintain electrical neutrality, chloride replaces the lost bicarbonate. (**C**) The P_{CO_2} level is close to the predicted level based on her HCO_3^- status, so that there is no additional respiratory acidosis. (**E**) There has been adequate respiratory compensation as explained.

59. Correct: Renal excretion of acid (C)

It has to be noted that all processes to maintain pH homeostasis start immediately after a disturbance is sensed. However, there are significant time differences for when the processes reach their maximal capacity. Renal excretion of acid takes by far the longest (typically several days) to reach its maximum, since new ammonia has to be generated to rid the body of H^+ in urine. (**A, B**) Chemical buffers are the first line of defense of pH (in the minute to hour range), with buffer processes in extracellular fluid being faster than cellular buffering processes. (**D**) Maximal renal excretion of base is faster than acid excretion, since it is regulated by the renal filtered HCO_3^- load and does not involve synthesis of new molecules. (**E**) The response of the lungs to induce hyper- or hypoventilation is the second fastest process after chemical buffering. Its maximal capacity is typically reached within 12 hours.

60. Correct: 5 (E)

The climber will hyperventilate in response to the hypoxia at high altitude, which lowers his alveolar and arterial P_{CO_2} and increases the ratio of HCO_3^- to P_{CO_2}. This causes a leftward shift in the Henderson-Hasselbalch equation ($H_2CO_3 \leftrightarrow H^+ + HCO_3^-$), resulting in a decrease in free H^+ and an elevation in pH. This is an uncompensated respiratory alkalosis, because pH increases due to changes in respiration, and the kidney does not compensate fully in this short period of time (will take about 2–3 days). (**A**) This point represents a person with respiratory acidosis, since the pH is reduced and the HCO_3^- is increased, and it is uncompensated since the point falls on the normal buffer line. (**B**) This point represents a person with metabolic acidosis, since the pH and HCO_3^- are both decreased, and it is uncompensated since the point falls on the normal P_{CO_2} isobar. (**C**) This is the normal acid-base status for a healthy person at sea level. (**D**) This point represents a person with metabolic alkalosis, since the pH and HCO_3^- are both increased, and it is uncompensated since the point falls on the normal P_{CO_2} isobar.

61. Correct: 7.51, 49, 38 (D)

The loss of gastric HCl due to vomiting leads to an increase in the plasma bicarbonate concentration (38 mEq/L) and a metabolic alkalosis. This makes the arterial blood pH alkaline (7.51). The increase in the pH will depress peripheral chemoreceptors and slow ventilation. The resultant increase in P_{CO_2} (49 mm Hg) will bring the pH closer to normal and at the same time increase renal H^+ secretion. If the patient rehydrates adequately, the pH will continue to approach normal pH, since the rate of HCO_3^- glomerular filtration will exceed the rate of H^+ secretion, and there will be a continuous loss of bicarbonate until all excess HCO_3^- has been excreted. Without rehydration, contraction alkalosis would maintain the pH disturbance. (**A, C, E**) Plasma pH will be alkaline, not acidic. (**B**) HCO_3^- and P_{CO_2} will be elevated, not decreased.

62. Correct: Metabolic acidosis (A)

The first look is always at the pH. Acidemia exists since the blood pH is abnormally low. Diarrhea causes a metabolic disturbance. Hence, next look at the HCO_3^- concentration. When its level is in the same direction as the pH (i.e., lower than normal), a metabolic acidosis is confirmed. Step three is to see whether the CO_2 level is in the same direction as the original disturbance (i.e., lower than normal). This is the case, indicating respiratory compensation. One could further ask whether the compensation has been as expected. Since HCO_3^- is about 12 mEq/L lower than normal, one would expect the P_{CO_2} to be about 13 (10 × 1.3) mm Hg lower than normal. This is the case, indicating a single acid-base problem. (**B, C, D, E**) These are incorrect, as explained.

Index

Note: Page numbers followed by *f* and *t* indicate figures and tables, respectively.

C

D

E

F

G

H

Q

R

T